Cold War in Psychiatry

Human Factors, Secret Actors

On the Boundary of Two Worlds: Identity, Freedom, and Moral Imagination in the Baltics
23

Cold War in Psychiatry
Human Factors, Secret Actors

Robert van Voren

Amsterdam - New York, NY 2010

Cover painting: "Noah" (oil on canvas) 2009, by Vytenis Lingys

The paper on which this book is printed meets the requirements of "ISO 9706:1994, Information and documentation - Paper for documents - Requirements for permanence".

ISBN: 978-90-420-3048-0
E-Book ISBN: 978-90-420-3047-3

Printed in the Netherlands

This book is dedicated to
Professor Pál Juhasz
who withstood the pressure of totalitarianism
and followed his own conscience

Table of contents

Foreword

The year 2009 marked the twentieth anniversary of the fall of the Berlin Wall. Even with a short look backward, 1989 appears to have been the year that was nothing short of a miracle. World War II, with its sinister and seemingly insurmountable divisions within Europe, appeared to leave no trace of the disbelief, despair and hopelessness that devastated Eastern and Central Europe for more than forty years. Instead, Europe was filled with joy and a sense of solidarity.

Adam Michnik, a hero of the Solidarity movement and a towering figure among public intellectuals and dissenters of Central Europe, commented that it is quite tempting nowadays to assume the role of having been the then-leading force and major inspiration behind the historic fall of totalitarianism in Europe. Therefore, it was with sound reason that Michnik called the year 1989 the "*annus mirabilis*," the miraculous year.

In the United States, it is taken for granted that it was the economic power of America that stripped the former Soviet Union of its potential, thereby inflicting on it a humiliating defeat in the Cold War. German politicians would proudly assert that their wise and patient *Ostpolitik* was a decisive factor in this historic struggle, rather than the direct force and bellicose stance of America. In Poland, nobody doubts that Pope John Paul II came to delegitimize Communism both as a world system and a major rival ideology. The Solidarity movement, itself, dealt a fatal blow to the mortally wounded Soviet system by showing that working class people can revolt against the Working Class State and deprive it of its legitimacy. In the Baltic states, it is widely assumed - and not without reason - that the living chain of the joined hands of Baltic people in 1989, followed by the exceptional role of Lithuania as the first rebellious and breakaway republic also played a role in the disintegration of the Soviet Union and the collapse of Communism in Europe. This role was much too obvious to need emphasis.

All these reasons and arguments are more or less correct. If a unique combination of forces and inspirations had not been possible, 1989 would never have become the decisive year that changed history beyond recognition. Yet one more human factor exists that seems to have been overlooked in Eastern and Central Europe. No matter how much passion and controversy this factor and its mention may arouse, I have to spell out its first and last names. This is Mikhail Gorbachev, the first and the last official President of the Soviet Union, the secretary general of the Communist Party of the Soviet Union, and the architect of the restructuring movement commonly known as *perestroika*. Needless to say, Gorbachev's personality was bound to bring a sharp dividing line between Eastern and Western Europe, probably nearly to the same extent as the assessment of 1968. The emergency of the New Left and of the student revolution in Paris and beyond engraved the memory of the West forming its new moral and political sensibilities. Yet this same year reminds us of how the Soviet Union killed the peaceful revolution of Czechoslovakia, thereby stripping Eastern and Central Europe of the last remnants of hope of creating a more humane version of its political modernity, the illusion known as socialism with a human face.

A Western European intellectual might view this as the Grand March of History stretching from the Latin Quarter of Paris to the rest of the globe, as the character Franz from Milan Kundera's novel *The Unbearable Lightness of Being* has it; but it was a tragedy and the jackboot trampling on the face of the human being in the way another character of the novel, Franz's mistress Sabina, a Czech artist in exile, describes it. Socialism and a promise of freedom as a theory in the West proved a horrible practice in the East in that same year of 1968. Memory politics, as well as opposing memory regimes, still divides Europe.

The same applies to Mikhail Gorbachev. A regrettable liar, coward and hypocrite in the eyes of Lithuanians who suffered most from the bestiality and brutality of Soviet troops in January 1991, Gorbachev is highly esteemed and cherished almost as a saintly figure in the unified Germany. On a closer look, however, he is more of a tragic figure straight from a Shakespearean play. Equally vilified in the Baltic countries as well as in Russia itself – the latter with its increasing nostalgia for the power and international prestige of the former USSR that is far beyond present-day Russia - Gorbachev is blamed for the collapse of the empire; he became a litmus test case of historical memory and political sensibilities. Yet the fact is that Gorbachev, whether a man of half-truth and of an inexorably doomed attempt to humanize totalitarianism, as the Lithuanian poet and literary scholar Tomas Venclova labeled him, proved far less driven by irrational impulses of power and blood-thirst than one could expect from the cornered head of the most dangerous and unpredictable state in the world. It is true that he misinterpreted nationalism of the occupied nations and misrepresented the real state of affairs of the USSR. More than that, he found himself totally confused and lost at a crossroads of the state whose very existence violated justice and all modern sensibilities. But there is a crucial point about the ambivalent gravedigger of the Soviet Union: Gorbachev willy-nilly allowed himself to be perceived globally as a rather weak and confused individual, which would have been unthinkable with his predecessors and successors. If anyone doubts that, let us try to imagine Yuri Andropov or Vladimir Putin in Gorbachev's shoes, let alone other ghosts of the Kremlin.

For lack of a better word for this phenomenon, I would call the reason behind Gorbachev's unwillingness to respond to his failure in the Baltics with massacre a form of decency and humanism, or at least human weakness and moral intuition that may have suggested to him that his story was over. Another epoch had begun, one in which he didn't belong. If one is able to step away from a powerful position and office without causing bloodshed and casualties in retaliation, it is a sign of decency and dignity. Therefore, sometimes it is worth celebrating not only the courage and resolve of those on our side, but the human weakness and confusion of our adversaries as well.

At the same time, we are witnessing how a sinister tendency is increasingly getting stronger in the United States and in Europe. Politicians find themselves preoccupied with two domains that serve as a new source of inspiration: namely, privacy and history. Birth, death, and sex constitute the new frontiers on the political battlefields. Politics is dying out nowadays as a translation of our moral and existential concerns into rational and legitimate action for the benefit of society and humanity, and, instead, is becoming a set of managerial practices and skillful manipulation of public opinion. Thus, it is not unwise to assume that a swift politicization of privacy and history promises the way out of the present political and ideological vacuum.

Suffice it to remember the hottest debates over abortion, euthanasia, and gay marriage over the past twenty or so years conclude that the poor human individual continues to be regarded as either property of the state and its institutions or, at best, a mere instrument and hostage of a political doctrine. This can be considered whether (s)he is born, or is dying, or consummating her or his marriage, etc.

Nothing new under the sky, though. If we are to believe such incisive dystopian writers as Yevgeny Zamyatin, Aldous Huxley, and George Orwell, or such groundbreaking social theorists as Michel Foucault and Zygmunt Bauman, modernity always was, and continues to be, obsessed with how to get as much control over the human body and soul as possible without physically exterminating people. The same is true with regard of society's memory and collective sentiment.

As we learn from George Orwell's *1984*, history depends on who controls those archives and records. Since human individuals have no other form of existence than that which is granted by the Party, individual memory has no power to create or restore history. But if memory is controlled or manufactured and updated every day, history degenerates into a justificatory and legitimizing design of power and control. Logically enough, this leads the Inner Party to assert that who controls the past controls the future and who controls the present controls the past. If the reader thinks that it does not make sense to refer to the Orwellian world any longer, please think about memory wars in present Europe. That Russia has already become a revisionist power is obvious. Moreover, it attempts to rewrite the history of the twentieth century rehabilitating Stalin and depicting him as merely a wise, albeit sometimes cruel, modernizer of Russia. As we can see, Stalin appears here to have been just another version of the Great Modernizer of the State, just like Peter the Great.

Needless to say, an attempt to outlaw what is regarded in Russia as historical revisionism has its logic; that is, criminalization of any effort to put into question whether the Soviet Union with its labor camps, overtly fascist practices and anti-Semitism (for those who have doubts about this, please do recall the Holodomor in Ukraine or methodical extermination of Russian Jews and Jewish culture under Stalin) was any better than Nazi Germany. By no means is it about the past. As early as under Mikhail Gorbachev, a plethora of decent and courageous Russian historians exposed the Soviet Union to have been a criminal state. Stalin was explicitly regarded as a criminal and paranoid dictator who committed horrible crimes against humanity. The fact that Vladimir Putin's Russia changed the interpretation of the past nearly overnight shows that everything is about the present, rather than the past.

Although the denial of the Holocaust is too complex a phenomenon to be confined to legal practices and administrative measures, Germany outlawed the denial of the Holocaust because of its firm commitment never to repeat its past. Russia cynically denies its occupation and annexation of the Baltic States, as well as its numerous crimes against European nations, because it sends a message to us that it would gladly repeat recent history restoring the past and rehabilitating political doctrine which Gorbachev's and Yeltsin's Russia regarded as overtly criminal and hostile to Russia itself.

Thus, the Baltic States and Eastern-Central European nations attempt to work out an antidote against Russia's revisionism. All in all, this attempt is understandable, but the idea of a political and moral equivalency of

Communism and National Socialism is highly debatable, to say the least. Western Europe and the USA will always take a deep exception to the claim that the Holocaust and Soviet crimes were of the same nature, and quite rightly so. Yet this is not merely a matter of dangerous political implications or morally repugnant conclusions that politicians tend to draw from our painful dilemmas.

The point is that history can never be left solely to politicians, no matter whether democratic or authoritarian. Like human beings and human rights that can never be reduced to a property of the state, history cannot be confined to the supplement of a political doctrine or relegated to the margins of a political regime it supposedly serves. History, if properly understood, is the symbolic design of our existence and moral choices we make every day. Like human privacy, our right to study and critically question history is a cornerstone of freedom.

Robert van Voren's remarkable study of the Cold War in psychiatry and of the political use and abuse of psychiatry in the name of law and order or for the sake of fostering a rival blueprint for a global social and moral order sheds new light on the attempt of Soviet psychiatry to marginalize, clinicalize, stigmatize, and, in effect, criminalize human rights activists and dissidents in the former Soviet Union. A valuable, intensely researched, well documented, provocative, and rich study, it covers an immense discursive, moral, and political territory stretching from a personal perspective and travel story, or an account of friendship and a moral autobiography, to in-depth exploration of the anti-psychiatry-based trend in North American and West European political philosophy, sociology, and psychology. This trend is, perhaps, best exemplified by Michel Foucault and his followers among French poststructuralists and historians of consciousness engaged in what the eminent American sociologist of Lithuanian background, Vytautas Kavolis, aptly described as resistance knowledge.

The book allows the point of entry into the aforementioned ambivalent and sinister tendency of modernity: namely, the conquest of the sphere of privacy and legitimate human secrets by power discourses and power politics. This is, hence, the added value and originality of this deeply personal, yet uniquely universalistic and humanistic book. Even putting aside its scholarly and overall intellectual value, the monograph serves as a potent antidote against a sort of moral and political amnesia from which Europe seems to suffer and also appears as a deeply symbolic and timely token of European solidarity. Van Voren's book reads as a *cri du cœur*, as a war cry, and as a rational political appeal to civilized humanity. It reaches out to a sensitive readership opening up for a dialogue with those who know little about the war that the Soviet system mercilessly waged on dissidents and human rights defenders through the network of mental asylums, and also through the means of instrumental "rationality" of psychiatry as a science and as an instrument to exercise power over the cornered individual and disciplined society.

A year ago, the book series on Baltic studies "On the Boundary of Two Worlds" offered to an English-speaking readership *On Dissidents and Madness: From the Soviet Union of Leonid Brezhnev to the "Soviet Union" of Vladimir Putin*, the book by Robert van Voren originally written in Dutch and published in The Netherlands, and then translated into English and published with Rodopi. It is with pleasure, then, that now I can present his new landmark contribution to Baltic and East/Central European studies.

This time the readership will be able to enjoy Robert van Voren's magnificent new book, *Cold War in Psychiatry: Human Factors, Secret Actors*. I wish this new book a long and happy life which it richly deserves.

Leonidas Donskis
Member of the European Parliament (MEP ALDE) and
Recurrent Visiting Professor of Politics at Vytautas Magnus University,
Kaunas, Lithuania

Introduction

> *Writing history, like any work on the past, never consists of establishing facts and nothing more. It always also involves selecting those facts that are more salient or significant than others and making connections between them. Selection and combination cannot only be directed toward truth; they must also always strive toward a good. Scholarship is obviously not the same thing as politics, but scholarship, being a human activity, has a political finality, which may be for good or bad.*[1]

Twenty years after the fall of the Berlin Wall, it is hard to imagine how the East-West confrontation dominated daily life, not only in Europe but also across the globe. Looking back, there are few elements of life that were not connected to it in one way or another. Clearly the most ostensible element was the political standoff between East and West, between NATO and the Warsaw Pact, but this was only the icing on the cake. Underneath, virtually everything was divided: an individual was either for or against, left or right, progressive or conservative. The political division dominated politics, daily life, and every other aspect related to it. In the West using "communist" symbols was an act of protest, expressing dissent, and many Western Communists purposely bought a Soviet *Lada* or a Czechoslovak *Skoda*. In the Soviet Union, anything "Western" was the closest you could get to being "hot." Plastic bags, ballpoint pins, plastic lighters and chewing gum were signs of bourgeois decadence, a small treasure, enough to bribe an official or to pay for a service rendered.

In my life it was no different. I grew up in the Dutch port of Rotterdam and in secondary school the majority of the kids was against the Vietnam War, especially those whose company you enjoyed. Those in favor of the war were considered to be nerds, dull creatures who studied hard and were keen to become productive elements of society: exactly the group in which I did not want to belong. Parents were usually against the USSR, even afraid of it, so adolescents were therefore automatically inclined to be in favor. I grew up in an environment that was definitely pro-American, even if only because I was born in Canada and my father lost his heart to that country. Throughout my youth, he longed to return so we frequented an

---

1 Todorov, Tzvetan: *Hope and Memory*, p.128

American church and had American friends. Until adolescence I looked like an all-American kid. Anti-Sovietism was mostly the result of reading about Stalinist terror: first Gulag Archipelago by Aleksandr Solzhenitsyn and then an avalanche of other books that unintentionally shaped not only my views but also the course of my life. By the end of the 1970s, I was heavily involved in human rights work on behalf of Soviet dissidents, with a special interest in prisoners that wound up in psychiatric hospitals for purely political reasons. In University in the early 1980s, most of my friends were against the American cruise missiles and in favor of unilateral disarmament and being against the Soviet SS-20s was 'not done' as it was almost heresy. I tried to refrain from political discussions, but as soon as they found out my political views some fellow students stopped talking to me because of my alleged "ultra-right attitude." University studies were dominated by Marxism-Leninism in all sorts and varieties, and criticism of the Soviet Union put you immediately on the wrong footing.

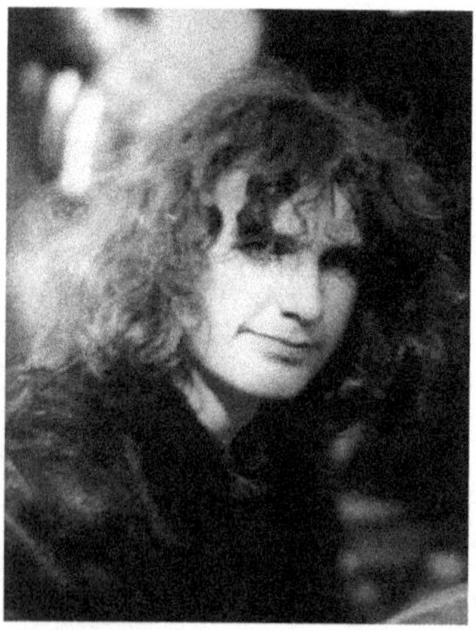
Robert van Voren, 1980

It all came to an end, quite suddenly, and somehow the issue was buried. People went on with their lives, and only a few returned to the past, to discuss the positions they had taken, how they interacted, why they made their choices and the associated implications. Yet this standoff inadvertently destroyed many relations, poisoned human interaction. It was a war, a psychological war, which victimized people on both sides and had long-lasting effects that still influence affairs today.

The first idea to write this book was formed during the throes of creation of another one, which consisted mainly of my own reminiscences of the past thirty years. One particular period seemed to offer more questions than answers, and when reading some documents and papers on the subject I became even more intrigued. I had been an active and quite centrally positioned actor in the events in question; however, it became increasingly clear to me that I had been living in a sort of mental cocoon, being part yet at the same time not knowing the full and maybe even the real picture. I let it be, for the time being, but promised myself to come back to it for further exploration.

The relevant period covered the years 1983-1989, when I was in charge of the International Association on the Political Use of Psychiatry (IAPUP)[2] and we "waged war" on the World Psychiatric Association (WPA). Our goal was to keep the Soviet All-Union Society of Neuropathologists and Psychiatrists (AUSNP) from being readmitted to membership of this international body, from which it had been forced to leave in early 1983 after it became clear that a majority in the General Assembly of the WPA would vote for its expulsion, because of the continued abuse of psychiatry for political purposes in the USSR. The campaign in favor of the expulsion of the AUSNP had been one of the main reasons for the founding of our organization in 1980. Automatically, GIP and the WPA were standing on opposite sides of the barricade.

I deliberately call it "waging war" because these were times when nuances were difficult to find. We were convinced that we were right, that the truth was on our side, and that the Soviets were deliberately using psychiatry as a tool of repression. The people within the WPA who tried to keep the issue off the agenda and, subsequently, wanted to bring the Soviets back into its fold were, in our view, "fellow-travelers" who ignored the pleas for help from the victims of political psychiatry and were not interested in defending ethics within their profession. I myself belonged to the hardliners.

Yet time has the tendency to soften views, to help reconsider positions and conclusions, and to make it possible to look at one's own behavior from a distance. Although I have never doubted that psychiatry was indeed used in a systematic manner as a tool of repression in the Soviet Union and in a number of other countries, I also have learned to see things from a different perspective. I became friends with Soviet psychiatrists, who had seemingly been on the "other side," including some who had been at WPA meetings as members of the Soviet delegation, and I started to understand their positions, their views on these events. It took a while, but gradually history lost its sharp edges and became more and more explorable.

The period 1983-1989 continued to intrigue, because there were too many hidden factors and open endings, questions to which I was seeking answers. I discovered that our organization had been infiltrated by the East-German secret service Stasi, with very unpleasant consequences. I also found out that one of the members of the Executive Committee of the WPA had been an informal agent of the Stasi, which made the picture even more complex.

2 In 1989 renamed into Geneva Initiative on Psychiatry (GIP), and in 2005 into Global Initiative on Psychiatry (GIP).

Undoubtedly, other intelligence agencies also had been engaged, yet their archives remained closed, either because the governments decided not to open them to the public or because no political change took place that would allow for disclosure. Although almost to the very end the Soviet AUSNP maintained that there had been no political abuse of psychiatry in the USSR, the Soviet press frequently wrote about such cases, thereby making the AUSNP look ridiculous and detached from reality.

The period did not end with the World Congress of the WPA in Athens in October 1989, where the Soviets managed to obtain a conditional return. However momentous that moment might have been to those of us so deeply involved in the issue, it was nothing in comparison to what happened on a global scale: less than a month after the WPA World Congress, the Berlin Wall came tumbling down, and before the end of the year communism had met its end in Eastern Europe. A few months later, in March 1990, Lithuania declared its independence as the first Soviet republic to make such a move and, although Soviet leadership resisted with armed force, the end of the USSR was an historical inevitability – and the consequences are still there today.

However, further exploration of the period 1983-1989 brought forth a very different picture than originally envisaged. It was not the main political events that triggered my attention but the people behind them, those who had "waged war" with me, on either side of the barricade. When discovering their lives, their backgrounds and convictions, history truly came to life and made it possible to see the political events from a human perspective. In particular, the lives of two members of the WPA Executive Committee intrigued me. One I had known, the other was only a vague image and name. Yet their lives gradually became like threads of DNA, circling around each other and intertwined at certain points, meandering through the history of the twentieth century with all its turmoil, horror and lost hopes. I traveled back with them into their past history and that of their parents, trying to bring back that was lost, or what was seemingly hidden under the dust of time. In addition, in the course of writing the book I met other actors, who became equally engaged and who also shared their reminiscences and views of what happened during those days.

The result of this odyssey is now in front of you. It is not a complete picture or the full story. Some parts were irretraceably lost, either because of inaccessible records (e.g. those of Western intelligence agencies, except for the FBI records on Mel Sabshin, which became available in the course of my research) or because the memories faded away with time. The objects of my research became researchers themselves, trying to recall what happened, looking for clues and documents, reading texts and commenting on them. What started as my own odyssey became a collective one, a collective effort to tell the story of our "war."

When I was a history student, a future Sovietologist, one of my favorite books was one by the German writer Heinrich Böll and the Soviet Germanist Lev Kopelev, *Why did we shoot at each other*? The book never reached a wide audience, yet the essence was majestic. It told their story during the Second World War, when both men were drafted into the army to fight each other, two peons in a war that engulfed the world and turned Europe into an endless graveyard. In time, the men became friends, engaged in the struggle for human rights in the Soviet Union, both on the same side of the barricade.[3]

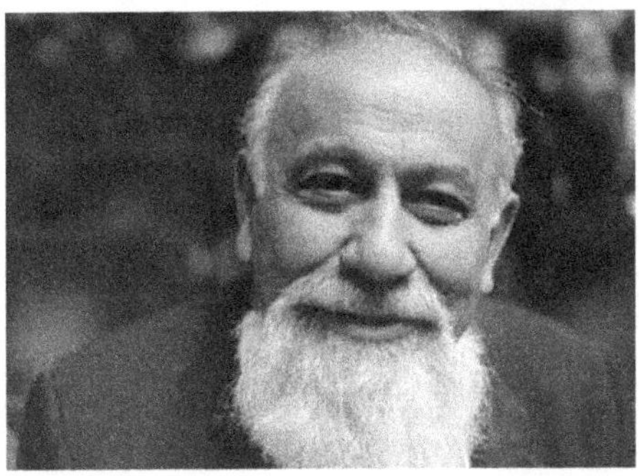
Lev Kopelev

This image of two former enemies becoming friends and companions stuck with me when writing this book. Also in my case, a friendship developed with one and deepened with the other. Even more important was the fact that I developed a deep respect for both, for their principles, and their roles in this particular history. I understood what they probably knew all along: that there was more that bound them than divided them, and that their different historical realities in no way prevented them from developing a friendship that survives until this very day.

There is nothing more complicated than history and the attempt to understand why things happened the way they did, what human interaction formed the chain of historical events. It is much easier to put people into boxes and to reduce them to simple stereotypes. It is more challenging to understand the full scope of human emotions, fears and desires, and external factors that determine whether a person winds up in history on the "good" or the "bad" side, or on both.

3 Böll, Heinrich, and Kopelew, Lew: *Warum haben wir aufeinander geschossen?* Lamuv Verlag, 1981

Yet probably the most difficult task is to develop a similarly distant view of oneself, to be able to evaluate one's own role and deeds critically, and with the same desire to put things in perspective. In a way it seems to go against human nature, against the desire to believe in your own importance and the importance of the activities that you undertook. In writing this book, I tried to look at myself, and at my role, from a distance. I tried to be critical, to understand. It is the reader who should judge whether I was successful. In some ways I may have been too lenient, in others too harsh; yet like all the other actors in this story I was shaped by my past, my environment, and by a limited view of what happened around me. Thus, unintentionally, this book became somewhat of an autobiographical one, an attempt to understand my own past activities and put them in a wider context.

For the above-mentioned reasons, this book is not a typical scholarly work[4]. It is based on archival research and on extensive interviews with many of the actors involved. It is equally based on personal recollections, both of myself and of others. And although the central historical event is the 1983-1989 struggle against Soviet political abuse, the book places these events against the backdrop of the turbulent history of the twentieth century. In mixing all these aspects into one story, I tried to maintain an acceptable level of clarity, and I hope I succeeded. This complexity doesn't make the book easier to read, but hopefully makes it more realistic: there is not one clear line in history; there is not *one* history. History is like a whirlwind of factors and actors, both hidden and overt; it is a concoction that never fails to attract and repel, an intriguing mix of what one learns and what will remain untold.

Odyssey

This book would never have been without Ellen Mercer, so my first and heartfelt thanks go to her. It was she who showed herself to be a real friend by maintaining contact with Jochen Neumann throughout the years, and who was the first to suggest to him that he should think of telling me his part of the story. Without her mediation, as Jochen confided to me later, this would never have happened and he would never have developed the trust in me that was needed to open up and tell me his life story. And it was again Ellen Mercer, who edited the manuscript, turning it into the form it has right now.

And that is when the odyssey began. My first intention was to do archival

[4] The book *Cold War in Psychiatry* was written as a dissertation for obtaining a doctoral degree in political science at Kaunas University, Lithuania.

research and interview both Jochen Neumann and Melvin Sabshin, the two main characters in the book. Yet gradually it got out of hand, and in the end I interviewed more than a dozen people in many countries, sometimes more than once, combining trips for my regular work with interviewing, and usually putting things to paper during the night, while sitting in my hotel room or at home when my wife and children were asleep and my time was my own.

Unforgettable events were the joint interviews of Jochen Neumann and Melvin Sabshin, later joined by Ellen Mercer as well, when, in a strange way, the Executive Committee of the WPA came back to life and the discussions provided a unique blend of memories that helped recreate the atmosphere as it had been years before. Also the long sessions with Costas Stefanis are lasting and dear memories. During these sessions, I had endless conversations with a man who initially seemed to be a main adversary but with whom, in many ways, took on the colors of a friend. Many thanks to those who agreed to be interviewed, in particular, of course, Jochen Neumann, Melvin Sabshin and Ellen Mercer, but also (in alphabetical order): Yosé Höhne-Sparborth; Andrei Kovalev; Valentinas Maciulis, Dainius Puras; Elena Raes-Mozhaeva; Norman Sartorius; Eduard Shevardnadze, Costas Stefanis and Antonis Vgontzas.

I want to thank Peter Reddaway, who provided me with a wealth of materials from his private archive; Sonja Süss, for giving feedback on her work in the Stasi archives and helped me get started there; Roswitha Loos of the Stasi archives, for preparing all my files so diligently and trying to answer my requests and questions; Helmut Bieber, who provided background information on the DVpMP; Mario Maj, for opening the WPA archives and allowing me to search for relevant materials; Loren Roth, for providing me with materials from his own records on the US delegation to the US and for giving ongoing feedback; Anatoly Adamishin and Richard Schifter, for their explanations on some of the issues of the US-USSR negotiations in 1987-1988; to Janos Furedi and Laszlo Tringer for helping to research the life story and fate of Pal Juhasz; to Elena Raes-Mozhaeva, for helping to find materials in Russia; to Vyacheslav Bakhmin, for sharing his memories from the 1980s; and to Leonidas Donskis, for his constant encouragement.

I thank all those who read my text, who commented on it and gave me critical feedback: my mother, a professional journalist who apart from being mother is also a critical listener and reader; Anatoly Adamishin; Rob Keukens; Andrei Kovalev; Ellen Mercer; Elena Raes-Mozhaeva; Dick Raes; Loren Roth; and, of course, Jochen Neumann and Melvin Sabshin.

Very special thanks go to Lela Tsiskarishvili, who was there from the very start, often the first (critical) reader of texts, sometimes still in their most rudimentary form, and whose comments and feedback fulfilled the role of the fictive audience I needed in order to retain my inspiration and to continue to be able to write.

And, last but not least, I thank my wife, Brigita, for her constant encouragement, for being there when needed, and for not being there when I needed space; for telling me I could manage and for believing that the end result would be worth the effort. The final judgment is up to you, the readers, but her support and belief in me was invaluable.

People say that writing a dissertation is hell. They are right. But if given the chance, I would do it all over again – it was a wonderful confrontation with my own past, with my own "holy houses" that turned out to be less holy than thought before. It also offered me the extraordinary opportunity of crossing bridges to alleged enemies who turned out to be altogether different than I imagined, and with whom I invariably developed a special bond. It was a unique experience.

Part I

Setting the Stage

Chapter 1 - Meeting Mel Sabshin

London has always seemed to me to be a combination of a wide variety of urban neighborhoods and majestic buildings in the city center, combined with endless rows of depressing brick homes and buildings lining the railroad tracks that travel to other places in the country. Yet London also has areas that are almost village-like, where the sense of being in one of the biggest European metropolis quickly fades away. One of those neighborhoods is where Mel Sabshin and his third wife live. They also maintain his home in the United States and, in spite of his old age, he continues to travel extensively. A small cobblestone street leads up to the row of townhouses where their home is found. When I ring the bell, he swings the door open with the typical broad smile on his face. We embrace. We haven't met for more than a decade and both have clearly aged. I have grown completely grey and am now wearing a beard; he has visibly shrunk. The once imposing physical stature has disappeared, yet I soon find that his imposing mental stature is still unchanged. He quickly takes the lead in the discussions, has clearly prepared himself for my visit and is full of excitement over our meeting. He slept badly, his wife Marion tells me. He is physically not well, has been seriously ill recently, yet also the prospect of returning to the past with me has filled him with excitement and kept him from sleeping.

My memory flashes back to the 1980s. Mel Sabshin is at the height of his career, as Medical Director of the American Psychiatric Association (APA) he leads the most powerful psychiatric empire in the world.[5] The APA has turned into an influential and extensive organization and is housed in a large multi-story building in the Washington, DC Metropolitan Area. The APA owns one of the largest psychiatric publishing houses and develops and publishes the classification of mental disorders, the Diagnostic and Statistical Manual (DSM). This DSM competes with the International Classification of Diseases (ICD) of the World Health Organization, and has been accepted as the main classification in quite a few countries around the globe. As Medical Director of the organization since 1974, Mel has

[5] The Medical Director of the American Psychiatric Association (APA) was actually not the chief executive officer of the organization. Formally this was the President of the APA, who was elected however for only a one year period and during his tenure as Medical Director Melvin Sabshin became in fact the intellectual leader of the psychiatric profession in the United States. His became in practice a more important function than that of the President of the APA, and during his years in power virtually no President challenged his authority. See also Sabshin, Melvin: *Changing American Psychiatry*, pp. 55-56

been instrumental in putting American psychiatry firmly on the world map, and, beginning in 1983, he also functioned as a member of the Executive Committee of the World Psychiatric Association, the main psychiatric body that unites psychiatric associations around the globe.[6] The latter was the main reason for my regular visits to his office, as I was in charge of the organization that coordinated the campaigns against the political use of psychiatry in the Soviet Union and which had been instrumental in forcing the Soviet member association out of the WPA in 1983.

The department that was crucial in putting the APA's vision of its role in world psychiatry into practice was the Department of International Affairs, led by Ellen Mercer. Ellen was not only one of Sabshin's key staff members, she was equally imposing in stature and presence. In the fight against political abuse of psychiatry, she was a key factor, as she had access to world psychiatric leaders yet, at the same time, she shared our views on how the abuse in the USSR should be brought to an end. In that sense, she formed a unique bridge between both worlds. She often attended meetings of the World Psychiatric Association, and regularly accompanied Mel Sabshin on his international travels. There she also met "the other side," the Soviets and their allies. She conversed with them and developed friendships, yet her heart was with us, and Mel Sabshin knew it. Her close relationship with our organization was at times a worry to him, as he told me every now and then in confidence; we should be aware how much her heart lies with us, and not abuse it. It was typically Mel: he was worried, warns us, yet at the same time he gave Ellen the freedom to make her own choices and to follow her convictions. And at moments when she brought him into trouble he stood by her, unwavering. That happened, for instance, in the summer of 1983, during the World Congress of the WPA in Vienna, when Ellen decided to allow our organization to use the APA-stand at the Congress to disseminate our materials. The WPA Executive Committee, and in particular its General Secretary Prof. Peter Berner[7] from Vienna, had banned us from the congress and forbid the distribution of our leaflets, and Ellen's action directly violated that ban. The reaction of Prof. Berner was one of extreme anger: he exploded, throwing the leaflets on the floor and Ellen was called before the Executive Committee for a disciplinary meeting. It was Mel who defended her, and made sure she remained untouched.

6 The World Psychiatric Association (WPA) is an international umbrella organization of psychiatric societies. For more information on the WPA and its structure see Chapter 15.

7 Peter Berner, born in Karlovy Vary (Czech Republic) in 1924, psychiatrist and neurologist, was from 1971 to 1991 university professor and head of the university psychiatric clinic in Vienna.

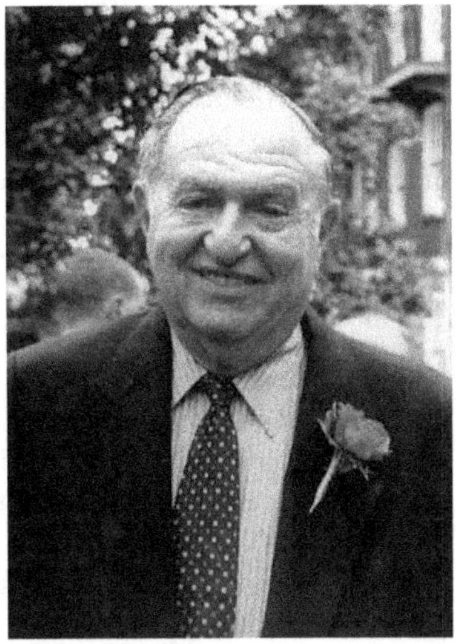

Melvin Sabshin, 2000

The same Mel Sabshin met with me in his office every time I was in Washington and he was also in town. We discussed strategy, the state of affairs in Soviet psychiatric abuse, and he questioned me about the policies of our organization. Mel is inquisitive, and needs to be convinced. He had no problem voicing his own opinion, or expressing his dissatisfaction when he thought we were following an incorrect course; yet, at the same time, he listened carefully to counter-arguments, enjoying the exchange of opinions and the clash of minds. In a fatherly manner, he challenged me to think more carefully about strategy, not automatically to follow a hard-line approach but to think how to deal with the existing situation in a strategic manner to obtain the maximum outcome. He is almost thirty-five years my senior, the difference in intellectual power and life experience is equally vast, yet he never gave me the feeling of being naïve, or "wet behind the ears," even though he must have winced regularly while listening to my youthful simplified outlook on the existing situation.

Now, almost twenty years after he ended his term as a member of the Executive Committee of the WPA, he is still his inquisitive self, sometimes making me wonder who interviews whom and who set the agenda for the meeting. He asks me my view on Chinese political abuse of psychiatry, listens to my answer and then says: "No, I think that is too simple. I think the answer must be more complex," and again forces me to dig deeper, to look behind the curtains for hidden answers. "And what do you think…" he continues, posing the next challenging question.

His excitement about the meeting has one clear focal point: it is his relationship with one of the other members of the Executive Committee of the WPA, Jochen Neumann. Neumann is the member of the Executive Committee I knew least about, and whom I never really met. The reason is obvious: Neumann was from East Germany, and by that fact alone in the "opposing camp." He supported the Soviet point of view, was the representative of the Eastern Bloc on the Executive Committee and, thus, for us "beyond reach." Yet at the same time I knew from Ellen Mercer that Neumann was intelligent, cultured, a very pleasant personality, and that gradually a friendship had developed between him and Mel Sabshin. It seemed the least logical combination: The East German Neumann, who not only voiced the views of the Eastern Bloc but also "aired" like an Eastern European, and Mel Sabshin, the exponent of American dominance in world psychiatry, very critical of Soviet psychiatric abuse and, in our view, a total ally in our campaigns.

These were the times of the Cold War, and sophistication and nuances in political views and outlooks did not flourish in those days. Black was black and white was white, and we made a clear distinction between those who supported our campaign against the political abuse of psychiatry in the Soviet Union (the good ones) and those who supported the Soviet position (the bad ones). It would not have been possible to combine friendship with a person from the "other side" while opposing psychiatry as a means of oppression.

Yet Mel did not have that problem. A reason why a friendship between the two supposed opponents developed was the fact that both were principled men. Neither was an opportunist, a career-seeker; both believed in what they stood for and put those convictions into practice. During the Executive Committee meetings, it was inevitable that they almost automatically disagreed on the Soviet issue; yet in most other respects they shared principles and had a common goal: to advance world psychiatry and to turn the World Psychiatric Association into an organization that would strengthen the profession worldwide.

Perhaps Mel's affection for Jochen Neumann was partially influenced by his own family background. His parents were born in what is now Belarus and what was then part of the Russian Empire. His father, Zalman Sabshin, was born in 1892 in Beshenkovichi, a Jewish shtetl near Orsha, close to what is now the border between Belarus and Russia.[8] He emigrated to the United States in 1910, two years before his future wife, Sonia Barnhard, made the same trip. She had been born in 1900 and came from the town of Slonim, not far from Grodno and 200 kilometer south of the Lithuanian capital of Vilnius, which was then called the "Jerusalem of the East." [9] In other words, Mel Sabshin's actual roots were in Russia, a country

8 His original surname is not known. His date of birth was April 26, 1892.

9 Sonia Barnhard was born on April 22, 1900. Her parents were Eli Sroliovich (later changed into Barnhard) and Chasha Zhuchlovitsky (which was later changed into Dillon).

that became part of the Soviet Union, with which Jochen Neumann was closely connected politically, but even more so culturally and emotionally. By growing up in a Jewish-Russian (and pro-Communist) environment, Sabshin became more receptive to Neumann's political background and his ways of perceiving things, his way of formulating his thoughts. It also strengthened the psychological connection with the world that Neumann represented.[10] However, an equally important factor that helped develop this bond was the fact that Neumann was ideologically not a hardliner but rather, as he later put it himself, "a cross between a bourgeois of the XIX century and an engaged communist." [11] Without this, Sabshin and Neumann would not have been able to cross the bridge and meet half way.

10 This is confirmed by both Neumann and Sabshin during a collective interview on July 29, 2009

11 Letter to Ellen Mercer, March 30, 2009

Chapter 2 – Melvin Sabshin's Roots

> *It was as if all the Jews of Russia were to be violently crowded in and piled on top of each other, like grasshoppers in a ditch; here they were miserably crushed together until the fruitless struggle for life should have done its work.*[12]

Melvin Sabshin's parents were part of a true exodus of Russian Jews, who left their country at the end of the nineteenth and the beginning of the twentieth centuries. While between 1820 and 1870 only some 7,500 Jews from Poland and Russia had immigrated to the United States, the numbers rose quickly after 1870. During the first ten years, 1871-1880, already 40,000 persons emigrated; in the following decade, the number increased to 135,000 and between 1891 and 1910 almost a million Jews found a new life across the ocean. Thousands of others went to Europe, Australia and South Africa.[13]

At the end of the 19th century, over five million Jews were living in Russia.[14] Virtually all of them lived in the Pale of Settlement, an area that corresponded to historical borders of the Polish-Lithuanian Commonwealth and included much of present-day Lithuania, Belarus, Poland, Bessarabia, Ukraine, and parts of western Russia. Additionally, a number of cities within the Pale were excluded from the permission to Jews to settle there. In the Pale, Jews constituted 11 percent of the total population; yet were often the majority in Byelorussian and Lithuanian cities.[15] Most of them were poor. In the 1890s, nineteen percent of Jewish families in Russia and over 22 percent in Lithuania lived in extreme poverty and had to ask for communal assistance to survive and be able to celebrate Passover.[16]

---

12 In *The Russian Jews* (1894), as quoted in Rischin, Moses: *The Promised City*, p. 19

13 Gitelman, Zvi: *A Century of Ambivalence*, p. 12

14 The census of 1897 showed that there were 5,2 million Jews in Russia, of which only 300,000 lived outside the Pale of Settlement. See Kochan, Lionel (ed.): *Jews in Soviet Russia since 1917*, p. 15.

15 According to the same census of 1897,over 50% of the population in towns in Lithuania and Belarus was Jewish. In Vilnius about half of the city's population was Jewish.

16 *The Promised City*, p.31. Alas, the immigration wave of the late nineteenth century and early twentieth century did not improve the quality of life for those left behind. Although the number of Jews went down, and one could assume this would decrease the economic pressure on those remaining, so did the number of consumers and potential clients for the remaining artisans, and thus the result was a further increased poverty.

Pogroms

The major reason for the sudden surge of emigration was the assassination of Tsar Aleksandr II on March 1, 1881, by a terrorist cell of the political movement "Narodnaya Volya." Although only one member of the group, Gesia Gelfman, was of Jewish origin, word soon spread that the Jews had killed the Tsar and a government inspired pogrom engulfed the country. One of the main instigators was the Chief Procurator of the Holy Synod, Konstantin Pobedonovtsev, also referred to as the "Grey Cardinal," who argued that the best way to deal with Russian Jewry was to force one-third into emigration, have one-third baptized and kill the remaining one-third.[17]

During the preceding decades, the Jews in Russia had actually gone through a period of relative tranquility. Over the past century, they had lived through cycles of relaxation and repression, often pressured by the Russian authorities to adapt and assimilate to their Russian environment. Within the Jewish community, various groups positioned themselves differently. The enlighteners, *maskilim*, wanted to bring the benefits of European culture to the Jews and advocated reforms in religion. They believed in the good will of the Tsar and thought he was working for their betterment. The *maskilim* were opposed by the more religious Jews, such as the *Hassidim*, who believed that the *maskilim* were undermining traditional authority in the Jewish community and were leading the Jews towards assimilation and integration into Russian culture.[18]

And while the majority of Jews remained firmly rooted in their traditional Jewish identity, a growing number turned to enlightenment in an attempt to connect their Jewishness with modernity, with progress. Some converted to Christianity, others became Russian in their way of life, or turned to socialism or internationalism. A growing number became politically active, not only trying to change the position of the Jews but with the goal of changing society and the political system as a whole.

---

17 Greenbaum, Masha: *Jews of Lithuania*, p. 187

18 See, among others, *The Jews in Soviet Russia since 1917*, pp. 18-19. More strict religious leaders such as the Vilno Gaon, who feared that Hassidic leaders themselves would become object of adulation, in turn, opposed the Hassidim. In particular they opposed the Hassidim's view that one could attain spiritual fulfillment not only through learning and intellectual efforts but also through sincere prayer and behavior expressive of the joy of drawing closer to God, including song and dance, often fueled by the use of alcohol. Slonim, coincidentally, was one of the centers of the Hassidim.

Most of the Jewish socialists were "narodniki," and based their hopes on an enlightened self-liberating peasant class. But when they finally met the peasants, they were bitterly disappointed, because "they beheld the peasants as most of them really were: a brutish, crude, boorish, superstitious lot, influenced by an obscanturist reactionary clergy. Theirs was a social class in which individuals brimmed with hatred and bitterness towards each other, their feudal lords, and all strangers, especially if they were not Russian Orthodox. Their priests taught them to hate Catholics because of the authoritarian hierarchy in Rome, Protestants for their individualism, and above all Jews, who had 'killed Christ.'"[19] Their political beliefs were further shaken when, during the 1881-82 pogroms, farmers actively participated in the witch-hunt against the Jews. Even more shocking to them was the fact that their fellow non-Jewish revolutionaries applauded the active participation of peasants as a first step towards political emancipation. The theory was that by striking at the Jews, the peasantry was learning to become self-assertive, to defend itself against its oppressors. They believed that eventually the peasants would learn that the Jews were not the real enemy, but, rather, the autocratic exploitative system. However, if some Jews had to be sacrificed in that process, so be it.[20] The *Narodnaya Volya* bulletin of 1882 summarized it quite directly: "Today the Jew, tomorrow the Czar and the kulaks."[21]

The pogroms of 1881-82 were followed by a set of laws of May 1882 in which it was stipulated that the Jews were no longer allowed to live outside the towns and shtetls. They were forbidden to do business on Sundays, and as Saturday was for them a holy day, it automatically meant that they were in an unfavorable position vis-à-vis their non-Jewish competition. In Russian schools a *numeris clausis* was introduced, which stipulated that in the Pale, only 10 percent of students in secondary schools could be of Jewish origin and 5 percent outside. [22] In 1890, the Moscow police ordered that all Jewish shops were required to have the owners' names in Hebrew, and a year later all the Jews were expelled from Moscow altogether. The May Laws have also been described as a perpetual administrative pogrom that remained on the books until the October Revolution of 1917.[23]

---

19 *Jews of Lithuania*, p. 195

20 *Century of Ambivalence*, p. 7-13

21 *Jews of Lithuania*, p. 196

22 In Moscow and St. Petersburg it was a maximum of 3 percent, which was later reduced even further

23 *Jews of Lithuania*, p. 190. The May Laws were introduced by Interior Minister Count Pavel Ignatiev.

The economic hardships, anti-Semitic pogroms and restrictive laws forced many Jews to leave their homes in search of a better life elsewhere. A mass migration started to develop, with many Jews from Lithuania and Byelorussia streaming south into Ukraine or westward to the industrialized cities of Poland. Urban centers developed almost over night. The Polish city of Lodz, a village with only 11 Jews in 1793, grew swiftly to a Jewish population of almost 100,000 in 1897 and 166,000 in 1910. Warsaw, which had 3,500 Jews in 1781, grew to have 219,000 in 1891.[24]

Because the restrictive laws banned Jews from owning or renting land, and later also from being innkeepers or restaurateurs, and the *numeris clausis* made access to educational institutions almost impossible, many tried to earn a living through artisanship. Workshops and sweatshops sprang up all over the towns and cities. Many Jews worked in the industries, thereby creating a new proletariat.[25] By the end of the 19th century, Jews constituted over 21 percent of the factory workers in the Pale, and in Poland the number was as high as 28 percent.[26] Jewish women had originally taken on many responsibilities in the family business in order to allow their husbands to devote time to religious study. In the 1870s, the introduction of the Singer sewing machine revolutionized Jewish homes, and wives and daughters were set to work making garments. In larger towns women started to work as tailoresses, seamstresses, sockmakers, etc. - trades that were very useful when they emigrated to the United States.[27]

Jews and socialism

The development of a Jewish working class in the cities also meant that Marxian Socialism achieved a much more widespread appeal. [28] As early as the 1870s, Jewish workmen resorted to sabotage and violence in strikes, driven by poverty and hardships. In 1888, the Social Democrats founded strike funds and strike treasuries in a variety of trades, setting off a more organized union activity.[29] Soon the first national trade union was organized in Russia,[30] and Jews formed the backbone of the organization.

24 *The Promised City*, p. 24
25 *The Promised City*, p.27
26 *The Promised City*, 28
27 *The Promised City*, p. 27
28 *The Promised City*, p. 43
29 In 1895 workers in the tobacco industry of Vilna managed to win several victories with their strikes, and in Bialystok thousands of textile workers set off a great labor upheaval.
30 The Universal Union of Bristle Workers in Russian Poland

Political activism among the Jews also resulted in higher numbers among political prisoners. Between 1901 and 1903, of the 7,791 persons imprisoned in Russia for political reasons, 2,269 were Jews. From March 1903 to November 1904, 54 percent of those sentenced for political reasons were Jews; of the women sentenced for political crimes, more than 64 percent were Jewish. In 1904, of an estimated 30,000 organized Jewish workers, 4,476 were imprisoned or exiled to Siberia.[31]

In 1897, a "General League – Bund – of Jewish Workingmen in Russia and Poland" was founded in Vilno, then a part of the Russian Empire, forming a national organization of social democratic and Marxist labor organizations. In 1901, Lithuania was added to the name.[32] Between 1897 and 1900, the Bund led 312 strikes that led to higher wages and better working conditions.[33]

In 1898, the Bund was instrumental in founding the Russian Social-Democratic Labor party (RSDLP) during a meeting Minsk, and it entered this party itself as "an autonomous organization, independent only in matters which specifically concern the Jewish proletariat." [34] However, at the Second Congress of the RSDLP in 1903, the Bund was expelled from the party because of its "nationalistic positions." [35] This expulsion only made the Bund even more Jewish in orientation. It formed self-defense groups against pogroms, and gradually the organization became a sort of "counter-culture," strongly promoting Jewish culture. This became even more so after the failed revolution of 1905, when political activity was heavily repressed. The Bund strongly promoted the use of Yiddish as a Jewish national language (and opposed the Zionist project of reviving Hebrew). It organized musical, literary and theatre societies, developed its own press, set up Yiddish schools, promoted Yiddish writers and was instrumental in developing a vibrant cultural life.

At the same time, Zionism was on the rise, based on the concept that for Jews there would never be place in Europe, emigration was no solution,

31 *The Promised City*, p. 45

32 In Yiddish "Algemeyner Yidisher Arbeter Bund in Lite, Poyln un Rusland"

33 *The Promised City*, p. 45

34 *Century of Ambivalence*, p. 15

35 The Bund formally rejoined the RSDLP when all of its faction reunited at the Fourth (Unification) Congress in Stockholm in April 1906, but the party remained fractured along ideological and ethnic lines. The Bund generally sided with the party's Menshevik faction and against the Bolshevik faction led by Vladimir Lenin.

and socialism would not be able to solve the Jewish predicament. It was believed that the only solution was to establish a Jewish state where Jews would find a home, free of persecution and anti-Semitism. One of the first adherents of this view, Leon Pinsker, argued that anti-Semitism was endemic to Europe, that its fundamental irrationality made it immune to education and rational arguments and, therefore, the Jews had no option but to leave the continent. At the beginning of the twentieth century, attempts were made to combine the ideologies of Zionism and socialism, and in 1906 the Poalei Zion Party was formed, professing this combination.

The Bund strongly opposed Zionism, arguing that emigration to Palestine was a form of escapism. Nevertheless, many Bundists were also Zionists, and the Bund suffered from a steady loss of active members to emigration.[36] Still, there remained a considerable portion of Jews that refused the concept that Europe was a hopeless territory and should be left behind. They believed that there was a place for them in Russia, as long as the political order could be reformed and liberalized. In 1905, 6,000 Jews signed a "Declaration of Jewish Citizens," arguing that Jews were human beings with the same rights as other people and that their rights should be respected accordingly.[37]

Anti-Semitism continued, however, and regular pogroms shocked the Jewish community. In 1903, a large-scale pogrom raked the city of Kishenev, killing 45 of the 50,000 Jewish inhabitants. More than 1,500 shops and houses were ransacked. Even liberal political leaders like Yusopov and Struve, "whilst expressing their sympathy with the suffering of the Jews and their repugnance at the instigators of the pogrom, violently attacked Jewish nationalism and the 'not too attractive character of the Jews'."[38] In 1905, a wave of pogroms enveloped the country after the Tsar had issued a manifesto granting the people a constitutional government. His decision was the result of mass protests and a general strike during the 1905 Revolution in October of that year, and anti-Semitic organizations used the occasion as a pretext to blame the Jews and organize pogroms in over 300 towns and cities. The worst pogrom took place in Odessa, where over 300 people were killed and 600 Jewish children orphaned. These events gave, of course, an extra impetus to the emigration of Jews. As the historian S. Ettinger concludes, "…the situation of the Jews was desperate; clearly, only the fall of the tsarist regime could save them."[39]

36 Many Bundists became later active in forming socialist parties in Palestine and, subsequently, Israel.

37 *Century of Ambivalence*, p. 20-21

38 *The Jews in Soviet Russia since 1917*, p. 19

39 *The Jews in Soviet Russia since 1917*, p. 20

In light of the above, it is not strange that, like so many others, Melvin's (grand) parents decided to emigrate in order to escape poverty and anti-Semitism, even though their political beliefs were socialist oriented.[40] For them, like for many other Jews, socialism provided the only hope for equality, for having their rights respected, for being accepted members of society. Zalman Sabshin had, in fact, been a Social Revolutionary activist before his emigration and only managed to avoid exile in Siberia by seeking a new life in the United States. His hometown, Beshenkovchi, had gradually become a regional center of development, involving surrounding *shtetls* such as Shiashnik and Sene. The town had the Lechwitscher school, a Lubavitch Schul[41] and another six synagogues, as well as chapter of various political parties: the Bund, the Socialist-Revolutionaries and the Zionists. The town experienced strikes as well as First of May celebrations. It also had a self-defense organization in the event of a pogrom and often sent helpers to nearby small towns whenever those had become the targets of a pogrom.

Zalman's father died at a young age and his mother was left with four children. Zalman's father had planned to send his son to a yeshiva, an action that was not possible after his death. A friend of the deceased father, Katshe Meisel, took Zalman into his business and along with an active role in his further development. Meisel's own children were highly intelligent and

40 See for instance *A Century of Ambivilence*, pp. 14-17 and pp. 59-64. Considering the fact that many Jews joined the socialist movement purely to escape from poverty and discrimination, hoping that this new revolutionary ideal of the equality of man that should bring freedom to Jews as well, it is even more tragic that on the eve of the Second World War this socialist orientation would lead to the general perception that Jews collaborated with the Soviet regime, which in turn led to a terrible backlash that was one of the factors that enabled the Holocaust to be so all-encompassing. Because in the end, the Jews were accused of having been instrumental in establishing communist power in Eastern Europe – yet they supported socialism only as a means of ridding themselves of century-long repression. It is one of the painful paradoxes of the twentieth century.

41 Chabad-Lubavitch is a Hasidic movement in Orthodox Judaism and one of the world's largest Hasidic movements, now based in Brooklyn, New York. Founded in the late 18th century by Shneur Zalman of Liadi, the movement takes its name from the town of Lyubavichi near Smolensk in Russia, which served as the movement's headquarters for over a century. It is about 100 kilometers to the East of Beshenkovichi. The movement thrived in Russia and Eastern Europe, despite persecution from the Bolshevik government and, later, the Nazi Holocaust. In 1940 the movement moved to the United States, and became a powerful force in Jewish life.

devoted Socialist-Revolutionaries. They introduced Zalman to the workers' movement and gave him free lessons. Zalman took studies seriously and studied during the nights and within several years he became a professional student. In 1910, he was arrested during the revolutionary strike in Vitebsk and was sentenced to several years of exile in Siberia. However, before he was sent into exile, he managed to escape to America.[42]

Slonim

It is like a time-machine trip back into history. The border is an easy one, much different than the border crossings I remember going into Russia. The guards are at ease, gentle, sometimes even pleasant and joking. Within eight minutes, I had passed the Belarus border.

Belarus is like a flash back into Soviet times. Although Western cars are around, many of the vehicles are still Soviet: Zhiguli's and Zaporozhets,' here and there an old Moskvich, and virtually all the trucks are Soviet-made Kamaz and MAZ, bulky concoctions that slowly crawl along the road exhausting dangerously black fumes. The latter are the standard trucks for collective farms, kolkhozy, that continue to dominate Belarus agriculture. The country's President Lukashenko is a former kolkhoz director and he clearly likes them very much. All along the way are signs of kolkhozy, combined with Communist symbols, monuments for the heroes of the Great Patriotic War (Second World War) and the occasional slogan like "Honor to Labor!" The occasional factory complex, with huge halls and banners urging the workers to work for a radiant future, complete the picture.

The road from Vilnius to Slonim is a straight one, from the border going down, passing Lyda, and then on to Slonim, in total about 200 kilometers. It meanders through gently sloping fields and pastures, intermitted by forests and every now and then the occasional village. Time seems to have stopped in some villages populated by old wooden houses that must have been there for more than a hundred years. Undoubtedly, many of the villages were Jewish shtetls, as this part of the country was the heartland of Jewish Eastern Europe. It belonged to many nations, including Lithuania, Russia and, between the two World Wars, Poland. Since 1944, it has been part of Belarus, now an independent country in the heart of Europe ruled by Europe's last dictator. The countryside is pleasant with kind and helpful people.

42 Mel Sabshin remembers that his father still had contact with the Meisel's in the early 1930s, when he was at around 5-6 years old.

The city of Slonim is located at the junction of the Shchara and Isa rivers, with a population of approximately 50,000 inhabitants. However, the place was much smaller when Melvin's mother left in 1912 to emigrate to the United States. The town then had probably about 18,000 inhabitants, of which two-thirds Jews.[43] The earliest record of the city dates back to the 11th century, although there may have been earlier settlement. The area was disputed between Lithuania and Kievan Rus' in early history and it changed hands several times. In the 13th century, Slonim became Lithuanian. Jewish settlement in Slonim appears to have started in 1388, following encouragement from the Lithuanian authorities. The Jews were credited with the development of local commerce in the 15th century; nonetheless, the Lithuanian Duchy temporarily expelled them in 1503.

In 1569, Lithuania and Poland united and Slonim became an important regional centre within Greater Poland. From 1631 to 1685 the city flourished as the seat of the Lithuanian diet. The Commonwealth of Poland-Lithuania was dismantled in a series of three military "partitions" in the latter half of the 18th Century and divided among its neighbors, Germany, Austria and Russia that took the largest portion of the territory. Slonim was in the area annexed by Russia.

The wars severely damaged Slonim, but in the 18th century, a local landowner, Graf Oginski, encouraged the recovery of the area; a canal was dug to connect the Shchara with the Dnepr River. In the late 19th century, Slonim's Jewish population had risen to 10,000.[44] The Slonimer Hasidic dynasty came from there, as well as Michael Marks, one of the founders of the department store chain Marks & Spencer's.

Russian control lasted until 1915, when the German army captured the town. Moshe Eisenstadt, a local resident at the time, described how the Germans were welcomed by the population: "What can I tell you? If we had seen the Messiah, the joy would not have been as great as when we saw the Germans marching through the town. Houses and stores immediately opened. People went out to walk in the streets, and everybody came out to greet the newly arrived Germans. In several parts of the town, old Jews came out of their houses and kissed the German soldiers. Everybody brought something to treat them with."[45] However, the joy did not last long

43 Memoirs of Moshe Eisenstadt, http://www.shtetlinks.jewishgen.org/slonim/Memoirs_of_Moshe_Eisenstadt.htm

44 According to the census of 1897, the total population was 15,893 of whom 10,588 were Jews.

45 Eisenstadt, p. 3

as Slonim found itself right in the middle of the front. Long barrages of artillery bombing followed, turning much of the town into rubble. Also the Germans turn out to be less civilized than expected, and repeatedly were seen stealing property.

The ending of the First World War did not end the war for Slonim. The area was disputed between the Soviet Union and the newly recreated state of Poland and suffered badly in the Polish-Soviet war of 1920; but in 1920 the Poles established control of the province. In 1939, the Molotov-Ribbentrop Pact between Nazi Germany and the Soviet Union resulted in the invasion of Poland by the two powers, causing a division of that country. Slonim was in the area designated by the Pact to fall within the Soviet sphere of influence. The Soviets placed that area within the Byelorussian SSR.

After a relaxing drive through the Belarus countryside, I entered Slonim, and the road led me up the hill, to the main street. It is a short one, a kind of central boulevard, that in Russian times was called Nievsky Prospekt; in Polish times was named after the writer Adam Mickiewicz and now, since Soviet times, is called May 1 Street. The Jews usually called it Paradne or Nievsk.[46] All the buildings on either side are new, either built after the war or in later days, Soviet style. But behind a row of buildings I almost immediately find the Great Synagogue, a baroque building dating back to 1642, and still towering over the adjacent buildings.[47] The building is dilapidated and unused; small buildings situated against the main corpus have caved in, often with only walls standing. Yet the main hall is still there. The building is surrounded by a fence, but I manage to get in through a crack and slide into the building. Emotion grips me when I see that it is relatively intact. The "Aron Kodesh" is still there, where the Torah Rolls were kept; Hebrew inscriptions were on the wall and some paintings can be discerned. The place is full of old bottles and cigarette butts, clearly used as a meeting place for alcoholics, friends and lovers, etc. but an eerie silence envelops me – the sound of silence. This was the main synagogue of Slonim, where, during the last two years of the war, 1939-1941, the number of Jews grew to almost 25,000 and when streams of refugees from Poland entered the city and stayed.

But nothing was left of Jewish Slonim. After the Nazi's occupied the city in the early days of the war, late June 1941, they started a campaign of terror that would last for more than a year. In three *Aktionen*, extermination

46 Alpert, Nachum: *The Destruction of Slonim Jewry*, p. 6
47 *The Destruction of Slonim Jewry*, p. 5

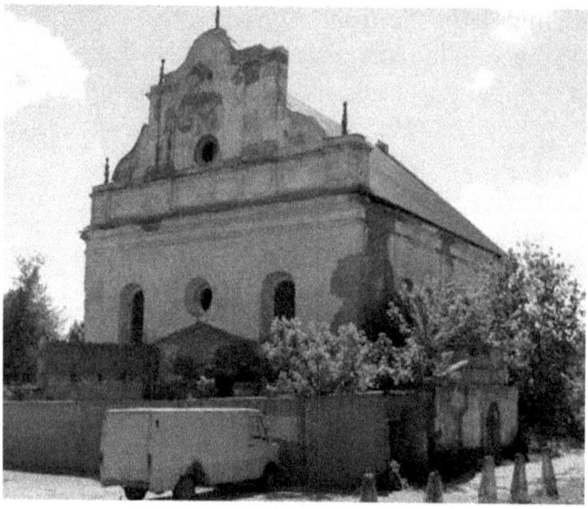

Synagogue Slonim

campaigns, virtually all the Jews of Slonim were killed in execution sites near the city.[48] The remaining 350 were kept alive in order to do slave labor for the Germans; eventually, they also were killed. Of the 25,000 Jews in Slonim, only a hundred returned.

I found myself in a city with a lost history, which had a flourishing Jewish community that was annihilated by the Nazi-German war machinery and local collaborators. Nothing is left, except the Great Synagogue slowly disintegrating next to what in Jewish times used to be the "Old Marketplace" and which was full of butcher shops, herring stalls, flour stores and workshops.[49] The Germans razed the Jewish cemetery during the war, tearing out the gravestones and sending the marble and granite to Germany. Even the ground was plowed under.[50] Most of the houses were burnt down during the third Aktion when 12,000 Jews were either burnt to death or rounded up and killed outside the city. I quickly leave the town; the sound of silence is too loud for me.

48 The first *Aktion* took place on July 17, 1941, and left 1200 Jews dead. The second *Aktion* of November 13, 1941, saw the murder of 9400 Jews. On June 29, 1942, a third *Aktion* resulted in 12,000 Jews killed. The fourth, killing the remaining 350, was on September 21, 1942.

49 *The Destruction of Slonim Jewry*, p. 5

50 *The Destruction of Slonim Jewry*, p.363

Chapter 3 - From Russia to the Statue of Liberty

> *"Despite their nostalgia for the scenes of their childhood and youth, having fled a despotic homeland to which there was no returning, they were quick to embrace America as their first true homeland."*[51]

> *"They felt themselves at the brink of a new era. In one swoop as it were, men stood liberated, naked of yesterday, aching for tomorrows fertile with limitless possibilities for human fulfillment in a world quit of ignorance, superstition, and despotism. (...) They unfurled the banners of common brotherhood on the highest plane of social idealism and pledged heart and mind to the promise of a new life..."*[52]

The fate of the Belarus town where Melvin's father came from, Beshenkovichi, was even worse than that of Slonim: after the war nothing was left, all the Jewish inhabitants were killed and acts of war had ravaged the shtetl.

In February 1994, Melvin Sabshin attended a conference of Russian psychiatrists in Smolensk, not far from the Belarus border.[53] Realizing that he is not far from his ancestor's birthplace, he requested help to go there and find his roots. "I picked him up in Moscow," remembers Elena Mozhaeva. "He had come to Moscow all alone, and from a friend I knew that he was not in good health and that recently his wife had died.[54] We agreed to meet at the hotel, and he would wait for me outside. When I came up to the hotel, he was already standing there: a tall lonely figure, with a huge cigar in the corner of his mouth. There was no doubt that this was Melvin Sabshin."[55] Together they traveled to Smolensk.

In spite of his request to get a car to take him to his father's birthplace, his Russian hosts initially did not organize anything. "He was all alone, and the bosses were not interested in him. There was another psychiatrist from Hamburg who was the center of attention, in particular of the Smolensk psychiatrists. They probably wanted something from him,

51 *The Promised City*, p. 110

52 *The Promised City*, p. 149

53 *Sotsial'naya i Klinicheskaya Psikhiatriya*, 2-1994, p. 158-9

54 Edith Sabshin died in 1992

55 Interview Elena Mozhaeva, June 6, 2009

because they were all around him, trying to make a good impression."[56] Eventually an angry Mozhaeva was able to make clear to the psychiatric leadership from Moscow that their behavior is despicable, and that something needs to be organized. In the end, together with the Chief Psychiatrist of Russia, Dr. Aleksandr Karpov, and the psychiatrist Georgi Kakayev who offered his car, Mozhaeva and Sabshin traveled to Belarus, yet they found no trace of his father's hometown. "Melvin was silent; it clearly made a deep impression on him. He was completely silent when we drove back to Smolensk, and when I looked at him I saw tears rolling down his cheeks." The next day Sabshin and his interpreter visited the memorial at Katyn, where in 1940 the Soviet secret police NKVD murdered approximately 22,000 Polish officers, policemen and intellectuals. The visit made an enormous impression on them. Back in Moscow, it was eventually Elena Mozhaeva alone who saw Melvin Sabshin off at the Moscow airport – the Russian psychiatric bosses and Chief Psychiatrist Aleksandr Karpov never appeared in the airport VIP-lounge to say goodbye, as intended.[57]

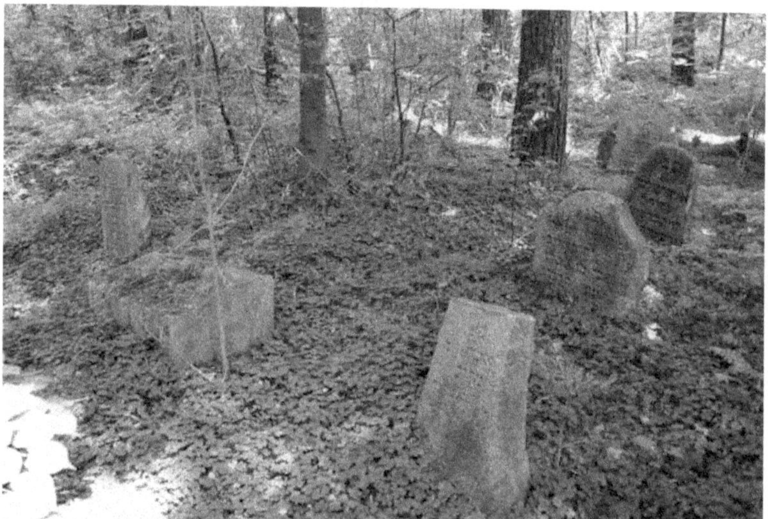

Jewish cemetary in Beshenkovichi, summer 2009

Still, it is not true that no trace was left of the Jewish shtetl of Beshenkovichi. Via the internet, I find the story of a former inhabitant of Beshenkovichi, who in the early 1990s returned to find his roots. He found no trace of

56 Interview Mozhaeva. The psychiatrist concerned was Dr. N. Koverk.
57 Interview Mozhaeva

the Jewish past in the town itself, but out in the forest he discovered the Jewish graveyard, with up to a thousand gravestones, silent witnesses of a past eradicated from the face of the earth.[58] A colleague from work visited the region and the town in the summer of 2009 since his grandmother coincidentally lived approximately fifty kilometers from Beshenkovichi. Indeed, while virtually no building in town was left standing, next to a leskhoz[59] he discovered a virtually untouched Jewish cemetery of unbelievable proportions, a total of 3 hectares full of headstones, partially sunk into the ground. It seems that either the psychiatrists traveling with Sabshin or the Belarus hosts decided to avoid the trouble of going all the way to Beshenkovichi, and instead reported that the town had ceased to exist. Or perhaps they meant that nothing was left of former Beshenkovichi?

The Promised City

Sonia Barnhard's father, Eli Sroliovich,[60] emigrated to the United States in 1910 in order to prepare the way for the rest of his family. His wife and four children – three brothers and Sonia – would follow two years later. A second sister was later born in the United States.[61]

Like so many other Jewish immigrants, he, and later the rest of his family, entered the country in New York and settled there. New York was a booming city in all respects. Between 1870 and 1915, the total population of New York more than tripled: from 1.5 million inhabitants to 5 million, and together with its suburbs it increased from 1.9 million to almost 7 million.[62] Many of these immigrants were Jews from Eastern Europe: between 1900 and 1914, almost 1.5 million Eastern European Jews emigrated to the United States, putting the total figure of emigrated Eastern European Jews

58 http://www.jewishgen.org/belarus/newsletter/frey.htm

59 A collective lumber farm

60 The name was later changed in Barnhard

61 Harry, Ray, Oscar and Davis, and the youngest daughter was Lilian.

62 *The Promised City*, p. 9-12. Equally, the New York harbor had become a main gateway, not only for immigrants but for goods as well. In 1874 seventy percent of all imports and 61 percent of all American exports passed through the port of New York. Between 1888 and 1908 the banking sector in New York grew almost 250 percent, tent times more than in the rest of the country. Forty percent of the largest corporation in the States had their seat in the city, and in 1914 New York produced almost 10 percent of the manufactures in the nation. And also within the State of New York, the city played this central role. In 1914, almost 68 percent of the state's factories were located in New York City. See *The Promised City*, pp. 5-8.

at well over two million.[63] This means that between 1870 and the First World War more than one third of the total Jewish population of Eastern Europe left their homes in search of a better future. And of these, 90 percent came to the United States, the majority settling in New York City.

Since the 1920s, New York boasted the largest concentration of Jews in history; in the 1930s and 1940s, over two million Jews were living in New York making up almost one-third of its population.[64] As a result, the ethnic composition of the city changed fundamentally over time. Since the middle of the nineteenth century, the percentage of foreign-born citizens and their children outnumbered those who were born in the country itself. By 1900, three quarters of the city were either foreign or children of foreign-born citizens. The most numerous nationalities were at that time German and Irish, but soon that position was taken over by (mainly Jewish) immigrants from Russia, Italy and the Austro-Hungarian Empire.

The Jews entering New York were mainly small-town Jews, from shtetls and towns across Eastern Europe, in search of an element that would bind them to their new life in North America. In the course of this process, they changed. Economically, physically and spiritually, they were on their way to become modern Americans.[65] However, their background also made them weary of venturing too far from New York, as the communities they came from were closely knit, and they were used to living in carefully maintained and intertwined social and religious environments. Yet the same background also gave them the urge to look beyond, to see their current position as workmen only as an intermediate step. In the shtetls and towns, economic individualism had been just as important as social and religious cooperation and, thus, they accepted their temporary degradation. "The Jews were fairly ravenous for education and eager for personal development (…) all industrial work was merely a stepping stone to professional or managerial positions."[66] Or as one fellow worker remarked: "…the Hebrew wage earner is only in the trade temporarily, hoping and praying that one day he will become a boss."[67]

The Lower East Side of Manhattan had become an immigrant Jewish

---

63 In the 1870s 40,000 Jews emigrated to the United States. In the 1880s this increased to 200,000, and in the 1890s another 300,000 followed.

64 *The Promised City*, p. ix. Only by the 1970s did the numbers go down, both in totals and in percentage of the population. By then approximately 15 percent of the population was of Jewish origin.

65 *The Promised City*, xi

66 *The Promised City*, p. 175

67 *The Promised City*, p. 186

cosmopolitan area, "a seething human sea, fed by streams, streamlets, and rills of immigration flowing from all the Yiddish speaking centers of Europe."[68] Life in the Lower East Side was not easy: it was crowded, dirty, with foul smells coming from garbage cans lined up on the sidewalks as if they were trees. Many people lived in "dumbbell tenements," houses that had six or seven floors and four apartments on each floor. The apartments on the front side usually had four rooms, the ones in the back, three; of all the rooms only one per apartment had direct access to daylight. Sometimes more than one family lived in such an apartment. In summer the heat became unbearable, the heat from the sun combined with that of boilers, gas lamps and coal stoves. Many tenants fled to the rooftops, balconies or sidewalks in order to be able to get some decent sleep. Two apartments shared a toilet, but as there were no public toilet facilities, the excrement and urine left behind in alleys and corners created a terrible stench. Every year, several hundred New Yorkers perished from the continuous heat.[69]

The situation improved a little in the early 1890s, when the construction of dumbbell tenements was prohibited and the worst situations in the existing buildings were corrected. Running water closets were installed in the existing buildings, and in new ones running water and toilets were obligatory.

Also, increasing numbers of Eastern Europeans started to venture outside the Lower East Side, looking for possibilities of employment that were compatible to their religious habits. In 1892, 75 percent of the city's Jews were still living in this part of town, but by 1903, the percentage had gone down to 50 percent and by 1916 the percentage had dwindled to just over a quarter.[70] Other areas that attracted large numbers of Jews were Brownsville, Williamsburg, South Brooklyn and the Bronx, where the Sabshin family settled. The development of rapid transit facilities and the construction of the underground transit hastened this process, as commuting became possible and hitherto distant areas became within reach.[71]

Life in America

Most Jewish emigrants from Russia decided to make a clear cut with their past. They had fled Russia because of poverty and anti-Semitism, and had

---

68 *The Promised City*, p.76. The five major varieties were Jews from Hungary, Galicia, Romania, Russia, and the Levant.

69 *The Promised City*, p.83

70 *The Promised City*, p. 93

71 *The Promised City*, p.93

no intention of reminding their children of those dark days. They often changed their names and avoided any discussion of where they had come from. Also in the case of the parents of Melvin Sabshin, much has been lost because of this intentional break with the past. It is, therefore, not strange that the descendents of Zalman and Sonia Sabshin know relatively little about their ancestors and their life in Russia, including the original names of Zalman Sabshin's parents.

Melvin's father, Zalman Sabshin, had been able to enter medical school in 1913, three years after his arrival in the United States. During the day he worked in a shop, but at night he would devote himself to his studies.[72] Although the family was rather poor, his siblings agreed to finance his study and helped him graduate from medical school in 1917. Zalman was certainly not the only one who managed to become a physician. For young immigrants who had come to the United States in order to fulfill their hopes and dreams of a professional education, the opportunities that New York provided were almost endless. Eager to learn, with inquisitive minds, they turned out to be excellent candidates for independent professions. Medicine proved to be the favorite study for them. A didactic medical school lasting two school years at propriety schools, with a school year lasting six months and with low tuition fees payable in installments, made entry into the medical profession much easier. [73] Between 1897 and 1907 the number of Jewish physicians rose from 450 to 1,000 in the borough of Manhattan and from 100 to 200 on the Lower East Side.[74]

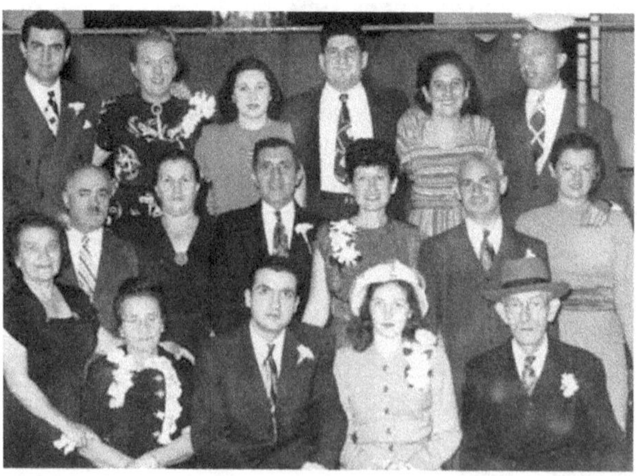

The Barnhards in the 1940s. Left upper corner Melvin Sabshin, under him his father Zalman

72 Preface to his collection of poems, by Daniel M. Brod

73 *The Promised City*, p. 71

74 *The Promised City*, p. 73

In 1920, Zalman Sabshin met Sonia Barnhard, who had entered the country in 1912. Her family was relatively well off. Her father had been in the lumber business in Russia, building rafts and sending them down the river to be sold. He had also helped Jews escape when they had been in trouble; one can assume that these were Jews who had been involved in one of the revolutionary parties and were threatened with arrest and deportation, very common in those days.[75] Most of Sonia's siblings managed to become middle class citizens in the United States. One brother became a lawyer, the other and engineer, the third a businessman. The elder sister did not have a professional career, while the youngest, Lilian, attended and graduated from Hunger College. Zalman and Sonia married soon after they met and their son Melvin was born in 1925.

The young couple moved to an apartment on Washington Avenue in the Crotona Park East section of the Bronx, a fairly new neighborhood that had developed in a relatively short time since the late nineteenth century and, by 1920, was home to a community of over 150,000 residents.[76] The apartments in this region were bigger and better in quality because of a Tenement House Law of 1901, which set rules for better fire protection, light and sanitation. The apartments ranged from "width from 40 feet to an entire city block and differing in quality from the unheated cold-water flat to the warm, roomy – often luxurious – elevator building. (…) When in 1920 the new Pelham bay subway made lower Southern Boulevard and Hunts point more accessible, the center of Hunts Point-Crotona Park East was already one solid mass of urban humanity."[77] The area was predominantly home to immigrants, of which 91 percent had foreign ancestry and 40 percent were actually foreign born; one-third of the population were Eastern European and Russian Jews of foreign birth.[78]

The Sabshins belonged to the Jewish medical community there, consisting of approximately twenty doctors (virtually all doctors in this part of town were of Jewish background)[79] with whom they formed a "Group for the Study of Art." Zalman Sabshin often wrote poems himself as well as scientific articles for a medical journal. In his later years, his poems would appear in a New York journal. He had developed his literary inclinations

---

75 Barnhard family archive.

76 According to statistics, there were just over 2,500 residents in Crotona Park East in 1892, with more than 150,000 in 1920. See Gonzalez, Evelyn: *The Bronx*, p. 69

77 *The Bronx*, p. 69

78 *The Bronx*, p. 69-70

79 Interview with Melvin Sabshin, July 29, 2009

at a young age, and liked to describe what he saw around him. In 1909, he wrote a play in four acts about the lives of Jewish "externikes." The play was to be printed in a Yiddish-Russian journal in St. Petersburg but his arrest and subsequent escape made this impossible.[80]

Melvin's mother was the "secretary" of the group and quite a forceful lady, with a strong influence on Melvin's upbringing. Both parents remained politically interested and leftist in their convictions. Although Zalman Sabshin had been more politically active in Russia than Sonia, he never talked much about politics to his son. His wife was in that sense the more active one, and even took young Melvin to the cinema to watch films about the wonderful life of children in the Soviet Union. Later, in spite of a few conservative outbursts during his adolescence, the young Melvin Sabshin continued to support communism or socialism during his early adult years.

As indicated earlier, this leftist attitude of Melvin's parents was shared by most Eastern European Jews in the United States, in particular those from Russia.[81] Since the late 1880s, socialism flourished in New York. Many of the Yiddish periodicals were socialist in nature, and by 1914 four dailies, including the socialist *Wahrheit* and *Forward* sold almost 450,000 copies.[82] Interestingly, the Yiddish socialist press managed to develop a new formulation of socialism, packaging it in a format that was understandable to its readers. "Scriptural invocations and preambles and the prophecies of Isaiah and Jeremiah gilded didactic texts, almost Talmudic in their tortuousness."[83] For many laborers, the socialist message was embraced with the same piety as with devotional exercises.

Between the early 1890s and 1905, the revolutionary fervor temporarily calmed down and disillusionment set in. Factional wars between the various socialists groups blurred the message. The need to earn money and build a future turned out to be stronger than the wish to build a socialist future. Joseph Barondess, a popular labor leader at that time, summarized it very nicely when he said: "Until the Ideal Society will be realized, I have certain duties to perform towards my clients, for which

80 Preface to his collection of poems, by Daniel M. Brod

81 Many of the immigrants from the Austro-Hungarian Empire maintained positive attitudes towards the political elite in their country, and many of their societies were named after the Emperor or his relatives.

82 *The Promised City*, p. 127

83 *The Promised City*, p. 157

they pay."[84] This all changed again in 1903, when pogroms ravaged the Jewish communities in Russia and the dream of revolution took on an almost unbelievable reality. The Yiddish press filled its pages with tales of horror, describing massacres and at the same time lauding the courage of revolutionaries in the former Motherland. On December 4, 1905, a crowd of more than 100,000 Jews marched up Fifth Avenue in commemoration of the dead of the 1905 uprising. Christian churches tolled their bells in sympathy for the mourners.[85]

The 1905 revolution resulted in the founding or resumption of socialist organizations. And there were many: Bundists, Zionists and Territorialists, Zionist-Socialists and Socialist-Territorialists, Poale Zion and Social-Revolutionary Territorialists. All groups did their best to support their endangered brethren overseas. Russian socialists came to the United States to attend meetings and speak to large audiences, including the pioneer revolutionary Nicholas Tchaikovsky and the writer Maksim Gorky. The Bund organized its first convention in New York.[86]

By the time Melvin's parents landed in New York, labor unrest had rocked the city several times. In 1912, a general strike rocked the garment industry, when some 10,000 workmen in the fur trade went on strike and managed to obtain a considerable number of concessions from their employers. Later that year, 50,000 workmen in the tailor industry called a general strike that was equally successful. A strike by women in the waist, whitegoods, dress and related industries in the early months of 1913 attracted wide sympathy; the memory was still fresh of a March 1911 fire in one of the waist factories, in which 146 women burned to death and many more were permanently maimed. [87] While the United Hebrew Trades union had only 5,000 members in 1909, by 1914 250,000 Jewish workers in 111 affiliated unions were members of this labor organization.[88]

Although they were Russian Jews, Melvin's parents were not active believers. To the contrary, religion played no major part in his upbringing. The only major aspect of this was the fact that the parents sent Mel to a Hebrew School outside of regular school hours, each week during one

---

84 *The Promised City*, p. 160. Joseph Barondess, "Kind of the Cloakmakers", came to New York in 1888 and developed from a peddler to a labor leader in the 1890s. In 1900 he was even appointed to the New York Board of education.

85 *The Promised City*, p. 163

86 *The Promised City*, p. 163-5

87 *The Promised City*, p. 253-5

88 *The Promised City*, p. 256

afternoon and on Sunday morning, to be educated in Jewish issues. This was very much in line with the general developments within the Jewish community in New York. While initially, in the 1980s and 1990s, the religious regimen of the old world had been maintained, gradually a certain relaxation settled in and people became less strict in their adherence. A sort of Americanization set in, in which many of the old traditions seemed to be obsolete or useless, and the urge to do business and to adapt the new way of life became a dominant aspect of life. In 1913, nearly sixty percent of the stores on the Lower East Side of Manhattan were open on the Sabbath, and the Keepers of the Sabbath Society failed completely in their attempts to maintain the old traditions. Their boycott of newspapers that sold on the Sabbath proved useless, and the Yiddish theatres were invariably sold out on Friday night and Saturday afternoon.[89] After the 1905 revolution in Russia, new holidays were added to the Jewish religious calendar, such as Socialist Labor Day on May 1.[90]

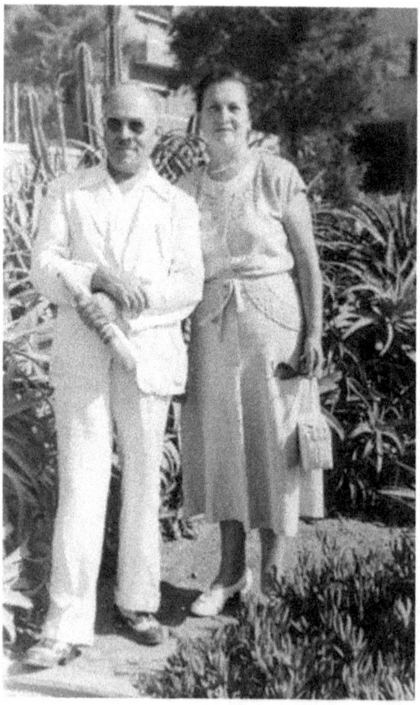
Sonya and Zalman Sabshin

Initially, Jewish immigration in the United Stares had found itself without its own language. Yiddish was considered a dialect, not acceptable as a tongue for those with intellect and seeking enlightenment. Yiddish was not more than a "jargon" that smelled of provincialism and backwardness. This changed in the course of the 1980s, when Yiddish became, instead, a tool of enlightenment and Americanization. Soon Yiddish periodicals started to appear, and between 1885 and 1914 over 150 daily, weekly, monthly and other regular publications appeared in Yiddish. An increasing number of authors started to use Yiddish as their language. In 1901, the Hebrew Publishing Company was

89 *The Promised City*, p. 146-7

90 This is not the same as the North American **Labor Day**, the first Monday in September, which is a creation of the **labor** movement and is dedicated to the social and economic achievements of American workers.

founded, which published pirated books in Yiddish translation, as well as Sholem Aleichem and Dr. Caspe's *Idishe Vissenshaftliche Bibliothek*. In 1912, a *History of the Jews in America* was published in both English and Yiddish, and three years after an *English-Yiddish Encyclopedia Dictionary* was published by the Jewish Press Publishing Company.[91] A Yiddish guidebook *Sholem Aleichem tsu immigranten* welcomed newcomers to the United States.[92]

Melvin Sabshin's parents sometimes spoke Yiddish, but they never taught their children to speak it. As with many other Jewish families, English was a language that stood for being part of their newly adopted land, their liberation from a despotic regime. It was important for them that their children integrated into this new homeland, and could develop themselves maximally. Yiddish as a main language would then be a burden, an obstacle, not an asset. However, when Zalman Sabshin had to discontinue his medical practice in 1938 because of malignant hypertension and was told he had only several years to live, he focused his attention on writing Yiddish poetry and eventually published a volume of poetry.[93] Having moved to Miami (Florida) for health reasons because of the better climate, he also became an active Zionist and was one the founders of a large Zionist district.[94] Zalman Sabshin died in 1955, much later than originally anticipated.

---

91 *The Promised City*, p. 132-133

92 *The Promised City*, p. 240

93 Published in January 1947 in Miami Beach "published by friends of the author". Most of the poems deal with the Second World War and applaud the Russians for beating Hitler. Some focus on all three Axis-countries Germany, Japan and Italy. One also voices anger at the British for restricting emigration to Palestine.

94 According to a preface in his book of poetry, Zalman Sabshin hoped to see a Jewish home in Erez Israel. His name was inscribed in the Golden Book of the Keren Kayemet (Zionist fund).

Chapter 4 - Meeting Jochen Neumann

It is not the first time we met. Our first meeting was more than twenty years before, in the fall of 1988 at a Regional Symposium of the World Psychiatric Association in Washington D.C. Then the meeting lasted not more than several seconds, the result of the fact that we both counted Ellen Mercer among our friends and bumped into each other in a corridor. An attempt of Ellen Mercer to introduce us was short lived – Jochen Neumann quickly disappeared among the psychiatrists present, clearly not keen to speak to the person who, for him, had become the personalization of the struggle against political abuse of psychiatry. I was at that meeting accompanying Dr. Anatoly Koryagin, the dissident Soviet psychiatrist who has been released a year earlier after six years of imprisonment for his protests against the political abuse of psychiatry in the Soviet Union, and Koryagin was the hero of the day at this meeting. Neumann avoided being seen in our neighborhood. "You can imagine what that would have meant politically for me," he reminiscences, "if I would have been photographed together with the two of you it would have been the end." He smiles; no further explanation is needed.

The first time we met again was in Berlin, coincidentally around the corner from the place where he lived as a student fifty years before. At that time, it was East Berlin, capital of the German Democratic Republic, the DDR. Now it was part of a reunified Berlin, where gradually the traces of the communist past disappear. We met in the lobby, and soon disappeared upstairs to talk in private and peace.

Jochen Neumann is 73 years old, and has been a "non-person" for almost twenty years now. After the fall of the Berlin Wall, he felt himself an outcast in his own country. Coincidentally, just before the Berlin Wall came down he had given up his position as Director of the Hygiene Museum in Dresden, but had not yet started a new job. He found temporary employment as director of an insignificant mental hospital and after a severe mental crisis, he lived for six years in Saudi Arabia, where he worked as psychiatric consultant and director of a 300-bed psychiatric hospital specialized in addiction issues.[95] He is still an outsider, feels not accepted in post-reunification Germany, and somewhat embittered by the fact that his career stopped at the age of 53 and that the society he helped built was overrun by Western Germany.

---

95 His stay in Saudi Arabia was during the period 1992-1997. There he was for five years Consultant Neuropsychiatrist and Medical Director of the Al-Amal Hospital in Riyadh as well as Clinical Assistant Professor for Medicine (Psychiatry) at the King Saud University in Riyadh.

He is no longer the firm Communist activist that he once was,[96] but he still believes that East German society was socially better and that the majority of ordinary people do not care whether they were not allowed to voice their opinions or not. "They want a job, a house, medical care, the Tageszeitung, and the possibility to travel."

Neumann still looks a bit East German, wearing a black shirt, reddish tie and wearing a pair of gold-rimmed glasses on a mostly balding head. Probably he would even like the idea that he still looks East German, because for him that was his homeland and it ceased to exist twenty years ago. I tell him the story of a woman I know in The Netherlands, who was born in East Germany, fled with her parents in 1953 at an early age, but always maintained her East German citizenship and still considers herself to be a citizen of that no longer existing State. Neumann nods, he recognizes the feeling, and - as I gradually understand - he fully shares it. For him the West Germans have taken over, obliterated all East Germany produced and stood for, and made it seem as if the German Democratic Republic never existed and if it did, it only produced bad things. Later he explains his position further: "If it had been the other way around, and East Germany had taken over West Germany, things would have been much worse."

Our conversation starts carefully, first downstairs with some persons nearby, clearly not to his liking, and later upstairs in my hotel room. Downstairs he clearly does not feel at ease, with other people around him, and he carefully makes sure they do not listen to what we are talking about. It is almost the world upside down: in the Soviet days I would be careful not to be listened to, watching the people around me and keeping my voice down, now it is almost the other way around – he wants to avoid people hearing about his Stasi past.

A principled man

In the course of time, a clearer picture emerges. Jochen Neumann is a bit of a loner, it seems. He suddenly appears at the hotel, exactly at the time

96 As he explained later, during an interview on July 29, 2009, "I am still a believer in communism, but I am no longer an activist or participant in what was called existing socialism. Socialism was wrong, it failed and I accept it. In the political dimension of my life I am no longer a participant in the leftist movement. But my heart is still at least Communist principled. What was called Communism in the East was contrary to the basic principles of Communism. But I considered at that time the forty years of socialism in the DDR as just a small part of what had to be a development over several centuries. "

of our appointment, briefcase in the hand, well organized. Within minutes we are already in a deep discussion, and I need to intervene and ask him to wait until I turn on the tape recorder. He is well prepared, knows what he wants to say, and too many questions in between are turned away – don't try to interfere with the course of his thought! He is keen to explain that he did his work out of conviction, and only did what he agreed to do. It is a fundamental issue, because the last thing Jochen Neumann wants is to be seen as a tool of a secret service, a man following and obeying orders. Yes, he wrote reports to them, informed them in detail of what was happening within the World Psychiatric Association, but never did he receive specific instructions with regard to the WPA.

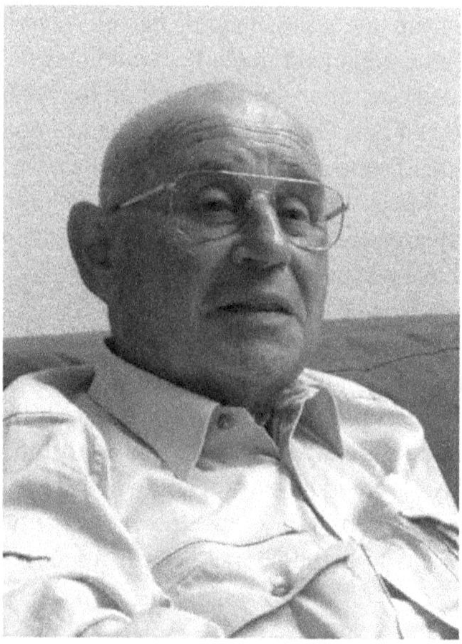

Jochen Neumann, July 2009

The day before our second meeting he sent me a document by e-mail, outlining his point of view. It is carefully worded, concrete, and allows no misconception. In the document he writes that "with regard to the influence [of the Stasi] on the Executive Committee and the WPA I would like to make the following specification. At no time did I receive any instructions with regard to the WPA from the MfS. They were only interested in knowing in detail what was happening within the WPA. In my reports I tried to the best of my (subjective) ability to create an image as realistic as possible of what was happening in world psychiatry and the WPA, also with regard to individuals involved. In doing so, I did not take into consideration any possible wishful thinking on the side of the recipient of the reports and have in these reports never answered any expectations involuntarily in order to stabilize my own position. My reports were (subjectively) uncompromising, honest, and reflected my knowledge and views of that time."

The document is short, but very precise. The italics and bold are used to emphasize important parts. Clearly, Jochen Neumann has a point to make, and he wants people to know that he acted on his own accord, according to his own beliefs and conscience, and takes full responsibility:

"With my Führungsoffizier[97], who was known under the name of Harry Kupfer,[98] I had come to a silent agreement, that I would not have to do, undertake or say anything that I would not do/leave/say spontaneously on my own accord and according to my own insights (already out of security reasons this should be the case). I have always taken the liberty to act according to this unwritten agreement and was in that respect free in my decisions, acts and verbal expressions (at least abroad). From that it should be clear that I did my work in the EC as an individual according to the best of my own knowledge and conscience. Concretely: Whatever I did or said, irrespective of whether it is now considered right or wrong, only I, Jochen Neumann, am responsible for this personally. I accept that responsibility."

Jochen Neumann finds it very difficult to lay any blame on other people, but also to say bad things about them. During our interviews, he regularly asks me to turn off the tape recorder, refuses to have less positive remarks on record. Initially I think this is out of reluctance to speak out, but soon I start to understand that this is part of Jochen Neumann's personality: he is a very principled man, takes responsibility for his actions, and hates bad-mouthing other people. His view on them is subjective; they should be responsible for themselves. It is not his task, or his right, to judge them.

The same counts for himself. He is very keen to make sure that he is seen in the right perspective. Again, this is not because of avoiding responsibility, to the contrary. He feels himself fully responsible, but wants to make sure that people understand he acted out of conviction, not personal gain. In the same document he writes (the bold and italics are Neumann's): "**During my time in the EC I have always considered and felt myself as a representative of the global community of colleagues and a servant of the WPA.** That I tried to get a justification for my responsibility in the context of my political convictions and experiences (that is, my clear communist political orientation) is another issue. If I should be judged, than I would like to be considered a perpetrator out of conviction and not as an empty-headed bastard and an adapting opportunist, who in the end tries to put the guilt on others."

And again he modifies the responsibility of others: "for reasons of fairness I have to remark that my *Führungsoffizier* strengthened me and always

97 For more information on the recruitment, tasks and work of the "Führungsoffizier" see page 134.

98 Real name Harry Sattler, see chapter 21.

approached me with understanding. (…). In spite of different cultural/ intellectual views and needs I have considered him until the last day of our collaboration as a buddy and a good comrade."

How principled Jochen Neumann is becomes clear a little bit later, when he pulls out an envelope from his briefcase. It is a letter that is twenty years old, from November 1989, and which he hid in a desk to make sure nobody would find it. He has pulled it out the evening before, and only remembers the contents in general terms. We open the letter and read. It is a letter to the successor organization of the Stasi, and to his *Führungsoffizier*, dated November 30, 1989. In the letter he expresses his indignation of what happened in the country, about what he learned about the methods in which they kept the country under control. He accuses them of incompetence, of not having been able to change the course of events and build a human socialist country. "Something one knew, a lot one assumed. But what the developments now bring to daylight supersedes however the psychological ability of every normal comrade to compensate. The security agencies had obviously secured everything institutionally and were equally obviously not able to convey the information coming from engaged and honest comrades – like myself – on what was happening in the country and in the Party to the leadership in such a way, that the now indelible shame and moral bankruptcy of the State and the Party could be avoided. (…) Like many others, I am overwhelmed by a mixture of anger and disenchantment, which are also based on very personal experiences. For that reason I am no longer able to collaborate further and withdraw my earlier written agreement for collaboration."[99] Being principled and precise, he also hands back the West-German Marks that were in his care as an advance and to be used for expenses during operational work.

The letter had its effect, undoubtedly, and Jochen Neumann was never contacted again. He smiles, a bit of a sad smile. He points out that the letter also means that he was excluded from being able to make use of the support mechanism that was quickly put in place and helped many of the people of the old regime survive and maintain themselves. Not that Neumann regrets his decision to break with the MfS and to express his views, he would not have taken anything anyway. He did his work out of conviction, not material gain. But it shows again how he paid for his principles, even when dealing with the Stasi.

My respect for Jochen Neumann took a new turn. A relationship is starting to build, that is hard to describe. Here is a man who was seemingly

[99] Letter from Jochen Neumann to the Stasi, November 30, 1989.

on the other side, defending the Soviet cause. Yet in talking to him, in understanding his actions and convictions, he gradually moves over to my side, to the category of people who stand for what they believe in, and take the consequences. Much later, when work on this book is already nearing its end and a relationship has developed between us based on trust and mutual respect, he sent me more reminiscences about his work in the DDR and his sometimes quite complex relationship with colleagues and senior officials. They also confirm the image of a man who is anything but an opportunist, but rather someone who has an almost stubborn tendency to stick to his own course in spite of the anger and irritation of people who could very well damage or even end his career. Interestingly, each time he may have been at risk, there was a senior psychiatrist or Party official who valued Neumann the way he was, and managed to mediate a compromise solution, thereby avoiding a catastrophe for Neumann himself.[100] Whatever one's political point of view, Neumann's behavior definitely fits in the category of principles, and even courageous.

My feelings of growing respect and affection appear to be shared by him. Formalities start to disappear, the "Sie" (respectful you) almost unnoticeably changes into "Du," and when I later send him the text of a speech I am planning to deliver a week later he quickly answers, with fatherly remarks how to improve. We have touched a common ground, have realized we are on the same wavelength, and his communist and my anti-Soviet past only make the interaction a more interesting one.

---

100 Some of these events are described by Neumann in the essay *Personen*, dated October 12, 2009, and will be described in Chapter 21.

Chapter 5 – Growing up in Post-War Germany

At the end of April or the beginning of May [1945] something happened that in one bolt structured the disorder and suffering in my head and developed my image of the world with big strides. (...) Within the period of one week, seamlessly, a child is turned into an unripe adult.

Jochen Neumann[101]

"My childhood was a happy one, in all respects," writes Jochen Neumann in one of his private essays, in which he reflects on his own life.[102] "It ended more or less abruptly in 1945, together with the turning of tides shortly before the middle of the century."

Indeed, the period 1944-1945 was a turning of tides, and so was actually the whole period of the Second World War. It is almost three quarters of a century later and hard to imagine the immensity of the destruction that befell the regions that quickly and unwillingly turned into battlegrounds. Millions of people were uprooted, became victims of acts of war, pillaging, rape and mass murder. In particular Eastern Europe was victimized, being caught between the military and ideological powers of two totalitarian regimes that, on one hand, collaborated extensively but at the same time plotted to overthrow the other. Much of the hardships of the second half of the twentieth century were a direct consequence of this war, which ended in a standoff between two military blocs. Central and Eastern European countries were either annexed or subjugated to a Soviet-oriented regime and Western Europe entered a prolonged period of political polarization, fear of a Soviet attack and a constant urge to profess its superiority.

Many thousands of books have been written about this Second World War, and about the ensuing Cold War, and many more will be written. However, no words will be able to capture the sheer horror that befell the people that had to live through it, or did not survive. Undoubtedly, the most ostensible

---

101 Neumann, Jochen: *Der Sozialismus und Ich*, pp. 2-3.

102 *Der Sozialismus und Ich*, November 29, 2008. Neumann wrote a considerable number of recollections, mostly during his life in Saudi Arabia in the mid 1990s and in the period 2005-2008, which were made available to the author. Although they were not intended for publication, they give an extraordinary insight in the development of Jochen Neumann as a person, and are sometimes quoted in this and other chapters with permission of the author. They are now located in the *Deutsches Tagebucharchiv* in Emmendingen, Germany.

victims in Europe were the Jews, who fell victim to a murdering machinery that, on one hand, was well-organized and systematic, but on the other hand based itself on existing anti-Semitic attitudes and made effective use of the desire of local populations to rid themselves of the people that evoked feelings of jealousy, fear and despise. The ensuing Holocaust resulted in the almost total annihilation of the Jewish presence in Eastern Europe and ended a rich history spanning almost six centuries. It also laid the base for the foundation of the State of Israel, the standoff in the Middle East and the continuous bloodshed in that region ever since.

The Soviet population undoubtedly lost more of its members than any other nation in the world, but not all can be ascribed to the terror of the Nazi war machine. Stalin, as ruthless a dictator as Hitler and as disinterested in the fate of his people, waged war on both the Nazi occupants and his own people, which is well symbolized by the existence of the special NKVD troops, the SMERSH, who were to shoot any Soviet soldier who tried to flee the battle front.[103] Accounts show that soldiers were sometimes more afraid of the SMERSH troops than of the Nazi enemy. Hundreds of thousands of Soviet troops would die purely because of unwise decisions of the Soviet military leadership or Stalin himself; just a few years before the war the Soviet leader had liquidated the top echelons of his military, which did not help his war effort.[104] And while Nazi troops attacked the country in the late days of June 1941, the Soviet authorities used much of their railroad capacity to ship prisoners from the European parts of the Gulag back to the East, away from the advancing troops, as free forced laborers. Those who could not be evacuated were shot to death, their corpses left to the advancing Nazi troops who tried to make use of the scenes for propaganda purposes.[105] Soon the ranks of the dead would be joined by the hundreds of

103 The main task of SMERSH was to secure the Red Army's operational rear from partisans, saboteurs, and spies; to investigate and arrest conspirators and mutineers, "traitors, deserters, spies, and criminal elements" at the combat front.

104 A personal account of this can be found in Adamishin, Anatoly: *Human Rights, Perestroika and the Cold War*, where former Soviet Deputy Foreign Minister Anatoly Adamishin describes how his own father disappeared during the first months of the war; p. 8

105 A well-known example is the Katyn massacre, a mass murder of thousands of Polish military officers, policemen, intellectuals and civilian prisoners of war by the Soviet NKVD. The number of victims is estimated at about 22,000. The victims were murdered in the Katyn forest in Russia, the Kalinin (Tver) and Kharkov prisons and elsewhere. About 8,000 were officers taken prisoner during the 1939 Soviet invasion of Poland, the rest being Poles arrested for allegedly being "intelligence agents, gendarmes, saboteurs, landowners, factory owners, lawyers, priests, and officials." Since Poland's conscription system required every unex-

thousands of Jews that were killed by the raging *Einzatstruppen* and their local collaborators.

End of childhood

For some Europeans, however, the war became only really visible in the end of 1943 or even as late as 1944, when military operations also reached their doorstep. This was particularly the case for children, whom the parents naturally tried to protect from any direct confrontation with the effects of war as long as possible. In many small towns in rural areas of Germany, the war seemed far away. The bombing of German cities and industrial sites by the allied air forces did not affect them, and probably the only direct proof that something was going wrong was the constant stream of notices of men gone missing or killed at one of the fronts. "The outer life was full of political symbolism, flags, images of the *Führer*, uniforms and posters, etc. But for me these were side issues that had no meaning. They were emotionally as important as the color of the leaves, the weather, and the daily childhood experiences. In our household, and in our further family life they played no role. In life at home, the Nazi clamor was cut out, even though my father in his position as teacher was visibly engaged on the outside, official, stage."[106]

Jochen Neumann was born in the town of Fischendorf, next to Leisnig, a small town in the central part of Saxony (Sachsen), Germany.[107] Leisnig, situated on the old road from Leipzig to Bohemia, was developed when some merchants settled at the foot of the Mildenstein Castle, which is over 1,000 years old. Coincidentally, the town was the birthplace of Friedrich Olbricht, one of the leaders of the famous July 20, 1944 plot to assassinate Adolf Hitler, for which he was executed.

---

empted university graduate to become a reserve officer, the Soviets were able to round up much of the Polish intelligentsia, and the Jewish, Ukrainian, Georgian and Belarusian intelligentsia of Polish citizenship. Nazi Germany announced the discovery of mass graves in the Katyn Forest in 1943. The revelation led to the end of diplomatic relations between Moscow and the London-based Polish government-in-exile. The Soviet Union continued to deny the massacres until 1990, when it finally acknowledged the perpetration of the massacre by NKVD as well as the subsequent cover-up. An investigation by the Prosecutor's General Office of the Russian Federation has confirmed Soviet responsibility for the massacres, yet does not classify this action as a war crime or as an act of genocide.

106 *Der Sozialismus und Ich*, p. 2

107 Fischendorf was then a separate town of approximately 1200 inhabitants; it is now part of Leisnig.

Jochen's father, Erhart, was a teacher who joined the Nationalist-Socialist Party NSDAP in the early days of the Nazi regime but was a Party member rather out of convenience, instead of national-socialist conviction. "My father was a "small Nazi," a member of the NSDAP who earlier also belonged to the SA.[108] With that you can without difficulty determine his position, and define at least his cooperative complicity and partial responsibility. And for this, he had to pay, amply, more than enough. And what else? What else could be noted? In our household there was, apart from the obligatory swastika flag, no objects or books that had a reference to the spirit of the times which outside dominated life with its omnipresent symbols. While my father was incarcerated ... I looked in all corners and angles for possibly implicating evidence. I only found a paperback edition of "Mein Kampf" hidden under a pile of books. From a dedication, one could deduct that it was given or donated to my father at God knows which event. As the only child, I was from an early age witness of everything that happened in our house. *Gross Deutschland*, or the *Reich*, the empire, or even the '*Führer*' played no role, not even during the psycho-euphoric times at the beginning of the war, when special reports on the radio were accompanied by the sound of a threateningly thundering Liszt (which even today sounds, or rather, rings in my ears) and which suggested enormous future perspectives for the Germany that was superior to all other countries."[109]

Later, in 2005, Neumann would look back in an essay and conclude that "... hypothetically, I come to the conclusion that my father slid into the fascist dirt superficially and lightheartedly, not sufficiently aware of his responsibility

108 In 1921 Adolf Hitler formed his own private army called Sturm Abteilung (Storm Section). The SA was instructed to disrupt the meetings of political opponents and to protect Hitler from revenge attacks. Captain Ernst Röhm became the SA's first leader. By 1934 the SA had grown to 4,500,000 men.
In the course of 1933, some of the Nazi leaders became increasingly concerned about the growing power of the SA and manufactured evidence that suggested that Röhm had been paid 12 million marks by the French to overthrow Hitler. Generals were afraid that the SA would absorb the much smaller German Army and industrialists were unhappy with Röhm's socialist views on the economy. Many people in the party also disapproved of the fact that Röhm and many other leaders of the SA were homosexuals. On 29th June 1934, Hitler, accompanied by the SS, personally arrested Ernst Röhm. During the next 24 hours 200 other senior SA officers were arrested. Many were shot as soon as they were captured but Hitler decided to pardon Röhm because of his past services to the movement. However, after much pressure Hitler agreed that Röhm should die and he was eventually killed by two SS men. The SA gradually lost its power in Hitler's Germany.

109 Neumann, Jochen: *Braun*, p. 2

but at the same time locked up in provincial-local dependencies, and just went along. During my adult years I never noticed with him downright opportunism, although he could have benefited from it more than once."[110]

Jochen Neumann also never noticed any anti-Semitism in his family.[111] "Anti-Semitic remarks were part of everyday life. For example, when things became a bit confused in school, people would call out 'Hey, we are not in a Jew school, are we!', and that was the mildest version of what occurred. Everything Jewish served as a characterization of something negative, primitive, incorrect and evil. My parents made very sure that these things did not become part of our daily language. Probably there were, in spite of the *Ariernachweis*,[112] on both parental sides some traces of Jewish roots, at least in the family of my grandmother on my mother's side, who was born Miska, and who came out of the Polish border regions next to Ukraine. In photos you can see some facial traits that point in that direction. Moreover, my mother used Yiddish words and expressions in abundance and was probably never aware of it, because she did this all her life, even in fascist times, with an open minded casualness. Only years later it became clear to me that these were Yiddish words. I considered this vocabulary at first to be slang from Silesia.[113] Ms. Neumann also managed to avoid becoming a member of the *NS-Frauenschaft,* a national-socialist women's organization, in spite of strong pressure from the wife of the mayor.

Also Jochen's grandfather showed an extraordinary naivety when it came to politics: "During the winter of 1944-45 (or was it 1943-44?) the *Winterhilfswerk*[114] gathered contributions. Depending on the sum donated, the donors received a small wooden pendant in form of an old-time locomotive with accompanying wagons in bright colors, hanging individually from a

110 Neumann, Jochen: *Wie Braun?,* February 2005, p. 3

111 Interview with Jochen Neumann, June 3, 2009

112 The "Ariernachweis" or "proof of being Aryan" was a document that proved that one was "Aryan". It was required by State and government authorities in the German Reich after April 1933 for officers and employees in public service, including scientists at German universities. With it began the exclusion of "Non-Aryans", especially Jews, Roma and Sinti by withdrawal of their civil rights and later through expulsions, ghettos, deportation and extermination in the Holocaust.

113 *Braun,* p. 2-3

114 The Winterhilfswerk (WHW) was an annual drive by the National Socialist People's Welfare Organization to help finance charitable work. Its slogan was "None shall starve nor freeze". It ran from 1933-1945 and was designed to provide food and fuel to Germans. Donors were often given small souvenir gratitude gifts of negligible value, somewhat similar to the way modern charities mail out address labels and holiday cards.

band as a mark on the garment or fixed together with a hook and an eyelet, and could to be put up on display. My grandfather received, as an exceptional donor, a complete set of this train in a costly display cupboard, which could be secured to the wall, and a personal thank you letter from the Saxon *Gauleiter* Martin Mutschmann.[115] The train set and the letter promptly received a place of honor over the desk. When, after the end of the war, again gifts were gathered for noble purposes, my grandfather again donated, with the same generosity, remarkable sums that resulted again in written thanks from the relevant authoritative. The bearer of this letter was astonished when he found the Mutschmann letter still on display. Thank God he was no bastard, and asked my grandfather quietly yet emphatically to remove *such* utensils as quickly as possible because the times had changed *fundamentally*."[116]

"From 1944 onwards there were more impressive signs and unusual situations, which I remember precisely (a plane crash near Naundorf and a bombing near Korptizsch, special reports on the radio, soldiers passing by or columns of refugees, relatives mourning those killed in action, various bottlenecks, air alarms, my father at the lowering of the flag, a visit to my father (as *Unteroffizierbewerber*) in the Brüx garrison and hiding in the air shelters for the rest of the night, even an air attack during a train journey through the Ore mountains.[117] But still the political shell around it was missing."[118] The young Neumann didn't even join the "*Pimpfe,*" the youth movement for the smallest that preceded the *Hitler Jugend.*[119] "I did not want to join the "*Pimpfe*" ... although that was unusual. All my contemporaries around me around were members. I just didn't like the group life there; for me it was a bit too rough (My whole life I never participated in a fight or similar robustness). My father, when I asked him, said he would leave it to me to decide, what I liked. The unusual, perhaps risky, aspect of this attitude I understood only years later."[120]

---

115 Martin Mutschmann (1879 - 14 February 1947) was the Nazi Region Leader (*Gauleiter*) of the state of Saxony (Gau Sachsen) during the time of the Third Reich. Mutschmann was made *Gauleiter* of Saxony in 1925. He was to maintain this position until the end of World War II and eventually sentenced to death and executed in Moscow. Generally his political activity concentrated on Saxony rather than on Germany as a whole. Mutschmann was passionately interested in the preservation of Saxon arts and crafts.

116 *Braun*, p. 1

117 *Erzgebirge*, the mountain range between Saxony in Germany and the Czech Republic.

118 *Der Sozialismus und Ich*, p. 2

119 The Pimpfen were the youngest subsection of the Hitler Youth (Hitler Jugend), prevalent in Nazi Germany from 1933-1945

120 *Braun*, p. 2

The house in which the Neumann's lived was only fifty meters away from the main road between the towns Grimma and Döbeln, where the bridge crossed the Freiberger Mulde River from Fischendorf to Leisnig. Soon the war was also on Jochen Neumann's doorstep. First a huge anti-aircraft gun was put up in the garden of their house, a wonderful attraction for the kids who were allowed to climb on it and managed to get some chocolate out of the soldiers manning it. Luckily the gun was removed before the Allied forces arrived; otherwise, the consequences could have been quite unpleasant.

A sequence of events followed, events that quickly ended Neumann's childhood and propelled him into adulthood. "Sometimes more, sometimes less consciously I registered things and became interested in things, the meaning of which I didn't yet understand one hundred percent but which, judging the mimics, movements and voice levels of the adult environment, were supposed to have the meaning of serious and threatening developments."[121] Jochen Neumann has some vivid memories of this turbulent period. One of them is when he and his mother visited his grandfather, who lived in the center of the town Rosswein. A neighbor of his grandfather informs Jochen's mother with a telling voice: "Mrs. Neumann, have you already heard, Küstrin has fallen." The way the message was put across made it clear to Jochen that something really bad had happened, even though "Küstrin" meant absolutely nothing to him and later that day it was explained to him that this defeat of the German troops sealed the fate of their home region.[122]

The following weeks were an endless series of war events. A nearby bridge was blown to pieces; chaos reigned and made normal daily and nightly life impossible. American troops reached the blown up bridge over the river Mulde, but within hours they disappeared again in the direction of Grimma. From the bathroom window, the Neumanns flew a white sheet, meant to represent a white flag. White pieces of cloth were flying from other houses as well, providing an unusual and eerie sight. "At the end of April or the beginning of May something happened that in one bolt structured the disorder

---

121 *Der Sozialismus und Ich*, p. 2

122 Before 1945 Küstrin (also spelled Cüstrin, Polish: Kostrzyn) was a town in Germany on the river Oder. After 1945 a new border was established along the Oder-Neisse line, and the city was divided between Germany and Poland. There was a big battle at Küstrin, and the fact that Küstrin had fallen meant that the Soviet troops had crossed the Oder. With that the states of Pomerania and Silesia had been lost (and that loss later turned out to be for ever), and Soviet troops had entered the state of Brandenburg. The fact that Jochen's mother originally came from Silesia made the effect of the remark even stronger.

and suffering in my head and developed my image of the world with big strides. With every day the final end of my childhood was sealed, punctually. Within the period of one week, seamlessly, a child was turned into an unripe adult. At the same time, this was the beginning of a still naturally formed and rather undifferentiated growing 'political' awareness and thought."[123]

Suddenly, Jochen smelled something unusual in the house. "I followed [the smell], and found our rolled up, stinking and smoldering swastika-flag in the kitchen oven. After a few clumsy and unsuccessful attempts to divert my attention my mother explained, stricken by panic, in a few very clear words what was happening, and what consequences were waiting for us. Immediately my senses were sharpened, my ears and eyes open. '*One*' was aware of '*one's responsibility.*' From then on with seismographic sensitivity, I registered the - also seemingly secondary - changes in the environment and an independent self-conscience developed itself, step by step. Whatever one thought or did, it all happened with a very clear understanding of danger and with great carefulness. Childish naivety and easygoingness were then a matter of the past."[124]

Uncertain times

The end of the war was also the beginning of a period of uncertainty, changing everything that seemed stable and a regular part of life. The American troops had withdrawn and, on the basis of an agreement between the Allied Forces, the village Fischendorf and the town Leisnig found themselves in the SBZ, the *Sowjetisch Besetzten Zone* (Soviet Occupied Zone). Life was unbearably difficult, and what was even more distressing was the absence of any clear vision of what would be next. Many people lost their zest for life; suicide was rampant. Some jumped from the bridge across the Mulde River: "Most of them [were] refugees from the former pioneer barracks. Also a mother and her child were among them. Too clever for our age, too early ripe and curious as we were, we kids tried to get a look at the dead brought into the mortuary of the cemetery in Tragnitz."[125]

School life returned, even though it would take a year before regularity had fully returned. Initially, the schoolchildren went to school in a café in the center of Leisnig, but after a while the school building itself reopened. By then, the Hans-Schemm-School was renamed Siegismund-Reschke-

123 *Der Sozialismus und Ich*, p.2-3
124 *Der Sozialismus und Ich*. P.3
125 Neumann, Jochen: *Die Brücke*, p.2-3

School, after a previous Leisnig mayor, and the bust of Hans Schemm, having been one of the national socialist idols, had been removed.[126]

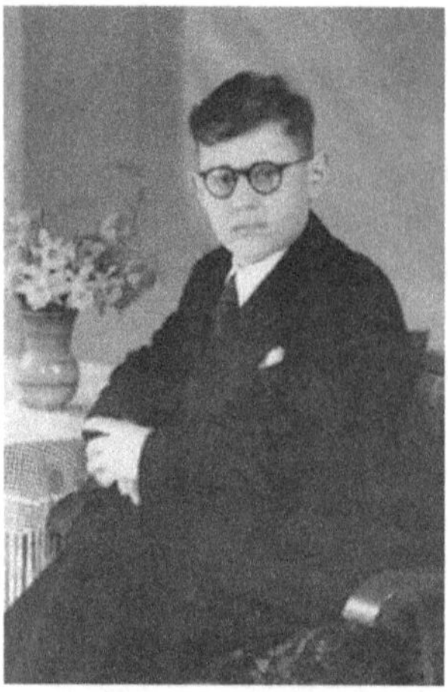

Jochen Neumann in 1950 when finishing school

The school was heated for only a few hours a day. Instead of glass they had put "Igelit" in the broken windows, "an opaque, milk-glassy plastic… as a result of which it was impossible to look outside. With time the Igelit colored brown and then disintegrated, but by that time glass was used again. You could look again out onto the square in front of the school. The protection trenches against shells were being filled up and the beautiful big and old linden trees were felled (…) because there was an urgent need of firewood. Metaphorically the deforestation on the square in front of the school represented the deforestation of the teaching at school."[127]

Many of the original teachers had been banned from work because of their alleged allegiance to the Nazi system. Also Jochen Neumann's father was for some time not allowed to resume his work as a teacher. The '*Altlehrer*' (old teachers) had been replaced by '*Neulehrer*' (new teachers), who often had no background in teaching whatsoever. Some were refugees from German areas from which they had been expelled, such as Prussia and Silesia, others were returning soldiers or people from the region who took any opportunity to get a job. "A dazzling group consisted of members of formerly nationalist-socialist families," Neumann remembers, "but because

126 Neumann, Jochen: *Schulspeisung*, p. 3. Hans Schemm, a teacher, worked during the First World War at a military epidemic hospital in Bayreuth where he became infected with tuberculosis. In 1919 he belonged to the Freikorps Bayreuth, which took part in the struggles in Munich. From 1923, Schemm had contacts with Nazi groups and in September 1923 he got to know Adolf Hitler. Schemm's political positions were clearly antidemocratic, anti-Semitic and anti-Communist. He founded the National Socialist Teachers' Federation in 1927 and a year later he became a member of the Bavarian Landtag. In 1928 and 1929, Schemm took over the leadership of several Nazi newspapers. Later he established several publications of his own. In 1930, Schemm became a member of the Reichstag. In April 1933, he was appointed by Hitler as the "Leader of Cultural and Educational Affairs of Bavaria." On 5 March 1935, Schemm died after an aircraft crash.

127 *Schulspeidung*, p. 3

of their youth they were still unblemished and had only just entered the job (a small part moved after a while to the Western occupied zone). The patchwork of the teachers collective after the war was completed with a small number of '*Altlehrer.*' Those were the teachers that had not been a member of the NSDAP. Often these did not have a clean conscience either, even though that would have been difficult to expect. But at least they guaranteed a certain level of professionalism."[128]

Having a father who used to be a teacher, Jochen Neumann was less affected by the low level of professionalism of his teachers. His father not only added his share to his son's education but also had a large number of schoolbooks dating back to both the time of the Weimar Republic and the Nazi period. Jochen studied them and found pleasure in showing off his knowledge, not only to his fellow schoolmates but also to the teachers. "It did not at all win over the new tutors for me since they all knew that I was the son of an *Altlehrer*, whom they anyhow mistrusted or to whom they ascribed negative attitudes. Unfortunately, I liked my little superiority and put targeted questions that the helpless teachers could not answer or to which they had no immediate answer on the very same day. Every now and then I played 'thick Wilhelm,' by precociously adding, for example, after each animal or plant name the scientific Latin name. In this period, my little soul was crumpled, filled with grief, fears and frustrations, and I compensated for this all during the lessons with the baffled teachers. While I impressed one with my knowledge (…), the other retained me like a hot potato."[129]

Jochen Neumann's equilibrium was, at that moment, rather shaky. At the end of 1945 the Soviet occupational forces had unexpectedly picked up his father, Erhart Neumann, who disappeared into the mist of the Soviet detention camps. For a long time, nobody knew what happened to him, and whether he was actually still alive. It was at first also unclear what the exact reason was for his arrest and of what he was accused, especially since he had merely been a petty party member and had not played any significant role in the Nazi regime. This initial uncertainty of his father's fate, the emotional distress of his mother and the uncertainty about the present and future must have had an enormous influence on the young Jochen.

Things got even worse for Jochen when a certain Getrud Beier becomes director of the school. She and her husband, Erich Beier, were originally from Leipzig, but moved to Leisnig after their hometown had been

---

128 *Schulspeisung*, p. 4

129 *Schulspeisung*, p. 4-5

massively bombed by the RAF.[130] Her husband taught at the Leisnig School, but was removed from teaching after the war because of his membership of the NSDAP. Mrs. Beier herself had not been a Party member and, after the war, clearly decided to play by the book. In spite of the fact that Erich Beier was a good friend of Jochen Neumann's father and that the couples visited each other, she decided to exclude Jochen from the school nutrition program with the argument that his father was a Nazi. This was a huge blow, because life was hard, hunger was all around and Jochen's mother was struggling to feed her son and herself by working as an agricultural worker. The additional food, provided class by class in Café Meißner in the *Chemnitzerstrasse*, was a welcome and necessary addition to the menu.

Suddenly, because of the director's decision, Jochen Neumann was excluded from this food program: "From now on, this was no longer for me, although I had no less hunger than all other students. Since nobody was allowed to stay unattended in school, when the time came, I had to march every day with the rest of the class to Café Meißner, but there I had to wait outside the window with a rumbling stomach and wait for my comrades to return to school again. After class, I banged my knapsack at home in a corner and immediately went to search for something edible. (…) Once I went shopping at the lower Schlossberg … and on the way back I could not control myself and while standing, I immediately ate everything that had been bought to last a whole week. Hunger is very painful, so roughly in the middle of the abdomen, buzzing about the skull. For me everything was already terrible. The trauma was further strengthened by the psychologically clumsy, sometimes impossible behavior of my mother, who, overwhelmed by hard work and worry (we did not know whether my father was still alive and where he was, we were afraid they wanted to take away our home) for the first time failed in her mother role. Instead of teaching me and punishing me for my own good in order to strengthen me, she made constant allegations and complained for weeks at a time that she had such a failing son."[131]

The school director, Getrud Beier, added oil to the fire by asking for a meeting with Jochen's mother and attacking her for not being able to raise her son in an acceptable way. This episode so much upset Jochen Neumann that it took him months to find his equilibrium again.

---

[130] During World War II, Leipzig was repeatedly attacked by British as well as American air raids. The most severe attack was launched by the Royal Air Force (RAF) in the early hours of December 4, 1943 and claimed more than 1,800 lives. Large parts of the city center were destroyed.

[131] *Schulspeisung*, p. 5-6

Chapter 6 – Shaken Foundations

Indeed, the arrest of his father was an unexpected turn of events that would seriously affect Jochen Neumann's sense of security. Initially everything seemed to be all right for Erhart Neumann; he survived the war and was not hurt. Near to the end of the hostilities, he had been drafted into the army as a reserve officer. While stationed in a garrison in Brüx, he underwent abdominal surgery, and subsequently retreated with German troops through the Ore Mountains. He remained otherwise unscathed, and after his decommissioning, he returned home. He had not been subjected to "*Entnazifizierung*"[132] because there was nothing substantial that could be brought against him. However, as an '*Altlehrer,*' he was not allowed to return to his former post at the Leisnig School. Luckily, he soon was given a position as teacher in the village Leipnitz, approximately 10-12 kilometers away from Leisnig, a distance he initially covered on foot daily. Soon he found accommodation with the Kirchhof family in Leipnitz. "Twice we transported brown coal briquettes in a huge borrowed cart," Jochen Neumann remembers. "[It was] a present from Mr. Kirchhof, a miner, along with the cut up remains of an apple tree from Leipnitz to Fischendorf. I remember vividly the nights in the little room, where my father and I slept in one bed, and the not-so-large Kirchhof property. If I had to pee during the night, then I did it straight from the window. Presumably it was this exhilarating experience of peeing out of the window that helped me store the daily experiences in Leipnitz so vividly in my memory."[133]

In the early summer of 1945, a sense of normal life started to develop in the SBZ. Initially some strange fellows appeared in town, one by one, who performed the role of executive official. At first, a certain Mr. Borchert appeared, who pretended to be a survivor of the concentration camps and allegedly couldn't move one of his arms because of a wound. He ruled the village as if he owned it, wore black suits and demonstratively a radiantly red tie. After a period of twenty-thirty days, he suddenly disappeared, from one moment to the next. It turned out that real former concentration camp inmates had recognized him as one of their guards, and the so-called wound on his arm was the result of a rather unsuccessful removal of his SS

---

[132] The *Entnazifizierung* (denazification) was a goal and a set of measures of the four-power after their victory over Nazi Germany, starting in July 1945 have been implemented. After the Potsdam Agreement, the German and Austrian society, culture, press, economy, judiciary and politics from all influences of Nazism be exempted. This should be done in the context of a comprehensive democratization and demilitarization happen.

[133] Neumann, Jochen: *Unterwegs*, p. 1

tattoo. Later, it was said that he had managed to escape to the Western Zone without any retribution.

The second temporary ruler was a Mr. Anders (or Albers). "He resided and ruled during maybe a month in Leisnig next to the Soviet command. What made him do this in particular, I forgot. Many saw him as a sort of mayor of Leisnig, others as a chief of police, which was more fitting to him. Anyway, he behaved as a sort of Satrap[134] (he seemed to master the Russian language as well), was feared and evoked an enormous respect because of the way he appeared in public. Only the occupation forces had access to cars and fuel. For that reason, he drove through the region, always at a gallop, in a carriage with white horses whom he mercilessly hit with his whip. Everyone jumped aside when Anders/Albers appeared on the horizon. On the streets partially covered with cobblestones, the heels of the horses and the metal-covered wheels of the carriage caused a characteristic fearsome noise that could be heard far into the distance."[135] This Anders or Albers also disappeared from one day to the next; nobody knew where he went nor did they miss him.

After the end of the war, father Erhart Neumann had gradually become part of daily life in Fischendorf again. He was generally known as a kind and unpretentious man, and, although a member of the NSDAP, he was considered not more than a 'small Nazi,' rather a sort of petty follower. At this time, an *Entnazifizierung* had not yet commenced, although one counted with every possible option, and the stories about confiscations, evictions from homes and the sort kept the family clearly alert. Still, the mayor from Nazi times, Franz Eifrig, had been able to return to his former profession of "bed feather cleaner" and only the *Ortsgruppenleiter*[136] of the NSDAP, Klaus, was interned in a detention camp. The new mayor, a Mr. Pöge, known as an old Social-Democrat, accepted the help of Mr. Neumann and the latter soon became in charge of the municipal accounts and helped the mayor with administrative work. Everything seemed to be slowly sliding back to normality, but this did not last long. The new authorities in the SBZ were preparing for a purge that would not leave the Neumann family untouched.

134 Satrap was the name given to the governors in the Median and Persian empires and in several of their successors. In modern literature the word usually refers to leaders or governors who behave as if they are rulers of superpowers or hegemonies.

135 *Unterwegs*, p. 2

136 The *Ortsgruppenleiter* is the political leaders of several towns or villages, or of part of a larger city, and including from 1500 to 3000 households.

Arrest

One day, Jochen Neumann was playing in the garden with a rabbit when a car stopped outside on the street. As this was an unusual event, Jochen decided to have a look. A group of eight armed men and a German interpreter jumped out of the car, rang the doorbell and asked for Jochen's father. He opened the door, and was immediately ordered to come along. "He was not even allowed to exchange a few words with us: crying loudly, while understanding nothing of what was going on, I ran after the small column. In front walked the German with my father and behind them were the eight Russians with their Kalashnikovs in alert positions. Then my father was pushed onto a truck and they drove off, to Leisnig and on to the castle, which housed the Leisnig prison since the beginning of the eighteenth century. My mother and I went the very same evening to the castle, but we received no permission to speak to my father."[137]

The family managed to hand over some clothing and shoes, as Jochen's father had left the house wearing slippers and without any warm clothing. Days passed without anything happening. It turned out that another person in the village had betrayed Neumann: he had been arrested first, but according to Soviet installed practice, he managed to buy his own release by denouncing two others. Still nobody really worried, because being only a "small Nazi," he would surely not be interned for a long time. It all seemed to be a mistake, and the mayor of Fischendorf promised to use his influence to obtain his release. "However the Fischendorf town elders, mainly Social Democrats with an anti-fascist touch, made clear to mayor Pöge that he [Erhart Neumann] was sorely missed, and that they needed him urgently to perform some bureaucratic acts. Some essential tasks had to be taken care of. Moreover, they knew from personal experience that my father never had been a bad guy and had done no evil to anyone. Somehow, they liked him. Therefore, they tried energetically to get him out from the prison, even though the German authorities did not actually have the authority to decide. But fate took its own course. They were introduced to the commander in the city and learned that the case of my father would be dealt with earlier than originally predicted. Unfortunately, though, on that day, a Thursday, some senior executives and higher-ranking officers in the command post were interrogated and prepared to be moved out. During that process, things got mixed up (which we learned only after years), mostly due to Babylonic language confusion.[138] In the end, all who were in the hall

137 *Unterwegs*, p. 3

138 Almost nobody spoke both Russian and German, so the Russians didn't understand the Germans and vice versa.

of the ground floor were selected for transportation without any further consultation. Circumstances forced me to be a witness of this transfer. Because we, my mother and I, had been informed that my father would probably be released, we stayed for hours in front of the command post in order to pick him up. Meanwhile, a truck drove up to the building. About a dozen men were led out of the entrance under guard; my father was among them. Disregarding the situation, I ran to my father and wanted to cling on to him. I was violently ripped aside by a guard and just managed to see how my creator was thrown onto the truck with a high arch (!).[139] The young Jochen Neumann was again shaken by this very traumatic event.

This group of prisoners, which mainly consisted of middle-rank Nazi officials, was first sent to the prison in Döbeln, where Jochen managed to see his father one last time behind the bars of his cell. The family tried to see their detained relative after that but to no avail. The doors remain closed and from that moment on, father Neumann vanished into a fog. The family was left in the dark, the typical feature of a totalitarian detention system.[140] "It was the end of the war, 1945. [On New Year's Eve] we are sitting in the living room at the Lorenz family home; there was punch. The mood is festive yet at the same time depressed. Paul Lorenz had been missing since Stalingrad. [My] father was incarcerated somewhere (…). Anna Lorenz and my mother had for hours kept their wedding rings dangling over the photos of their husbands on twine threads. It was also possible to do that over a glass of water. Depending on whether the rings swayed or circled (or didn't move at all, which was a catastrophe), it was allegedly possible to learn whether those absent were still alive and were in good or bad shape. The entire procedure was not very clear, however, and in any case not unambiguous. Somehow unrest started. Anna Lorenz gave 10 marks. Rosel Quaiser, an old spinster and mill owner who had gone broke, was a respected card player, probably the best in the vicinity. She had supported herself by prophesying over water … on this occasion, she had been invited for a drink and, of course, had to bring her cards along in order to clarify the fate of those absent. The outcome was: both husbands were still alive, but it was impossible to provide more exact information. (They never heard of Paul Lorenz again and he was declared dead in the 1970s.) The evening was rescued. One could, even if with hardly concealed unrest, enter the new year."[141]

Later it turned out that Erhart Neumann was sent to the detention center in Bautzen, generally known by the ominous name of "The Yellow Misery."

139 *Unterwegs*, p. 4

140 *Unterwegs*, p. 4

141 Neumann, Jochen: *Silvester*, p. 1

Bautzen

Special camp N. 4 in Bautzen, "The Yellow Misery," was one of the camps used by the Soviet authorities. Many minor Nazis and war criminals were kept in this camp, but gradually an increasing number of political opponents of the new regime were interned there as well. Some of those interned would have to wait until 1956 before they were finally released.

Originally, the prison had been built with reformist ideas about penitentiary facilities in mind. However, considering the nickname, little of that remained. In May 1945, the Soviets took over the prison and developed the special camp for detained former functionaries of the Nazi regime. In Bautzen itself, a smaller prison was turned into a pre-trial investigation prison, Bautzen II.

Within several weeks, approximately 6,000 people were incarcerated in Bautzen. Between May 1945 and 1956, approximately 27,000 prisoners passed through the gates.[142] At least 3,000 of them died while being imprisoned, due to the bad living conditions and other non-natural causes.[143]

Bautzen was not a labor camp. The only goal of the institution was complete isolation. Bad hygienic conditions resulted in many infectious diseases and in the death of a considerable number of prisoners. Each prisoner received two liters of water a day, to be used both for drinking and washing. Soap was insufficiently available; prisoners were wearing the clothes in which they were arrested. To curb the spread of vermin, clothes were disinfected regularly, but still lice were all over the place.[144] Food consisted mainly of three-quarters of a liter of watery soup and 250 grams of bread. The bread was usually handed out in loaves of one kilo, which then had to be shared by four prisoners. Self-made weights ensured that the division was equal. Spoons also had to be shared, due to insufficient availability. Irregularly salt, sugar and marmalade was added to the ration. In spite of the bad health condition, the ration was sliced in half during the winter of 1946; as a result, the mortality rate went up quickly.[145]

---

142 After the founding of the DDR in October 1949, the special camp was officially closed in February 1950, and the majority of those interned were released. However, people convicted by the Special Military Tribunals continued to stay in Bautzen until 1956, now guarded by the *Volkspolizei* (People's Police).

143 Hattig, Suzanne, et.al.: *Geschichte des Speziallagers Bautzen*, p. 10-11

144 *Bautzen*, p. 96

145 *Bautzen*, p. 93

Father Neumann had a terrible time in Bautzen, which lasted several months. Neumann remembers: “We never really learned what my father (and others) encountered there; he almost never spoke about it. He only indicated that the detainees were sometimes terribly beaten, and even that he told only with the maximum resistance, although we constantly asked him questions. When only the word “Bautzen” was mentioned, my father slid back in years and into himself, became ashen grey and had tears in his eyes.”[146] Yet at that time, during the winter of 1945-1946, the Neumann’s still had no idea whether father was still alive or not. In March 1946, a person appeared on the doorstep, claiming to have met the father in Bautzen and asserting that all is OK. Out of gratitude the Neumanns feed and cloth the messenger, who cling on to the hope that father is alive. Then, the man quickly disappeared again. Only later did they discover that he was a swindler and that he never met their husband and father.

Mühlberg

Later, Erhart Neumann was transported to the *Mühlberg Speziallager Nr. 1*, another main Soviet detention center, and originally a camp for prisoners of war.[147] In the summer of 1945, the Soviet secret service, NKVD, used some of the barracks of Mühlberg to house groups of Vlasovites, Soviet soldiers who joined the Russian Liberation Army of General Vlasov and fought the Red Army after they were taken prisoner by the Germans. Most of them were either sent to the Soviet Gulag or executed.[148]

On September 10, 1945, the Mühlberg camp was formally taken over by the NKVD and prepared as a special camp for internees from the SBZ. In mid-September, groups of prisoners were moved there from various cities all over the SBZ, and at the beginning of October 1945, a transport of 2,400 prisoners was delivered from Bautzen. However, Jochen Neumann’s father was probably transported later, as according to Neumann’s memory, his father celebrated Christmas in Bautzen.[149]

---

146 *Unterwegs*, p. 4

147 The Mülhberg camp was originally established by the German army in September 1939 as a camp for Prisoners of War and named Stalag IV B. After the Red Army liberated the POW’s there on April 23, 1945, the camp had remained empty for a while.

148 For more information on General Vlasov and his army see, among others, Fröhlich, Sergej: *General Wlassov; Russen und Deutsche zwischen Hitler und Stalin*, Köln, 1987

149 Jochen Neumann clearly remembers his father telling him how they celebrated Christmas, one of the few stories he shared, and that one of the prisoners was

When the camp was established it was in a desolate state. The period between the end of the war and September had been enough for the population living in the proximity to remove anything that could be used. Everything had been taken out of the barracks: not only all the furniture was gone but also the heating system had been removed, the glass had been taken out of the windows and even the wooden floor boarding was gone. Only the water pipes had remained untouched.[150] The prisoners were set to work, removing all the debris and cutting trees in the proximity to get wood for construction. A special "Jauchekommando" (sewage commando) was set out to work to clean out the sewage with their own hands in order to de-clog it and make it function again. This commando was notorious for the number of prisoners dying as a result of strenuous labor and infections. The prisoners were also told to enforce the perimeter with a doubled fence of barbed wire, watchtowers and a security strip, a forbidden zone, in which a prisoner would be shot without warning if he entered it. In 1946, an electric fence was added.

Prisoners in Mühlberg had no communication with the outside world. They were not allowed to correspond with their relatives, and since the spring of 1946, no new construction was needed in Mühlberg, the possibility of smuggling messages via people on the outside also disappeared. Even in the case of death, relatives were not notified: there was total isolation. This isolation was relaxed a little in the fall of 1947, when newspapers were allowed in. In particular, the newspaper "*National Zeitung*" of the national democratic party of Germany formed an important communication channel for prisoners and relatives on the outside would publish small advertisements hoping that their imprisoned relatives would find them.[151]

The camp was managed in the form of "self-management," prisoners in charge of

---

beaten to death because he stole something from the prison warehouse for the Christmas "party."

At the end of 1945 approximately 10,000 people were interned in Mühlberg. Of these, 54% were interned because of their membership of the NSDAP; 78% of the prisoners were considered to be Nazi criminals. See: Morré, Jörg: *Speziallager des NKWD*, p. 60.

On average 11,800 prisoners were held in Mühlberg, and in total almost 22,000 prisoners entered its gates. Of these, 6,725 prisoners died of starvation, illness or cold, be almost one-third of its total population. Of these, 40% died during the hunger winter of 1946-1947. After a first wave of releases in July 1948 the camp was finally closed in November 1948. The remaining 3,600 prisoners were transferred to the special camp in Buchenwald, where most would remain interned anther two years.

150 *Speziallager des NKWD*, p. 52

151 *Speziallager des NKWD*, p. 60

control and organized by a strict military order. Most of the leading positions were taken over by people who had "management-experience," most often acquired during their work in Nazi organizations. As a result, the leadership consisted mainly of high functionaries from the Hitler Jugend and the Bund Deutscher Mädel, which gave the camp the nickname "Nazilager" (Nazi camp).[152]

The prisoners in Mühlberg suffered from chronic malnourishment. In the beginning, the daily allowance was 500-600 grams of bread, 15-20 grams of butter and every fifth day 20-30 grams of sugar or marmalade. In the morning, each prisoner would get half a liter of coffee, and in the evening, half a liter or three-quarters of a liter of thin potato soup with some slivers of meat. However, during the first half of 1946, the potato soup was changed into a pulp soup, with pulp being leftovers from the production of potato starch. As a result of the pulp, many prisoners suffered from edema. In addition, at the end of 1946, the daily allowance was reduced by half, and the soup then consisted only of water.

Also about Mühlberg, father Neumann remained mainly silent, hardly ever telling what he had gone through. And almost as unexpected as he had been arrested, he was released, most probably in the summer of 1947.[153] "One day I went home from school … when somebody from Fischendorf shouted at me across the street: 'Hey, Neumann, your father is back.' I didn't hurry very much. So much had been told before that turned out to be untrue, why should it be different this time. Finally I arrived home. Instead of my father an emaciated person in rags and full of dirt was sitting on the sofa in the kitchen, hardly moving a finger. My mother was already on her way back from her work at a farm far away, as she returned only in the evenings; she boiled a large pan of potatoes and prepared hot water to wash him. It was my father, indeed, who was hanging there, but who had changed beyond recognition. He raised himself to say hello with great difficulty. I stayed aside a bit, because there was nothing that connected me to this person. Only gradually, I realized what had happened. From those days, I kept a strange unpleasant image of my father. He had physically changed, had become a skeleton and had thick legs from fluids, and mentally he had grown old. Who was before an interested and bright person, was now a man sitting around for days, mute and clearly with orientation problems in surroundings that had become strange to him. (…) What shocked me as his son was how slow he was and completely disinterested in everything around him."[154]

152 *Speziallager des NKWD*, p. 56

153 Could also have been a year later, in 1948, but this is not clear from the available data.

154 *Unterwegs*, p. 6

Chapter 7 - Political Turmoil at Tulane University

The blacklist was a time of evil and... no one on either side who survived it came through untouched by evil.
Dalton Trumbo[155]

... Men become Communists out of the best of motives and some of them cease to be Communists for the same motives once they learn that those who accept the pernicious doctrine of the end justifying the means will inevitably find that the means become the end.
Richard M. Nixon[156]

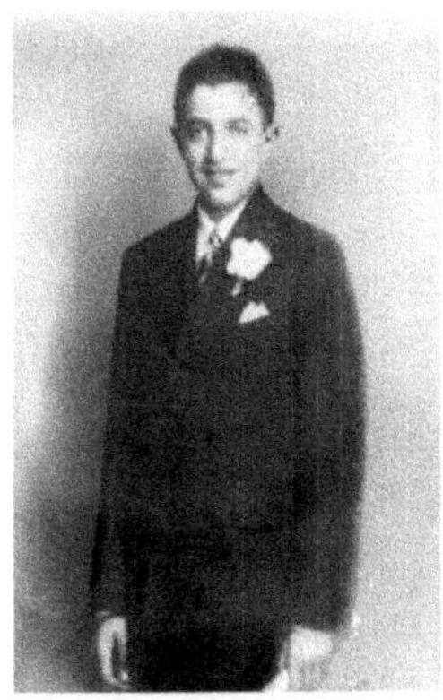

Melvin Sabshin as a student at Townsend Harris High School, 1937

On the other side of the Atlantic Ocean, Melvin Sabshin had done what his parents expected from him and had made his first steps to what would become a brilliant career. In 1936, at the age of ten, he was admitted to the prestigious Townsend Harris High School, located in the downtown location of the New York City College on Lexington Avenue, Manhattan.[157] He traveled there on the Pelham Bay subway from the station at East 174th Station down to Lexington Avenue, a ride of more than an hour each way.[158] While skipping one grade after the other, he graduated in 1940, shortly after having turned fourteen years of age. Then, at the young age of 14, he was admitted to the University of Florida,

155 From: *Additional Dialogue: Letters of Dalton Trumbo 1942-1962,* in Bentley, Eric (ed.): *Thirty Years of Treason*, p. xxi

156 Richard M. Nixon, former member of the HCUA and former U.S. Resident, in *Plea for an anti-Communist Faith*, in *Thirty Years of Treason*, p. 570.

157 Townsend Harris High School is a high school in the borough of Queens in New York City and consistently ranks as among the top 100 High Schools in the United States. The school is named for Townsend Harris, who besides his many diplomatic accomplishments had helped found the Free Academy of the City of New York, later to become City College, and was a strong proponent of free education. The Free Academy's introductory year gradually evolved and in 1904 became a full fledged, 3-year high school, housed on three floors of what is now Baruch College. In 1942 it was closed by mayor Fiorello La Guardia.

158 Interview Melvin Sabshin, July 29, 2009

from which he graduated in 1943 at the age of seventeen – quite an educational feat, to put it mildly.

His parents had moved in 1940 to Miami, Florida, in order to accommodate the failing health of father Zalman Sabshin, and Gainesville proved to be not too far away. All in all, the support of Melvin's parents was important, both in the emotional sense and in getting access to educational institutions at a very young age. In particular, Melvin's mother made sure that her son received adequate attention from the faculty staff, and it was the University's President, John Tigert, who, after several letters from Mrs. Sabshin, agreed to write a letter of recommendation to the Admission Committee of the Tulane University School of Medicine.

In 1944, Melvin Sabshin entered Tulane University in New Orleans, Louisiana, after having spent one year in the US Army. One of the main reasons for joining the army as a volunteer had been the fact that he was having difficulties in getting access to medical school because of his Jewish background. Since the late 1910s, anti-Semitism had been on the rise in the United States. The First World War resulted in an anti-foreign hysteria that did not leave even New York unaffected. Hospitality for the stranger turned into rejection and a climate of intolerance. New York, being the main entry point in the United States, became the focus for anti-immigration sentiment. Increasing numbers of "undesirables" were barred from entering the country. Religiously rooted prejudices slid into racist forms, and being the most numerous of the newer immigrants, the Jews easily became victims of this changed mood. Economic discrimination became overt. Advertisements with available job positions clearly indicated that only "Christians" were sought, thereby excluding Jews, and offers of apartments for rent made clear that Jewish tenants were not desired.[159] Still, apart from having difficulty in finding a place in medical school, Melvin Sabshin does not recall other instances of outright anti-Semitic behavior towards him personally.[160]

---

159 *The Promised City*, p. 260-265

160 Interview Melvin Sabshin, April 29, 2009. In Gainesville, Melvin Sabshin was a member of the Pi Lambda Phi Fraternity, which had originally been set up in 1895 at Yale University by a group of men who were denied the right of admission into college fraternities because of their religious and racial (Jewish) backgrounds. They had a vision of a fraternity where neither sect nor creed should ever act as a bar to admission for any man. In 1941 Pi Lambda Phi merged with the Phi Beta Delta Fraternity, who shared the same views and values, and these two merged fraternities were those where Jews were accepted as members. In that sense anti-Semitism may have been much more noticeable to Melvin Sabshin than he now remembers.

At first Melvin was stationed at Camp Blanding in Florida, which, in 1940, had been put to use by the US Army as an active duty training center,[161] but he was soon moved to Fort McPherson outside Atlanta, Georgia, where he started working as a postman in the post office.[162] In 1944, Melvin was sent to the US Army City College in New York, where they determined that he should take advantage of the fact that he had been admitted to Tulane Medical School; he was then sent to LaGarde General Hospital in New Orleans to enter Medical School at Tulane University.

In 1944, the climate of political intolerance and anti-Communism was still at a low. At most universities, the political debate came to a standstill between 1941 and 1945, while the country was waging war in both Southeast Asia and Europe, but it would resume as soon as the war was over. Like all other university institutions, Tulane had become increasingly dependent on federal financial support, including military funding for scientific research. This dependence would severely threaten the intellectual freedom of the university staff and its students, and would soon lead to a number of serious conflicts, in which Melvin Sabshin also played a part.

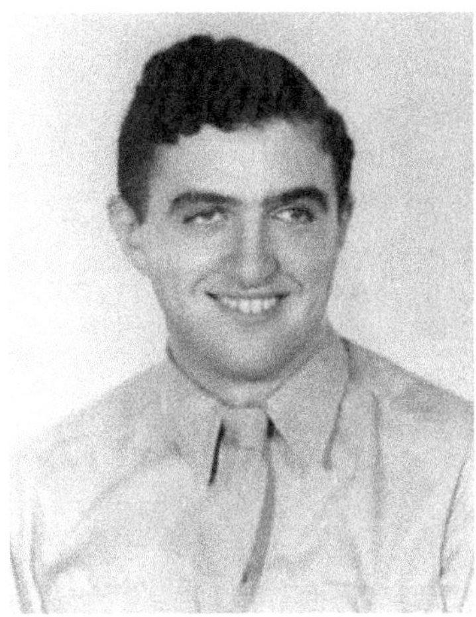

Private Mel Sabshin 1944

The onset of the cold war, during which the political beliefs of private citizens were increasingly scrutinized, led to a spirit of intolerance and distrust. This crusade very much focused on intellectuals, as their ideas were often considered to be unconventional and, therefore, threatening to the "American spirit." This often resulted in accusations of "un-American behavior" by anti-Communist zealots and over-active politicians. In particular, in the south of the United States this had a strong effect, as the mood there was determined by a

161 Originally, Camp Blanding was used by New England and Southern troops preparing for deployment overseas. However, during the course of the war, Camp Blanding served as an infantry replacement training center, an induction center, a German prisoner of war compound, and a separation center.

162 Fort McPherson had been greatly expanded after the outbreak of World War II, and in addition to serving as a general depot, a reception center was established to process thousands of men for entry into the service. McPherson also served as a major hospital center.

combination of anti-Communism and issues related to civil rights and the segregation of blacks in society. There white supremacists used the issue of Communism as a tool to discredit civil rights supporters, and this anti-Communism would have a lasting effect on academic life. In addition, the rising tide of anti-Communism in the late 1940s and early 1950s further strengthened the anti-Semitic mood in the country. The connection was not such a strange one, because many members of the Jewish community often looked at issues from a different perspective. "As political liberals, Jews articulated positions that many Americans considered suspect. Not only advocacy of civil rights and civil liberties, but support of the United Nations, federal aid to education, and efforts to take religion out of public schools – a key issue for American Jews – set them apart from many, possibly most, Americans. Jews responded differently to the political events of the period than did most other Americans. According to a 1952 Gallup Poll, for example, 56 percent of all Catholics and 45 percent of all Protestants considered the anti-Communist tactics of Senator Joseph McCarthy acceptable. In contrast, 98 percent of all Jews polled disapproved."[163] The American Jewish Committee commissioned a sociological study on the interconnection between the two, which "pointed to a strong and chilling connection between the two, propelling this defense organization and others to strategize."[164] The study was carried out in connection with the fervor following the trial and June 1953 execution of Ethel and Julius Rosenberg, a Jewish couple accused of spying for the Soviet Union.[165] The fact that the two were of Jewish origin had a profound effect on the Jewish community.

Charity hospital

Tulane University would become strongly involved in the cold war controversy in 1948, when law professor Mitchell Franklin agreed to serve on the campaign of presidential candidate Henry A. Wallace, who was

163 Diner, Hasia R.: *The Jews of the United States*, p. 277

164 *The Jews of the United States*, p. 278.

165 Julius Rosenberg (1918 -1953) and Ethel Greenglass Rosenberg (1915 -1953) were American communists who were convicted on March 29, 1951, and on April 5 were sentenced to death. The conviction helped to fuel Senator Joseph McCarthy's investigations into anti-American activities by U.S. citizens. The Rosenbergs denied the espionage charges even as they faced the electric chair. They were executed on June 19, 1953 for conspiracy to commit espionage. Since the execution, decoded Soviet cables have supported courtroom testimony that Julius acted as a courier and recruiter for the Soviets, but doubts remain about the level of Ethel's involvement. The decision to execute the Rosenbergs was very controversial at that time and is still debated.

running for president as leader of the Progressive Party. A decade earlier, in the mid-1930s, the university had been singled out as a bulwark of "un-American ideas" when four of its professors were indicted on charges of "un-Americanism." One of them, historian Mary Allen, was accused of having visited the USSR on a regular basis and of being friends with W.B. Binkley, who was the New Orleans secretary of the Communist Party. A second, Herman C. Nixon, was one of the South's leading academic liberals, founder of several political movements that supported the New Deal and equal civil rights. The attack on the four professors in 1936 was part of a much larger national campaign against Communist influence at universities. This campaign started with legislative actions against Communism at the universities of Wisconsin and Chicago and ended in 1940-1942 with hearings by a Rapp-Condert committee, resulting in some thirty instructors of the New York City higher education system being sacked because of their pro-Communist convictions.[166]

In the years between 1936 and 1948, most of the political activities of liberal academics at Tulane were channeled through an off-campus organization, the Louisiana League for the Preservation of Constitutional Rights. This organization, of which Herman Nixon was the first president, dealt with most of the issues in a rather indirect manner, while trying to maintain an image of being a respectable organization supported by prominent New Orleans families. Under Nixon's successor, Harold Lee, the league even adopted a more "conservative" stance by excluding Communists and blacks from its membership and separating the issues of intellectual freedom and civil rights. In a radio interview in May 1940, Lee bluntly stated, "Negroes had no rights that the police felt obligated to respect".[167]

When the war started in December 1941, the political debate at Tulane came temporarily to a halt. The university was placed on a wartime footing. But when the war ended in 1945, the tension and the pressures on intellectual freedom soon returned as a result of the onset of the cold war. The main issues now became anti-Communism and civil rights, whereby the first was often used to discredit those who fought for civil rights and other liberal reforms. At this time, Melvin Sabshin was already in his first year as an intern in psychiatry at Charity Hospital in downtown New Orleans.

Melvin Sabshin had been moved to LaGarde General Hospital in New Orleans in 1944 and started his medical studies at Tulane University.

---

166 Mohr, Clarence L., and Gordon, Joseph E.: *Tulane*, p.53-55

167 *Tulane*, p. 61-62

Normally he would have entered the Army Special Trainings Programs (ASTP), a program designed by the military to increase the number of doctors. However, the war was coming to an end and policy was changing. Instead he was honorably discharged from the army, with the first two years in medical school paid from the GI Bill of Rights program.[168]

At LaGarde, Melvin became friends with Bill Sorum and James Rogers. Rogers came from Georgia, a quiet fellow who was "exceedingly intelligent."[169] Bill Sorum was a lifeguard at the swimming pool and a member of the football team, like Rogers. Sorum, who had flunked out of the Officers Training Program but had remained a corporal, had a great influence on Melvin Sabshin. His influence was still noticeable when interviewing Melvin Sabshin in April 2009; several times he reiterated: "Sorum had a great influence on me."[170] The group of friends also became politically active. "Sorum, Rogers and I were influenced by several soldiers who had strong pro-Communist leanings. For the next seven or eight years, I remained interested in these activities in New Orleans, only to change my political opinions radically by events in the mid 1950s."[171] Both Sorum and Rogers are mentioned many times in Sabshin's FBI file, as we will see later.

The friendship between the three deepened further when Bill Sorum started his three-year residency at Tulane, one year later than Melvin and James Rogers, who were at that time roommates. Sorum was married to Monica Fusilier, who later became a relatively well-known psychiatrist and psychoanalyst and who was also politically active. Sabshin remembers a trip to a political gathering, where they traveled in one car: he, Bill Sorum, his wife Monica and several blacks. On the road, they were stopped by the police; a frightful experience that he still vividly remembers sixty years later. He only later realized that it must have been even scarier for Monica Fusilier, because for a white woman to sit in a car with blacks was as big as a political sin could get.[172]

It is also the time that Sabshin fell in love with a girl "with beautiful

[168] *Sabshin*, p. 22

[169] *Sabshin*, p. 22

[170] Interview Melvin Sabshin, April 21, 2009. Bill Sorum was later actively involved in activities of the American Psychiatric Association (APA). Ellen Mercer, then Director of International Affairs of the APA, remembers him as a very kind and intelligent man. He died in the 1990s.

[171] *Sabshin*, p.23

[172] Interview Melvin Sabshin, 21 April 2009

red hair, a deep southern drawl and a very strong interest in the children hospitalized at that time," Bettye Smith.[173] They had an intense romance, ending with them eloping to Mississippi for a quick wedding. Parents on both sides were not amused. They soon had a son, Jim Sabshin, who was born in November 1950 and named after James Rogers (who in turn named his own son after Melvin[174]). However, by the time the parents accepted the marriage, their relationship was already faltering and the couple finally divorced in 1952.

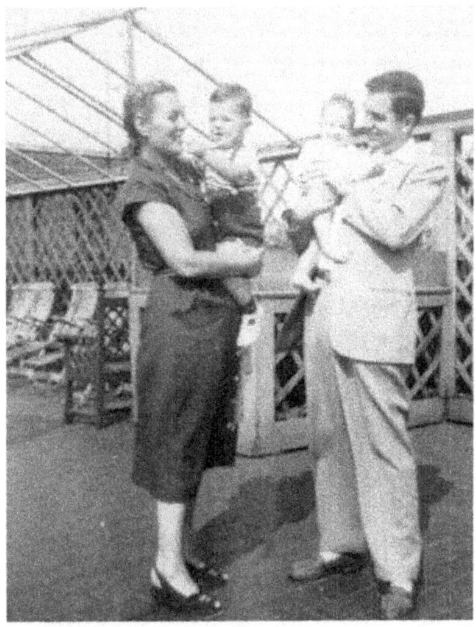

On the right Mel Sabshin with son Jimmy, 1951

Apart from his professional medical development, Melvin Sabshin also took an active political role during his first year in as an intern in psychiatry at Charity Hospital, both inside university and outside. Charity Hospital had been quite recently relocated to a newly constructed building, the "New Charity Hospital," that replaced a one hundred year old structure that was dilapidated, overcrowded and not fit for its task. However, also the "New Charity" had a distinct problem: since its construction in 1939, it had gradually sunk into the swampy delta soil. By 1943, the central part of the complex had officially sunk almost half a meter. There were even rumors that a whole floor had disappeared in the ground: "You know, (…) when you go to New Orleans you will find that the new Charity Hospital constructed by those Louisiana politicians has sunk one entire story. What is supposed to be the first floor is now the basement… So when you enter Charity, you really walk into what was planned to be the second floor."[175] The fact that the hospital was slowly sinking in the soft sediment of New Orleans was not so strange: it turned out that too few and too short poles had been used for its foundation, some of which had completely disappeared in the ground even after one blow by the pile driver.[176]

173 *Sabshin*, p. 26

174 Jim Rogers was less successful in his medical career that the others. He eventually moved back to Georgia and died at a young age.

175 Salvaggio, John: *New Orleans Charity Hospital*, p. 141-143

176 *New Orleans' Charity Hospital*, p. 142

Shortly before Sabshin and his friends commenced their internship at Charity Hospital, work started on the reconstruction of the hospital's psychiatric department. Until then, it had been primarily one big ward. The chairman of the psychiatry and neurology department at Tulane, Dr. Robert Heath, described the facilities: "The entire Charity psychiatry ward was similar to a giant cage: the patients were all fenced or caged in one large area; there was not even a door. It was infrequent that doctors even went in there... Most patients were strapped to the beds, and they had to be untied in order to examine them."[177] Now the entire floor of the psychiatric department was renovated, and completed in 1952. It had eighty beds, some private and semi-private rooms, four dining rooms, two solaria and special observation and hydrotherapy facilities.[178]

Like most if not all other public facilities, all services at Charity Hospital were segregated and divided into "W" departments (for whites) and "C" departments (for colored). In 1942, during a financially very difficult period, the W(hite) part of the facility had even been closed, and white and "negro" clinics had been held on alternate days, with the white part opening again only in March 1947.[179] When the hospital developed plans in 1948 to segregate the Blood Bank of the hospital where Sabshin was working at that time, he led a campaign against these plans. The Blood Bank, one of the first in the country to be founded in 1942 and the largest in the South of the United States,[180] was the only part of the hospital that was not yet segregated. Melvin's campaign was successful; the segregation was not carried out.[181] Not a small feat, considering the political climate at that time.

Anti-Communism on the rise

As noted before, Tulane had become a center of political debate in 1948 when law professor Mitchell Franklin agreed to serve on the campaign of presidential candidate Henry A. Wallace, who was running for president as leader of the Progressive Party.[182] Wallace, who had been a prominent "New

177 *New Orleans' Charity Hospital*, p. 162
178 *New Orleans' Charity Hospital*, p. 162
179 *New Orleans' Charity Hospital*, p. 157
180 *New Orleans' Charity Hospital*, p. 151
181 *Sabshin*, p. 25
182 Melvin Sabshin actively participated in the collection of 55,000 signatures needed for him to run for Presidency. Interview with Ellen Mercer, Jochen Neumann and Melvin Sabshin, December 1, 2009.

Dealer," was accused by his opponent, President Truman, as being "parlor pink," and because of Franklin's positioning as one of his campaigners the university was immediately attacked as having sympathies for "un-American" ideas and activities.

The issue received a national spin-off in April 1948 when Franklin, under strong pressure to resign from the University, was offered a job as a temporary legal consultant at the United Nations Secretariat. He decided to accept the offer knowing that after his work at the United Nations, he would have a Guggenheim scholarship in New York. He immediately resigned from the Wallace campaign, and left for New York. However, the damage was already done. Right-wing critics of Tulane alerted allies in Washington D.C., in particular Congressman F. Edward Hébert, at that moment a member of the House Un-American Activities Committee.[183] This is the type of information Hébert was looking for, and it immediately put him into action. Using a session of the Committee on another case,[184] he lashed out against Tulane University: "I am from Tulane (…) and to my chagrin there are more Communists who infest that place than Americans." He continued by saying that there was "one man named Franklin, who taught the Communist line to the students of Tulane, and who is now on leave from that university on an appointment to the United Nations and I cannot find out who put him there."[185]

The result was increased activity in Louisiana, in particular orchestrated by a group of Tulane alumni who circulated a petition against the alleged

183 The House Committee on Un-American Activities (HCUA, 1938-1975) was an investigative committee of the United States House of Representatives. In 1969, the House changed the committee's name to "House Committee on Internal Security". The prestige of HCUA began a gradual decline beginning in the late 1950s. By 1959, the committee was being denounced by former President Harry S. Truman as the "most un-American thing in the country today." When the House abolished the committee in 1975,its functions were transferred to the House Judiciary Committee.
Interesting in the context of this book is a bill to be adopted by the Senate and House of Representatives that was proposed by a Mr. Arthur Hays on February 10, 1948, to a sub-committee of the HCUA chaired by Richard M. Nixon, to eliminate "the Communist nuisance" by determining that "all suspected Communists or people we don't like be submitted to a mental test" and that a commission be set up to "invent a mental reading machine which when applied will say 'Communist' when the individual is not a loyal citizen." Also, "all Communists must wear boots, red shirts, fur caps… and grow beards…" until such a machine would be developed. See: *Thirty Year of Treason*, p. 252

184 The espionage case of Alger Hiss, on July 31, 1947

185 *Tulane*, p. 71

Communist influence at Tulane where "faculty members and particularly students (…) are doing apostolic work in the party line."[186] The petitioners demanded that all literature to be used during teaching be screened beforehand, and that membership lists, bylaws, and the "programs" of campus organizations should be submitted before they are allowed to operate. Also, all access to the campus should be denied to organizations and groups with interests that are "antagonistic to those of the University and the American government," while "all faculty members who openly profess sympathy with Communism and discontent with the American form of government" be dismissed.[187]

The petition forced the University's President, Robert Harris, to take a much clearer position than he desired. A year earlier, he had been able to avoid taking a sharp position by stating that "as an American university, Tulane asserts that the democratic form of government is the only tolerable system," but also that "false ideologies chiefly attract the uninformed" and therefore it was necessary that "foreign ideologies be examined critically and objectively by scholars who comprehend their falsity."[188] However, this time there was no escape. Harris now flatly stated that Tulane had no faculty members who professed "sympathy with Communism and discontent with the American form of government." He went further by stating that Tulane was in fact "one of the most conservative University campuses in the country (…) with only two persons on the faculty … that anyone has called Communistic and they are not accused of being Communists but of following the party line. As a matter of fact, I know they are not Communist." One of the persons mentioned was Mitchell Franklin, whose participation in the Wallace campaign had caused the stir; the other was "silly Field," being Art Department chairman Robert Field who was considered by Harris as a "sort of Hindu Mystic." [189]

Even though the support for Wallace among students turned out to be very limited, (according to a straw poll only 5 percent of the faculty and students supported him, while 41 percent favored Republican presidential candidate Thomas E. Dewey)[190] the damage was irreversible. Hébert was not re-elected to the House Un-America Activities Committee for lacking the necessary law degree, but the stage had been set for a much more radical anti-Communist campaign.

---

186 *Tulane*, p. 72

187 *Tulane*, p.72

188 *Tulane*, 67-68

189 *Tulane*, p.73

190 *Tulane*, p. 74

Initially Tulane president Rufus Harris tried to regain the space needed for intellectual freedom. In a speech delivered twice, in April and June 1949, he made his case very clear by stating that higher education "cannot make progress if it must encounter the witch hunts, and explain and apologize for every wild and malicious rumor. It has no chance if it must first and constantly overcome the clutches of those who fear that every teacher who has a view different from his own is a chat or a crackpot if not indeed a Communist. It cannot succeed if we employ in America the totalitarian concept that disagreement is unlawful..(…) Investigation of all ideas new and old must be permitted. Mistakes in judgment must be tolerated. That is not inconsistent with American tradition, is it, as long as the motive is honest and the purpose objective? (…) We must decide realistically whether we will really tolerate the search for the truth," he concluded, or otherwise "the only course left is to blow out the light and fight it out in the dark."[191] However, it was already too late; the space for liberal thinking within the academic community had become extremely limited. The House Un-American Activities Committee had already sent out a letter to eighty-one educational institutions, including Tulane, demanding a list of all the textbooks used in courses in, for instance, literature, economics, political science and history.

Harris's statements about academic freedom were all the more remarkable, considering the fact that only several months before Tulane had been rocked by yet another scandal. The cause was a party organized by a first semester graduate student at the School of Social Work, attended by approximately sixty-five persons. The meeting was racially mixed, thirty-six whites and twenty-nine blacks attended the meeting that was either sponsored by or organized in support of the Young Progressives interracial party. When the meeting did not end after a warning by the police, all those present were arrested. An inter-racial meeting was at that time "not done" in this part of the United States, and what was worse was the fact that it was organized by or in support of an organization that would soon wind up on the list of subversive organizations. The gathering resulted in an uproar, and ended all attempts by Harris to maintain some level of academic freedom. In response to outcries that Tulane had become Communist, Harris had no choice but to make exactly the statement he had so much tried to avoid. In a "Letter from the President" he wrote: "Tulane does not and will not tolerate Communism. We appoint no Communists to the faculty. The greatest precautions are observed. There is no place for a Communist here. We do not believe there are any… The acclaimed or proven Communistic affiliation of no one will be tolerated."[192]

191 *Tulane*, p. 77
192 *Tulane*, p. 81

However, there were Communists at Tulane. The Communist Party in New Orleans had, at that time, a following of between two and three hundred persons, of which probably one third were actual members. Most members were among workers at the waterfront, but it also had a "professional branch" that included students and physicians of medical faculties.[193] One of them was Melvin Sabshin. In an interview in April 2009, he gives the first hint that he was, in fact, a Party member. In his typical inquisitive way, he asks me what I think about it. I tell him that you can be a technical member, or a member in heart and soul. "In my case you can say I was both," he says, with a big smile on his face. For the first time after sixty years, he fully and unequivocally discloses his political affiliation in the late 1940s and early 1950s.

First FBI surveillance

Melvin Sabshin's involvement in the Communist Party of Louisiana and related organizations certainly did not go unnoticed by the FBI. To the contrary, his activity resulted in an avalanche of reports, either by "confidential informants" or by agents of the Federal Bureau of Investigation (FBI). The total file on Melvin Sabshin covers almost 400 pages covering the period from 1951, when the first investigation was initiated, to 1974, when Sabshin was appointed as Medical Director of the American Psychiatric Association in Washington D.C.

On September 15, 1951, the FBI Office in New Orleans requested permission of the Director of the FBI to carry out an investigation into Melvin Sabshin about whom, according to the request, it was determined that "Sabshin was known as subversive on the Tulane campus and that he always followed the Communist party line."[194] Several weeks later the FBI in New Orleans received authorization to "conduct an investigation regarding Melvin Sabshin, who is at the present time an assistant in the psychiatric Department of Tulane University."[195]

According to the investigation report, Melvin Sabshin was by then heavily involved in politics. He was allegedly a member of the Civil Rights Congress of Louisiana, which had been designated by the Attorney General "as within the purview of Executive Order 9835 (in other words, to be a

193 *Tulane*, p. 79

194 New Orleans file 100-14602, regarding Melvin Sabshin, Security matter C, addressed to the Director FBI, and dated September 15, 1951.

195 Authorization to SAC New Orleans, dated October 8, 1951

"subversive organization" which seeks "to alter the form of government of the United States by unconstitutional means").[196] Also, he appeared on the list of individuals who declared that they were qualified voters of the City of New Orleans … who wished to organize a new political party to be recognized as such under the laws of the State of Louisiana under the name 'Progressive Party.' According to another source, both Melvin Sabshin and his wife were active in the affairs of this party[197] which was founded in 1948, had been "characterized as a Communist Party front" and had "Communist Party members who played an important part in its organization. Although the Progressive Party was infiltrated by Communist Party members, it was not dominated and controlled by them."[198]

The Communist Party of Louisiana, to which Melvin Sabshin was associated (and of which he says he was a member), had decided on November 25, 1951, to divide itself into "separate Negro and white groups," which was apparently not to the liking of Sabshin, because the latter "announced … that they were not going to attend any further meetings until this dispute was 'cleared up.' They did not specify the identities of the organizations whose meetings they would not attend,"[199] but for the FBI it was clear that this concerned the Communist Party. The "they" in this case must have been Melvin Sabshin, along with Bill Sorum and James Rogers, who repeatedly are mentioned the FBI file as being close friends of Sabshin's with a strong influence over him; although their names are crossed out from the text, it is clear that the documents refer to the two of them.

The interracial issue very much concerned Melvin Sabshin, as we know from his resistance against the separation of the blood bank in Charity Hospital, and according to a 1953 report by the FBI Sabshin organized "an interracial social gathering" at his home in 1948 or 1949, apparently shortly after his marriage to Bettye Smith.[200] "Confidential informant T-22" reported that Sabshin had a lot of literature available that the informant considered to be of a Communist nature. "He recalled one piece of literature [that was] a pamphlet on intermarriage of a question and answer nature. He could not recall the details but the general tenor was that Russia favored

196 According to the document, it was established that Sabshin was registered as a member on June 30, 1950.

197 Information provided by "Confidential Informant" No. T-5 and T-4; FBI investigation report file 100-14602, pp. 5-6

198 FBI Investigation report file 100-14602, p. 6

199 FBI Investigation report file 100-14602, p. 7

200 FBI Investigation report of June 30, 1953, in file 100-14602, p. 11

intermarriage."[201] How detailed the FBI reports on Sabshin were, and how much they tried to find incriminating evidence against him can be seen from the following information provided by the same informer: "He said that Sabshin had a collection of Russian records in his apartment consisting of an album by Paul Robeson singing Russian music of the Communist era and other records of Russian music of the Communist era rather than the Russian masters. (…) In a discussion over the loss of an American plane over Russia, Sabshin stated that the United States papers only gave one side of the story and Sabshin expressed a definite uncertainty as to which nation he would fight for."[202] Also another informant added that Melvin Sabshin had indicated that "he was not certain which side he would fight on. He said he might fight on the Russian side."[203] The latter remark was of course exactly the type of information the FBI was looking for.

The FBI documents lists many allegations provided by "confidential informants" with regard to Sabshin's Communist inclinations, such as the fact that he was a close friend of [name deleted] who "always had Communist literature and apparently continuously agreed with Communist party doctrines and current policies in his statements."[204] Another "confidential informant" reported that Sabshin "followed the Communist Party line" and that "all three… were believed to be card holders in the Communist Party,' although the witness could not 'prove it'."[205] A bit further the report indicated that "Melvin Sabshin 'traveled around' with [two names deleted][206] and 'were known on the campus as subversive.' It could not be said that Sabshin was actually a Communist Party member, but with [two names deleted] 'he advocated the Communist line.'[207] Investigation also disclosed that Sabshin was a subscriber to the newspaper *Daily Worker*, an East Coast publication linked to the Communist Party.[208] Most of the informants were neutral with regard to Sabshin's positioning, or at least their opinions didn't show in the reporting; one, however, is quite clear: he referred to Sabshin as one of the "traitors for Russia."[209] Another

201 FBI Investigation report of June 30, 1953, in file 100-14602, p. 13

202 FBI Investigation report of June 30, 1953, in file 100-14602, p. 13

203 FBI Investigation report of June 30, 1953, in file 100-14602, p. 14

204 FBI Investigation report file 100-14602, p. 8

205 FBI Investigation report file 100-14602, p. 8. It is clear that the deleted names are those of Sorum and Rogers.

206 Most probably Bill Sorum and James Rogers

207 FBI Investigation report file 100-14602, p. 8. It is clear that also in this case the deleted names are those of Sorum and Rogers.

208 Report by FBI New Orleans, dated July 31, 1952.

209 FBI Investigation report of June 30, 1953, in file 100-14602, p. 14

informer, who knew Sabshin from 1944 onwards, discontinued his "close friendship with the subject because Sabshin would 'follow the Communist party line'."[210]

The 1951 investigation focused not only on Melvin Sabshin himself. Also his parents were screened, and according to the report their names 'appeared in the official files of the Progressive Party, Miami, Florida. It could not be stated whether or not they were members of the Progressive Party or whether their names were merely on the Progressive Party mailing list in Miami."[211] The name of Sabshin's mother, Sonia Sabshin, "appeared on a card which appeared to be a list of members of the Miami Council of the American-Soviet Friendship, Inc. Mrs. Sabshin's card bore the number 7812, the date August 1, 1945..."[212] The investigation involved their neighbors, and, of course, credit and arrest information.

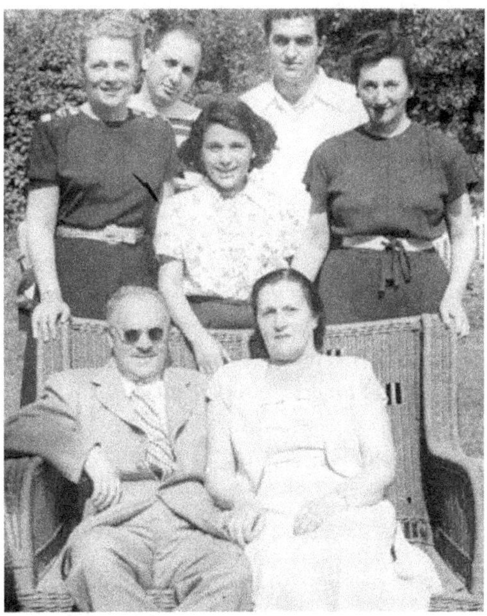

The Sabshin family 1940s

From then on, Sabshin was subject to intense surveillance and all his activities were scrutinized. In 1952, the FBI reports that on April 19, 1952, "Melvin Sabshin... attended a meeting... in New Orleans. The meeting was also attended by numerous members of the Communist Party. The purpose of the meeting was to view a movie concerning the Peace Conference held in Warsaw, Poland. The movie was made in 1950."[213] Apparently, also a representative of the 'National Committee for Justice in the Rosenberg Case' spoke at the meeting. A year later, a New Orleans FBI surveillance report of June 30, 1953, indicates that Sabshin had been "identified as a Communist Party member by

210 FBI Investigation report of June 30, 1953, in file 100-14602, p. 15
211 FBI Investigation report file 100-14602, pp. 10-11
212 FBI Investigation report file 100-14602, p. 11
213 FBI Investigation report of March 4, 1952, in file 100-14602, p. 2

3 former Communist party members. Subject [is/was] also a member [of the] New Orleans Youth Council, Labor Youth League and Students for Wallace. Attended gatherings sponsored by [the] National Committee to Secure Justice in the Rosenberg Case. Subscribed to *The Worker.*"[214]

The same year, in August 1953, Melvin Sabshin is discharged from the U.S. Air Force as a reserve. He had been called up as a reserve in connection with the Korean War and was assigned to the Robins Air Force Base in Georgia while continuing to live in New Orleans.[215] A lengthy document on First Lieutenant Melvin Sabshin from the Headquarters of the U.S. Air Force indicates that on September 1, 1953 a hearing was held to discuss whether there was "reasonable doubt" that Sabshin's continued membership of the U.S. Air Force could be viewed as a "good security risk." The documents lists all the reasons for the hearing, summarizing the information in the FBI file on his membership in Communist or Communist-affiliated organizations, wrong contacts and hostile beliefs.[216] According to a second document, a Board of Officers was convened at Robins Air Force Base later that year.[217] A 1971 FBI file indicates that Melvin Sabshin did not wait for the conclusion of these investigations and was honorably discharged from the Air Force on March 11, 1954, after his own resignation.[218] As he later sadly remarked: "because of my past political activities, the commission was taken away from me."[219]

Still, the extensive 1953 surveillance report makes clear that Melvin Sabshin was not a very vocal member. According to "confidential informant T-4" ("a self-confessed former member of the Communist Party"), Sabshin "seemed to stay in the background," but did "take part in the discussion."[220] "Confidential informant T-7" reported that Sabshin "was active in recruiting new members into the Communist Party,"[221] and according to "confidential informant T-16," Sabshin, Sorum and Rogers "attempted to interest students… in Communism and had gotten at least one to attend

214 Report by the New Orleans FBI, dated June 30, 1953.

215 As shown in a letter from Robins Air Force Base of October 31, 1953, announcing the formation of a Board of Officers to determine whether Sabshin formed a "security risk".

216 Document 21-40348-50 of the Department of the U.S. Air Force, dated August 8, 1953.

217 Letter from Robins Air Force Base of October 31, 1953

218 FBI report no. SL 140-NPRC-C, Bureau file 121-40346, August 30, 1971, p. 2

219 E-mail from Melvin Sabshin, February 12, 2010

220 FBI Investigation report of June 30, 1953, in file 100-14602, p. 4

221 FBI Investigation report of June 30, 1953, in file 100-14602, p. 5

open meetings of some sort with them. (...) ...They were 'almost open' in their beliefs and ... on numerous occasions they had tried to convince students in favor of 'the Marxist doctrine'."[222]

However, also "confidential informant T-8" found Sabshin not to be particularly active and "two other Communist Party members of the Youth Group... were constantly being sent to see Sabshin in order to interest and activate him in the Youth Group..." The informant stated that the Youth Group... consisted of about twenty members who were directly under the influence and direction of [name deleted] of the Communist Party in Louisiana. The informant recalled that during the middle of 1949, there was some question as to whether Sabshin could be signed up again as a Communist Party member for the following year."[223] Another "confidential informant" added that "Sabshin seldom spoke and that it was difficult to have any clear idea as to how he felt on any issue other than his professional work."[224]

The 400-page file painfully shows how extensively and detailed the FBI scrutinized Melvin Sabshin's life. Former friends, colleagues, neighbors of Melvin Sabshin himself as well as of his parents were questioned. Apart from collecting "political information," a full "neighborhood watch" was carried out, whereby neighbors and landlords were questioned as to whether they had noticed anything suspicious. The files bear a stunning resemblance to the Stasi files that I researched for this book, the main difference being the absence of denunciations regarding alcoholism, adultery and possible homosexual tendencies. However, this is replaced by rather vague remarks regarding political views, or allegations of interracial contacts. For instance, one informant mentioned that it seemed strange to her that the Sabshin residence had "a succession of colored maids who had lived with the Sabshins permanently in the home and had shared a bedroom with the Sabshin's child."[225] Some informants clearly felt uneasy, not wanting to have their identities disclosed to the object of investigation ("I would prefer to appear only before a loyalty hearing board and not in the presence of Sabshin")[226] or refused to sign any statement ("Both of

222 FBI Investigation report of June 30, 1953, in file 100-14602, p. 11

223 FBI Investigation report of June 30, 1953, in file 100-14602, p. 5. According to T-7 Sabshin "held some office in the New Orleans Youth Council, such as Secretary or Treasurer." FBI Investigation report of June 30, 1953, in file 100-14602, p. 6

224 FBI Investigation report of June 30, 1953, in file 100-14602, p. 10

225 A 29-page FBI Investigation Report on Melvin Sabshin, October 17, 1952, p. 4

226 Statement by a witness, October 25, 1952

these informants declined to furnish a signed statement, and they will not appear before a Loyalty Hearing Board").[227] Yet some revealed themselves to be zealous contributors to the investigation; for instance, one added that he "cannot recommend him for a position within the United States Government because he believes that the appointee was during this period a member of the Communist Party."[228]

The case of Robert Hodes

One of the factors that not only strongly influenced Melvin Sabshin's career but also his political positioning was the case of Dr. Robert Hodes. Hodes was a well-known neuro-physiologist, a native of New Jersey and a Harvard graduate,[229] who had come to the faculty of psychiatry of Tulane in February 1949, just at the moment when Tulane president Rufus Harris had issued his statement that there were no Communists at Tulane and that none would be tolerated. Hodes was a pioneer in the field of clinical nerve conduction studies and had been recruited to come to Tulane to participate in an investigation into the biological basis of schizophrenia. He and his wife Jane were actively involved in the Communist Party, although Hodes didn't advertise this. He was said to be a leader of the Communist Party in New Orleans, although the source was the head of the pediatrics department who also was a member of the medical school's executive faculty, and might have said this just to damage Hodes.[230] Dr. Robert Heath, chairman of the psychiatry and neurology department, described Hodes as "extremely to the left in his political views." He also alleged that one of the followers of Hodes was secretary of the Communist Party for Louisiana and had been sent to medical school by the American Communist Party to become a special agent working among the blacks in Mississippi and Louisiana to build the strength of the party in the southern United States.[231]

Whatever his link to the Communist Party in New Orleans, Hodes' leftist leanings soon became public knowledge. He openly expressed his dislike of the segregationist policies, socialized with blacks and publicly embarrassed the university and his colleagues when he encouraged black scientists to attend the American Physiology Association meeting in New Orleans in 1951 and then challenged Tulane's segregated cafeteria that refused to feed

227 FBI report from New York, November 5, 1952

228 FBI Investigation report, NY 121-15707, no date provided.

229 Brown, Sarah Hart: *Standing against Dragons*, p. 112

230 *Tulane*, p.97

231 *New Orleans' Charity Hospital*, p. 164

the visiting black scholars.[232] He also held gatherings at his home where politics and social philosophy formed the core of the discussions. These discussions also continued during weekly gatherings with medical school associates. Melvin Sabshin was one of the Tulane students who frequented these gatherings.[233]

The positioning of Hodes resulted in a lot of friction, and eventually in a conversation with the Dean, Maxwell Lapham, he was asked to resign. Hodes refused, and was subsequently reappointed for another year, however according to Dean Lapham it was with the understanding that he would use the year to find employment elsewhere. When Hodes subsequently tried to enlist some medical students to support him in his conflict with Lapman and the university, he was told that his tenure would end much earlier, on January 31, 1953. The Tulane President openly accused Hodes of being "arbitrary, stubborn and egotistical to the point of being determined to have his own ideas prevail in everything," but that was not all. Hodes was also accused of having attended or organized a meeting where money had been collected for Communist China, which militarily supported North Korea with which the United States was at that time at war, and which had entered the Korean conflict itself in October 1950. At the said meeting, a presentation had been given by the China Welfare Appeal, a group that had been listed by the Attorney General as being subversive.[234] "In connection with these attitudes it became known that Dr. Hodes was actively sympathetic with the political cause of Red China and the North Koreans – those against whom this country is presently engaged in war. (…) One member of the Department later expressed the belief that Dr. Hodes was instrumental in getting money and aid to North Korea. I reported this information to the Federal Bureau of Investigation. Dr. Hodes' political activities aggravated, if they did not provoke, this dissension in the department."[235] When exactly Harris informed the FBI is not exactly clear, but this seems to have led to the recruitment of some of Hodes' students as informers.[236]

Dr. Hodes responded by demanding a dismissal hearing and solicited Benjamin Smith as his lawyer. Smith, a friend of former Tulane law professor Mitchell Franklin, was well known for his defense of blacks and had been much involved in court cases involving black workers,

---

232 *Standing against Dragons*, p. 110

233 Interview Melvin Sabshin, April 21, 2009

234 *Standing against dragons*, p. 110; The Attorney General's list of subversive organizations was published on the *Federal Register 13* on 20 March 1948

235 *Tulane*, p. 94

236 *Tulane*, p. 97

among others from the New Orleans local representation of the Maritime Union. According to the FBI, he had also attended political gatherings at Hodes' home.[237] Because the university had not cited "incompetence" or "moral turpitude" as reasons for the dismissal, the American Association of University Professors (AAUP) supported Hodes' demand and asked that the board of administrators of Tulane University formally review the matter.[238] A group of medical students, of which Melvin Sabshin was an active member, played a central role in organizing Dr. Hodes' defense.[239] According to the FBI, Sabshin also testified as a witness for Hodes, and "was standing 100 percent behind" him.[240]

The Board of Administrators went along with the demand, and from February through April 1953 the dismissal hearings took place. The hearings themselves were more a melodrama than a sincere attempt to uncover the actual political views of Dr. Hodes and the behavior that had led to the decision to dismiss him. The university avoided the real issue, with the Board of Administrators asserting that Hodes had caused "friction" in the department. Benjamin Smith responded that Hodes was not a "frictionable person" and in his brief he noted that only "insubordinate and incompetent technicians" had accused Hodes. He concluded that the charges were Tulane's "immoral and disreputable attempt" not only to rid itself of a professor "with unpopular political views" but also to discard "its very strength and virtue… academic freedom and scholarship." [241]

Hodes himself equally refused to mention his Communist beliefs and pointed out that he had been scientifically successful at Tulane and that he was being dismissed for political reasons.[242] He claimed that he had been told that the university was afraid their fundraising campaign would be hurt and that a number of wealthy alumni would discontinue their financial support. He added that Dr. Heath had told him to ignore the problems facing Negroes and concentrate on curing schizophrenia. That would help the Negro people more."[243]

Some colleagues, when interviewed by the committee, confirmed that Hodes' dismissal was, in fact, for political reasons. One witness, Dr. Ervin,

---

[237] *Standing against dragons*, p. 108

[238] *Standing against dragons*, p. 109

[239] Interview Melvin Sabshin, April 21, 2009

[240] FBI Investigation report of June 30, 1953, in file 100-14602, p. 12

[241] *Standing against Dragons*, p. 109-110

[242] *Tulane*, p. 95, *Standing against Dragons*, p. 110

[243] *Standing against Dragons*, p. 111

said that it was "my impression that the general conclusion, the only reasonable explanation, for this occurrence was in terms of Dr. Hodes' unpopular political and social views and that there was no other explanation that seems to suffice at the time to explain what happened." Dr. Smith, another witness, was even clearer when stating that he "was going to be dismissed because he was a Communist." A the statement also was made that he was not only a Communist but was a leader of the Communist Party in New Orleans, and that evidence for this was said to have been obtained from two medical students who were FBI agents."[244]

How Robert Hodes tried to avoid exposing his true political beliefs himself can be seen in the following exchange during one of the cross-examinations:

"Answer: this was a gathering in my home in the spring of 1951, sometime. I don't remember the date, at which some money was collected by a man who happened to be in the city, and old friend of mine, who came to our house… to collect some money to purchase books and medical supplies for China.

Question: What China? 'Red' China?

Answer: Quote, China.

Question: Free China. I think you said 'Red' China?

Answer: I was quoting Dr. Heath.

Question: What was it for?

Answer: For collecting money for China.

Question: Was it 'Red' China?

Answer: You can call it 'Red' China. It was not Chiang Kai Shek.

Question: It was the same Chinamen fighting in Korea, wasn't it?

Answer: Right."[245]

In the end, the dismissal of Hodes was upheld. A full transcript of the hearing was made available in the library of the medical faculty, at the request of the Tulane chapter of the American Association of University Professors, chaired by chemistry professor Hans Jonassen.[246] The farewell party organized by Hodes and his wife was attended by Melvin Sabshin.[247]

Hodes left New Orleans and, after a short stopover in Britain and the Soviet Union, he traveled with his family to the People's Republic of China in 1954. The family stayed in Beijing for five years where, according to his wife,

244 Lewis, Lionel S.: *Cold War on Campus*, p. 56

245 *Tulane*, p. 96

246 *Tulane*, p. 100

247 FBI Investigation report of June 30, 1953, in file 100-14602, p. 12

Robert Hodes "laid the basis for modern neurophysiology in Peking."[248] When the Hodes felt they were no longer needed in China, they decided to return to the United States. By then they had become disenchanted with Chinese communism, and they also did not want to raise their children in a foreign country.[249] An additional factor that made them come back was the fact that McCarthyism was already on the wane. By 1959, they were back in New York where Hodes became a professor of physiology at Mount Sinai Hospital, thanks to his brother who was on the staff of there.[250]

In the early 1960s, Robert Hodes actively participated in a campaign to upgrade the opportunities for blacks in his profession, while his son became an activist for civil rights in Mississippi and briefly worked in the legal offices of Benjamin Smith, the same lawyer who had defended his father in 1953. Hodes also actively opposed the war in Vietnam and eventually died in 1966; his scholarly legacy was donated by his family to the medical library at Meharry, one of the top black medical schools in the United States.[251]

The Hodes case clearly showed that Tulane President Harris was able and willing to follow up on his assertion of February 1949 that "there is no place for a Communist" at Tulane. The dismissal had a strong demoralizing effect on the medical school of Tulane and resulted in lowered morale among junior-level medical faculty and student trainees. There was no mass exodus of professors, but for Melvin Sabshin the outcome was reason enough to continue his career elsewhere. He has a strong feeling of betrayal by Hodes, who had left for China unannounced while leaving his dedicated supporters behind. Combined with his divorce from Bettye Smith, the desire to leave and start anew somewhere else became too big to resist. He applied for positions at two places elsewhere in the country, the Western Psychiatric Institute of the University of Pittsburgh and the Psychiatric and Psychosomatic Institute of Michael Reese Hospital in Chicago. In spite of warnings by the FBI about his political beliefs, Melvin Sabshin was accepted as a salaried staff member of the latter institution by its director, Dr. Roy R. Grinker, Sr.[252] His decision to take him on board played a decisive role in Melvin Sabshin's further career.

---

248 Schrecker, Ellen W.: *No Ivory Tower*, p. 295

249 *No Ivory Tower*, p. 295

250 *Standing against Dragons*, p. 112; *New Orleans' Charity Hospital*, p. 164

251 *Standing against Dragons*, p. 112

252 *Sabshin*, p. 28.

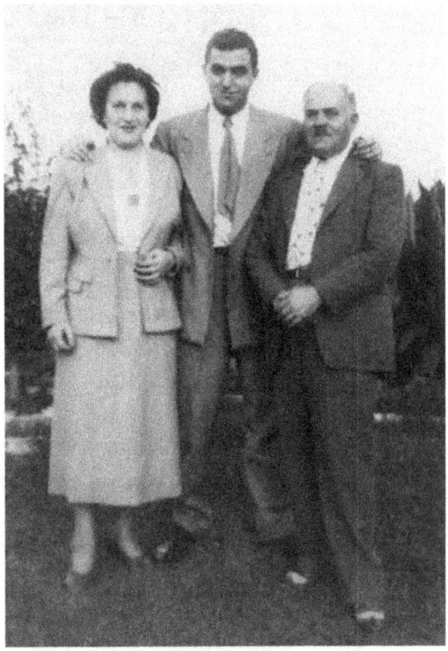

Melvin Sabshin with his parents, Sonia and Zalman Sabshin

When Melvin Sabshin moved to Chicago, the FBI's interest in him did not cease. To the contrary, the FBI followed his trace and on September 18, 1953, the FBI in New Orleans reported to the FBI in Chicago that Sabshin has moved to their city and was lodging in the Hotel Versailles. The transfer file adds that he was regarded as a Communist and a security risk.[253] An investigation report made by the Chicago FBI on February 19, 1954, repeated most of the information provided earlier, yet added one interesting issue: the fact that Melvin Sabshin made a false statement in 1951 when he "executed an affidavit with the U.S. Public Health Service under an arrangement whereby he would receive U.S. Public Heath Service aid on a training grant. (…) This affidavit contains the statement, 'I do hereby certify that I do not advocate nor am I a member of any political party or organization that advocates the overthrow of the Government of the United States by force or violence…'."[254] Sabshin's New Orleans file was closed on March 22, 1954,[255] yet this last issue would certainly play a part in later contacts between Melvin Sabshin and the FBI in 1957-1958, as we will see in a later chapter.

---

253 FBI internal notification from SAC New Orleans to SAC Chicago, September 18, 1953, and memorandum of SAC New Orleans to the Director of the FBI of December 29, 1953, FD-128 (3-4-52).

254 Memorandum of the New Orleans FBI to the FBI Director, December 29, 1953, FD-128 (3-4-52), p. 6

255 Document stating: "since all information in the possession of the New Orleans Office has now been forwarded to Chicago, this case is being placed in a closed status…" Document dated March 22, 1954.

Chapter 8 – The Formation of a Communist

"I had the image, still very ornate, of an ideal, just society with equal opportunities for all, which avoided all the mistakes made in previous times. A heaven on earth, free from oppression, peaceful and humane..."

Jochen Neumann [256]

The war's end and the subsequent arrest and internment of his father had a profound influence on Jochen Neumann and to a large degree determined the course he took in life.

In an essay titled "Socialism and Me," coincidentally written several months before our first contact in 2008,[257] he summarized the effect very vividly: "After the return of my father from the military and his arrest shortly thereafter, followed by his subsequent internment in Bautzen and Mühlberg, family life consolidated itself somewhat. The harshness of the time, the general living conditions and those specific for our family (among others my father's professional ban) did not allow much cheerfulness, but the family was a conflict-free zone, and was on the inside balanced. After the precipitated end of my childhood, my emotional development continued discordantly and jerkily, dependent on external factors. Like many of my contemporaries, I was deprived of a 'youth' in the proverbial sense of the word. We were forced into a three quarters adulthood created by outside factors, one that logically would not yet have been able to develop. The childlike personality was, so to speak, stretched to adult size on the Procrustean bed of contemporary history at the expense of mental dilution. The result was an unfortunate mixture of an insecure, impertinent and premature precociousness with, for that age, an inadequately advanced but factually thoroughly correct knowledge of the general world events around you and social conditions and their backgrounds in one's direct environment. A side effect was an early social consciousness with immature "political" insights, positions and desires. I experienced the oppression and social uprooting of my father unrestrictedly, because it also concerned me indirectly. These experiences catalyzed my critical thinking on the one side and complicated it on the other. The world at home and the world out there, such as in school, were at times objectively and emotionally diametrically opposed."[258]

---

256 *Der Sozialismus und Ich*, p. 5

257 Work on this essay, *Der Sozialismus und Ich*, started in 2005 and finished in November 2008.

258 *Der Sozialismus und Ich*, p. 3

While gradually recovering from his years of imprisonment, father Erhart Neumann tried to understand what had caused the fate that had befallen him, and the events that had led to his painful personal downfall (including the period of internment in Bautzen and Mühlberg, as well as his professional ban). At the same time, he tried to look at the course of history in Europe in a more 'objective' manner and gradually created a new world image for himself. While doing so, he involved Jochen in that process as part of his education; a relationship developed between the two, of both buddy and teacher. Father Neumann blamed his situation on the "Communists," very much in line with the thoughts expressed on the Western radio stations at that time, which the family secretively listened to at night. "With pleasure, even too readily, we would have lived then in the Western occupation zone."[259] In addition, Jochen had his own experiences, which helped him form his own views and convictions independent from his father.

Gradually the influence of Jochen's school became stronger. Some of the teachers with democratic convictions tried to provide their students with an education that enabled them to develop their own political thinking and views. "Some of my classmates were 'young pioneers'[260] and talked about collective meetings of the sort of the *Wandervogel* movement,[261] and about friendly contact among the boys as well as within the group. For me, as an only child with a parental home that I experienced as socially fragile, this sounded appealing and so I also became a member of this youth organization that was just taking shape and which gradually took a mainly political direction."[262]

Joining the communist movement

Initially the pioneers were banned from school, as it was a political organization and schools were supposed to be neutral territory, so they met in a sort of barracks. The main goal was to form a counterweight against

259 *Der Sozialismus und Ich*, p. 4

260 The *Ernst Thälmann Pioneer Organization*, consisting of the Young Pioneers and the Thälmann Pioneers, was an East German youth organization of school-children aged 6 to 14. They were named after Ernst Thälmann, the former leader of the Communist Party of Germany who was murdered in Buchenwald concentration camp

261 W*andervogel* is the name adopted by a popular movement of German youth groups from 1896 onward. The name can be translated as migratory bird and the ethos is to shake off the restrictions of society and get back to nature and freedom.

262 *Der Sozialismus und Ich*, p. 4

the national-socialist ideology with which the children had been brought up during the period prior to 1945. In the case of Neumann, this resulted in a conflict situation at home, as he gradually developed an antifascist (or "early communist") conviction, while at home anti-communist and bourgeois attitudes prevailed. Neumann started to avoid telling the truth and started hiding his views at home, pretending they did not differ from those of his parents. At the same time, he developed a fundamentally socialist or communist worldview. When he joined the *Freie Deutsche Jugend* (FDJ)[263] in 1950, he presented this at home as a necessary step for his future career, although, in fact, his convictions were more or less in line with those of the FDJ (which, as Neumann writes, was then still mostly focusing on anti-fascism).

During his years in secondary school, Jochen deepened his political convictions; yet the basis was "a non-dogmatic and humanistically interpreted socialist attitude whereby the accents lay more on justice, equal opportunities for all, the right to education, healthcare etc. Fundamental questions such as private property, production ratios, and class struggle were a basis for convictions yet without any relevance. They were rather gradually forced upon us from outside, by sometimes overactive zealots such as our school director Streller."[264] Jochen's political development was, in this period of his life, constant and without breaches, with no direct conflicts with his parents, who did not interfere with his political positioning. His father had found a new job outside his original profession as a bench worker at the textile factory, "VEB Textima" in Leisnig, and had accepted the new political order although, as Neumann puts it, this was more an issue of understanding what his allegiance to the NSDAP had caused rather than the development of an anti-capitalist or pro-communist belief. In the second half of 1950, he was allowed to return to his original profession.[265]

---

263 The *Freie Deutsche Jugend* (FDJ), Free German Youth, was the official socialist youth movement of the German Democratic Republic and the Socialist Unity Party of Germany. The organization was meant for young people, both male and female, between the ages of 14 and 25 and comprised about 75% of the young population of former East Germany. The FDJ was intended to be the "reliable assistant and fighting reserve of the Worker's Party," and the political and ideological goal of the FDJ was to influence every aspect of life of young people in the GDR, distribution of Marxism-Leninism and the indoctrination of socialist behavior. It arranged thousands of holidays for young people through its *Jugendtourist* agency, and ran discos and open rock air-concerts

264 *Der Sozialismus und Ich*, p. 5

265 Neumann, Jochen: *Kraut und Rüben*, p. 1-2. His father died in 1974.

The people who greatly influenced Jochen Neumann during this period were the families of Dr. Max Findeisen, a lawyer and notary, and of Johannes Rossberg, a factory owner. Findiesen had traveled extensively before the war and brought home many interesting and unusual objects from the colonies. Rossberg had been a pilot and had flown a wide range of planes, of which parts were decorating his home, such as a lamp made out of a propeller of a plane he had once flown. The end of the war had been perceived by both as a complete disaster and the only son of the Findeisens, Helmut, who had been with the Waffen-SS,[266] shot himself on May 8, 1945, when it was absolutely clear that the war was lost. The family had lost its fortune when the brewery owned by Ms. Findeisen was nationalized by the government. Also the Rossbergs had lost their property and, as a result, had become non-entities in a new society, which they viewed with hate and distrust.

At home, the relationship between Jochen's parents was faltering. Later, in 2002, he writes: "I experienced the growing apart and [subsequent] separation of my parents as a disaster that influenced my life deeply and continuously."[267] With all this disenchantment, unhappiness and despair around him, there was a force that drove him to "the other side" - that side considered by his immediate environment to be hostile and the root of all that went wrong. Jochen's father belonged to the middle layer of the small-town society, where he didn't feel himself very much at home. Jochen felt more attracted to the intelligentsia, which, however, was politically conservative. Yet politically he was more attracted to the lower class, which didn't appeal to him intellectually. This dilemma resulted in a sort of in-between state, belonging neither here nor there.

This situation did not last too long. The marital crisis between his parents and the resulting disintegration of the family and his feeling of being out of place with the upper class of Leisnig radicalized Jochen; in addition, his desire to take a position against his original environment strengthened this process. On the other hand, the social environment was rather small and included only a few dozen families belonging to the upper class; thus, it was almost impossible for Jochen to avoid mingling with them even though internally his distance from them grew unabat-

266 The Waffen-SS was the combat arm of the SS, an organ of the Nazi Party. The Waffen-SS saw action throughout World War II and grew from three regiments to a force of over 38 divisions, which served alongside the regular army, but was never formally part of the Wehrmacht. They were involved in many wartime atrocities.

267 Letter by Jochen Neumann, November 21, 2002

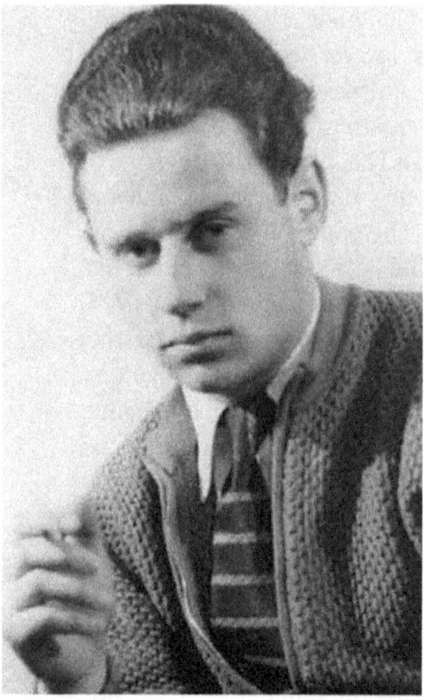

Jochen Neumann as student, 1956

edly. A new group in his school started to form consisting of boys interested in culture and intellectual development but at the same time with a clear leftist orientation. "I managed to keep a balance within myself of my protest against the micro-bourgeoisie in Leisnig, to which I felt culturally attracted and even subjected, and my honest leftist political views including the desire to belong to a social group as a replacement of the family."[268]

In 1954, Jochen applied for membership of the "Party of the Working Class," the Socialist Union Party (SED), and in March or April of that year, he was accepted as a candidate member. He didn't even inform his parents, and as he soon after he reached the age of 18 and became an adult, there was no need to do so anyway. "From now on, the formation of my ideological opinions and views were dominated by the Party."[269] The Party environment had a profound influence on Neumann, since among the membership were many people who had fought in Spain during the civil war, who had been in the underground during the Nazi regime or who had survived the concentration camps. Their examples were important sources of inspiration for Neumann.

University

Having grown up in a rural environment, throughout his younger years Jochen had gradually developed an interest in botany and biology. His father made a press so he could dry leaves and flowers, and, as a next step, a herbarium was developed. Gradually his interest developed more towards zoology and anthropology, and the young Neumann even managed to trigger a reaction from the director of the Leipzig Zoo. This director sent him some literature and even offprints and, for a while, corresponded with the young boy, whose hunger for information

---

268 *Der Sozialismus und Ich*, p. 6

269 *Der Sozialismus und Ich*, p. 7

was hard to quench. In secondary school, Neumann chose the natural science package and gradually started to cherish the ideal of becoming a veterinarian. However, art and culture also were high on his list of interests and some teachers had considerable influence on his desire to learn more and explore the fields of art, architecture and art history. Life was difficult, living conditions quite bad and the effects of war visible and noticeable in every area of daily life. Good books were hard to get, and Jochen managed to collect information of interest only by writing to places like the Vatican Museum.

After considering various possibilities, Jochen eventually decided to go for an education as a veterinarian and applied for studies at the University of Leipzig. However, his political convictions and determination clashed for the first time when a representative of the *Kasernierter Volkspolizei* (KVP)[270] visited the school in order to recruit new officers. Neumann, who recently joined the Party, was put under pressure and advised to take his responsibility as a Party member and join the KVP. He was told that as an officer, he could always do his studies on the side: "In our ranks, we need a lot of diligent comrades in all professions, and, of course, also animal doctors."[271]

His career in the military was a disastrous one, not because he was unfit to be a military man but, rather, because he always felt pushed in a different direction. Even though they told him that the KVP would be in need of veterinarians, he was sent to be trained for the East German Navy in August 1954. His training began with, among others tasks, cleaning toilets that were indescribably filthy. Jochen's discomfort turned into anger and a refusal to be pushed around, and eventually "the borders of my willingness to adapt and my ability to accept suffering had been crossed and I had enough of it. Angrily I told them that I wanted to be discharged and that I was no longer willing to have military training. As the angry and flabbergasted gentlemen did not want to have a scandal on their hands, I received a certificate of discharge and a train ticket to Leisnig…"[272]

Eventually, it was the army command in Jochen's home region that helped him enter the university. "After a week, [the commander] told me resignedly that it was out of the question that I could still be placed at the studies

270 Kasernierte Volkspolizei (KVP, German for Garrisoned People's Police) were the military units of the Volkspolizei (police). These units became basis of the National People's Army established in 1956.

271 *Der Sozialismus und Ich*, p. 7

272 *Kraut und Rüben*, p. 5

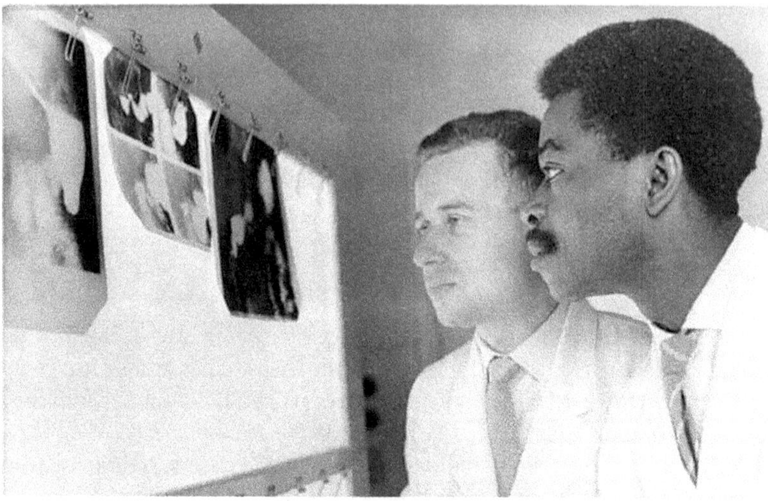

Jochen Neumann as assistant in II. Medical Clinic of Charité, 1960

of veterinary medicine. (…) If I agreed, I could report already the next morning to the *Ritterstrasse* in Leipzig and start my studies of medicine. I did that without hesitation. During the third week of September, I was registered and became a student."[273]

273 *Kraut und Rüben*, p. 5

Part II

The Curtain Opens

Chapter 9 – Origins of Soviet Political Psychiatry

"Sakharov is objectively a mentally ill person. The complication with regards to operational consequences lies in the fact that for political reasons he cannot be committed to a psychiatric hospital."
Lieutenant General F.D. Bobkov, KGB, 1976[1]

The other day I was watching a film starring Angelina Jolie and John Malkovich, *Changeling*, a film set in the mid-1930s in California. In the film, a mother whose young son has gone missing and who is desperately trying to find him, refuses to accept a boy s brought to her by the Los Angeles Police Department (LAPD) and presented as her son. She knows the boy is not her own, but the LAPD insists that he is, because they need to show a disgruntled public that they are able to resolve cases. When the mother persists and maintains it is not her son, the police become angry, and eventually she is locked up in the psychiatric department of a Los Angeles hospital. She can leave, but only after she signs a statement that she was wrong and acknowledges that the LAPD did whatever they could and were right in having her hospitalized for her own safety. It eventually takes a public campaign to have her discharged and to reveal the abuse by the LAPD.

I was watching and, without realizing beforehand, the film made me move back to the issue that has dominated my life for more than thirty years. I was watching clear-cut political abuse of psychiatry, maybe not as a governmental policy, but clearly as a policy instituted by lower-level authorities showing how easily psychiatry can be used to get rid of bothersome persons. This

1 BstU, HAXX 2941, pp. 97. Fillip Denisovich Bobkov was Head of the Fifth Directorate of the KGB since 1967 and retired from the service before the demise of the USSR in 1991, being deputy chairman of the KGB and in rank a general of the service. After this he became advisor to Vladimir Gusinsky, owner of the Most Corporation and one of the most influential persons in Russian politics in the early 1990s. Bobkov brought many former KGB officers to his "security service" at the Most corporation, including his former deputy Ivan Abramov, who succeeded him as head of the Fifth Directorate of the KGB after Bobkov had succeeded Vladimir Chebrikov as deputy chairman of the KGB in 1985 (who, in turn, succeeded Yuri Andropov as KGB Chairman, as Andropov became the new General Secretary of the CPSU). For more on Bobkov and his political machinations see *The Age of Assassins* by Yuri Felshtinsky and Vladimir Pribylovsky, a.o. pp. 15-8

is how it all starts; in a climate of totalitarianism with a single ideology to which all must adhere and nobody can challenge. In such settings, the barrier to using psychiatry as a means of repression is a thin one, very thin. That is probably one of the factors that explain how the practice developed in the Soviet Union as well. What started as an expedient way of getting rid of bothersome people gradually turned into a government policy of locking up political opponents in psychiatric hospitals.

The political abuse of psychiatry in the Soviet Union clearly originated from the concept that persons who opposed the Soviet regime were mentally ill, as there seemed to be no other logical explanation why one would oppose the best socio-political system in the world. The famous Soviet dissident Vladimir Bukovsky, himself a victim of the political abuse of psychiatry, wrote in his memoirs: "Khrushchev figured that it was impossible for people in a socialist society to have antisocialist consciousness ... Wherever manifestations of dissidence couldn't be explained away as a legacy of the past or a provocation of world imperialism, they were simply the product of mental illness."[2]

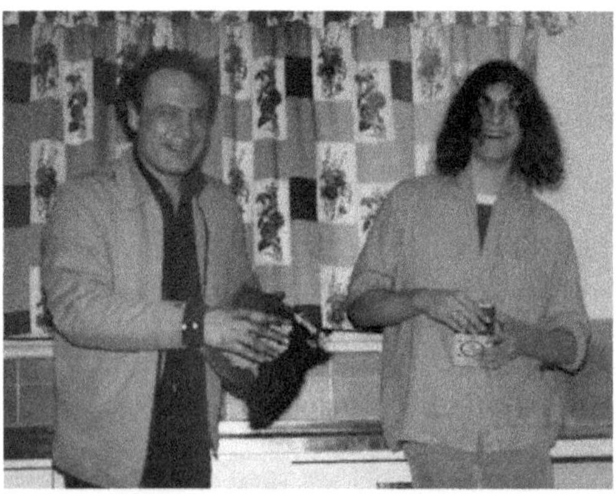

Vladimir Bukovsky and Robert van Voren, 1979

Soviet leader Nikita Khrushchev himself worded this in a speech: "A crime is a deviation from the generally recognized standards of behavior frequently caused by mental disorder. Can there be diseases, nervous disorders among certain people in Communist society? Evidently yes. If that is so, then there will also be offences that are characteristic for people with abnormal minds ... To those who might start calling for opposition to Communism on this basis, we can say that ... clearly the mental state of such people is not normal." [3]

The diagnosis "sluggish schizophrenia," developed by the Moscow School of Psychiatry and, in particular, by its scientific leader Academician Andrei Snezhnevsky[4] provided a very handy framework to explain this

[2] *To Build a Castle*, p. *156*

[3] *Pravda*, May 24, 1959.

[4] Andrei Vladimirovich Snezhnevsky, born in 1904 in Kostroma, graduated

behavior. According to the theories of Snezhnevsky and his colleagues, schizophrenia was much more prevalent than previously thought because the illness present with relatively mild symptoms and progress to more serious symptoms later. As a result, schizophrenia was diagnosed much more frequently in the Soviet Union than in other countries in the *World Health Organization Pilot Study on Schizophrenia* reported in 1973.[5] In particular, sluggish (slowly progressive)[6] schizophrenia broadened the scope because, according to Snezhnevsky, patients with this diagnosis were able to function almost normally in the social sense. Their symptoms could resemble those of a neurosis or could take on a paranoid quality. The patient with paranoid symptoms retained some insight in his condition, but overvalued his own importance and might exhibit grandiose ideas of reforming society. Thus symptoms of sluggish schizophrenia could be "reform delusions," "struggle for the truth," and "perseverance."[7]

In an interview with the Soviet newspaper *Komsomolskaya Pravda,* two Soviet psychiatrists, Marat Vartanyan and Andrei Mukhin, explained in 1987 how it was possible that a person could be mentally ill while those around him did not notice it, as could happen in case of "sluggish schizophrenia." What did mentally ill then mean? Vartanyan: "… When a person is obsessively occupied with something. If you discuss another subject with him, he is a normal person who is healthy, and who may be

---

from the Medical faculty in Kazan in 1925 and started working in the psychiatric hospital in his hometown. In1932-1838 he was chief doctor of this hospital and became active in the field of research. In 1938-1941 he was senior scientific associate and deputy director of the Moscow Gannushkin Psychiatric Research Institute and in 1947 he defended his dissertation on psychiatry for the elderly under the title *Senile Psychoses*. During the war he was first linked to a battalion and then became chief psychiatrist of the First Army. In 1945-1950 he worked as a lecturer at the psychiatric faculty of the Central Institute for Continued Training of Physicians and for almost two years (1950-1951) was Director of the Serbski Institute. Until 1961 he was head of the psychiatric faculty of the Central Institute for Continued Training of Physicians. In 1962 he became head of the Institute for Psychiatry of the Academy of Medical Sciences of the USSR a position he held until his death on July 17, 1987. In addition, from 1951 onwards he was chief editor of the Korsakov Journal of Neuropathology and Psychiatry. In 1957 he became a candidate Member of the Academy of Medical Sciences, in 1962 a full member.

5 *The International Pilot Study on Schizophrenia*. World Health Organization, 1973.

6 In Russian: "vyalotekushchaya shizofreniya"

7 See Bloch, S., *Soviet Psychiatry and Snezhnevskyism*, in Van Voren, R. (ed.), *Soviet Psychiatric Abuse in the Gorbachev Era*, pp. 55-61.

your superior in intelligence, knowledge and eloquence. But as soon as you mention his favorite subject, his pathological obsessions flare up wildly." Vartanyan confirmed that hundreds of persons with this diagnosis were hospitalized in the Soviet Union. According to Dr. Mukhin, this was because "they disseminate their pathological reformist ideas among the masses."[8] A few months later the same newspaper listed a number of symptoms "a la Snezhnevsky," including "an exceptional interest in philosophical systems, religion and art." The paper quoted from a 1985 *Manual on Psychiatry* of Snezhnevsky's Moscow School and subsequently concluded: "In this way any – normally considered sane – person can be diagnosed as a 'sluggish schizophrenic'."[9]

There are several people who analyzed the concepts of sluggish schizophrenia in the USSR, and the scientific writings focused on this diagnosis. One of the first to tackle the issue was the Canadian psychiatrist, Harold Merskey who, as early as 1986 analyzed a number of scientific articles published in the *Korsakov Journal of Neuropathology and Psychiatry*, together with neurology resident Bronislava Shafran from New York.[10] They took two sample

8 *Komsomolskaya Pravda*, July 15, 1987

9 *Komsomolskaya Pravda*, November 18, 1987

10 Harold Merksey, who initially worked in Britain but later emigrated to Canada, is mentioned in a 1975 document in the *Mitrokhin Archive* as one of the most active opponents of the political abuse of psychiatry in the USSR. The document mentions also that an anonymous letter should be prepared by the KGB in Moscow and mailed to him via the Soviet Embassy in London. In the letter a person should warn this "'honest patriot' of England" that he is in danger and that a physical attack on him is being prepared. See: Mitrokhin Archive, Woodrow Wilson International Center for Scholars, Cold War International History Project, folder 28, *Practicing Psychiatry for Political Purposes*, document 5. The plan to send Merskey an anonymous threat was indeed enacted. As Merskey himself writes: "I did receive an anonymous letter which I took to be from an anti-Semitic crank. It came in the first part of 1976 on lined paper in a cheap brown envelope to my home address and the postmark was from S.E. London. The letter was nasty but did not seem very dangerous but I took the precaution of telling my wife Susan and then secretary Marge Zietsman to be careful on opening letters. Our children at that time were between 4 and 10 years old. At the time I had no idea it was from the KGB and simply thought it was from an un-educated hostile person." (e-mail from Harold Merskey, April 10, 2010). One explanation why Merskey was particularly targeted might be the fact that he was also active in other ways. "Besides my psychiatric stance I was also working for Jews to emigrate to Israel. It started in 1972 when I was one of four Jewish doctors who responded to a call to try and help get Jewish doctors out of the USSR in accordance with their desire to leave for Israel. I was late to the founding meeting of the Medical and Scientific Committee for

years, 1978 and 1983, and found a total of 37 and 27 articles respectively focusing on schizophrenia. In their article, they concluded that "the notion of slowly progressive schizophrenia is clearly widely extensible and is much more variable and inclusive than our own ideas of simple schizophrenia or residual defect states. Many conditions which would probably be diagnosed elsewhere as depressive disorders, anxiety disorders, hypochondriacal or personality disorders seem liable to come under the umbrella of slowly progressive schizophrenia in Snezhnevsky's system."[11] In addition, they also questioned the quality of psychiatric research in the Soviet Union, at least as far as the articles they analyzed are concerned. "If the articles we are considering had been submitted in English to a Western journal, most of them would probably have been returned for radical revision. As noted above, the original writing is diffuse and cumbersome: we have attempted to make some of it more readable in translation. At times the writing is also disturbingly incomprehensible, even to readers who grew up speaking Russian and received a Russian medical education. Furthermore, the articles are often not arranged in a conventional pattern."[12]

Two years later, Semyon Gluzman carried out even more extensive research, while sitting in the Lenin Library in Moscow and going through the publications step-by-step including, in particular, dissertations and other scientific studies by staff members of the Serbski Institute. His results were not less shocking. In his analysis, he quotes a large number of works by well-known associates of the Serbski Institute like Margaretha Taltse,[13] Yakov Landau,[14] and Tamara Pechernikova.[15] In some of these studies, the

---

Soviet Jewry and in my absence the other three left the "plum" for me to be chairman." (E-mail from Harold Merskey, April 11, 2010).

11 Merskey, H, and Shafran, B.: *Political hazards in diagnosis of 'sluggish schizophrenia,* p. 249. Published in the British Journal of Psychiatry, 1986, 148, pp.: 247-256

12 *Political hazards in diagnosis of 'sluggish schizophrenia*, p. 251

13 Margarita Feliksovna Taltse, head of the Fourth (Political) Department of the Serbski Institute after Daniil Lunts (died 1977), involved in quite a few cases, including Yuri Shikhanovich, Ivan Yakhimovich, Vyacheslav Igrunov, Iosip Terelya

14 Yakov Lazerevich Landau, associate of the Serbski Institute, involved in the cases of, a.o., Pyotr Egides and Gederts Melngaitis. In 2001 Dr. Landau said on Polish television that "the organs [KGB] burdened us with very responsible work (…) They expected us to do what they asked us to do, and we knew what they expected." See Van Voren, R., *Comparing Soviet and Chinese Political Psychiatry*, in: Journal of the American Academy of Psychiatry and Law, 30: 131-5, 2002

15 Tamara Pechernikova, associate of the Serbski Institute, involved in cases such as Natalya Gorbanevskaya, Vyacheslav Igrunov and Ivan Yakhimovich

political "illness" was far from being camouflaged, such as patients who were considered to be ill because of "excessive religiosity."[16] Another study concludes that "compulsory treatment in an ordinary psychiatric hospital may be recommended for patients with schizophrenia with delusional ideas of reform, who show a diminished level of activity and in whom we can observe a difference between their statements and behavior." However, others showed an "extreme social dangerousness and [this formed] the foundation of the recommendation for compulsory treatment in a Special Psychiatric Hospital"[17] A 1982 study by Serbski psychiatrists Landau and Tabakova[18] was chillingly direct: "Previously conducted study of patients [by Landau and Tabakova] with delusions of reform showed that the content of such delusional ideas extends beyond the realm of their interpretational relations, it always involved various aspects of the life of society as a whole... These patients wrote numerous appeals and complaints to various organizations... The clinical aspects of the patients' pathological state as described above, coupled with their sense of psychological ('offensive') urgency, and, with their outwardly intact and orderly behavior ... determined the greatest degree of their social dangerousness and made it necessary to refer them to special psychiatric hospitals..."[19]

Andrei Snezhnevsky

Andrei Snezhnevsky, who dominated Soviet psychiatry for almost forty years, can best be described as a very controversial figure who, on one hand, was heavily implicated in the political abuse of psychiatry and very close to the Soviet leadership, yet at the same time was often described as a modest man, a good clinician and certainly not a standard apparatchik. His office was decorated with a large portrait of Ernest Hemmingway, not a regular feature in a Soviet nomenklatura office. Yuri Novikov, a department head of the Serbski Institute who defected to the West in 1977 and knew Snezhnevsky personally, describes him as cold, distant, yes also ascetic, serious, and often shy. He also recalls that Snezhnevsky sometimes stuck out his neck for others. In the late 1930s, Snezhnevsky was deputy director of the Moscow Gannushkin Psychiatric Research Institute and, thus, unable to avoid the arrest and deportation of a well-known colleague, Erich Sternberg, a German communist of Jewish origin who had fled from the

16 *On Soviet Totalitarian Psychiatry*, p.42

17 *On Soviet Totalitarian Psychiatry*, p. 43

18 Anna Iosifovna Tabakova, associate of the Serbski Institute, involved in the cases of, a.o., Yuri Shikhanovich and Ivan Yakhimovich

19 *On Soviet Totalitarian Psychiatry*, p.44

Nazis to the USSR in 1933. However, immediately following the death of Stalin, Snezhnevsky brought him back to Moscow and gave him a position at his Center. Considering the prevailing anti-Semitism in the Soviet Union, this was far from regular behavior.[20]

The role of Andrei Snezhnevsky in the political abuse of psychiatry has been subject to much debate. Some consider him as one of the main architects of the political abuse, a cynical scientist who served the authorities and willingly developed a concept that could be used to declare political opponents of the regime to be mentally ill. Others have defended Snezhnevsky and have pointed out that he was not the only person who believed in the concept of "sluggish schizophrenia" and that his ideas were abused by a regime without his active involvement. However, it is known that Snezhnevsky himself participated in some of the examinations of dissidents, and thus a complete whitewashing of his role is thereby impossible. How did he become such an important figure and a dominant force in Soviet psychiatry for so many years?

In the mid-1990s, two psychiatrists working in his research center wrote an analysis, which they requested never be published and remained in the archives of the Geneva Initiative on Psychiatry.[21] Fifteen years later, the text is still of great interest, and provides a unique insight into Soviet psychiatry and the central role of Snezhnevsky. The authors' names, known to the author but kept anonymous for reasons of confidentiality, put the role and position of Snezhnevsky against the backdrop of a totalitarian Stalinist society, where each and every branch of society was dominated by one leader, one school, one leading force. "We assume that [Snezhnevsky's school became the leading one] first of all because one or the other direction in Soviet psychiatry had to fulfill that role as a consequence of the general conditions [in society]." The authors point out that the leading role of Snezhnevsky's school was imposed after a joint session of the Academy of Sciences and the Academy of Medical Sciences on June 28 – July 4, 1950 and, subsequently, during a session of the Presidium of the

20 Novikov, Jurij, *Andrei Sneznevskij – seine Wege und Irrwege in der sowjetschen Psychiatrie.* Erich Sternberg (1903-1980), born in Prussia and educated in Berlin, worked at the Charité in Berlin and in Dresden before he lost his positions because of his Jewish background when Hitler assumed power in 1933 and fled to the USSR.

21 Initially the book, titled *Psychiatry, psychiatrists and society,* was to be published by Geneva Initiative on Psychiatry, but subsequently shelved because the authors had reason to believe that publication would be followed by repercussions that would affect their careers.

Academy of Medical Sciences and the Board of the All-Union Society of Neuropathologists and Psychiatrists on October 11-15, 1951.[22]

The centerpiece of the attack on all other directions in Soviet psychiatry was a lecture during these sessions by four authors, A.V. Snezhnevsky, V.M. Banshchikov, O.V. Kerbikov[23] and I.V. Strelchuk. "In principle there were four psychiatrists that could claim that position [of the leader]… It is clear that these four formed a sort of clan, amongst whom the pie had to be divided…. Maybe Banshchikov and Strelchuk left the ring because they were professionally clearly secondary to Snezhnevsky and Kerbikov.[24] But the latter two were quite equal. What caused the decision as to who of the two would be on top, we don't know."[25]

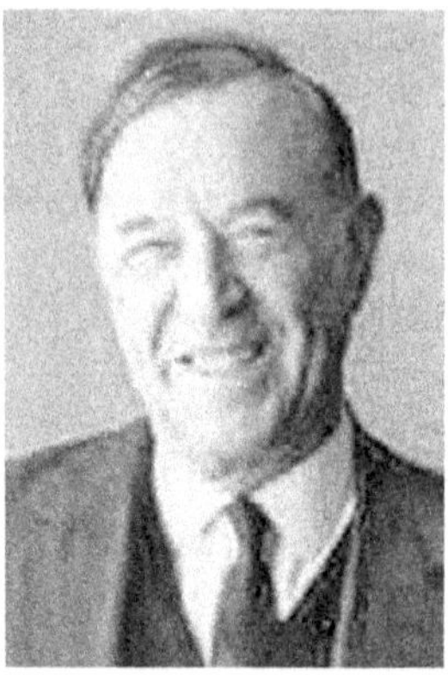

Prof. Andrei Snezhnevsky

The authors describe Snezhnevsky as a competent scientist, yet also as a person who met all the requirements imposed by the state and avoided everything that could have a negative effect on his scientific work.

22 *Psychiatry, psychiatrists and society*, p. 58. The joint session of the USSR Academy of Sciences and the USSR Academy of Medical Sciences met in compliance with an order of I. V. Stalin to institutionalize the theory of higher nervous activity of I. P. Pavlov. The session decreed that annual scientific conferences should be held to consider problems related to Pavlovian physiology. In response to this call, a year later a session of the Presidium of the Academy of Medical Sciences and the Board of the All-Union Society of Neuropathologists and Psychiatrists on the 'Physiological Teachings of the Academician I. P. Pavlov on Psychiatry and Neuropathology' was convened. A number of influential Soviet psychiatrists - V. A. Giliarovskii, M. O. Gurevich and A. S. Shmaryan —were condemned for adhering to anti-Marxist ideology and to psychiatric theories conceived by Western psychiatrists. The named psychiatrists acknowledged the correctness of the accusations, admitted their 'errors,' and promised in the future to follow Pavlov's teachings on psychiatry. The session's Presidium urged the development of a "New Soviet Psychiatry" based upon experimental and clinical findings and consistent with the Pavlovian conceptualization of higher nervous activity, which considered psychiatric and neurotic syndromes in terms of the dynamic localization of the brain's functions.

23 Oleg Vasilievich Kerbikov (1907-1965), Head of the Yaroslavl Medical Institute and Professor of psychiatry in Yaroslavl, in 1952 became Head of the Department of Psychiatry of the Second Moscow Medical Institute and a member of the Academy of Medical Sciences in 1962.

24 Both V.M. Banshchikov and I.V. Strelchuk were narcologists by profession.

25 *Psychiatry, psychiatrists and society*, p. 88

"He chaired the session of the shameful 'trade union meeting' in 1973 that was organized to 'discuss' (as a form of harassment) Dr. V.G. Levit, who had decided to immigrate to the United States.[26] It is hard to understand how this all could be part of the biography of one and the same person. He was a talented scientist, whose goal in life was clearly to find the scientific truth, and at the same time he was an amoral politician, who made this same truth secondary to the demands of the authorities. … Such a submission was the price he had to pay for the leadership position of both himself and his school."[27]

"We witnessed how, with a sense of dependence and willingness to submit, he talked with any official of the party apparatus," the authors continue. "Therefore, we are convinced that he was not an ideologist, not an architect of psychiatric repression. He was a submissive implementer of that policy and agreed to look the other way, because he preferred to do so and not leave to do some regular job. … Exactly that – scientific work – was the goal in the life of Snezhnevsky and for that he paid his share all his life. That is not something new. Already doctor Faust sold his soul to the devil; there were people before him, and after him. Snezhnevsky was one of them."[28]

They describe one occasion when, under leadership of Nikolai Zharikov, a psychiatrist who would later become President of the All-Union Soviet of Neuropathologists and Psychiatrists (AUSNP), a research group was formed to investigate social factors that influenced the illness of the patient. "However, it is unclear why the 'internal censor' betrayed Zharikov, who planned to carry out this work without permission from Snezhnevsky. Whatever the reason, he had made a major mistake." Snezhnevsky became furious and immediately forbade the work in the current form. It had to be reworked, and in the end every reference to "social factors" was taken out. "For Snezhnevsky even such work seemed to be unacceptable. It touched upon social life. He could not allow that to happen."[29]

Equally swift was the response by the Soviet psychiatric nomenklatura to an article published by Dr. Etely Kazanets in *Archives of General Psychiatry* in July 1979. In this article, Kazanets strongly criticized the current use of the diagnosis of schizophrenia in the Soviet Union, directly referring to the theories of the Moscow School of Andrei Snezhnevsky: "Particularly troublesome are cases of psychosis that lack the characteristic

---

26 In March 1989, Dr. Levit was a member of the US Delegation to the USSR to investigate the political abuse of psychiatry, see chapter 27

27 *Psychiatry, psychiatrists and society* p. 96

28 *Psychiatry, psychiatrists and society* p.97

29 *Psychiatry, psychiatrists and society* p. 113

clinical progression of schizophrenia. Some psychiatrists contend that a listing of the schizophrenias should include so-called transient, periodic or time-limited schizophrenia, which manifests after exogenous stresses but, during periods of transmission, leaves 'hardly any changes in personality, ... signs of psychic weakness having been exhausted' and can in fact follow a relapse course."[30] Kazanets criticized not only what he saw as an overly broad use of the diagnosis of schizophrenia, but also the fact that once a person had a diagnosis of schizophrenia, it was almost impossible to have this diagnosis revised. "This resulted in long and unfounded retention of patients on the dispensary list... Keeping these people on dispensary lists for long periods constitutes a real threat to their individual rights." This should be altered, he concluded, "especially in persons who have made good social vocational adaptation."[31] The reaction of Kazanets employer, the Serbski Institute in Moscow, was immediate: Kazanets lost his job.

Snezhnevsky was not only a leader who fulfilled all the requirements set by the authorities and, as indicated above, personally participated in the examination of dissidents.[32] He was also a totalitarian leader. "The atmosphere in the collective was far from ideal. In fact, in the Institute the same totalitarianism prevailed as in the rest of the country ... His opinion was decisive in all questions, from setting priorities in scientific work to hiring new associates, their promotion or dismissal. The scientific council... had no real meaning. Decisions were prepared beforehand in "the corridors of power."[33] As a result, the prevailing attitude became one of pleasing the chef, not of finding scientific results. "This excluded the development of new and original ideas."[34]

The two authors conclude: "Stalin was 'Leader, Father and Teacher' (all three with capital letters); beyond doubt that is also how he really regarded himself. Is it then strange, that that image was transferred to all large and small leaders who were raised by him? And Snezhnevsky was one of them...."[35]

---

30 Kazanets, E., *Differentiating exogenous psychiatric illness from schizophrenia,* p. 740

31 Kazanets, E., *Differentiating exogenous psychiatric illness from schizophrenia,* p. 745

32 Among the persons he personally examined are Zinovyi Krasivsky and Leonid Plyushch.

33 *Psychiatry, psychiatrists and society* p. 113

34 *Psychiatry, psychiatrists and society* p. 114

35 *Psychiatry, psychiatrists and society* pp. 114-5

Ridicule

The dominance of the Moscow School and its concept of schizophrenia was all pervasive, and only few dared to resist. However, behind closed doors it also led to ridicule, which was clearly illustrated by an essay written in 1974 but disseminated in *samizdat* only in the late 1980s.[36] The author, who remained anonymous at the time for obvious reasons, was Dr. Viktor Gindilis, who admitted his authorship in 1989 and agreed to its wider dissemination.[37] However, only in 1996 was the article published.[38]
As Gindilis explains: "Before writing an article, one should pass through a not very difficult but intensive preparation phase. It would be ideal if the author managed to get a job as a researcher at the Institute of Psychiatry of the USSR Academy of Medical Sciences because then the chances of success would be much better. (…) Try to put yourself into a special mood, or, as the actors say, into the condition of 'scenic inspiration.' To do so, one should temporarily fill oneself with holy trepidation for the great doctrine developed by A.V. Snezhnevsky and his collaborates.

The essence of this 'New Testament' is as follows. Long, long ago, when nothing existed on this Earth, including the Earth itself, there was but one schizophrenia. Nobody could see it because it was 'obscured,' 'masked' or 'latent,' a kind of schizosis. Centuries passed, pathos changed into nosos, and a model institute was established at the territory of the Kashchenko Hospital. All the patients of that hospital were, naturally, schizophrenics, though the similarities between them resembled the similarities between a woman's brooch and a plain toilet, but all of them had one thing in common: they had the same 'process.' This process just varied in course, manifestations, onset and outcome, it had different causes and different mechanisms, but these minor things should not discourage you, my young friend. Keep in mind that your main task is to have your product published in the Korsakov Journal. Thus, schizophrenia is all around. Neither neurosis, nor psychopathy, neither

---

36 The essay is dated January 1974. *Samizdat* stands for "self-publication" and relates to the unofficial publications of the dissident movement in the USSR. Apart from samizdat there was also *magnitizdat* (after *magnitofon*, cassette recorder), which referred to the habit of copying music cassettes with often illegal or unofficial concerts and songs by singers who were critical of the Soviet system, such as Vladimir Vysotsky and Yuli Kim.

37 Viktor Mironovich Gindilis, born 1937, was head of the Genetics Laboratory of the All-Union Research Institute in Moscow, of which Andrei Snezhnevsky and later Marat Vartanyan were directors. In 1992 he immigrated to the United States and died in 2001.

38 *Mental Health Reforms*, issue 1, 2000

reactive psychosis, nor chairs, nor couches, neither cats nor dogs exist by themselves. They are only the essence of clinical variants of schizophrenia, which sometimes neatly and cleverly disguise themselves. To uncover these masks, to discover 'developmental environment,' those are the noble acts of the knights of psychiatry, who have already accomplished so much that doctors are no longer able to name things after themselves."

Gindilis then went on making some concrete recommendations to future authors of the Korsakov Journal: "Come to like and use such capacious and informative words as 'atypical,' 'pseudo-' and '-like.' For example, 'pseudocyclothymic-like,' 'atypical pseudopuberty shift,' 'neurotic-' and 'psychopathic-like', 'pseudooligophrenic-like,' etc. (...) While calling something 'pseudo-' or '-like', you should formally (only formally) recognize the presence of the other part, but in order to emphasize that what you really mean is schizophrenia, a comparison with some ideal and non-existent characteristics is needed. It does not really matter that real psychopathia, neurosis or manic-depressive psychosis will move from the area of mental pathology to the normal spectrum, even supernormal. Then you will have more grounds to assume that schizophrenia is the only thing existing in psychiatry."

Gindilis concluded his essay with a final warning: "Send us your article, if it meets the requirements described, perhaps we shall have it published. However, do not be surprised if you, by chance, see your article with your spelling mistakes in our journal, but without your name as the author. Anyway, it does not matter who the author is, since the author is actually always one and the same."

Who knew, who understood?

Of course, the core group of psychiatrists that developed this concept on the orders of the Party and the KGB knew very well what they were doing; yet, for many Soviet psychiatrists, the diagnosis of mental illness seemed a very logical explanation, because they could not explain to themselves otherwise why somebody would be willing to give up his career, family and happiness for an idea or conviction that was so different from what most people believed or forced themselves to believe. In a way, the concept was also very welcome, as it excluded the need to put difficult questions to oneself and one's own behavior. And difficult questions could lead to difficult conclusions, which in turn could have caused problems with the authorities for the psychiatrist himself.

The onset of political psychiatry can probably best be seen as the result of a combination of factors that were only possible to mature under a totalitarian regime. The decision in 1950 to give monopoly over psychiatry to the Pavlovian school of Professor Andrei Snezhnevsky was one crucial factor. Here there was a scientist with a vision, who believed he could make history by proving his view of psychiatry, and the totalitarian climate made it possible for him to implement his plans unobstructed. Well-known psychiatrists who disagreed with him lost their positions; some were even exiled to Siberia.[39]

Needless to say, Soviet society had become a centrally ruled totalitarian State. Everything, even hobby clubs and sports clubs, was politicized and nothing was possible without the will and support of the Communist Party. The purges of the 1930s, 1940s and early 1950s made this perfectly clear; when suddenly in one night, for instance, all Esperantists in Leningrad were arrested with another group or sector of society targeted the next time. Doctors had been subordinated to the Party by having them swear the Oath of the Soviet Doctor instead of the Hippocratic Oath. And the Oath of the Soviet Doctor was very clear: the ultimate responsibility was to the Communist Party, and not to medical ethics.[40] According to the two authors mentioned earlier, "the main priority of the Soviet state was always itself. The interests of the individual were viewed as being secondary, and this general notion was reflected in many aspects [of psychiatric practice]. … The political abuse of psychiatry started much earlier than is generally assumed. It started when the State used the paternalistic tradition of Russian psychiatry and forced the psychiatrists to impose a certain way of life on their patients."[41] To illustrate this, the authors provide the example of a doctor discharging a patient before treatment is actually completed, not because the patient can go home, but because otherwise the patient stays away from work too long and that has a negative effect on the statistical "success-rate" of the mental health institution; and this, of course, goes against the "interests of the State."[42] Elsewhere in their manuscript, the authors give another example, in which one of them received a phone call from the local Party organs, asking to postpone the discharge of a patient for two weeks "because we don't want to run the risk of having a Communist festivity disturbed." In that case, the authors conclude, it is very hard for a psychiatrist not to fulfill this seemingly innocent request.

39 *Russia's Political Hospitals,* pp. 220-223.

40 The Oath of the Soviet Doctor was adopted by the Presidium of the Supreme Soviet of the USSR on March 26, 1971. Vedemosti Verkhovnogo Soveta SSSR, 1971, no. 13, p. 145

41 *Psychiatry, psychiatrists and society*, p. 38

42 *Psychiatry, psychiatrists and society*, p.38

Also the dissident psychiatrist and former political prisoner Anatoly Koryagin mentions this pressure from judicial organs. "At the beginning of the 1960s, working as a young psychiatrist in Siberia, I personally experienced the kind of pressure that is exerted on doctors by the KGB, by the procurator, and by officers of the Ministry of the Interior. Lawyers and officers of the Ministry tried to impress on me many times the nature of the psychiatric illness from which this or that person was supposedly suffering – and I was a psychiatrist! They assured me that to give a psychiatric examination to such a person was a tedious formality from their point of view. In each case, in order not to become a compliant party to the official organizations, I had to refuse categorically to make individual judgements, and to demand that these 'psychiatrically ill' people be examined by a medical panel or by a panel of forensic psychiatrists. ... Many yielded to this pressure... and people were placed in psychiatric hospitals without a proper forensic psychiatric examination."[43]

And of course, Soviet psychiatrists had little chance to escape the all-pervasive control by the Communist Party and its organs because they were in fact three-fold dependent on the Soviet state, scientifically dependent, politically dependent, and economically dependent. They were scientifically dependent because their possibility to work in the field of their science and do research was dependent on their allegiance to the Soviet authorities; they were politically dependent and had to organize their professional life and interaction with authorities in such a way that they would not loose their support; and they were economically dependent, as private practice did not exist, they were all employees of the State.[44] People in leadership positions did not only need to have the capacity to fulfill their leadership role and be successful in it: "that success... depended on other conditions; those who were able to maintain the necessary interactions with the authorities had the biggest chance of making a career. For that they had to fulfill a multitude of requirements. Next to specific personal qualities that were necessary to be able to maintain contacts with specific party officials, there were also other demands, in particular having a character by the book."[45]

Another factor that helped to impose the political abuse of psychiatry on the psychiatric community and root out potential opposition against it was the fact that "for many years there was an unchangeable yet informal hierarchy of mental health institutions. This looked more or less as follows: the highest step on the ladder formed the scientific research institutes, then the psychiatric

43 Koryagin, A., *The involvement of Soviet psychiatry in the persecution of dissenters*, p. 336

44 *Psychiatry, psychiatrists and society*, p. 86

45 *Psychiatry, psychiatrists and society*, p.87

faculties, then Moscow and Leningrad psychiatric hospitals, then oblast and city psychiatric hospitals, then oblast and city outpatient clinics and, at the lowest step, came the regional psycho-neurological outpatient clinics and cabinets. If a doctor who worked in a dispensary would change a diagnosis, it was usually considered as an "attack" on the institution that was higher up on the hierarchical ladder. For many years, a "lower institution" was obligated to follow a diagnosis established by a "higher institution." [46] In other words, if the Serbski Institute in Moscow declared a dissident to be mentally ill, no lower-placed psychiatrist would dare go against it.

The authors conclude: "As a result, traditional Russian paternalism combined with the traditions of Soviet bureaucracy caused a deep conflict between society and psychiatric services: patients in psychiatric institutions changed into a formal social group that was subject to discrimination; many principles of professional ethics became distorted; the stimuli to improve the professional level of psychiatrists were to a large degree lost."[47]

Finally, one should not forget that the Soviet Union had become a closed society, a society that was cut off from the rest of the world. World psychiatric literature was unavailable, except to the politically correct psychiatric elite. "Western psychiatric literature became rare: the number of periodicals that came was limited and a large part wound up in the 'special holdings' (*spetskhran*) of the Lenin Library [in Moscow] and where access was impossible."[48] The power of the Party seemed endless, whether you believed in their ideals or not. Thus, any person who decided to voice dissent openly ran a high risk of being considered mentally ill. As a result, the political abuse of psychiatry that primarily affected intellectuals and artistic circles grew into an important form of repression with approximately one-third of the dissidents in the 1970s and early 1980s being sent to psychiatric hospitals rather than to a camp, prison or exile.

Dissident psychiatrist Dr. Anatoly Koryagin, who served six out of a total sentence of fourteen years of camp and exile for having been a member of a "Working Commission to Investigate the Political Abuse of Psychiatry," examined seventeen victims or potential victims of political psychiatry. His diagnoses were used as a defense against being declared insane or as a means to show the outside world that a hospitalized dissident had been incarcerated for non-medical reasons. On the basis of his sample, Koryagin came to the interesting conclusion that the length of hospitalization seemed to correspond

46 *Psychiatry, psychiatrists and society*, pp. 41-42
47 *Psychiatry, psychiatrists and society*, p. 43
48 *Psychiatry, psychiatrists and society*, p. 58

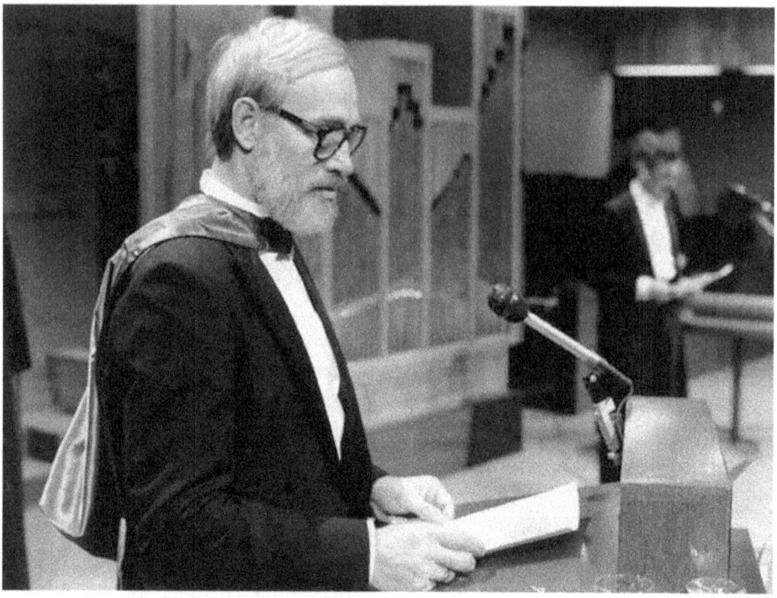

Koryagin receives Honorary Doctorate, 1988

to the length of a sentence a political prisoner would have received. In other words, a political prisoner charged with "slandering the Soviet state" usually was hospitalized for about three years (the maximum term under that article of the USSR Criminal Code) while a person accused of anti-Soviet agitation and propaganda usually stayed in for much longer - seven years or more (again the maximum sentence under that article). Cynically, one could say that the crazier a person was, the more serious his damage to the Soviet state![49]

Dissidents had the theory that mentally weaker persons were more often sent to camps, while the mentally strong and unbreakable faced an uncertain future in psychiatric hospitals without a specific sentence and being tortured with neuroleptics and by other means. All in all, it is safe to conclude that the victims of political repression were carefully selected; this form of punishment seemed to be the most fitting for them.

However, it is important to note that the Soviet Union was certainly not the only country where these abuses took place. Over the years, a great deal

[49] See Koryagin, A, *Unwilling Patients*, in Van Voren, R. (ed.), Koryagin: A Man Struggling for Human Dignity, Amsterdam, IAPUP, 1987, pp.43-50. A very interesting book on the origins and scope of political abuse of psychiatry in the Soviet Union is Korotenko, A., and Alkina, N., *Sovietskaya Psikhiatriya – Zabluzhdeniya i Umysl*, Kiev, Sphera, 2002

of documentation on other countries passed the desk of the International Association on the Political Use of psychiatry (IAPUP).[50] One of the countries where systematic political abuse of psychiatry appears to have taken place was Romania. In 1997, IAPUP organized an investigative committee to research the situation in that country. [51] The group also received information on cases in Czechoslovakia, Hungary and Bulgaria, but all these cases were individual and there was no evidence of any systematic abuse. Later, information appeared on the political abuse of psychiatry in Cuba, which was, however, short-lived.[52]

An extensive research on the situation in Eastern Germany came to the conclusion that no systematic abuse of psychiatry for political purposes had existed in this socialist country, although politics and psychiatry appeared to be very closely intermingled.[53]

In the 1990s, Geneva Initiative on Psychiatry was involved in a case of political abuse of psychiatry in The Netherlands when the Ministry of Defense tried to silence a social worker by falsifying several psychiatric diagnoses. The case took many years to be resolved and although the victim was compensated and even knighted by the Dutch Queen, it is still not

50 The International Association on the Political Use of Psychiatry (IAPUP) was set up in Paris in December 1980 as a confederation of national groups who were involved in the campaign against the political abuse of psychiatry. The author became General Secretary of the group in 1986. Since, the name changed into Geneva Initiative on Psychiatry and, in 2005, Global Initiative on Psychiatry (GIP).

51 See *Psychiatry under Tyranny, An Assessment of the Political Abuse of Romanian Psychiatry During the Ceausescu Years*, Amsterdam, IAPUP, 1989

52 Brown, Ch.A., and Lago, A., *The Politics of Psychiatry in Revolutionary Cuba*, New York 1991

53 Süss, S., *Politisch Missbraucht? Psychiatrie und Staatssicherheit in der DDR*, Berlin, Ch. Links Verlag, 1998. One of the factors that prevented a political abuse of psychiatry in the DDR might have been the fact that German psychiatrists, both in East and West, had a heightened awareness with regard to the possibility of their profession being abused for political means because of the Euthanasia program of the Nazi regime, as a result of which tens of thousands of mental patients and mentally disabled people were murdered. On top of that, many of the founders of the DDR had been victims of the Nazi regime and established their state with the goal to make sure the past would never be repeated; thus the idea that psychiatry would again be used for political purposes was alien to them. According to the Berlin psychiatrist Hanfried Helmchen at least equally important was the fact that "the DDR was not as closed as the Soviet Union because almost all citizen of the DDR had access to Western media, mostly radio and television. Nevertheless, at least two people recently described in the *Deutsches Ärzteblatt* political abuse of psychiatry in the DDR experienced by themselves." (e-mail from Prof. Helmchen, April 17, 2010)

fully resolved.[54] The issue of political abuse of psychiatry in the People's Republic of China emerged again in recent years and has caused repeated debates within the international psychiatric community.

Early cases of political psychiatry

Generally speaking, the systematic use of psychiatry to incarcerate dissidents in psychiatric hospitals started in the late 1950s and early 1960s. However, there are cases of political abuse of psychiatry known from a much earlier date. In 1836, the Russian philosopher Pyotr Chaadayev published a critical article on the backwardness of Russian society in a journal, which immediately triggered the wrath of Tsar Nicholas I. The latter explained Chaadayev's critical remarks by asserting that the philosopher was suffering from mental illness: "… the thoughts expressed in it have aroused feelings of anger and repugnance in all Russians without exception. But the horror quickly turned to sympathy when they learned that their unhappy compatriot suffers from derangement and insanity. Taking into consideration the unwell state of this unfortunate person, the government … forbids him to leave his house and will provide free medical care…"[55] Chaadayev remained under house arrest for a year but continued writing and published his works in France instead of Russia.

In early Soviet times some attempts to use psychiatry for political purposes took place; yet these cases, as well as the Chaadayev case, can be compared to the Spijkers case in The Netherlands: giving a psychiatric diagnosis seemed to be the easiest option.

In the 1930s, the political abuse of psychiatry took on a more systematic form. According to a series of letters published by a Soviet psychiatrist in The *American Journal of Psychiatry*, it was one of the leaders of the Soviet secret police, Andrei Vyshinsky, who ordered the use of psychiatry as a means of repression.[56] According to the author of the letters, whose name was known to the editor but otherwise remained anonymous, the first Special Psychiatric Hospital in Kazan was used exclusively for political cases. Half of the cases were persons who indeed were mentally ill, but the other half were persons

---

54 For the case of Fred Spijkers see Nijeboer, A., *Een man tegen de Staat*, Breda, Papieren Tijger, 2006

55 Medvedev, Z. and Medvedev, R, *A Question of Madness*, London, Macmillan, 1971, pp. 196-197.

56 *American Journal of Psychiatry*, 1970, vol 126, pp. 1327-1328; vol. 127, pp. 842-843; 1971, vol. 127, pp. 1575-1576, and 1974, vol. 131, p.474.

without any mental illness, such as the former Estonian President Päts who was held in Kazan for political reasons from 1941 till 1956.[57]

The Serbski Institute for General and Forensic Psychiatry in Moscow also had a political department, headed by Professor Khaletsky. However, according to Soviet poet Naum Korzhavin, the Serbski was at that time a relatively humane institution with a benevolent staff.[58] However, the atmosphere changed almost overnight when, in 1948, Dr. Daniil Lunts was appointed head of the Fourth Department, which was later usually referred to as the Political Department. Previously, psychiatric hospitalization had been considered a "refuge" against being sent to the Gulag, but from that moment onwards this policy changed.[59]

Additional cases of political abuse of psychiatry are known from the 1940s and 1950s, including that of a Party official, Sergei Pisarev, who was arrested after criticizing the work of the Soviet secret police in connection with the so-called Doctor's Plot. As mentioned elsewhere, this was an anti-Semitic campaign developed at Stalin's orders that should have led to a new wave of terror in the USSR and probably to the annihilation of the remaining Jewish communities that had survived the Second World War. Pisarev was hospitalized in the Special Psychiatric Hospital in Leningrad, which together with a similar hospital in Sychevka had been opened after the Second World War. After his release in 1955, Pisarev initiated a campaign against the political abuse of psychiatry, concentrating on the Serbski Institute that he considered to be the root of all evil. As a result of his activity, the Central Committee of the Communist Party established a committee that investigated the situation and concluded that the political abuse of psychiatry was indeed taking place. However, the report disappeared in a desk drawer and never resulted in any action taken.[60]

---

57 *Kaznimye sumasshestviem*, Frankfurt, Possev, 1971, p. 479.

58 *Russia's Political Hospitals*, p. 53-54.

59 Van Voren, R, *Daniil Lunts, Psychiatrist of the Devil*, unpublished manuscript, 1978; Van Voren, R., *Soviet Psychiatric Abuse in the Gorbachev Era*, Amsterdam, IAPUP, 1989, p.16. According to Boris Shostakovich, "D.R. Lunts was unhappy in life, with very complicated family circumstances, innerly lonely, weak, and absolutely not a bad person. Understanding of this came much later, when after the death of his wife an eldest daughter, he married S.L. Taptatova. He became completely different: more calm, soft, started to dress elegantly and thawed. Unfortunately, he was only able to live not long like this by fate. (…) His widow … writes, and somehow correctly, about his conviction that for those people it was better to stay in a psychiatric hospital than to be sent to prison." Biography of D.R. Lunts, in *Ocherki Istorii*, published on the occasion of the 75th anniversary of the Serbski Institute, pp. 202-204

60 Pisarev, S., *Soviet Mental Prisons*, Survey, London, 1970, pp. 175-180

Until the mid-1960s, the political abuse of psychiatry in the USSR went mostly unnoticed, including among Soviet dissidents who had not yet realized that a dangerous new form of repression threatened them. In his memoirs, Vladimir Bukovsky writes about his stay in the Serbski Institute: "We were absolutely not afraid to be called lunatics – to the contrary, we rejoiced; let these idiots think that we were lunatics if they like or, rather, let these lunatics think we were idiots. We remembered all the stories on lunatics by Chekhov, Gogol, Akatugawa and, of course, also *The Good Soldier Schweik.* We roared with laughter at our doctors and ourselves."[61] But it was only later that they realized that the old woman who cleaned the ward reported everything to the doctors, who used the information to prove their mental illness. In 1974, Bukovsky wrote together with the imprisoned psychiatrist Semyon Gluzman a *Manual on Psychiatry for Dissenters*, in which they gave guidelines to potential victims of political psychiatry on how to behave during investigation in order to avoid being diagnosed as mentally ill.[62]

On the basis of the available evidence, one can conclude that in the course of the 1960s, political abuse of psychiatry in the Soviet Union became one of the main methods of repression. By the end of that decade, many well-known dissidents were diagnosed as being mentally ill. According to F.V. Kondratiev, an associate of the Serbski Institute, between 1961 and his research (which was published in 1996), 309 people were sent to the Fourth Department of the Serbski Institute for psychiatric examination after having been charged with anti-Soviet agitation and propaganda (art. 70 of the RSFSR Criminal Code),[63] and 61 with a charge of "slandering the Soviet State" (art. 190-1 of the RSFSR Criminal Code).[64]

---

61 *To Build a Castle,* p. 199.

62 *Russia's Political Hospitals*, pp. 419-440.

63 "Anti-Soviet propaganda" was one of the articles of the Criminal Code that were used against Soviet dissidents. Each Soviet republic had its own Criminal Code. In the Russian Criminal Code, usually quoted, it was article 70 and read: "agitation or propaganda carried on for the purpose of subverting or weakening Soviet power or of committing particular, especially dangerous crimes against the state, or the circulation, for the same purpose, of slanderous fabrications which defame the Soviet state and social system, or the circulation or preparation or keeping, for the same purpose, of literature of such content, shall be punished by deprivation of freedom for a term of six months to seven years, with or without additional exile for a term of two to five years, or by exile for a term of two to five years."

64 Like "anti-Soviet agitation and propaganda" (article 70 of the RSFSR Criminal Code) this article was used widely against Soviet dissidents and read: "circulation of fabrications known to be false which defame the Soviet state and social system. The systematic circulation in an oral form of fabrications known to be false which defame the Soviet state and social system and, likewise, the preparation or circula-

However, he admits that 'politicals' were also charged with other crimes, such as hooliganism, and, therefore, the numbers might be higher.[65]

Interesting data are also provided in a December 15, 1969 report by Lieutenant-General S. Smorodinski of the KGB in Krasnodarski Krai showing that people who were sent to the Serbski Institute were only the tip of the iceberg. The mentioned document was sent by KGB Chairman Yuri Andropov to the Politburo in January 1970 in order to discuss measures to register and isolate mentally ill persons in the country more effectively. Among those who to be registered and isolated were those "who had terrorist and other intentions dangerous to society."[66] Smorodinski listed a number of these dangerous criminal acts, including people who tried to escape from the Fatherland (for instance, a P.A. Skrylev who tried to flee to Turkey with an Antonov AN-2 plane and was shot down by the Soviet Air Force, according to the report), people "fanatically trying to meet with foreigners," as well as those who tried to found new parties or persons suggesting control mechanisms with regard to the Communist Party. According to Smorodinski, one person suggested establishing a "council to control the activities of the Politburo of the Central Committee of the CPSU and local party organs," which was considered to be an especially dangerous act; others were accused of spreading anti-Soviet leaflets. Smorodinski concluded in his document that the Krasnodarski Krai had only 3785 beds available, while 11-12,000 persons should be hospitalized. Andropov added to Smorodinski's document: "Similar situations occur in other parts of the country." In other words: the number of beds in the USSR needs to be increased considerably in order to meet this urgent demand.

How extensive the abuse had become in the early 1970s is also well illustrated by a report on a high-level meeting between MfS and KGB in Berlin in April 1976, with data on the situation a few years earlier: "The increased stability of society in the USSR is also clear from the fact that in 1974 fewer people were

---

tion in written, printed or any other form of works of such content shall be punished by deprivation of freedom for a term not exceeding three years, or by correctional tasks for a term not exceeding one year, or by a fine not exceeding 100 rubles."

65 *Ocherki Istorii*, published on the occasion of the 75th anniversary of the Serbski Institute, pp. 140-141.

66 Letter of Yuri Andropov to the members of the Politburo, No. 141-A, dated January 20, 1970, "Secret". It is accompanied by the report by Smorodinski addressed to Yuri Andropov. The document is part of a much larger collection of documents from the Politburo, the Central Committee of the Communist Party of the Soviet Union (CPSU) and the KGB that were scanned by Vladimir Bukovsky during his research for the planned trial against the CPSU (which never took place) and which he subsequently put on the internet. See: *www.bukovsky-archives.net*

convicted of slandering the state or anti-Soviet propaganda than in previous years. For example, in 1973 a total of 124 persons were arrested for these crimes compared with 89 persons in 1974, in the context of which it is important to note that 50% of these people were mentally ill."[67] In the same report, the question is raised as to why the prominent human rights activist and Nobel Peace Prize laureate Andrei Sakharov, a "three time Hero of Socialist Work and the discoverer of the Soviet nuclear weapons" had become a dissident. The report quoted Lieutenant General Bobkov, head of the Fifth Directorate of the KGB: "Sakharov is objectively a mentally ill person. The complication with regards to operational consequences lies in the fact that for political reasons he cannot be committed to a psychiatric hospital, as it would turn him into a martyr. Lieutenant General Bobkov stressed that Sakharov should not become a 'hunted figure'."[68]

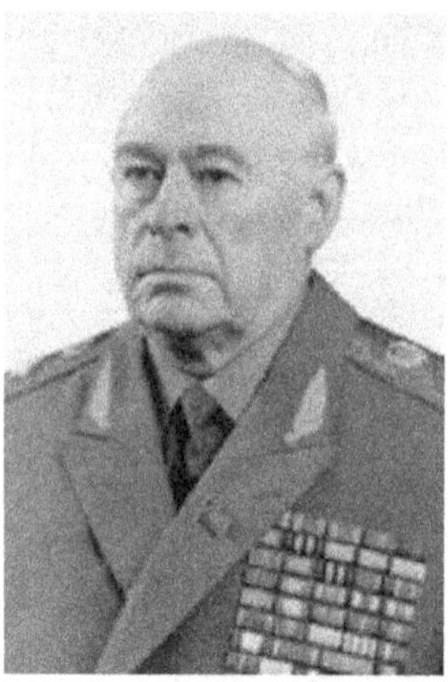

KGB Lieutenant General Filip Bobkov

The use of psychiatry as a means of repression was not only used against individual persons, but sometimes also to separate larger groups of "undesired elements" from society for a certain period of time; for instance, during Communist festivities or special events like the 1980 Olympic Games in Moscow. In some cases they were delivered en masse, such as in 1971 in Tomsk: "At a ceremonial meeting of the hospital staff in 1971 [in Tomsk], which I attended, [hos-

67 MfS-HAXX, 2941, p. 93.
In a memorandum by KGB Chairman Yuri Andropov to the Central Committee of the Communist Party, dated December 29, 1975, more interesting figures are provided. According to Andropov, in the period 1967 until 1975 in total 1583 people were sentenced on basis of articles 70 and 190-1of the RSFSR Criminal Code, while in the preceding eight years (1958-1966) the total had been 3448 persons. However, later in the document he notes that during the period 1971-1974 63,108 persons had been "profilaktizirovano" (prevented), in other words, had been convinced by various means not to continue their anti-Soviet behavior. Memorandum by Yuri Andropov, no. 3213-A, December 29, 1975, p. 3

68 MfS-HAXX, 2941, p. 97. The Fifth Directorate of the KGB was responsible for censorship and internal security against artistic, political, and religious dissension; renamed "Directorate Z", protecting the Constitutional order, in 1989. The same Filip D. Bobkov attended in 1987, together with among others Minister of Health Evgeni Chazov, a Politburo meeting where they were instructed by Mikhail Gorbachev to prepare the transfer of Special Psychiatric Hospitals from the Ministry of Internal Affairs (MVD) to the Ministry of Health. See *Human Rights, Perestroika and the end of the Cold War*, p. 157, and correspondence with Anatoly Adamishin, November 4, 2009

pital director Dr. Anatoly] Potapov[69] said literally the following: 'We expect to register a great number of patients on November 4-7. There'll be a special mark on their papers. They are suffering from 'paranoid schizophrenia.' We are to accept them all no matter how many there are..."[70] In 1980, KGB Chairman Yuri Andropov was quite explicit in a "top secret" memorandum to the Central Committee of the Communist Party with regard to the preparations of the Olympic Games. In his 6-page report he quite explicitly wrote that 'with the goal of preventing possible provocative and anti-social actions on the part of mentally ill individuals who display aggressive intentions, measures are being taken, together with police and health authorities, to put such people in preventive isolation during the period of the 1980 Olympics."[71] His deputy Viktor Chebrikov and Minister of Internal Affairs Nikolai Shchelokov referred to them as "mentally ill with delusional ideas."[72] This use of mental hospitals to separate undesirable elements during Communist holidays and special events was not limited to the USSR, however. Similar practices were reported from Romania under Ceausescu and in the People's Republic of China.[73]

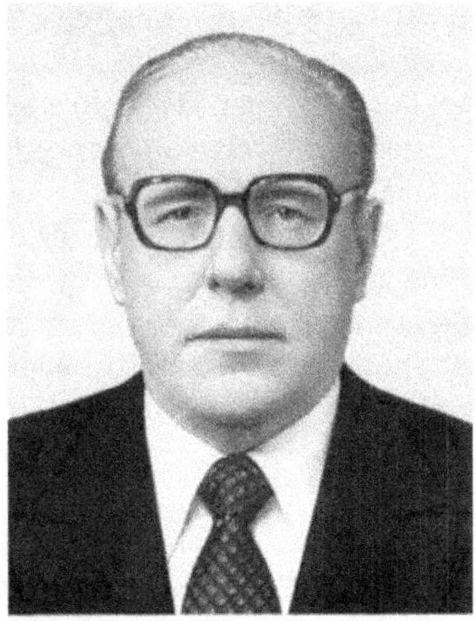

Chebrikov, official State portrait, 1985

---

69 Anatoly Potapov, a psychiatrist by profession, was from 1965 to 1983 director of the psychiatric hospital in Tomsk. He would later become Minister of Health of the Russian Soviet Republic.

70 *Moscow News* no. 37, 1990, reprinted in *Documents* 38, September 1990.

71 *Regarding the main measures to guarantee security during the period of preparation and implementation of the XXII Olympic Games in Moscow*, signed by KGB Chairman Yuri Andropov, document 902-A, dated May 12, 1980, p. 3.

72 *On the measures of the MVD of the USSR and the KGB of the USSR to guarantee security during the period of preparation and implementation of the XXII Olympic Games in Moscow*, "top secret" memorandum to the Central Committee, signed by Nikolai Shchelokov and V. Chebrikov, p. 2. Viktor Chebrikov was Deputy Chairman of the KGB in 1962-1982 and Chairman in 1982-8. Nikolai Shcholokov, Minister of Internal Affairs and a personal friend of Soviet leader Leonid Brezhnev, was accused of corruption in 1988 and committed suicide.

73 For Romania see: *Psychiatry under Tyranny*, p. 9. In China, in preparation of the Olympic Games of 2008 the Beijing police defined a grading standard for mentally ill persons who could cause incidents and accidents and are moderately disruptive. Security brigade chiefs, civil police chiefs and the secu-

Keeping up appearances

While to the outside world, the Soviet authorities maintained that the Western criticism of Soviet psychiatry was nothing more than "a slanderous campaign organized by reactionary and Zionist circles in England and the USA" and the main focus of their counter efforts was to explain the "humanist nature of Soviet medicine,"[74] internally and behind closed doors they were actually far more critical of the prevailing situation in psychiatry. A whole set of documents, copied by Vladimir Bukovsky in 1992 in the archives of the Central Committee of the CPSU, including reports by the KGB, primarily concerning themselves with this issue. Already in 1971, Minister of Health Boris Petrovsky[75] reported to the Central Committee that the living conditions in the Special Psychiatric Hospitals did not meet the standards necessary for adequate treatment of the mentally ill. The reason for this remark was an investigation of the situation under which two dissidents, Viktor Fainberg and Vladimir Borisov, were being held in the Special Psychiatric Hospital in Leningrad. The investigation was carried out after Academician Andrei Sakharov had complained about their situation to the Minister of Health in a telegram in March 1971. In the ensuing report, both men were of course described as being mentally ill,[76]

rity directors of all police branches in all the incorporated districts and county councils of Beijing were trained according to the "Beijing City mental health ordinance". Also a thorough investigation of basic information regarding the mentally ill of Beijing was carried out. The Beijing Police used the above-mentioned professional training and basic investigation to determine a grading standard to rate the risks posed by mentally ill persons. See www.legaldaily.com.cn April 4, 2007

74 Report on the VI World Congress of Psychiatry marked "secret" to the Central Committee of the CPSU, October 21, 1977, p. 1-3

75 Boris Vasilievich Petrovsky was a general surgeon who made several major contributions to cardiovascular surgery, transplant surgery, and oesophageal surgery. He organized and headed the All-Union Research Institute for Clinical and Experimental Surgery. After his retirement in 1989 he remained the director emeritus of the institute and died in its intensive care unit. For more than 15 years (1965-80) Petrovsky was minister of health in the former Soviet Union.

76 According to the document Viktor Fainberg was suffering from personality disorder with psychopathological disorders (paranoid development of the type of social reform delusions), Vladimir Borisov from personality disorders (infantilism, paranoia). Borisov was eventually forced to emigrate from the USSR. When he refused to cooperate with the authorities regarding his emigration, they made his brother prepare the necessary documents, who maintained an "operational contact" with the KGB. See Mitrokhin Archive, Woodrow Wilson International Center for Scholars, Cold War International History Project, folder 28, *Practicing Psychiatry for Political Purposes*, document 4

yet, at the same time, the Minister confirmed that measures had to be taken to improve the living conditions.[77]

Petrovsky's criticism did not stand alone. Three years earlier, decree 517 of the Central Committee and the Council of Ministers of July 5, 1968 stated, "On measures to further improve health care and the development of medical science in the country," and outlined that 125 psychiatric hospitals each with at least 500 beds should be built before 1975, and indeed the Five Year Plan of 1971-1975 included the construction of 114 psychiatric hospitals with a total capacity of 43,800 beds.[78] However, the situation continued to be unsatisfactory. In 1971, the Ministry of Health together with the Ministry of Internal Affairs (MVD) and the KGB sent a plan to the Council of Ministers for the further improvement of medical assistance to persons with mental illness. The fact that the MVD was involved in the writing of this plan is not surprising, as the Special Psychiatric Hospitals fell under the jurisdiction of that Ministry.[79] However, what is clear from all relevant documents is the fact that also the KGB was continuously involved in the matter.[80] The plan was discussed by the Presidium of the Council of Ministers on January 26, 1972, and the decision was reached to establish a working commission under chairmanship of comrade Rakovski.[81]

A few weeks later, the commission received a highly critical four-page report by the Department of Science and Education of the Central Committee, addressed to the Central Committee, which provided much detail about the prevailing situation. The report mentioned that for several years, special attention had been paid to mental health care services in the country, but that the Central Committee was still receiving "complaints from the population with regard to serious shortcomings in mental health care services in the

77 Report by B. Petrovsky to the Head of the Department of Science and Education of the Central Committee of the CPSU, March 25, 1971.

78 *On the situation of psychiatric help in the country*, p. 3

79 The Special Psychiatric Hospitals were transferred to the Ministry of Justice only in 1988.

80 Their interest was probably connected to the fact that incidents with persons with mental illness fell automatically within the domain of the KGB's task to provide internal security, but also because these incidents or crimes involved those with a political connotation – such as outlined in a KGB report to the Politburo in 1969 and quoted earlier in this chapter.

81 Excerpt from the minutes No. 31, paragraph 19c of the session of the Central Committee of the CPSU of February 22, 1972. Among the members of the commission is a comrade Tsvigun, probably referring to Semyon Kuzmich Tsvigun, Deputy Chairman of the KGB 1967-1982 and husband of Leonid Brezhnev's sister-in-law.

country" and that "the state of psychiatric help continues to be unsatisfactory. According to the report, the number of people in need of psychiatric help had grown enormously; while in 1966 just over two million citizens were on the psychiatric register, the number had grown by 1971 to 3.7 million.[82] In many of the hospitals, the report continued, patients had only 2-2.5 square meters at their disposal, although the norm was 7 square meters. "Cases in which patients are sleeping in pairs in one bed and even on the floor are not rare. In several hospitals, double bunk beds have been made."[83] The report continued: "As a result of overcrowding of hospitals, sanitary-hygienic norms are being violated, unacceptable conditions are created for living, diagnosing and treatment of mentally ill persons as well as for the work of the personnel. Often patients are discharged prematurely."[84] In the Russian Soviet Republic, the number of available beds in social care homes was less than half of what was needed.[85]

---

82 In 1988 the number of persons on the psychiatric register had grown to 10.2 million. See: Ogonek (no. 16, 15-22 April, 1989, p.24) According to the authors of the book *Psychiatry, psychiatrists and society* during the 1960s-1980s the total number of registered mental patients in the USSR increased by tenfold. The growth concerned in particular the lighter form of mental illness, because it was not because more and more people fell ill but because more and more people turned for psychiatric help. New mediation appeared, treatment by doctors became more and more effective, and people for whom before it didn't make any sense to go to the dispensary now went as well. (…) However, the instructions did not take these changes into account. The number of social sanctions (and they increased in number) concerned, like before, everybody who was on the psychiatric register…and could exclude the possibility of being involved in various forms of professional life, driving a car, go to a sanatorium, buy a hunting rifle, go abroad on a business trip or as a tourist, etc." *Psychiatry, psychiatrists and society*, pp. 39-40

83 *On the situation of psychiatric help in the country*, Report to the Central Committee, February 18, 1972, signed by the Head of the Department for Science and education S. Trapeznikov, p. 1

84 *On the situation of psychiatric help in the country*, p. 1. One of the problems that aggravated the situation was the fact that while more hospitals were being built, also the number of hospitalizations increased, and persons with mental illness were increasingly not only hospitalized in time of crisis but also when outpatient treatment would have been sufficient. "This is quite clearly reflected in the epidemiological data. The number of ill people who were never hospitalized decreased over time, and the number and regularity of hospitalizations increased. For instance, among the Moscow outpatient clinics that were part of the study in 1967 a total of 18,3% of the patients had never been hospitalized, while in 1981 that percentage had decreased to only 4,9%. See: *Psychiatry, psychiatrists and society*, p. 30

85 At the end of the 1980s – beginning of the 1990s the USSR had 284 psychoneurological outpatient clinics, in 1983 of which there were beds, and 491

The report continued with criticism regarding the state of affairs of outpatient psychiatric services and pointed out that no scientific research institute for child psychiatry existed in the country. In addition, "Psychiatric scientific research institutes insufficiently concern themselves with the improvement of the quality of treatment of the mentally ill using new effective psychotropic drugs. The list of available psychotropic drugs in the country is very limited."[86]

Still, in spite of all the efforts, the living conditions in mental institutions remained unsatisfactory. Several years later, in October 1976, Deputy Minister of Health of the USSR, S. Burenkov sent an outline to the Central Committee of the package of plans to "expose the mendacity and incompetence of bourgeois propagandists, who try to use the misfortune of mentally ill people for purposes of political speculation." As one of the proposed activities, he mentions: "The Ministry of Health of the USSR continues to carry out jointly with the MVD of the USSR regular inspections of special hospitals, where persons with mental illness are undergoing compulsory treatment, with the purpose to end existing insufficiencies and to carry out proposals to improve the provision of psychiatric care to this category of patients."[87] The same plans are outlined in a joint document from the Departments of Science and Education and of Propaganda of the Central Committee, to which is added the remark: "The KGB of the Council of Ministers of the USSR is informed in detail of these activities … December 13, 1976."[88]

---

psychiatric hospitals. The total number of bed in the USSR was 380,604. On top of that the Ministry of Social Affairs had 261,000 beds at its disposal. See: *Psychiatry, psychiatrists and society*, p. 29

Social care homes, the so-called "internaty", are institutions for chronic mental patients usually located outside the cities. The population consists not only of chronic mental patients but also persons with intellectual disability and often also social outcasts. Also as of 2010 many of such institutions exist on the territory of the former USSR and the living conditions are in general very bad.

86 *On the situation of psychiatric help in the country*, p. 3

87 *On measures to counter the anti-Soviet campaign in the West concerning "the use of psychiatry in the USSR for political purposes"*, report to the Central Committee by the Ministry of Health, October 22, 1976, p. 4

88 *On measures to counter the anti-Soviet campaign concerning the so-called "abuse" of psychiatry in the USSR*, report of the Heads of the Departments of Science and Education (S. Trapeznikov) and Propaganda (M. Nenashev), December 9, 1976, p.3

Chapter 10 - Meeting Ellen Mercer

In a way it is as if time stood still. There is an American movie, "Groundhog Day," in which a television weatherman, during his assignment to cover the annual Groundhog Day event, finds himself repeating the same day over and over again. I repeatedly get the feeling that I am part of a similar situation. Ellen Mercer's apartment is unchanged; most of the furniture and oriental art positioned at various places around the room is exactly as I remembered. The small garden downstairs is somewhat overgrown, but still very much the "Alhambra Gardens," as we jokingly called it, after having seen the real Alhambra gardens in Spain during a Regional Symposium of the WPA in the spring of 1989. Instead of two cats in the house, six are now residing in different rooms, although two are said to be only "temporary residents." The cats immediately remind me of Anatoly Koryagin, the dissident Soviet psychiatrist and former political prisoner, who used to stay at Ellen Mercer's place when visiting Washington D.C. in the late 1980s. He would drive Ellen nuts by making jokes about the cats, in particular by making a move with his hand as if he would grab one of her cats by the tail, swing it around and then throw it in the air. It was a joke, of course, but invariably had the desired effect every time he made the gesture.

The house is full of memories, and the unchanged surroundings evoke them immediately. Within no time we are sitting at the dining table, ready for long talks about the past and present. The only difference with twenty years ago is the fact that both of us have laptops on standby (to be used later to send documents back and forth, the modern form of human interaction) and, this time, I didn't bring my portable fax machine, which was my faithful companion in those days. But just as it was back then, the living room is turned into an office.

Ellen Mercer has been so much part of the story of the fight against the political abuse of psychiatry that she is almost a personification of it. She was involved in the American Psychiatric Association's international activities since 1979, when the new Medical Director, Melvin Sabshin, offered her the opportunity of developing this new program that subsequently evolved into the Office of International Affairs. She became the Director of the office and the epitome of international psychiatry. With her humor, loud and contagious laugh, and her radiant white hair, she was and is a person not to be missed, loved by many, and feared by others because of her strong opinions, sharp tongue and inability to stay silent when something happened that went against her convictions. Hence her stance regarding the political abuse of psychiatry in the Soviet Union, and on human rights in psychiatry in general. She never hid her views, even in communication with those who disagreed with her fundamentally.

The first time we met was in spring 1983 at a dinner in Geneva, Switzerland, at the home of Professor Charles Durand, one of the most prominent Swiss psychiatrists at that time who was involved in the international campaign against the political use of psychiatry. She had traveled to Geneva for another meeting and, coincidentally, our group met almost at the same time, and so she was asked to join our strategy-planning meeting. From that moment onwards, Ellen Mercer became increasingly involved in the planning and execution of the campaign and gradually turned into our "secret weapon. "What the others did not know, however, was that she was our secret service, our ears and eyes. As Director for International Affairs of the APA, she participated in most meetings, had direct access to internal documents of the WPA and knew exactly who was taking which position."[89]

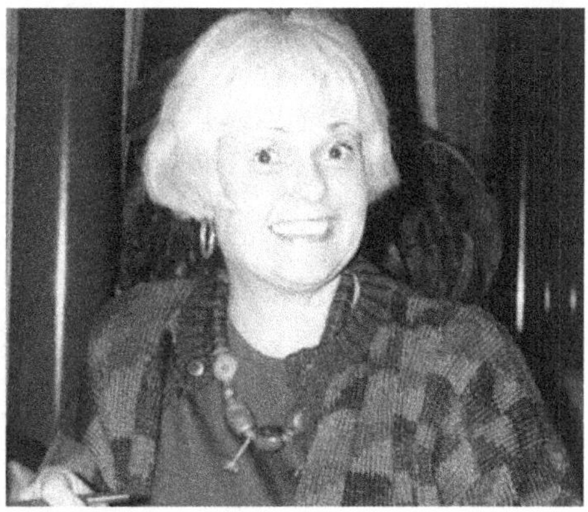
Ellen Mercer 1983

Ellen Mercer joined the American Psychiatric Association in 1975, about half a year after Melvin Sabshin became Medical Director. Until then she had been working for the U.S. Agency for International Development, which was actually a front for the CIA. She had been recruited while a student at Florida Southern College, and subsequently lived abroad for four years, first in Laos and then in Taiwan, as a CIA operative.[90] Upon coming back to

89 *On Dissidents and Madness*, pp. 64-65

90 Ellen Mercer never mentioned her work for the CIA openly, although quite a few people suspected it. The way I found out was when we went out for a walk in the mid-1990s, and when driving past the gates of the CIA complex at Langley she said: "My, have I passed these gates often." However, WPA General Secretary Fini Schulsinger knew about the fact that Ellen Mercer had been with the CIA and warned Jochen Neumann from the very start that Ellen Mercer had a CIA connection. The question is from which source he had this information. Interestingly, the second warning that Mercer had a CIA connection (in the past) came from the Stasi, and Neumann always assumed that was still the case. Interview Ellen Mercer, Jochen Neumann and Melvin Sabshin, December 2, 2009.

the United States she left the CIA, not something they particularly liked. "I was supposed to go through all kinds of psychological tests and debriefing programs, but I just told them I wouldn't and that was it."[91] After looking around a bit she applied for a job at the American Psychiatric Association (APA), which was meant to be a temporary one to help her reorient herself. "I never worked in a non-governmental organization before," she recalls, "and I had no idea what was expected of me, how things worked."[92] Her experience of living abroad was probably one of the reasons Melvin Sabshin hired her in the first place, because he had been instrumental in helping the Thai to set up a Medical School in Chang Mai, Thailand, and so here was a common interest. In fact, Ellen was the first person Melvin Sabshin hired when his tenure as Medical Director started.[93]

With Ellen Mercer as Director of the Office of International Affairs, Melvin Sabshin had a very dedicated associate; she was hardworking, committed, energetic, and determined to do things one hundred percent. Yet having her on staff undoubtedly caused some difficult moments as well, when expressing her views openly or when her views were contrary to those of Melvin Sabshin. The only time they really clashed, though, was in 1990 when the Soviets were preparing to send a psychiatric delegation to the United States and Ellen found the names of some psychiatrists on the list that were alleged to have been involved in psychiatric abuse issues. She objected to them being invited, but Melvin asked her not to interfere. She couldn't resist telling him, though, and also expressed her concerns about the composition of the group when a reporter asked her about her opinion. The man explored the issue, wrote an article, and the result was that one of the main donors pulled out, leaving Mel Sabshin livid.[94] The delegation still came to the U.S. but without those of suspicious backgrounds. It was a clash, but didn't alter their relationship based on trust, friendship, and him allowing her to follow her conscience and deal with human rights issues whenever she deemed necessary.

It is a rare quality, when a person is able to be direct and outspoken, not afraid to say things that might not be popular, and still be liked by all sides. In Ellen Mercer's case, this was reality: all sides considered her to be a friend, an ally. Marat Vartanyan, the skillful lobbyist of Soviet psychiatry and the Number One apologist of Soviet psychiatric abuse, circled around her like a Don Juan, charming and flirting, trying to show the world how

91 Interview with Ellen Mercer, June 27, 2009
92 Interview with Ellen Mercer, June 28, 2009
93 Interview with Ellen Mercer, June 27, 2009
94 Interview with Ellen Mercer, June 27, 2009

close they were, although time and again Ellen would tell him how much she disagreed with the things he stood for. One time he complained to her, after some people had visited him in Moscow and had informed him that Ellen had told a lot of bad things about him. "Why are you telling people bad things about me," he lamented, putting up an innocent face. "I don't know who you are talking about," Ellen responded. "Besides, I tell so many people bad things about you that I can't keep track of them." She admitted, however, that she was fascinated by his ability to navigate the criticism and to play all sides in his favor.[95] Also within the WPA, Ellen Mercer was respected, and was on good terms with most of the members of the Executive Committee. Even in one of the Stasi reports, she is mentioned as a "highly intelligent, good looking and charming woman with an enormous persistence…" as well as the person who is "responsible for the foreign policy of the APA."[96]

Among the global circle of psychiatrists, Ellen was the face of American psychiatry. Foreigners visiting the APA Annual Meetings all flocked to her hospitality suite, where she would welcome the foreign guests, help them out when problems occurred, feed them lunch and drinks at the end of the day. The hospitality suite was the place where the action was, where you could meet people from all parts of the world – and all saw Ellen Mercer as their friend. Even now, over ten years after Ellen left the APA, wherever you go many middle- aged psychiatrists will start smiling when they hear her name, and remember the days the Annual Meeting of the American Psychiatric Association was the main event in world psychiatry.

When Melvin Sabshin left the American Psychiatric Association in 1997, Ellen Mercer stayed on, but not for long. Sabshin's successor, Steve Mirin, had no interest in international affairs and, in general, tried to make a clean break with Sabshin's legacy. In establishing his control over the organization, he removed everybody who had been part of Sabshin's team, and Ellen was no exception. In November 1999, she was told to clear out her desk and be gone before the end of the year. Many organizations and persons protested, including the Geneva Initiative on Psychiatry, of which I was General Secretary. In a letter to Dr. Mirin we wrote: "For many - if not most - international contacts of the APA, the organization's values were embodied in the person of Mrs. Mercer, who not only shared but also empowered this commitment to strive for a humane and ethical psychiatry. Her presence at international psychiatric meetings (and certainly not only at APA Annual

95 Interview with Ellen Mercer, June 27, 2009

96 HAXX 1386/1 p. 41

Meetings) gave this conviction a face and a voice and I am convinced that many people credited the APA for their support during difficult moments because Mrs. Mercer was there, ready to help and support, whenever needed. ... The main issue is, that an organization capable of dumping a person just a few months away from the 25th anniversary of employment with the organization in the rudest possible manner and without even offering the chance to negotiate a fair and generous compensation, is clearly an organization that no longer values human beings and human dignity - and is certainly not the organization that played such a prominent role in the fight against the political abuse of psychiatry."[97]

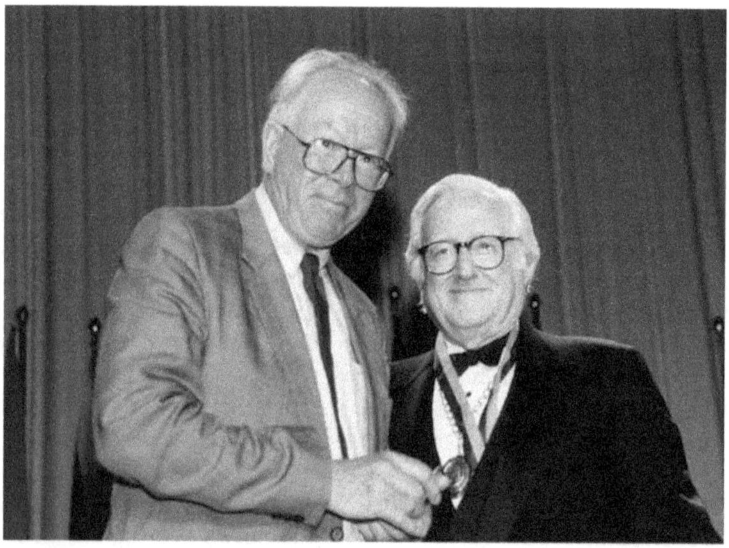

Jim Birley receives his Distinguished Medal from APA

For Jim Birley, a Past President of the British Royal College of Psychiatrists and at that moment Chairman of the Geneva Initiative on Psychiatry, the decision of Steve Mirin to dismiss Ellen Mercer was reason enough to send back his Medal as a Distinguished Fellow of the APA, a move that left a lot of people flabbergasted. He was one out of many who were appalled by the decision, and who had seen and admired Ellen Mercer's work in the international arena.

[97] Letter to Dr. Steve Mirin, December 1, 1999

Chapter 11 - The Shield and Sword of the Party

I will repeat once again: we need to know everything! Nothing should go unnoticed by us.

Erich Mielke, 1981

The German Democratic Republic (Deutsche Demokratische Republik, DDR) was founded in October 1949 in a fundamentally hostile environment and was, from the very start, in need of a service that would guarantee its security. The Eastern part of Germany had been considerably pro-Nazi during the national-socialist regime of 1933-1945, and many of its citizens saw the demise of the Third Reich as a failure, not as liberation from Fascism. Thus, the relationship between the government, which mostly consisted of people who themselves had been traumatized by their incarceration in concentration camps under the Nazi regime or who had survived the Holocaust, and a population that did not share their sense of victory, was tense. This is probably one of the explanations of how it is possible that former victims of a dictatorial Nazi regime eventually became rulers of a dictatorial state.[98]

Also, the Eastern German zone fell under Soviet rule, and the Marshall Plan that was pumped into the American, British and French zones in order to get Germany back on its feet, was inaccessible to them.[99] The difference in poverty and economic growth increased considerably, with Eastern

98 The almost automatic reaction is to call the DDR a totalitarian state, like the other state in Eastern Europe and the USSR. Yet many of my interlocutors, former citizens of the DDR, do not fully agree that it just totalitarian; for them it was a state that was designed to be democratic but that because of both external and internal circumstances became dictatorial, "paranoid". The system of involving citizens in all levels of society soon became a system of total control over its population, yet they assert that this was not the original goal of this system of government. The outcome, though, had all the elements of a totalitarian state.

99 The Marshall Plan was the primary plan of the United States for rebuilding and creating a stronger foundation for the countries of Western Europe, and repelling communism after World War II. The initiative was named for Secretary of State George Marshall. The reconstruction plan, developed at a meeting of the participating European states, was established on June 5, 1947. It offered the same aid to the USSR and its allies, but they did not accept it. The plan was in operation for four years beginning in April 1948. During that period, some USD 13 billion in economic and technical assistance was given to help the recovery of the European countries that had joined in the Organization for European Economic Co-operation. By the time the plan had come to completion, the economy of every participant state, with the exception of Germany, had grown well past pre-war levels.

Germany lagging more and more behind especially because the Soviets, instead of rebuilding the economy, dismantled much of what was left of the German economic power and shipped the machinery to the Soviet Union as war reparations. During the early stages of the occupation (in particular 1945 and 1946), the Red Army seized around a third of the remaining industrial equipment from Eastern Germany to be shipped back to the Soviet Union, with a further 10 billion dollars in reparations extracted by the early 1950s in the form of agricultural and industrial products. [100]

In the perspective of the East German leadership, the Western allied zones became increasingly hostile. Travel between the Western and Soviet zones was unrestricted and large numbers of citizens living in the Soviet zone (*Sowjetische Besatzungszone*, SBZ) made their way to the Western zones, ridding the Eastern part of many of its skilled laborers and higher educated people. And, of course, Western infiltrations into the Eastern part became more and more frequent, thereby contributing to the sense of unsafety and thus the desire to arm itself against foreign influences. The result was a state that craved a system that would keep the enemies at bay, and the Ministry of State Security (*Ministerium für Staatssicherheit*, MfS, or Stasi) had to provide that service.

With the above in mind, it is not strange that almost from the very start the DDR depended heavily on a wide network of informers and secret agents. Undoubtedly, the fact that the country had not known any democratic state structure since 1933 also played a role. In particular, the population showed its widespread discontent on June 17, 1953 with an uprising caused by an increase of labor production quotas by 10%. This uprising resulted in a paranoid atmosphere, in which the DDR State declared itself as being good and progressive with the opposing side being bad, reactionary and asocial. The State tried to establish a society in which there was no conflict, where all shared the same values. The result was a collective regression, with a State that centered its attention on the division between Good ("us") and Bad ("they") and the fear that Bad would penetrate its society and cause this much-feared conflict. In the eyes of the ruling Party the only way to defend society against this outer threat was by building an ever-expanding system of spying on its on citizens.

The Stasi

When the *Ministerium für Staatssicherheit (*MfS, or Stasi) was founded in February 1950, it was immediately instituted as the "*Schild und*

[100] *The Russians in Germany*, p. 167-9

Schwert der Partei" (the Shield and Sword of the Party) and was directly responsible to the SED, the ruling Socialist Unity Party. As it was not subordinate to any Ministry, it fell also outside Parliamentary control. At the beginning, approximately 1,000 agents staffed the organization, but that number grew very quickly, in particular after the June 1953 uprising that resulted in more than a million DDR citizens on strike and demonstrations in 700 communities. This came quite unexpectedly for the Stasi and the SED leadership. The Soviet Army quelled the uprising, and thousands of people were imprisoned. Following this event, which clearly showed the lack of control over society, the MfS was temporarily subordinated to the Ministry of Internal Affairs and carefully reorganized before being turned into a separate Ministry again two years later. Erick Mielke would lead the organization from 1957, when it became independent again, until 1989, when the Berlin Wall came down.[101]

The number of persons involved with the Stasi grew enormously over the years, as a result of the ever-expanding spying system, and eventually reached more than a quarter of a million. In the middle of the 1950s already 20-30,000 persons were registered as "*Inoffiziele Mitarbeiter*"(unofficial agents, IM).[102] In 1989, with a total population of approximately 16 million citizens,[103] 91,000 persons were working full-time for the Stasi, while 174,000 persons were functioning as unofficial agents (IM). The maximum number of persons working as IM for the Stasi was in 1975, with approximately 180,000 persons spying for the organization. In total, about 600,000 persons worked for the Stasi during the forty years of its existence.[104] In addition, the MfS had a near-perfect system of controlling communications between DDR-citizens and communication with foreigners. It systematically checked letters and parcels, telephone calls and telegrams, in particular in case of communication with individuals abroad. In 1989 in East Berlin alone, 20,000 phone conversations were tapped simultaneously.[105]

101 Kerz-Rühling, I., and Plänkers, Th., *Verräter oder Verführte*, p.11. This book is authored by a group of psychoanalysts and probably the most interesting and insightful book on the issue that I read in preparation of this book.

102 Gieseke, J.: *Der Mielke Konzern*, p. 112

103 The East German population declined steadily throughout its existence, from 19 million in 1948 to 16 million in 1990.

104 ibid. Gieseke mentions 173,000 IM in 1988/1989. *Der Mielke Konzern*, p. 115

105 *Der Mielke Konzern*, p. 158. Jens Gieseke also compared the size of the East German security agencies with that of West Germany, including border control, police, etc. He reports that the intelligence agencies in total had 15,500 people working for them, while the MfS had 91,000 official agents employed. In total, taking all agencies together, the security agencies had one agent for 77 citizens in East Germany, and one agent for 241 citizens in West Germany. See

The Stasi had multiple tasks, including those that in other societies would be delegated to the police or other institutions. The organization was responsible for control over the economy, over mail and other means of communication, passport control at the borders of the DDR, control of tourism, fighting terror, espionage and counter-espionage, and the control of (potential) enemies of the state and hostile organizations.[106] At the same time, the MfS infiltrated most sectors of society, including the police, army and other services that were supposed to be part of the system to maintain control over society. The only part of society that was "off limits" to the MfS was the leadership of the SED, a ban that was established unequivocally in 1954.[107]

Who worked for the Stasi and why?

The network of *Inoffizielle Mitarbeiter* (IM) formed an essential part of the control system that the Stasi had in place in the DDR. According to guideline 1/79 of December 1979 they formed the "main weapon against the enemy."[108] In a thesis for the MfS University in Potsdam-Eiche, three Stasi officers explained why the IM were so important: "The ability to penetrate into the thoughts of others can only be accomplished by other human beings. In the time of modern technology there is, in spite of highly developed machinery and mechanisms that facilitate the physical and mental tasks of human beings, nothing that nears the ability of man to research the train of thoughts of other human beings. ... There is no equal replacement of the *Inoffizielle Mitarbeiter* who are active in this direction, and there won't be either."[109]

The term "*Inoffizieller Mitarbeiter*" was part of the "clean" vocabulary that had been developed, and which "cleansed" the actual work from its unpleasant features. In the early days, collaborators of the service had been called "*Geheimer Informator*" (secret informer, GI), or "*Geheimer Mitarbeiter*" (secret collaborator, GM). The task of the GI was to keep his or her ears and eyes open and report anything suspicious; the GM

Der Mielke Konzern, p. 107. As far as the KGB is concerned, for instance, its size of official agents and collaborators remains unclear, and the same counts for its successor Federal'naya Sluzhba Bezopasnosti (FSB). The number of personnel and its budget remain state secrets; according to unconfirmed sources the budget jumped nearly 40% in 2006.

106 *Verräter oder Verführte*, p.12

107 *Der Mielke Konzern*, p. 149

108 Müller-Engbergs, *Inoffizielle Mitarbeiter*, p. 305

109 *Der Mielke Konzern*, p. 112

also carried out "active" secret tasks. In 1968, this all changed and the vocabulary was altered. Instead of "advances in career" or "financial advantages," they now referred to "personal or material interests;" instead of being forced to collaborate, it was now called "implementation of the desire to compensate."[110]

Although an unexpectedly high number of DDR-citizens worked officially and unofficially for the Stasi, it seems that many of the IM did not realize at that time how large the organization actually was. In fact, after *Die Wende,* they were just as surprised as the rest of the population.[111] Also, many of the IM downplayed the effect of their work. For the psychoanalytic study, *Verräter oder Verführte,* twenty former Stasi agents were interviewed, and their answers carefully analyzed. Many indicated that they either did not realize the consequences of their informing upon others, or had the feeling that they belonged to the "chosen ones" and, hence, had a sense of superiority or importance. One former IM even says: "By the way, the Stasi, I have to admit, did not seem like a secret service to me, for me it was more like a hidden arm of the Party. And everything I would have talked about anyway, I told them as well. Only this time one had to write it down, that was the only difference."[112]
At the same time, even though the number of people involved in Stasi work was enormous, it was all very carefully regulated. The Stasi was allergic to "spontaneous" spying by DDR-citizens, information that came to them directly without any structured basis of collaboration. This "allergy" grew over the years; at first "spontaneous denunciations" were still used. In 1955, 60% of the cases were still the result of "spontaneous denunciations," while only 20% were the result of IM activity.[113] Still, many of the spontaneous denunciations were probably not coming from the general population, as the distrust towards the Stasi was huge. In a report from Neubrandenburg, it is written that "the work of the Ministry of State Security is, at this time, very much hampered by the distrust of the people, who compare the MfS with the Gestapo and the SD. The distrust directed towards the power structures of Fascism is transferred to the MfS."[114]

In Nazi-times, the Gestapo had worked quite a bit with such "spontaneous collaboration," which often constituted information by neighbors or others in the environment of the victim who used this means to settle old scores

110 *Der Mielke Konzern*, p. 112-113
111 *Verräter oder Verführte*, p.13
112 *Verräter oder Verführte*, p. 62
113 *Der Mielke Konzern*, p. 124
114 *Der Mielke Konzern*, p. 124-125

or problems at work or in the family. In fact, the Gestapo had never been a large organization and very much depended on collaboration with other bodies, e.g. the police and the NSDAP and its daughter organizations. Approximately 60-80 percent of the "cases" initiated against citizens were the result of spontaneous denunciations by citizens (quite similar to the figure in the DDR in 1955, ten years after the war). Often these were based on citizens using the Gestapo to settle disputes with others, for instance a renter against his landlord, a worker against his boss, or inter-family disputes. On the basis of research, experts conclude that in Nazi-Germany, 5-10 percent of the population was either willing to denounce fellow-citizens, or actually did so in practice. It was this low threshold for people to denounce others that made the Gestapo terror so successful: everybody was a potential victim, one never knew who would be next. [115]

The Stasi eventually worked quite differently, carefully selecting its collaborators and, only after careful screening, signed a contract stipulating the conditions of its "collaboration." Why the Stasi did not make use of "spontaneous denunciations" is a matter of debate. Some say it was because it was a highly organized system, others maintain that the distance between the regime and the population was much larger than in Nazi times and the support for the regime much less. As a result, there needed to be a formal way to connect people to the service and make sure they would deliver the necessary information to keep the population under control.[116] This argument seems a strange one, though, considering the fact that the main reason for working with the Stasi appears to have been the political convictions of the persons concerned. As Gieseke notes in his book, the majority basically believed in the essence of the socialist idea, in the legitimacy of defending the system against outside enemies and in assisting peace within society and between nations through the unofficial collaboration with the MfS. [117] In 1967 in Potsdam, 60% of the IM questioned during an internal investigation mentioned the "recognition of societal obligation" as main reasons for collaboration, while 49% mentioned a "sense of moral duty and conscience."[118] And, finally, also in the field of State security the plan economy did its work and defined targets had to be met. With the goal of increasing the number of agents (for instance in the mid 1970s), many people were recruited who were actually not of very high value. It was the numbers that counted, not the quality.[119]

115 *Der Mielke Konzern*, p. 117-119
116 *Der Mielke Konzern*, p. 121
117 *Der Mielke Konzern*, p. 126
118 *Der Mielke Konzern*, p. 127
119 *Der Mielke Konzern*, p. 122

The organization issued a large number of internal directives regulating the acquisition of unofficial collaborators, as well as the way they should be prepared for their task and how communication should be maintained. The latest version of this directive dates from 1979, in which the unofficial collaborators (IM) were described as "The main arm in the fight against the enemy," who should contribute to "the warranty of the DDR and the strengthening of socialist society."[120] In the same year, a profile for the IM was developed in order to form the basis of future acquisition of Stasi collaborators. This profile discussed all aspects, such as age, professional position, family circumstances, personal abilities as well as issues dealing with political convictions and the person's character. Interestingly, it specified that important character traits of the future IM should be **honesty**, **reliability** and **flexibility**, while at the same time it stipulated that in order to be an effective spy, the person should be dishonest and betray. [121]

The latter is of great importance, as the service seems to have been very effective in disconnecting the spying, in general, from the effects of the spying on other people.[122] By doing so, they limited the possibility of a conflict of conscience, but also helped their informers create for themselves the impression that what they did was not so important. Some believed in the system and saw it as their duty to defend Socialism against attacks from the capitalist West; others were critical of the system as such but still found for themselves an excuse to downplay their secret activities. One of the interviewees in the study *Varräter oder Verführte* says, that there "was a huge difference between my memories and what was written [in his Stasi file]..." he continues: "I didn't know my cover name anymore, and I didn't know what would happen [with my information] after that? With a written statement, signed or not, I read it for the first time in my file. … And there was at that moment a huge shock."[123] Other interviewees indicated that they had no idea what happened with the information they provided, and when they found out, they either felt a deep sense of shame or tried to rationalize the consequences: "When something came from any useful conversations, I told that they could also have found that out in a café where they might be sitting."[124]

---

120 *Verräter oder Verführte*, p. 13

121 *Verräter oder Verführte*, p.14

122 According to the authors of *Verräter oder Verführte* about half of the interviewees had no idea what happened with the information they gathered and also did not try to find out. See page 143.

123 *Verräter oder Verführte*, p. 77

124 *Verräter oder Verführte*, pp. 65, 143.

Other agents started feeling inner conflicts when they developed sympathy for the persons they had to spy on which, in some cases, became a strong complicating factor. "...When we started to like each other, it became, of course, even more difficult. I liked him, and he liked me. ... As the months went by, an attitude developed – and I thought to myself: shit, you now have problems in both directions. Because of the man opposite me, I have a conflict of conscience because what I am doing is not good and, in the other direction, I have fear. It was a funny mixture of feelings." The situation became even more complicated when the person this IM had to observe started sharing forbidden literature: "For me getting to know this man opened new worlds to me that I had not known before, and that actually fit quite nicely in my own political thinking with regard to this system."[125] In some cases, the change of heart caused the IM agent to start defending the person he was supposed to inform upon, hiding the real state of affairs and filing reports with useless information.

Recruitment

In recruiting agents, the MfS was able to make use of a number of important factors. First of all, the people who grew up in the Nazi period of 1933-1945 or, after, in the DDR, had no experience of living in an open and democratic society where developing one's own opinion and position would have been possible. The nature of the system prevented many, if not most, people from developing their own autonomous and self-confident personalities. In addition, since in all sectors of society a culture of dependence was promoted (school, youth movement, army, work place), it was therefore easier for a DDR citizen to follow the instructions of a "*Führungsoffizier,*" a Stasi agent who worked as a case-manager for the unofficial associate, the IM. This "*Führungsoffizier*" had received special education in operational psychology and had the task of developing a relationship of trust. He was supposed to become a friend and helper, and in many cases became a father figure, often filling the gap of an absent parent. Much time and effort was put in the development of such a relationship. "They weren't the types that one might imagine now, vulgar and despicable people, who only want to dig into bad things," one former IM said in an interview. "Instead they sometimes took a lot of time to talk with me about politics and life and about studies, and what I expected from life and so on. For me it was also a possibility to have interesting conversations."[126] Also, many of the recruited agents came from broken families, often with a father absent as a result

125 *Verräter oder Verführte*, p. 201-202

126 *Verräter oder Verführte*, p. 134

of the Second World War or because of divorce, and many were under considerable psychological pressure. In the analysis of twenty former Stasi IM agents, Ingrid Kerz-Rühling and Tomas Plänkers found a whole series of traumatic experiences among the interviewees, including sexual abuse, physical abuse during youth, alienation from one or both parents, and/or insufficient care during childhood. Even among those who were not traumatized in such a way, the authors found that more than half of them suffered from disturbances in the ability to develop full relations with other people.[127] It does not need much argumentation to conclude that as a result of these factors, recruitment became much easier, as the defense mechanism of the persons concerned was either damaged or virtually absent.[128] The Stasi case-managers very cleverly made use of these factors during the implementation of their task. The fact that the Stasi officer fulfilled this "parent role" was also a factor in limiting the feelings of shame or guilt.

Finally, fear of what the consequences would be if one refused to collaborate completes the set of factors that made people agree to collaborate. According to the available data, approximately one-third of the IM candidates turned down the offer to collaborate, and quite often without any serious consequences. The easiest way to get out of an attempt by the Stasi to be recruited was by disclosure, telling the environment what happened. But in some cases even that did not prove enough to get the Stasi off one's back.[129]

However, there was also the category of MfS associates who were proud of the task they had been given and who saw it as their contribution to the Socialist state. They did not suffer from inner conflicts about the work they had been doing. As one former IM put it, "I wanted to do something to help my country, to defend the DDR, to do something against the inhumanity of capitalism, against the warmongering."[130] For them the recruitment by the Stasi was a sign of importance, of recognition of their value to society. It was only logical that they would provide their service to the State.[131] Among those who worked for the HVA, the foreign service of the MfS, these feelings of guilt or conflicts of conscience seemed altogether absent, as they were not spying on people in their own country but recruiting and managing spies abroad.[132]

---

127 *Verräter oder Verführte*, p. 139

128 *Verräter oder Verführte*, p. 231-237

129 *Verräter oder Verführte*, p.14, 17; *Der Mielke Konzern,* p. 132

130 *Verräter oder Verführte*, p. 124

131 *Verräter oder Verführte,* p. 121

132 *Verräter oder Verführte*, p. 127, 140, 143

Also in the case of Jochen Neumann, this appears to have been the case. In our conversations, he makes a major distinction between the work he did as a foreign agent, and the "sniffing around in other people's business" that the IM in the country were doing. With a condescending show of his hands he makes clear what he means: their job was a dirty one, one he doesn't want to have anything to do with.[133]

After a trial period or the fulfillment of a concrete task, the "candidate" became a full-fledged IM. In some cases, this didn't work out either because the person turned out to be dishonest, or untrustworthy, or the information was not of sufficient quality. In the period between 1985 and 1989, about ten percent of the persons initially recruited were not maintained by Stasi, but about the same number of new persons were recruited to fill the empty places.[134]

The Stasi and the medical community

Special attention was given to several sectors of society, which were considered to be of "heightened risk." These included the churches, youth and health care. They all fell under department XX of the MfS. Health was of particular interest, as doctors were considered to belong to a rather conservative and bourgeois sector of society. On top of that, a large number of doctors had fled to the West, so early detection of such plans was of vital importance to the East German health care system. Only when a new generation of "socialist" doctors entered the health care system did the situation improve a little, yet the interest of the MfS remained big and collaboration between the health sector and the Stasi via unofficial agents close.[135] It is, therefore, no miracle that three to five percent of the physicians functioned as IM for the MfS, a considerably higher percentage than the rest of the population.[136] Many of the leading psychiatrists in the DDR were connected to the Stasi.

A thorough study of IM-activity among doctors brought attention to the files of 493 physicians who worked as *Inoffizieller Mitarbeiter*. On the basis of that research, one can conclude that, in most of the cases, the *Führungsoffizier* wrote the reports for the Stasi files based on notes made during meetings with their agents or taped conversations. Apparently, the Stasi understood that

133 Interview with Jochen Neumann, March 26, 2009

134 *Verräter oder Verführte*, p.17

135 *Der Mielke Konzern*, p. 146

136 *Zielgruppe Ärzteschaft*, p. 20

demanding written reports from physicians could be problematic.[137] Studies by the MfS University in Potsdam revealed that the majority of physicians in the DDR were critical or even negative about the concept of a "socialist medical sector" (*sozialistische Ärzteschaft*). Many kept away from politics, even though the medical sector had become "nationalized" like any other sector of society, and, politically, physicians refused to subordinate to the dictates of the Party and officials who did not belong to their profession. According to the same study, the difficult work conditions for doctors in policlinics, as well as the stress caused by insufficient personnel, resulted in a hostile attitude towards the State and the Party.[138]

An important issue in the work of physicians for the Stasi was the issue of medical confidentiality. Legislation in the DDR was not very different than in West Germany, except for the fact that among the crimes that physicians should report to the authorities in case they received information also included "serious political crimes" such as "subversive human trade," serious cases of "subversive agitation" and preparation for "illegal border crossing."[139] However, in the beginning of the 1970s, DDR-lawyers argued that by now a new society had been established in which a "socialist physician" had been formed, whose functioning was based on "a combination of Marxist-Leninist attitude, humanitarian convictions, the use of exact science and a socialist drive to perform." This changed concept of the role of a physician also led to a new view on medical ethics. They argued that the Hippocratic Oath had become particularly important among DDR physicians, because it provided an exemplary model for the socialist physician.[140] In that sense, the position of physicians was still different than in the USSR, where the Hippocratic Oath had been replaced by the Oath of the Soviet Doctor, in which he pledged his first allegiance to the Communist Party and only second to medical ethics.

Still, almost 28 percent of the agents whose cases were studied in "*Zielgruppe Ärzteschaft*" breached the code of medical confidentiality. Some provided detailed reports on their patients or even full medical files. Many of those who delivered these extensive reports were psychiatrists or chief physicians.[141] A very small percentage agreed to work for the MfS

137 *Zielgruppe Ärzteschaft,* p. 31

138 *Zielgruppe Ärzteschaft*, p. 33

139 *Zielgruppe Ärzteschaft*, p. 185-6. Medical confidentiality in the DDR was regulated by article 225 StGB-DDR, comparable to article 138 of the StGB-BRD; The duty to report crimes was regulated in article 226 StGB-DDR.

140 *Zielgruppe Ärzteschaft*, p. 185

141 *Zielgruppe Ärzteschaft*, p. 187. In total 116 of the 418 IM-physicians whose files could be studied breached medical confidentiality.

but stipulated that they could not report on their patients because of the allegiance to the Hippocratic Oath.[142] One doctor informed the Stasi three years after signing an agreement to collaborate that he could not fulfill his obligations because of his professional ethos.[143] Others discontinued their collaboration because of a conflict of conscience, but that was a small percentage.[144] Still, the number of *Inoffizieller Mitarbeiter* who discontinued their collaboration on their own accord was considerably higher than in other professional circles.[145]

One particular case of a physician who had seemingly no problem sharing confidential information on her patients with the Stasi was that of Dr. Gisela Otto, the East-Berlin gynecologist who many years worked for the MfS and infiltrated both the *Deutsche Vereinigung gegen politischen Missbrauch der Psychiatrie* (DVpMP) and the Moscow Working Commission to Investigate the Use of Psychiatry for Political Purposes, with far reaching consequences.[146] She had been a personal acquaintance of Lieutenant Colonel Eberhard Jaekel, head of MfS Chief Directorate XX/1.[147] Their acquaintance dated back to not later than 1973, when they had a conversation about a colleague of hers who had committed suicide; during the conversation, she provided intimate details about the life of the deceased. They together visited the person's office and, at the end, Otto handed Jaekel the complete medical file that she had kept on the deceased. From that moment onwards, Jaekel himself functioned as her *Führungsoffizier*.[148] However, even before,

142 *Zielgruppe Ärzteschaft,* p. 202

143 *Zielgruppe Ärzteschaft*, p. 203

144 *Zielgruppe Ärzteschaft*, p. 219

145 *Zielgruppe Ärzteschaft*, p. 225

146 See chapter 10

147 Eberhard Jaekel, born in 1937 in East Prussia (now Kaliningrad region), since 1955 employed by the MfS, in 1971-1989 head of the Chief Directorate XX/1 of the MfS, member of the SED since 1958. His highest achieved rank was that of lieutenant colonel. See *Politisch Missbraucht*, p. 176. Jaekel was specially interested in the field of medicine and its sub-specialty psychiatry, as can be seen from the title of his dissertation in 1974 when he obtained his degree at the University of the Ministry of State Security (MfS Hochschule): *Regarding some peculiarities to be taken into account during collaboration with unofficial collaborators from the medical intelligentsia in order to heighten the efficacy of their deployment in the fight against subversive attacks by the enemy*". Jaekel maintained close relations with the Minister of Health of the DDR, Dr. Ludwig Mecklinger, the head of the health policy department of the Central Committee Prof. Karl Seidel and the Deputy Minister of Health of the DDR Dr. Rudolf Mueller, all three connected to the MfS in their own right.

148 *Zielgruppe Ärzteschaft*, p. 131

Otto had been functioning as a "contact person," feeding the Stasi for quite some time information on people within the central State apparatus, about extra-marital affairs and marital difficulties. Initially, she had expressed her concern that her violation of medical confidentiality would become public knowledge, but soon she had accepted the provision of information to the Stasi as part of her "work" and urgently and ambitiously asked for a mission.[149] This mission would be the infiltration of the DVpMP and the Moscow Working Commission on the Use of Psychiatry for Political Purposes, a mission she carried out with much success. Her Stasi files show, however, that she herself was recruited because of an extra-marital affair, and was thus hooked, and subsequently found herself sliding into a cycle of deceit and deception. Her seeming enthusiasm was, thus, the result of coercion, rather than conviction.

149 *Zielgruppe Ärzteschaft*, p. 131-2

Chapter 12 – Opposition at Home and Abroad

A scholar, contemporary of Galilei
Was intellectually as smart
He know the world was turning round
But the family had his heart [150]

It seems that evil, the moment it has made itself visible, easily reproduces itself, while good remains difficult, sporadic, fragile. Yet possible.
Tzvetan Todorov

Solid public awareness in the West that Soviet psychiatry might be subject to political abuse came in 1965 with the publication of the book *Ward 7* by Valery Tarsis. Tarsis, a writer born in 1906 in Kiev, wrote his book based on his own experiences in 1962-1963, when he was hospitalized in the Moscow Kashchenko psychiatric hospital for political reasons. In 1966 he was allowed to emigrate to the West, and was soon stripped of his Soviet citizenship.[151]

Soon after the publication of *Ward 7*, a second case of political abuse of psychiatry raised public attention in Britain. A young Moscow interpreter, Evgeni Belov, became friends with a group of four British students by whom he had been contracted as an interpreter. Although at first positive about the Soviet system, he gradually became more critical, and started to voice demand for more freedom. He called for free trade unions, a free press, and started writing letters to the Party. As a result, his Party membership was suspended and he was called to appear before a committee. He refused, and instead sought justice higher up, writing letters of protest to Leonid Brezhnev himself. When the British students returned from a short visit to Tokyo, Belov had disappeared. To their shock, it turned out that he had been interned in a psychiatric hospital. A campaign to get him out provided no results. Instead, in a letter to a British newspaper, Belov's father asserted that his son was really ill, and the campaign slowly ground to a halt. However, the public interest had been triggered.[152]

Also the case of Aleksandr Volpin raises awareness in the West. Volpin, a son of the famous Russian poet Esenin and born in 1924, was first hospitalized

---

150 From *Kak Byt' Svidetel'em* (how to be a Witness), Vladimir Albrekht, a manual how to behave during a KGB interrogation.

151 *Soviet Psychiatric Abuse - Shadow over World Psychiatry,* p. 65-66

152 *Soviet Psychiatric Abuse - Shadow over World Psychiatry*, p. 68-69. The case of Belov was also mentioned in the Soviet propaganda booklet *S Chuzhogo Golosa*, published in Moscow in 1982, p. 39-40

in 1946 in the Leningrad Special Psychiatric Hospital for writing a poem that was considered to be anti-Soviet. Under Khrushchev's reign, he was subsequently hospitalized three times: in 1957, in 1959-1960 again in the Special Psychiatric Hospital of Leningrad and, eventually, in 1962-1963. In 1968, he was hospitalized again, and this time his case reached the attention in the West. After a wave of protests he was released, and allowed to immigrate to the United States, where he became a professor of mathematics.[153]

The case of Volpin also resulted in the first organized protest against the use of psychiatry for political ends. In February 1968, a group of 99 Soviet mathematicians and scientists signed a protest letter to the Soviet authorities, demanding his release. Shortly before, a group of Soviet dissidents had sent an appeal to a conference of communist parties in Budapest, in which they called on the participants "to consider the peril caused by the trampling on human rights in our country." Among the means of persecution, they specifically mentioned political abuse of psychiatry: "the most shocking form of reprisal – forcible confinement in a mental hospital."[154] Some of the signatories to the appeal became founding members of the first organized group of dissidents, the Action Group for the Defense of Human Rights, which was set up in May 1969.

Among the members of the Action Group were people who later fell victim to psychiatric abuse themselves: the poetess Natalya Gorbanevskaya, who in 1968 demonstrated on Red Square against the invasion of Soviet tanks into Czechoslovakia; Vladimir Borisov, the partner of Irina Kaplun,[155]

---

153 *Soviet Psychiatric Abuse - Shadow over World Psychiatry*, p. 70-71. In January 1976 the Central Committee of the Communist Party of the Soviet Union (CPSU) claimed that he had been hospitalized in a psychiatric hospital in Italy during a visit to that country in a message to "fraternal parties", issued to counter "anti-Soviet propaganda". See minutes 201`of the session of the Politburo of the CPSU on January 14, 1976, p.8. The claim was repeated, among others, by Soviet press agencies TASS and Novosti as well as the periodical of the American Communist party *Daily World*, who were subsequently sued by Esenin-Volpin. The case again reached the agenda of the Politburo in January 1977, where it was decided to use diplomatic channels to solve the case and not allow correspondents of TASS or Novosti to show up in court. Report to the Central Committee by Yu. Andropov, V. Kuznetsov, L. Zamyatin and L. Tolkunov, of January 24, 1977.

154 *Soviet Psychiatric Abuse - Shadow over World Psychiatry*, p. 73

155 Irina Kaplun was one of the founding members of the Moscow working Commission to Investigate the Use of Psychiatry for Political Purposes, see later in this chapter

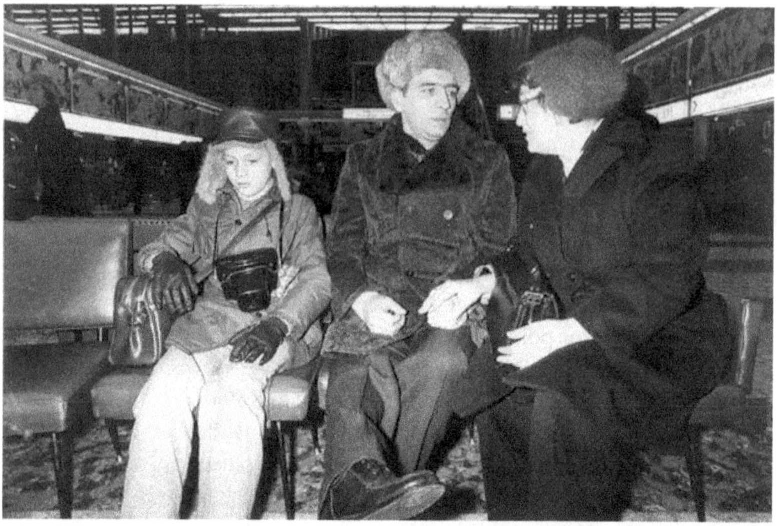

Leonid Plyushch and his family short after his arrival in the West

who later was one of the founders of the independent labor movement in the USSR; Yuri Maltsev, a translator; and Leonid Plyushch, a Ukrainian cyberneticist who later was hospitalized in the Special Psychiatric Hospital of Dnepropetrovsk and was horribly tortured with neuroleptics.[156]

[156] Leonid Plyushch, born in 1939, a Ukrainian cyberneticist, became a dissident in 1968. He was arrested in January 1972 on charges of anti-Soviet activity, and was jailed for a year before his trial began. During his trial, the court sat in camera and in the absence of the accused. Although no expert witnesses of any kind were called, Plyushch was declared insane, and was ordered to be "sent for treatment in a special type of hospital." He was locked up in a ward for severely psychotic patients. In the Dnepropetrovsk Special Psychiatric Hospital where was administered high doses of haloperidol, insulin and other drugs, which temporarily made him incapable of reading and writing. Three commissions that examined him after a year of detention, one of which was chaired by Andrei Snezhnevsky, found him suffering from "reformist delusions" with "Messianic elements" and "sluggish schizophrenia." After strong international protects and an intervention by the French Communist leader George Marchais he was allowed to leave the Soviet Union together with his family in 1976. The involvement of the French Communist Party in the case of Plyushch, as well as the concerns voiced by the Italian Communist Party over the persecution of dissidents in the USSR, led to a memorandum of KGB Chairman Yuri Andropov to the Central Committee asking for active measures to explain the fraternal French and Italian parties their misunderstanding of the real situation. Memorandum 3213-A of December 29, 1975, signed by Yuri Andropov and marked "top secret."

The international community becomes involved

In the late 1960s-early 1970s, several well-known cases resulted in a further increase in public concern over the issue. Within a relatively short period of time, the West was informed about a number of psychiatric hospitalizations of well-known dissidents: first of General Pyotr Grigorenko in 1969, and then of the well-known biologist Zhores Medvedev in 1970. Grigorenko had earlier been hospitalized in 1964 after criticizing the Soviet Politburo for having wandered away from the real Marxism-Leninism. In May 1969, he was again arrested during a short stay in Tashkent because of his dissident activity and accused of "slandering the Soviet state" (art. 190-1 of the Criminal Code of the RSFSR). Although at first a commission of psychiatrists in Tashkent declared him mentally healthy, he was subsequently transferred to the Serbski Institute in Moscow and declared to be of unsound mind. He spent 40 months in the Special Psychiatric Hospital in Chernyakhovsk and in an ordinary psychiatric hospital outside Moscow.[157]

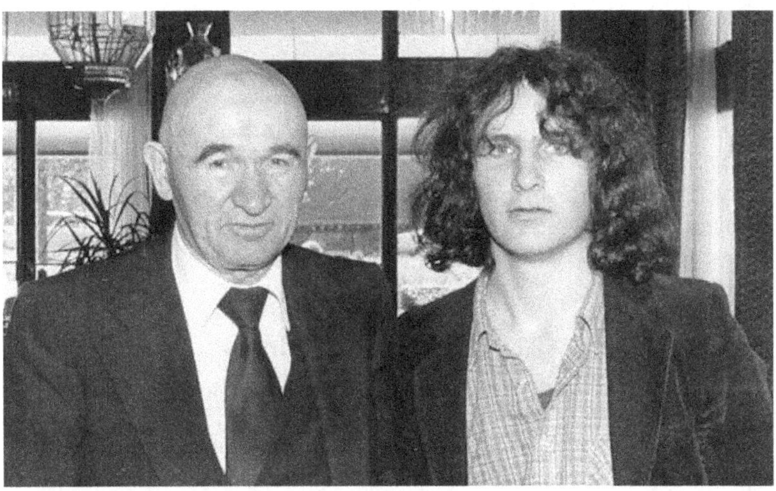

Pyotr Grigorenko with the author, 1981

Zhores Medvedev spent only nineteen days in involuntary confinement, but the fact that well-respected scientists like Andrei Sakharov and Pyotr Kapitsa

[157] Grigorenko's second arrest and hospitalization was mainly because of his defense of the Crimean Tartars, a nation that had been deported from the Crimea by Stalin because of its alleged ": collaboration with the Nazi Germans." A full account of the Grigorenko case can be found in Grigorenko: *Errinerungen*, pp. 352-376 and pp. 484-496.

leapt to his defense and the wide publicity surrounding it did the Soviet authorities much damage.[158] And, to make things worse, in the summer of 1970 the American broadcasting corporation CBS aired an interview with Moscow dissident Vladimir Bukovsky, who himself had been a victim of political abuse of psychiatry and who for the first time tried to explain why dissenters were put in psychiatric hospitals: "The fact is that the inmates, the patients in the hospital, the prisoners, are people who have done things which from the point of view of the authorities are crimes but which are not criminal from the point of view of the law. And in order in some way to isolate them, to punish them somehow, such people are declared insane and are detained as patients in these prison mental hospitals."[159]

As a result of the growing numbers of dissidents winding up in psychiatric hospitals the protests in the West grew and eventually culminated into a campaign to end this abuse of the psychiatric profession. In 1971, Vladimir Bukovsky sent a file of 150 pages documenting the political abuse of psychiatry to the West. For the first time, Western psychiatrists could study copies of the psychiatric diagnoses by Soviet psychiatrists involved in the abuse and learn the details of their diagnostic methods. The documents were accompanied by a letter by Bukovsky asking Western psychiatrists to study the six cases documented in the file and say whether these people should be hospitalized or not. A group of British psychiatrists examined the file and concluded: "It seems to us that the diagnoses of the six people were made purely as a consequence of actions in which they were exercising fundamental freedoms..."[160] They suggested that the issue be discussed during the upcoming World Congress of the WPA in November 1971 in Mexico.

However, such discussion was not to take place. Although the President of the Congress, Dr. Ramon de la Fuente, referred to documents that had been received about some places in the world where political opposition was treated as mental illness, and he argued that "to keep silent about such an ignominious situation would weigh heavily on our conscience",[161] his words found no echo in the WPA General Secretary, Dr. Denis Leigh.[162] Leigh had

---

[158] See Roy and Zhores Medvedev: *Wie is er Gek (Who is Crazy)*. Andrei Sakharov (1921-1989), famous Soviet dissident and the 1975 recipient of the Nobel Peace Prize; Pyotr Kapitsa (1894-1984), physicist and Nobel laureate, member of the Presidium of the Soviet Academy of Sciences)

[159] *Soviet Psychiatric Abuse - Shadow over World Psychiatry*, p. 77

[160] *The Times*, November 16, 1971

[161] *Mexico City News*, 13 November 1971

[162] Dr. Denis Leigh (1916-1998) qualified from Manchester in 1939 and became

already informed Snezhnevsky of the complaints and had sent the latter the "Bukovsky Papers," and laid out his position with regard to the WPA's obligations: "Nowhere in the statutes is there any mention of the WPA making itself responsible for the ethical aspects of psychiatry, nor is there any relevant statute or by-law relating to complaints made by one member society against another member society. I think it is legally quite clear that the WPA is under no obligation to accept complaints from one member society directed against another member society."[163] According to him, the only thing the WPA could do was to refer the cases to the relevant member society, in this case the Soviet All-Union Society of Neuropathologists and Psychiatrists, which is exactly what he had done.

Leigh's interpretation of the WPA Statutes was tendentious, to say the least, because one of the purposes of the organization as set out in its statutes was "to promote activities designed to lead to increased knowledge in the field of illness and better care for the mentally ill." However, the Committee did not dispute Leigh's interpretation of the statutes, and, as a result, it was clear that there would be no debate in the WPA's General Assembly.[164] Three days later, Leigh suggested establishing a committee to

---

Medical Doctor in 1947. Two years later he was appointed consultant to the Bethlem Royal and Maudsley Hospitals in London. During the Second World War he served first as a regimental medical officer and then specialized in neurology. By the end of the war he was adviser in neurology to the eastern army in India. He maintained his military connections and served as Honorary Consultant to the British Army until 1980. Dr. Leigh is author of over 300 scientific publications, and his interest in the history of psychiatry led to him early psychiatric books and manuscripts. In 1961 he wrote The *Historical Development of British Psychiatry,* which deals with the 18th and 19th centuries. From 1966-78 he was Secretary General of the World Psychiatric Association. Leigh was one of the strongest defenders of the Soviet All-Union Society and actively fought the condemnation and subsequent isolation of Soviet psychiatry, making himself quite unpopular with his brusque behavior. Melvin Sabshin remembers how appalled he was when he overhead Leigh making anti-Semitic jokes with some Russian psychiatrists (interview with Ellen Mercer, Jochen Neumann and Melvin Sabshin, December 2, 2009). In the IAPUP files I coincidentally found letters from Leigh dating back to 1988, ordering books on the issue of Soviet psychiatric abused published by the organization, showing his continued interest in the issue.

163 Minutes of the WPA Committee Meeting, November 28, 1971

164 A document by the KGB dated June 2, 1972, to fraternal intelligence services and marked "SECRET", reports that the Soviets effectively managed to block the "provocation" at the Mexico World Congress of the WPA. "At a press-conference, our psychiatric experts convincingly proved that not one mentally healthy person could be interned in a psychiatric hospital in the USSR; in de-

consider the ethical aspects of psychiatric practice, but also in this case no mention was made of the issue of political abuse of psychiatry in the Soviet Union. Soviet psychiatrist Marat Vartanyan, by then already one of the main apologists of Soviet psychiatric abuse, was even elected as associate secretary of the Executive Committee. A day after the Mexico Congress, he stated publicly "the nature of our [socio-political] system is such that this could not possibly happen."[165]

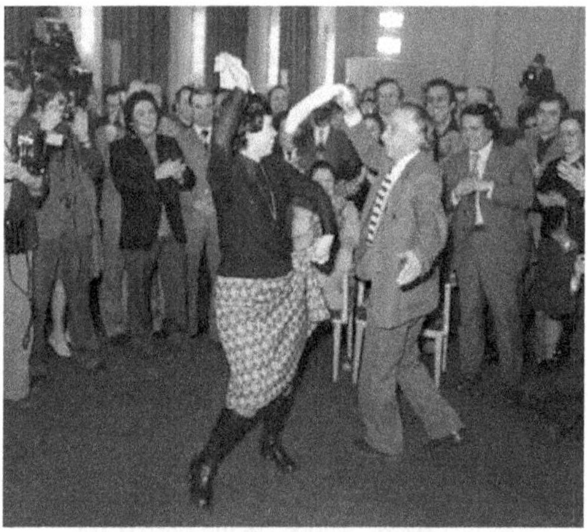

Luis Corvalan dancing the tango in East Berlin, early 1977

The failure to discuss this issue opened the door for the Soviet authorities to sentence Vladimir Bukovsky to twelve years in camp and exile, and to increase the use of psychiatry as a means of repression. In the 1970s, approximately a quarter to one-third of Soviet dissidents were sent to psychiatric hospitals rather than to prison, camps or exile. Vladimir Bukovsky himself was eventually exchanged for the Chilean Communist Party leader Luis Corvalan.[166]

Opposition at home

By the middle of the 1970s, dozens of dissident groups had been set up in the Soviet Union. Since 1975, when the Helsinki Accords on European Security and Cooperation were signed that formalized détente and at the same time guaranteed the human rights of all citizens in Europe and North America, a whole mosaic of dissident organizations was formed in the USSR.[167] In

tail the fundamentals of Soviet legality in connection with the hospitalization of mental patients were explained, in other words the essence of the anti-Soviet propaganda was exposed." See MfS-HAXX, 2941, pp. 9-14

165 Reuter report, Mexico City, December 2, 1971. For more information on Marat Vartanyan see chapter 19, "Soviet Actors".

166 The exchange took place at Zürich airport on December 18, 1976, and was the first high-level exchange between a Soviet political prisoner and a figure imprisoned in the West that was of sufficient interest to the Soviet authorities. Bukovsky currently lives in the United Kingdom.

167 The Helsinki Accords had a "Third Basket" hat focused entirely on human

some republics, such as Estonia, Latvia, Lithuania and Ukraine, dissident groups often had a nationalist character, with the goal of either defending their cultural autonomy or striving for their lost independence. Other groups defended the rights of the disabled, of religious denominations, free trade unionism or feminism. The Helsinki Groups, founded in 1975 in many of the Soviet republics, specifically focused on the implementation of the Helsinki Accords. That year, 1975, turned out to be a special one for the dissident movement, as Academician Andrei Sakharov, its unelected but also undisputed leader, was honored with the Nobel Peace Prize.

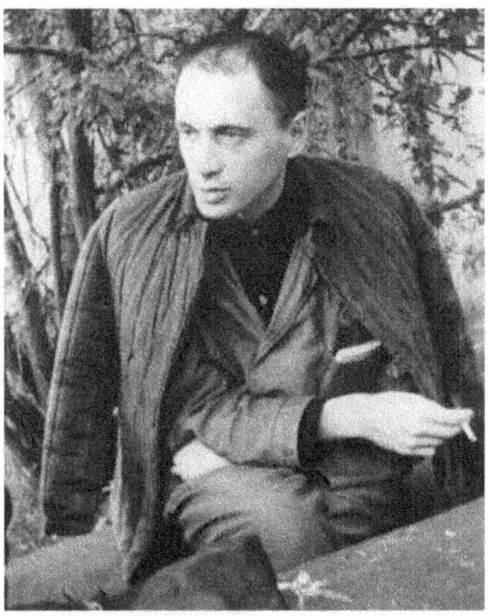

Semyon Gluzman in exile, 1979

One of the Moscow dissidents, 24-year old auxiliary doctor Aleksandr Podrabinek, was particularly interested in the issue of political abuse of psychiatry. He meticulously researched the issue, which eventually resulted in his book "Punitive Medicine" that was smuggled out of the USSR just in time to be summarized in a special 25-page document that Amnesty International issued on the eve of the 1977 WPA World Congress in Honolulu. A few years earlier, Vladimir Bukovsky and the psychiatrist Semyon Gluzman had written a Manual for Dissenters on how to behave during psychiatric evaluation in order to avoid being diagnosed as mentally ill. Both knew the subject very well, as Bukovsky had been hospitalized several times for political reasons, and Semyon Gluzman had written a diagnosis in absentia of General Pyotr Grigorenko, for which he had received a sentence of seven years of camp and five years of exile. Both were serving time in a political labor camp in Mordovia.[168]

---

rights. The Commission for the Cooperation and Security in Europe (CSCE) was supposed to monitor the implementation of the Accords, and later, after the end of communism, was renamed into Organization for the Security and Cooperation in Europe (OSCE).

168 For the Manual see *On Soviet Totalitarian Psychiatry*, pp. 70-87. Semyon Gluzman, born in 1946, was arrested in 1971 and spent ten years in camp and exile for his "in absentia" diagnosis of General Pyotr Grigorenko. He currently lives in Kiev, Ukraine.

Together with a self-educated worker of 47, Feliks Serebrov, his friend Vyacheslav Bakhmin, a 30-year old computer programmer, and one of Bakhmin's friends, Irina Kaplun, Aleksandr Podrabinek founded, in January 1977, the Working Commission to Investigate the Use of Psychiatry for Political Purposes.[169] The group was formally linked to the Moscow Helsinki Group, and former victim of psychiatric abuse General Pyotr Grigorenko functioned as a sort of liaison person. During the four years of its existence, the Commission published over 1,500 pages of documentation, among which 22 Information Bulletins documented the political abuse of psychiatry in great detail. In total, more than 400 cases were documented.[170] Also, the Information Bulletin was used to inform the dissident movement about Western protests against the political abuse and, for instance, the developments concerning the World Psychiatric Association (WPA).[171] Summaries of the Information Bulletins were also published in one of the main *samizdat* publications, the *Chronicle of Current Events*.[172] The Information Bulletins were sent to the West, where human rights activists used them during their campaigns, but also to the Soviet authorities,

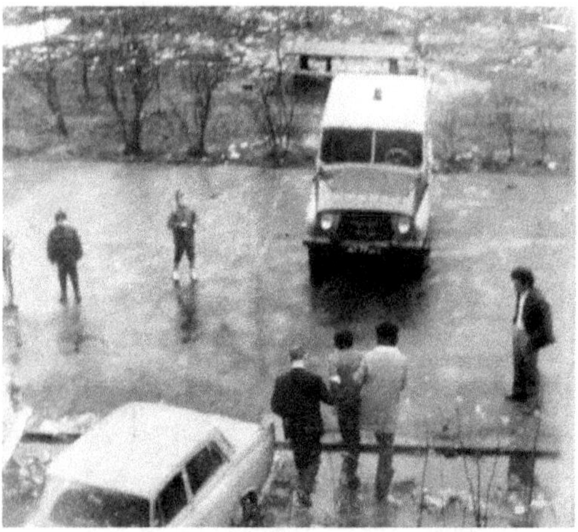

Arrest Aleksandr Podrabinek, 1977

169 Vyacheslav Bakhmin, Irina Kaplun and a third Moscow dissident, Irina Yakir, had previously been arrested in 1969 because of planning protests against the celebration of the 90th birthday of Soviet dictator Iosif Stalin. Both Bakhmin and Kaplun had been charged with anti-Soviet agitation and propaganda, but for unclear reason the case was dropped after ten months' of pre-trial investigation. Feliks Serebrov was first arrested in 1947 for taking part in the theft of salt from a railway station. He was sentenced to death but the sentence was commuted to ten years of imprisonment. He was released in 1954, after the death of Stalin, but arrested again in 1958 for "excessive use of self-defense". He spent 19 months in camp working as a lumberjack.

170 *Soviet Psychiatric Abuse in the Gorbachev Era*, p. 27

171 *Soviet Psychiatric Abuse - Shadow over World Psychiatry*. P. 81

172 The information bulletin Chronicle of Current Events (*Хроника текущих событий*) was one of the longest-running and best-known samizdat periodicals in the USSR dedicated to the defense of human rights. For fifteen years from 1968 to 1983, a total of 63 issues of the Chronicle were published.

with the request to check the information and inform the Commission if mistakes were found.

The productivity of the group was extraordinarily high and, apart from documenting the political abuse of psychiatry, they also set themselves the task to aid victims of the abuse and their families, and to work for a general humanization of living conditions in psychiatric hospitals, which were pretty bad by all standards. Even one of the architects of Soviet political abuse, Academician Andrei Snezhnevsky, acknowledged a few years earlier that the conditions were unacceptably bad and had organized inspections by commissions from the Ministry of Health. "The inspectors were appalled by what they saw. Their general conclusion was: a prison is a prison, and nothing else. Their recommendation: to convert the prisons into hospitals. The result was that on 16 February 1973 the Ministry of Internal Affairs issued Directive No. 022-S, which contained the order to 'change the whole appearance of the hospitals from looking like prisons to looking like hospitals."[173]

Throughout its existence, the Commission continued to speak out against the conditions in the psychiatric hospitals. In its view, the hospitals should be handed over to the Ministry of Health, whereas now they were administered by the Ministry of Internal Affairs (MVD), which also administered the penitentiary system.[174] Sometimes the Commission would approach the directors of the psychiatric hospitals where political abuse of psychiatry had occurred, informing them of what was happening in the international arena (such as the Honolulu Congress of the WPA, where Soviet psychiatric abuse was condemned by the General Assembly) or asking them to assist the Commission in its work: "If it should be that inaccuracies appear in these reports, we ask you to let us know and to send appropriate corrections to the address below. Corrections and additions to published material are published by us in subsequent issues of the Bulletin."[175] Of course, the Commission never received any response. However, if mistakes were found, corrections would be published in the next issue of the Information Bulletin.

---

173 *Soviet Psychiatric Abuse - Shadow over World Psychiatry*, p. 288. In practice, however, not much changed and the conditions remained inhumane. The author saw this with his own eyes in the early 1990s when the Soviet Union collapsed and gradually the doors opened. Often the living conditions were horrendous. See, for instance, *On Dissidents and Madness*, p. 144

174 Only in 1988 the hospitals were transferred to the authority of the Ministry of Health, although the security remained the domain of the Ministry of the Interior and, later, the Ministry of Justice.

175 *Soviet Psychiatric Abuse - Shadow over World Psychiatry*, p. 87

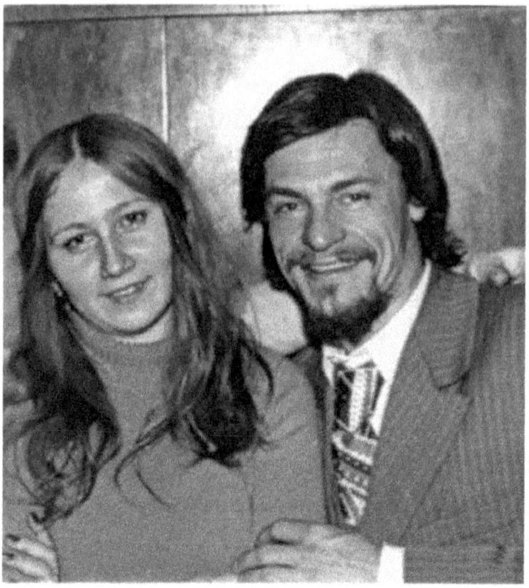

Aleksandr Voloshanovich with the wife of Aleksandr Podrabinek, 1980

The Commission stated its task was not primarily to diagnose people or to declare persons who sought help mentally healthy or mentally ill. However, in certain cases "a psychiatrist, who renders invaluable help to the Commission, examines persons who come for help to the Commission and gives an accurate diagnosis of their mental condition. The Commission uses these reports in its work and publicly refers to them when this is essential."[176] Initially it was psychiatrist Aleksandr Voloshanovich from Dolgoprudny, a Moscow suburb, who provided these diagnoses. But when he was forced to emigrate in early 1980, his work was continued by the Kharkov psychiatrist Anatoly Koryagin. Also some foreign psychiatrists helped in diagnosing former or potential victims of psychiatric abuse.[177]

Opposition abroad

Bukovsky's appeal of 1971 resulted in the formation of the first groups to campaign against the political abuse of psychiatry in the USSR. In France, a group of doctors formed the "Committee against the Special Psychiatric Hospitals in the USSR," while in Britain a "Working Commission on the Internment of Dissenters in Mental Hospitals" was formed. Among its founding members were Dr. Sidney Bloch, a South-African born psychiatrist, and Professor Peter Reddaway, a Sovietologist and lecturer at the London School of Economics and Political Science. They would later be the authors of one of the most important books on Soviet psychiatric abuse, "*Russia's Political Hospitals,*" that for the first time documented the abuse in every detail. The Working Commission published an analysis

---

176 *Soviet Psychiatric Abuse in the Gorbachev Era*, p. 26

177 Among them were the British psychiatrist Gery Low-Beer and Swedish psychiatrist Dr. Harald Blomberg.

of Bukovsky's documents, which turned out to be a very helpful tool in developing an international campaign.[178]

In response to the Western campaigns and the mounting pressure on the Soviet authorities, the latter decided to alter their strategy. Instead of hospitalizing well-known dissidents, they now avoided any public scandal by changing course. Initially they still hospitalized known dissidents in Ordinary Psychiatric Hospitals, and no longer in Special ones, yet soon they stopped their hospitalization altogether and used the "psychiatric tool" only for lesser and unknown dissidents. Often as soon as a victim of political abuse became known, the person would be released or re-diagnosed as being mentally health and sent to non-psychiatric places of detention. Also, the Soviets started to react much stronger to protests from the West by boosting the image of Soviet psychiatry and particularly institutions like the Serbski Institute that were heavily involved in the political abuse, and by deliberately misquoting Western psychiatrists who allegedly had said they saw no proof of any abuse or found Soviet psychiatry to be highly respectable.[179] For instance, the British psychiatrist John Wing was quoted as having said: "I admire the Soviet system because in the USSR everything is done to restore the patient to normal life... I cannot find anything to criticize. I find everything is beautiful."[180] When later asked whether he said any such thing, he denied having ever made any such statements.[181] In particular, Marat Vartanyan turned out to be a very skillful distorter of expressions by Western experts, and masterfully turned things upside down whenever necessary.

In addition, the Soviets launched a sort of counter attack by lobbying the WPA (of which Marat Vartanyan was at that time one of the members of the Executive Committee) and the American Psychiatric Association (APA). The APA was important as a national psychiatric association, as it was the largest psychiatric association in the world, highly influential and on top of that linked to the National Institute for Mental Health (NIMH) in Washington D.C. This Institute was, for the Soviets, of the utmost importance. In 1971, an agreement had been reached for joint US-USSR

178 *Soviet Psychiatric Abuse - Shadow over World Psychiatry*, p. 282-3

179 In late 1971 the Serbski was awarded by the Government of the USSR the Order of the Red Banner of Labor, and the Institute and its Director, Dr. Georgi Morozov, were portrayed in the most positive manner.

180 *S Chuzhogo Golosa*, pp. 57-8. The chapter on psychiatry in this book provides a whole range of alleged positive remarks by Western visitors to the Soviet Union, in particular on pages 57-59.

181 *Soviet Psychiatric Abuse - Shadow over World Psychiatry*, p. 285

Research on Schizophrenia, the result of the blossoming détente and President Nixon's visit to Moscow, and NIMH was the institution had was commissioned to administer the implementation of this agreement.

In the period between the World Congresses in Mexico in 1971 and in Honolulu in 1977, a growing number of national psychiatric associations expressed their concern over the issue, but not more than that. The World Psychiatric Association did not study any of the evidence it received, nor did it interview former victims of Soviet psychiatric abuse. At the same time, however, they continued to maintain friendly relations with the Soviet psychiatrists that were closely involved in the political abuse of psychiatry. In November 1972, Secretary General Denis Leigh and Treasurer Professor Linford Rees even accepted an honorary membership of the Soviet All-Union Society. Professor Rees would later change his position and become an active opponent of Soviet psychiatric abuse.[182]

The Soviets continued to win their Western colleagues over. In October 1973 a WPA Congress on schizophrenia was held in Moscow, with among the main speakers Andrei Snezhnevsky and Serbski Institute director Georgi Morozov. After the conference, a group of psychiatrists were invited over to the Serbski Institute, where they were shown the case histories of six dissidents including the well-known victims General Pyotr Grigorenko, Ukrainian dissident Leonid Plyushch and Moscow biologist Zhores Medvedev, accompanied by a short English summary. Subsequently, they were shown an examination of a person who was said to be a dissident, and they ascertained that the man was indeed suffering from schizophrenia. The foreign visitors refused to sign any document, but this did not stop Marat Vartanyan from issuing a statement that five of the six cases that had undergone forensic psychiatric examination were, in the opinion of the WPA Committee, suffering "from a mental illness at the time of their respective commissions of enquiry."[183]

---

182 Professor Linford Rees (1914-2004) graduated from the Welsh National School of Medicine in Cardiff and moved rapidly to psychiatry. In 1938 he became an assistant medical officer at the Worcester and City Mental Hospital at Powick, and took the diploma in psychological medicine and his MD in 1943. In 1947 Rees became deputy physician superintendent of Whitchurch Hospital, Cardiff, and regional psychiatrist for Wales and Monmouthshire. He then returned as a consultant psychiatrist to the Bethlem and Maudsley Hospitals in 1954. He was appointed lecturer and then Professor of Psychiatry at St Bartholomew's Medical College (London University), where he remained until he retired in 1980. He was the author of *A Short Textbook of Psychiatry* in 1967 and numerous papers on all aspects of psychiatry.

183 See *Russia's Political Hospitals*, p. 317

The WPA Committee refused to accept this statement, but that didn't keep Vartanyan from publishing it in the leading Soviet psychiatric journal.[184] It was to be repeated several times in the following years.
A month after the meeting at the Serbski, the British Royal College of Psychiatrists adopted a motion in which it deplored the political abuse of psychiatry and condemned the doctors who participated in it. For the first time, the College discussed whether it should withdraw from the WPA if the Soviets remained among its membership. This caused Dr. Leigh to "associate himself and the WPA … with the decision to consider more deeply than hitherto the whole matter of psychiatric abuse and to seek ways of bring pressure to bear on countries where abuses occur."[185] Although he voiced his opinion that the WPA did not have the resources to examine complaints about misuse of the psychiatric profession, he suggested that the WPA should make a declaration at the next General Assembly of the organization on "the general principles underlying the ethical practice of psychiatry," and then it would be up to national associations "whether or not to draw up a detailed code on matters affecting practice in its own country. Thus, we avoid problems connected with religion, national policies, political belief and so forth, and can concentrate on the principles."[186] Dr. Leigh's evasive moves triggered a response from the Royal College, that it would do everything possible to have the next General Assembly of the WPA condemn the systematic political abuse of psychiatry in the Soviet Union. This was quickly followed by a request from the American Psychiatric Association that a special session be held on concrete abuses of psychiatry at the World Congress of the WPA, to be held on Hawaii in August 1977.[187]

A report on a meeting of Dr. Leigh with Professor Karl Seidel on May 20, 1977, written by his Stasi *Führungsoffizier* Eberhard Jaekel after their debriefing session, sheds an interesting light on the positioning of Leigh. According to the report, Leigh was convinced that "the Soviets have behaved often very clumsily in connection with negotiations, discussions and announcements with regard to the issue of the alleged political abuse of psychiatry in the USSR. As a result, the USSR has provided to certain forces a basis for their attacks. According to his opinion, some of the dissidents who have left the USSR are not mentally ill, even though they were incarcerated in a Soviet psychiatric hospital and Soviet propaganda

184 *Zhurnal Nevropatologii i Psikhiatriii imeni S.S. Korsakova*, 1974, Vol. 74, No. 3, p. 471-472

185 See *Russia's Political Hospitals*, p. 335

186 *WPA Newsletter* 31. October 1975

187 *News and Notes*, Royal College of Psychiatrists, November 1976; *Psychiatric News*, October 1, 1976.

refers to them as mentally ill. D. Leigh mentioned, for instance, the former General Grigorenko, who in his view is just a querulant. Also Bukovsky, expelled from the Soviet Union, is considered by him to be a 'smart guy' with a completely 'normal behavior,' who is also not spreading blunt anti-Soviet views…"[188] Also, Leigh did not buy the Soviet definition of schizophrenia, Seidel reported, which in his view is far too broad.[189]

At the same time, however, Leigh was convinced the CIA was behind all the campaigns against the political abuse of psychiatry. "He knows the work of secret services, as he had been a psychiatric consultant to the Army." On top of that, Leigh was convinced that "American Jewry" dominated the WPA. "Proof of this is the fact, that the Presidents of the World (sic!) Association are usually American Jews, like for instance Marmor, Weinberg, Freedman, Gibson, Speigel, etc." In addition, Leigh strongly expressed his dislike for rich Americans, who think they can buy anything. "More than once he expressed his conviction that the political campaigns were organized by the CIA."[190]

188 MfS 13788/83, pp. 119-120

189 MfS 13788/83 p. 120

190 MfS 13788/83 p. 121-3. Here either Seidel or Jaekel made a mistake: the persons mentioned were Presidents of the American Psychiatric Association, not the World Psychiatric Association.

Chapter 13 – A Secret Actor

"...The candidate is very suitable for legends and varieties and is able to hide her goals and feelings and to deceive her environment. This character trait turned out to be very promising for the collaboration."
Eberhard Jaekel, MfS

The other wolves would tear me to pieces if they knew
that my howling is in fact weeping.

Octavian Paler[191]

Only because of the fact that the DDR collapsed and was subsequently taken over by its West-German neighbor did the Stasi archives remain, to a large degree, intact and accessible to the public. In most other former East Bloc countries, accessibility is either much more limited or non-existent (such as in Russia, where the KGB archives were open to researchers for a short while in the early 1990s). The archives of Western intelligence agencies also remain inaccessible and, thus, it is unclear which intelligence agencies were actively engaged in the affairs of the World Psychiatric Association or, at least, monitoring the involvement of both the WPA and organizations such as IAPUP in the issue of political abuse of psychiatry in the Soviet Union. We noted earlier that WPA General Secretary Fini Schulsinger knew about Ellen Mercer's former employment by the CIA. He was also well informed about the backgrounds of other people, and it remains unclear from which source he had this information. It is, however, safe to assume agencies from both sides were involved; yet to what extent will almost certainly remain unknown.

For many years, we wondered if our organization was infiltrated and, if so, by whom. It was not a hypothetical question, we knew, because being the main organization that campaigned against the political abuse of psychiatry in the Soviet Union, we were sure that the Soviet KGB, either directly or via Eastern European secret services, would target us. In the Netherlands, we prepared ourselves for such an event and it was our policy not to employ anybody whose origins were in Eastern Europe, even though they might persistently offer to assist us: we'd better be sure and not take the risk.[192] All of these years, we wondered where the "leak" was, how our organization had

191 Paler, Octavian: *Poems*. Albatros. Bucuresti, 1998

192 *On Dissidents and Madness*, p. 140

been infiltrated. Until 1999, when the book "*Psychiatrisch Missbraucht*?" by Dr. Sonja Süss was published and we learned that our organization had been infiltrated via our West German member organization, the DVpMP, chaired by the Starnberg psychiatrist, Dr. Friedrich Weinberger.[193] It might not have been the only leak, but it sure was a damaging one.

Paradoxically, the initial information was upsetting but, in a strange way, also comforting. At least we finally knew what had happened. In my 2009 book, "*On Dissidents and Madness,*" I wrote: "It could have come straight out of a cheap espionage novel. Friedrich [Weinberger] was single and admired Porsches and blond women. From the Stasi archives, it appeared that one of his ladies was a colonel of the Stasi, a Dr. Gisela Otto, who was designated with the codename "Jutta," and who was selected to draw Friedrich out. Considering the fact that she was described as being good looking and very convincing with men, there is little doubt she succeeded in using all her charms on Friedrich, who promised to share all his information with her."[194] What I didn't know then, was the fact that Otto was neither blond nor a Stasi colonel, but a dark-haired gynecologist from Berlin who had been recruited by the Stasi in a rather devious manner.

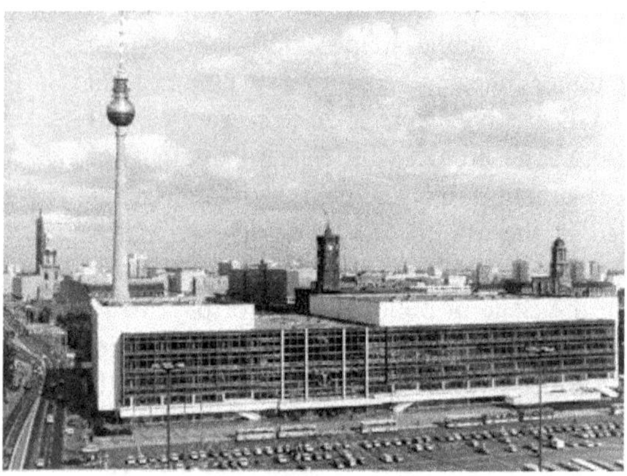

Palast der Republik, Berlin

Dr. Gisela Otto, born in 1935 was, from 1970 until her defection to the West in January 1986, medical director of the policlinic in the *Haus der Ministerien* in East Berlin, housed in the building of the former Aviation Ministry of Herman Göring.[195] She was a personal acquaintance of

[193] Friedrich Weinberger M.D., a neurologist and psychiatrist, now retired and currently living in Garmisch-Partenkirchen, Bavaria (West Germany), was founder of the *Deutsche Vereinigung gegen politischen Missbrauch der Psychiatrie* (DVpMP),

[194] *On Dissidents and Madness*, p. 140

[195] Dr. Gisela Otto (maiden name Sarnow, 1935-1995), was trained as a doctor in 1959-1964 in Rostock and the hospital of the People's Police in Berlin, and since 1965 worked in the Haus der Ministerien. On December 11, 1985, she received the recognition as "Merited Physician of the People of the DDR".

Lieutenant Colonel Eberhard Jaekel, a lawyer who since 1964 worked with the Stasi and had achieved the position of head of the Chief Directorate XX/1.[196] As indicated earlier, he had become Otto's *Führungsoffizier* after she had been recruited to work for the Stasi. As noted above, the recruitment was not an altogether voluntary affair; actually, to the contrary, and reading Gisela Otto's Stasi file was one of the most painful moments of my research for this book.[197] Personal circumstances lead in April 1973 to a situation where Otto had to agree to collaborate in order to save her own skin. Initially, she provided the MfS with confidential information on some of her patients and a year later, in March 1974, she agreed to collaborate as an *Inoffizieller Mitarbeiter*.[198] Apparently, she never signed any statement to that effect but gave an oral commitment. A few years later she was given a special mission by the MfS.[199]

Jaekel described Gisela Otto as a "very intelligent, art-loving and ambitious physician. ... Characteristic for her is a high level of productivity in her functioning as medical director of the policlinic, as physician in this clinic, as lecturer at the Academy of Continued Education of Physicians and in her desire for her own academic continued education. She works every day very intensively and long hours, both in her institution and at home. ... Another evident character trait of the candidate is her ability to develop a relationship with another person within a short period of time, as a result of which the other is triggered to talk with much openness about all the existing problems. ... The candidate is very closed and tries above all to shield her private life from outsiders. ... In this respect the candidate is very suitable for legends and varieties and is able to hide her goals and feelings and deceive her environment. This character trait turned out to be very

196 According to the Stasi files, Gisela Otto was also acquainted with the wife of Professor Seidel, who worked as a physician in the Palast Hotel in East Berlin, coincidentally the place where Neumann had his first meeting with the Stasi. See BstU, 10707/86, 2, p. 112. As the Neumann's were also acquainted with the Seidels, Jochen Neumann vividly remembers the shock among them when Gisela Otto decided not to return from a foreign trip but instead to defect to the West in 1986.

197 BstU, 10707/86, Band 1 and 2. For moral and ethical reasons, I deliberately remain vague with regard to the reasons why Dr. Otto agreed to collaborate with the Stasi. Although she spied not only on our German branch and Moscow dissidents, but also on many of her patients, it became clear to me that she was trapped and found herself in a downward spiral of deceit, which probably was a heavy burden on her conscience.

198 According to a report by Eberhard Jaekel, written after Otto's defection to the West in 1986. BstU, 10707/86, 1(I), pp. 255-256

199 *Zielgruppe Ärzteschaft*, p. 132

promising for the collaboration. With respect to the MfS the candidate is of extraordinary openness with regard to all existing problems. She herself states in addition that apart from the MfS, there is no other person who is so well informed about her person, her views and her emotional life. ... The candidate is, in addition, a good looking, modern and, for men, definitely an attractive woman, who is dressed in a very advantageous and modern way."[200]

Between the WPA World Congresses of 1977 and 1983, Jaekel also dealt with the issue of political abuse of psychiatry in the USSR. Special attention was directed at the German association against the political abuse of psychiatry (*Deutsche Vereinigung gegen politischen Missbrauch der Psychiatrie*, DVpMP), which had been founded in March 1977 and in December 1980 would be one of the founding organizations of the International Association on the Political Use of Psychiatry.[201] The organization became one of the main objects of attention in the ongoing collaboration between Stasi and KGB, and quite a few detailed reports on the surveillance can be found in the archives of the Stasi.[202] Two agents were put into action, one of them being Dr. Hans Eichhorn (code name "Grabowski") and the other Gisela Otto (code name "Jutta").[203]

Why the Stasi was so interested in the issue of political abuse of psychiatry in the USSR can easily be explained. A prime target for the Stasi were "hostile organizations" operating from the territory of the *Bundesrepublik Deutschland* (BRD, West-Germany), and one of those organizations – the DVpMP - was specifically set up to combat the political abuse of psychiatry in the USSR. Also, quite a few former Soviet dissidents were living in the BRD (for example the Germanist and close friend of Andrei Sakharov, Lev Kopelev, and the former political prisoner, Kronid Lubarsky), and one should not forget that Munich was the seat of Radio Free Europe/Radio

200 *Zielgruppe Ärzteschaft*, p. 132. *Politisch Missbraucht*, p. 640-1

201 For extensive information on the DVpMP see Marlies Onken: "*Als Arzt wie als Staatsbürger...*". The Stasi reported the founding of the DVpMP for the first time in an internal document of July 5, 1978. See MfS-HAXX, 2941, pp. 34. The DVpMP is the main subject of several other Stasi reports that focus on the campaign against the political abuse of psychiatry in the USSR and specifically describes the background to the founding of the international Association n the Political Use of Psychiatry, pointing out that at the founding the General Secretary of the organization, Gérard Bles, stated that it was supported both by the French President François Mitterrand and the French Communist leader George Marchais. See HA XX 1386/2, pp. 243-247, as well as pp. 281-285

202 For instance HAXX 1386/1 pp. 209-210

203 *Politisch Missbraucht*, p. 638-639. *Zielgruppe Ärzteschaft*, p. 132-3

Liberty, which regularly paid attention to the issue in their broadcasts to Eastern Europe and the USSR. This made the political abuse of psychiatry in the USSR automatically an important issue at the annual working meetings between the Stasi and the KGB. The other socialist countries did not have such a specific interest, and if the archives of the intelligence agencies in other former socialist countries were as open as the former Stasi archives, I doubt such a wealth of material would be found. It should be remembered that the KGB had a good and effective ally in the Stasi – the service was considered to be one of the most effective secret services worldwide.

The plan to infiltrate the DVpMP through *Inoffizieller Mitarbeiter* had been developed by the head of Directorate XX/1 of the Stasi, Eberhard Jaekel. On May 11, 1978, Jaekel presented a plan for the infiltration of the DVpMP to his staff. He outlined the history of the organization, its goals and objectives, and named the organizations with which it collaborated. He further stipulated what measures should be implemented against the DVpMP. The Chief Directorate VIII of the Stasi should, the plan indicated, try to find compromising material against its members and find out more about their political and moral positions. Two agents were to be deployed, being the above-mentioned "Grabowski" and "Jutta."[204]

Of course, Jaekel did not act alone, and his plans were coordinated with the KGB in Moscow, as can be concluded by the reports on the working meetings between the two agencies.[205] The collaboration between the MfS and fraternal intelligence agencies was an ongoing affair. Within the context of my research, I found many documents related to collaborative work with both the KGB and the Bulgarian and Hungarian secret services, particularly with regard to the surveillance of citizens traveling to each other's countries (e.g. Bulgarians traveling to the DDR) or former Soviet citizens now living in West-Germany. On top of that, the MfS and KGB held joint working meetings on the operational level, as well as annual high-level meetings to discuss the state of affairs with regard to the enemies of socialism and other issues of common interest.[206] For example, in April 1976, top officials of both services met in Berlin for five days, among them being the deputy chairman of the KGB, Vladimir Chebrikov (who was at that time Lieutenant General and would later become Chairman of the KGB and member of the Politburo) and, during certain parts of the

204 *Politisch Missbraucht*, p. 638-9

205 See, for instance, HA XX 1386/2, pp. 253-242 on the working meeting between the KGB and Stasi on 11-15 May 1982.

206 Such meetings took place, for instance, in Berlin April 1975 and in April 1976, and in May 1978 and November 1980 in Moscow.

meeting, MfS Director Erich Mielke. A 56-page report describes in detail the issues discussed, including the names of individuals in whom the KGB is interested or on whom they would like to get further information from the MfS.[207] In a report on a four day meeting between the KGB and Stasi in May 1982, in which also Eberhard Jaekel participated, the DVpMP, Friedrich Weinberger and Kronid Lubarsky, are a repeated subject of discussion.[208] In that sense, it is clear who is in charge here: it is mainly the KGB that decides the agenda and after the meeting a whole list of MfS departments are issued instructions to satisfy the requests from "our friends," as the KGB is usually referred to in Stasi documents.[209]

The deployment of "Grabowski" was not successful. In 1981, he was appointed as director of the psychiatric hospital Ueckermünde in eastern Mecklenburg-Vorpommern, near Germany's border with Poland. The hospital, where in Nazi times hundreds of mentally handicapped children had been killed as part of the "Euthanasia" program,[210] was in terrible condition and urgently needed reconstruction. As a result, the deployment of Grabowski would "at least be postponed with five years," as his *Führungsoffizier* reported in a report of early December 1980.[211] With Stasi agent Gisela Otto, things would go much more successfully.

Infiltration

Gisela Otto contacted the chairperson of the DVpMP, Dr. Friedrich Weinberger, for the first time in 1978. Weinberger was then living and working in the town of Starnberg, near Munich, and had been one of the founders of the organization in 1977.[212] Apparently the contact had been established via

207 Among the persons that are of special interest to the KGB in 1976 are the Germanist and dissident Lev Kopelev, the Georgian singer Bulat Okudzhava, Taganka Theater Director Yuri Lyubimov, cellist Rostropovich and painter Oskar Rabin. Interestingly, the issue of political abuse of psychiatry is then only indirectly mentioned in connection with the cases of Zhores Medvedev, Leonid Plyushch and General Pyotr Grigorenko (wrong named in the document as General Karenkov). Later, the issue becomes one of the main items of discussion, pretty much dominating the agenda of the meeting.

208 HA XX 1386/2, 235-242.

209 BVfS Potsdam, BstU 1071, pp. 48-60 and 117-172

210 See for instance Regina Scheer: "*Störend, Verstörend*" in *Freitag* 14, March 31, 2000.

211 *Politisch Missbraucht*, p. 639

212 According to the Stasi files, Weinberger was born around 1930 (HAXX 1385 p. 155) and fiercely anti-communist. According to document HAXX 1385

a certain Dr. Teodorowitsch, a retired psychiatrist and a founding member of the DVpMP, as well as a member of the Russian Orthodox community in Munich.[213] According to the Stasi files, Otto decided to try to establish contact with Weinberger indirectly by selecting a woman with a Russian sounding name in the telephone directory and establishing contact with her. The reason for this complicated approach

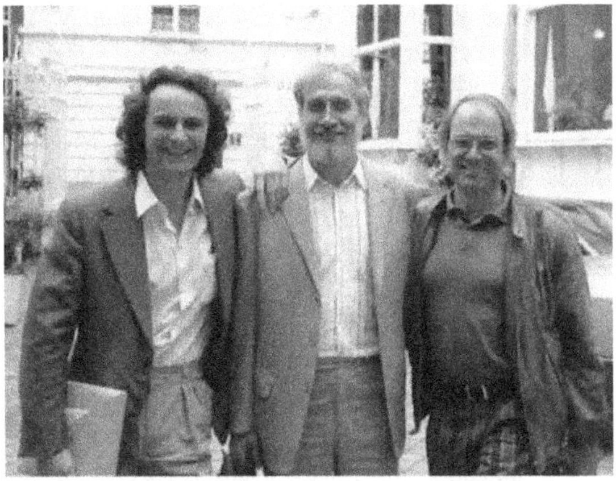

l.t.r. Robert van Voren, Anatoly Koryagin, Friedrich Weinberger, 1988

2226, he had been in the DDR ten times between mid-November 1964 and early September 1966. Since, he had not been in the DDR (MfS 10707/86 II, pp. 15-6). In one of the documents (HAXX 1385, p. 397), it is asserted that he had his practice as psychiatrist purely for financial reasons, that is to earn himself a living, and that his fight against communism was a driving force for him. "Weinberger has an anti-socialist attitude and is an enemy of the Soviet Union. Weinberger sees as main task for his organization the collection, assessment and dissemination of information from the USSR, the DDR and other socialist countries concerning cases of alleged abuse of psychiatry in the fight against the 'civil rights movement'." (HAXX 2941, p. 36)
Dr Otto also mentions his close connections with the political party CSU in her reports.

213 *Rundbrief,* 1-1999, p. 9 In a letter dated June 25, 2009, Dr. Helmut Bieber writes: "Dr. Nedeshda Theodorowitsch (a retired psychiatrist) ... was one of the more elderly members of our association, who in 1976 signed with us the Open Letter in the *Deutsches Ärzteblatt*, and was active as a founder of DVpMP in the same year. In the early times, our members would meet at her apartment in central Munich - that apparently belonged to the Russian Orthodox Church, of which she was a member – a few times. The lady was among the first people who told us about the abuse of psychiatry..." Also Peter Reddaway remembers her well (e-mail, July 9, 2009). The Stasi describes her in a memorandum of July 5, 1978, as a person who "plays a central role in the network of the organization. It became known that Theodorowitsch receives handwritten information and reports from the USSR, which she translates and edits for publication. She is also editor of the monthly information service *Religion and Atheism in the USSR*, which is waging a campaign against the USSR." According to the same document Theodorowitsch was originally from Minsk, and a "political enemy of the USSR." See MfS-HAXX, 2941, p. 38

was that Otto felt she "couldn't contact Weinberger directly as I could not know that he is one of the leading persons of the group."[214]

Teodorowitsch indeed introduced her to Weinberger, as Otto reported upon return to East Berlin: "I presented myself very shyly as a specialist in gynecology and obstetrics, and told him where I worked. He fully understood that it was a conversation that had to remain between the two of us, as establishing contact with him was extremely dangerous. I told Dr. W[einberger] that I was also in Munich illegally, as a guest of Professor V., with whom I was close friends. I talked about my scientific work, my international recognition, but very modestly and that for this reason I had the liberty to receive further education in the capitalist foreign countries and participate in congresses. He welcomed this very much and said that we should be very careful because in our countries punishment is not stopped when it concerns a well-known scientist. He would be very sorry if his organization would have to concern itself with obtaining my release."[215]

In order to increase Weinberger's confidence in her, Gisela Otto also involved two other physicians from Munich, one of whom was the earlier mentioned Professor V., the other a Dr. M. "who very enthusiastically reported on my scientific work and my dissertation. It was also Dr. M. who told Dr. W[einberger] that I [Gisela Otto] had become a much demanded speaker at international meetings. That was a big advantage, because it is impossible to paint a picture of yourself the way somebody else can do it. I explained my interest in political abuse of psychiatry by telling him the reason I became a doctor. I highlighted the ethical problems. I told him that I had learned about the subject of psychiatry in the Soviet Union for the first time from Dr. H, whom I had met in Moscow. Since that moment the issue had not left me in peace, and I had tried in all possible ways to get materials on the issue."[216]

Between 1978 and 1983, Otto met Weinberger repeatedly. How often they met is not known, and cannot be exactly retraced. Weinberger himself gives the figure of approximately six meetings, and denies he met her also at congresses in Marseille and Strasbourg, as she reported to the MfS, and where, according to reports, she was one of the speakers.[217] Dr. Helmut

---

214 *Politisch Missbraucht,* p. 641

215 *Politisch Missbraucht,* p. 641

216 *Politisch Missbraucht,* p. 642

217 *Rundbrief,* 1-1999, p. 9. The Stasi files confirm in fact that they met in Strasbourg and in Marseille. BstU, 10707/86, Band 1 and 2. Further reports on

Bieber, who was a member of the DVpMP and quite close to Dr. Weinberger, was not kept informed and had no idea what was going on. According to him, "nobody of our group ever met her. I remember, however, Fritz W[einberger][218] mentioning mysteriously that he stayed in contact with a woman doctor (psychiatrist) from East Berlin but he would not let out any details."[219] Also from the Stasi archives, it is clear that Weinberger behaved rather conspiratorially. In his correspondence with "Jutta," he made use of a pseudonym and also a different mailing address; over the phone, he spoke only in general terms and constantly told her to be careful.[220] Several times they used a messenger in West Berlin, who traveled to East Berlin in February 1979 to pick up materials that "Jutta" had taken back with her from Moscow (e.g. Information Bulletins of the Moscow Working Commission).[221]

However, at the same time Weinberger was much less careful when he put Otto in touch with Peter Reddaway (and they spoke over the phone at least once). He also organized at least two meetings in a Munich hotel between her and Kronid Lubarsky, a Munich-based former Soviet political prisoner who led one of the main centers for the collection of information on repression in the USSR and published in his weekly *USSR News Brief*, which contained short telegram-style information on KGB-activities against the dissident movement.[222]

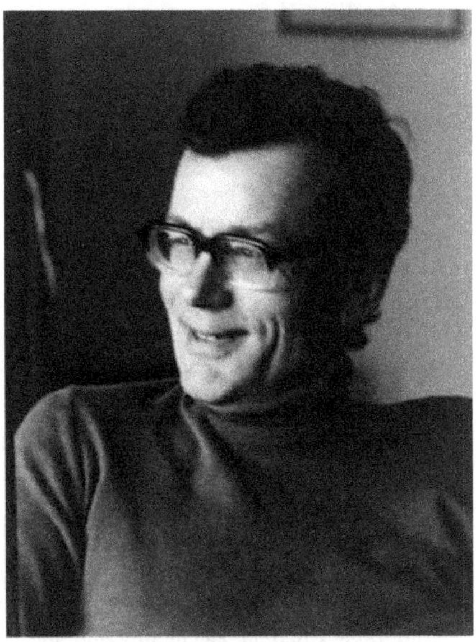

Kronid Lubarsky, 1981

Jutta's meetings with Weinberger can be found in file HA XX 2MA 3304 and in MfS 10707/86 II.

218 Fritz is short for Friedrich

219 Letter from Dr. Helmut Bieber, April 25, 2009. Apparently Otto presented herself as a psychiatrist, although she was not.

220 *Politisch Missbraucht*, p. 642

221 MfS 10707/86 II, pp. 3

222 BstU, 10707/86, 2(II), p. 145

The Stasi file on Gisela Otto makes very clear that over the years, a special relationship developed between her and Friedrich Weinberger, at least as far as he was concerned. As she reported: "The *IM* 'Jutta' feels that she succeeded through her conversations with Weinberger to make the relationship more intimate. Because of the *IM's* adaptation to the attitude of Weinberger with regard to the functioning of his organization, Weinberger feels himself very closely connected to the IM. Weinberger clearly plans to integrate the IM deeper into the organization."[223] All documents show that he actively tried to develop a relationship with her, explaining how special their connection was to him, although there was no indication it went beyond an intellectual connection, or maybe a platonic (love-) relationship.[224] On one hand, the files show that Weinberger courted Otto, taking her to expensive restaurants and – according to Otto - proudly showing her around in public (which does not really conform to his otherwise conspiratorial behavior); but, at the same time, he never made any direct attempts to seduce her. Instead, he invited her to his home to have dinner and listen to classical music and following one of their meetings, he took her on a wine-trip through the wine regions of West Germany.

To her *Führungsoffizier,* Otto reported that "Dr. W[einberger] trusts me, and is willing to hand over all the materials he has access to. ... He sees me as a comrade in arms."[225] Indeed, that seems to have been the case. Even worse, Weinberger suggested that she contact Vyacheslav Bakhmin and Irina Kaplun, founding members of the Moscow Working Commission to Investigate the Use of Psychiatry for Political Purposes during her next

223 BstU, HAXX 2941, p. 77. In HAXX 1385, p. 205, Otto writes about her rather perfidious tactics to win the confidence of Weinberger: "We talked about the feelings that move me, that I am emotionally willing to contribute to the struggle against the abuse of psychiatry in the USSR and the fight against the so-called lack of freedom. The feelings I analyses on basis of my basic convictions with regard to ethics, respect, personal dignity, feeling of justice, compassion, courage. I had a clear feeling and am quite convinced that the sometimes very intensive conversations, that were intermingled with jointly experienced impressions of beautiful buildings, paintings or sculptures, resulted in an absolute confidence in me on his part." Also in HAXX 1385 p. 386 it is stressed that "the sympathy of Weinberger for the IM is not based on interest of W. in an intimate relationship with the IM, but is apparently based on seemingly similar existential experiences, cultural interests and in particular on the joint ethical attitude towards the so-called abuse of psychiatry that the IM pretends to have."

224 See for instance HAXX 1385, p. 213. Otto says: "He never used our being alone together in any form that I would have felt as not being totally comfortable."

225 *Politisch Missbraucht*, p. 642

business trip to Moscow in December 1978.[226] She should deliver material aid, pick up materials from the Working Commission, and help them where necessary.

As soon as Jutta informed her *Führungsoffizier* about this request, the latter contacted the KGB in Moscow, organized a business trip to Moscow for himself in order to make sure that a connection was established between Jutta and the KGB.[227] "The KGB reported in briefs number 1507/78 and 1630/78 that the mentioned persons were under active operational surveillance because of their anti-Soviet activity. In accordance with the request of the KGB to deploy the IM of Chief Directorate XX and her contribution to the operational surveillance of the concerned persons, it is planned to put IMV "Jutta" during the period of 6/12 to 10/12/1978 with a legend into action in Moscow and to instruct her to establish contact with Kaplun/Bakhmin. In doing so, the IM should follow the instructions and positions that have been given to her by Weinberger. ... It is planned to have a meeting with the IM in Moscow on December 7, 1978, in order to give her specific orders in connection with her task based on a meeting in the Fifth Department of the KGB on the same day."[228]

During this visit to Moscow, "Jutta" met several times with members of the Working Commission, who welcomed her with open arms in their apartments and provided her with information both orally and in written form.[229] The information was immediately handed over both to the KGB and to *Führungsoffizier* Jaekel, who subsequently wrote in his report: "The Soviet comrades were informed of the achievements after each visit and gave instructions for the behavior of the IM. All the materials that had been handed over to the IM were given to them to study... During a closing meeting on December 10, 1978, the following request was received from the Soviet comrades: in the interest of the establishment of a trusting relationship between the IM on one hand and Weinberger and the hostile groups in Moscow on the other, to pass on all the materials the IM had been given, to make photocopies of all the materials for transfer to the KGB, to send a detailed report to the KGB on the reached goals of the IM, to prepare information on Weinberger

226 At that moment Irina Kaplun probably already left the Working Commission, but continued to maintain contact with the Commission members.

227 *Zielgruppe Ärzteschaft*, p. 133

228 *Politisch Missbraucht*, p. 643

229 An extensive report on her meetings with Irina Kaplun and several others, including Working Commission member Irina Grivnina, can be found in HAXX 1385, pp. 184-200

for the KGB, to send a photo of Weinberger to the KGB. ... The IM was during her deployment in Moscow reliable and disciplined. She carried out all orders carefully and responsibly. She considered the tasks as the main reason for her stay in Moscow and put the implementation of the orders above everything else."[230]

At the beginning of 1979, the Fifth Department of the KGB thanked the director of Chief Directorate XX of the Stasi in writing for the help in their surveillance of Bakhmin and Kaplun, as well as for the materials received via "Jutta" and suggested "with the purpose of secretly keeping our joint efforts ... to continue the operation under the name 'Cascade'."[231] According to information in the file of "Jutta" and directorate XX/1, Dr. Otto maintained close contact with Friedrich Weinberger, in part via intermediaries in West Berlin.[232]

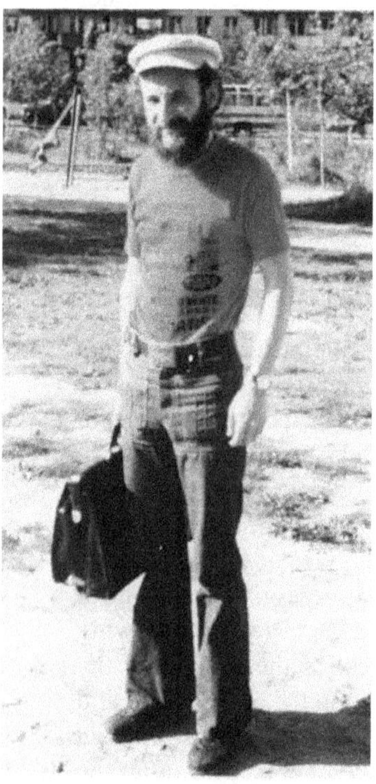

Vyacheslav Bakhmin, 1979

In the course of 1979, Eberhard Jaekel developed his future plans for operation 'Cascade' and in September 1979 he finalized a conceptual plan "on basis of the directions of the Fifth Directorate of the KGB of the USSR in their letter of August 27, 1979, to give the following goals and instructions to the IM for a meeting with Weinberger: on basis of the repeated urge from Weinberger by telephone. The directions continued that the IMV[233] "Jutta" definitely should undertake a trip to Moscow in order to re-establish contact with the hostile groups around Kaplun and Bakhmin, the IM should ask Weinberger for a concrete task as well as an indication how to position herself, in order to get to know the hostile goals and objectives of Weinberger and his supporters against the USSR and the involvement of the Soviet dissidents in the

230 *Politisch Missbraucht*, p. 644

231 *Politisch Missbraucht*, p. 644

232 *Politisch Missbraucht*, p. 644

233 IMV: *Inoffizieller Mitarbeiter* who is directly involved in the surveillance and uncovering of persons involved in hostile activities. Later The IMV was renamed into IMB

activity of his organization. … The IM will inform Weinberger that the possibility for such a trip will occur in October 1979, during which she is ready to establish again contact with Kaplun and Bakhmin."[234]

And indeed, in September 1979 Jutta traveled again to Munich to meet with Weinberger, who welcomed the possibility of having again the possibility for direct contact with Moscow and during which he told her that "the main task should be to collect the most recent materials and information on the activity of the Working Commission in Moscow and their cases of internment of political opponents in psychiatric hospitals and to smuggle it out of the USSR."[235] He gave her medication, food products and clothes that the dissidents needed, and asked her to hand this over to the Working Commission, together with some letters. On her next trip to Moscow, she was again accompanied by MfS lieutenant colonel Jaekel.[236]

Having traveled to Moscow four times a year as a courier for the dissident movement between 1980 and 1985, and having known the members of the Working Commission personally, I can very well imagine how Gisela Otto was received. What always amazed me was the fact that as soon as you would ring the doorbell of a dissident, the door would swing open, you would be pulled inside, asked to task off your shoes, shuffled into the kitchen where a table would be filled with food and anything else they could find in the refrigerator. Only then they would ask you why you were there.[237] Having been sent by the DVpMP, Jutta must have had received the same treatment, and considering her characteristics as previously described by Jaekel, she probably quickly obtained the trust of the members of the Working Commission, and abused it maximally.

For Jaekel the trip was again a success: "According to the collaboration plan between HA [Chief Directorate] XX and the Fifth Directorate of the KGB, in the period of 21-28 October 1979 the deployment of IMV "Jutta" in Moscow succeeded in carrying out certain measures in the implementation of the operation 'Cascade.' At the instruction of the chairman of the hostile organization … Dr. Weinberger, Friedrich the IM established contact with hostile objects Kaplun, Irina and Bakhmin, Vyacheslav, and carried out several meetings with them. According to the established operational goals, the IM succeeded in strengthening the

---

234 *Politisch Missbraucht*, p. 644

235 *Zielgruppe Ärzteschaft*, p. 133

236 *Zielgruppe Ärzteschaft*, p. 133. *Politisch Missbraucht*, p. 645.

237 See, for instance, *On Dissidents and Madness*, pp. 17-22

confidential relations with both persons and obtain further confirmation of their hostile attitude and activity against the USSR."[238]

All the materials and information she received was handed over to the KGB immediately. The materials were used during the trials against members of the Working Commission, who were arrested one after the other in 1980-1981 and sentenced to various terms of imprisonment. With the arrest of the last member in freedom, Anatoly Koryagin in February 1981, the Working Commission ceased to exist.[239]

One can only speculate as to the extent Otto knew the damage her actions would cause. Being an intelligent woman who consciously and deliberately traveled to Moscow to infiltrate a dissident group and hand over documents to the KGB, she must have realized it was not a holiday outing. Weinberger writes that "with regard to the arrest of the members of the Commission, who had welcomed her so lovingly and whom she betrayed so coldly to the KGB, Otto showed herself during a next meeting ... as being deeply shocked."[240] The question is whether that was just part of her act in which she was, according to Jaekel, so good.

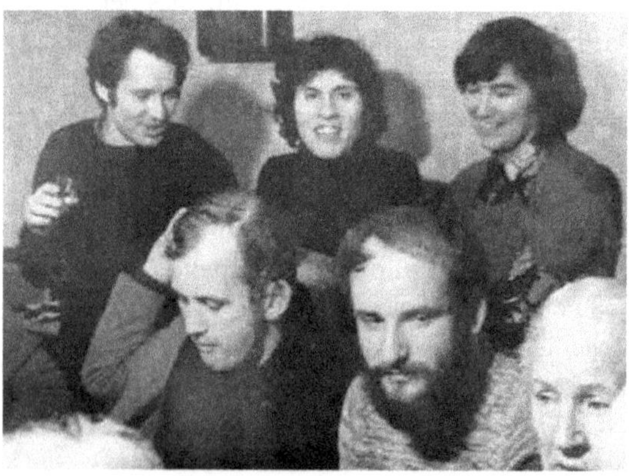

Back row on the left Vladimir Borisov, middle Irina Kaplun. In the front row in the middle Vyacheslav Bakhmin

One can also wonder why Friedrich Weinberger decided to use Jutta for this purpose, and never shared the information with other members of the DVpMP, or with fellow members of

238 *Politisch Missbraucht*, p. 645

239 For more information see the next chapter. Vyacheslav Bakhmin does not remember Jutta, nor were there - logically - any references to her work as a spy during his trial. Communications with V. Bakhmin, July 2009. At least part of the materials that Jutta received from the members of the Working Commission can be found in the Stasi archives (HA XX 6659 and probably also in HA XX 6657). They include copies of the *Information Bulletins* of the Moscow Working Commission, as well as personal letters addressed to a.o. Kronid Lubarsky (including one from Irina Kaplun, who would soon die in a car accident) and notes with addresses and instructions.

240 *Rundbrief* 1-1999, p. 9

IAPUP (of which he had been a member of the coordination council since December 1980). He himself wrote later that "already from the very start there was the suspicion that, with Otto, an informer was trying to slide into our midst. However, none of us in IAPUP had secrets. In the first place, the dissidents wanted the world to learn about the abuse of psychiatry and the KGB to learn of the worldwide opposition against it. In that sense, the issue as to whether she was a spy or a sympathizer made no difference. The person concerned [FW] [241] happily told the lady, that within the context of the opposition [against the political abuse] had been put in motion, but did not tell how weak this [opposition] in reality actually was. If Otto was a spy, then the costs that those in power incurred in order to get information from her, without putting it into figures, was also a form of feedback for the urgency of the work. What Otto, a scientific heavyweight who had travel possibilities both in East and West, learned was ... carefully selected. In the course of the approximately six meetings between 1978 and 1983, as can be seen afterwards from the files, he [FW] made some careless moves. However, Otto did not learn anything about the members of the Commission that was not yet generally known and should not have become known." And Weinberger continues: "that the KGB would need spying by the Stasi and the support of a German physician, and for that purpose would use a lot of time, money and effort, that is something that the person concerned [FW] did not count with. The effort seems even today not only devilish, but also pretty much absurd."[242]

The question of how Otto managed to get so deep into our organization regularly haunts me, as most of the members of the Working Commission were my friends and I know what their subsequent fate was. On top of that, I was a courier myself, regularly sent people to members of the Commission, and never knew that Weinberger was making use of an East German "psychiatrist." My guess is that Weinberger wanted to increase his importance within the international campaign against the political use of psychiatry, and in doing so became reckless. A remark in one of the Stasi files clearly points in this direction: "Weinberger expressed himself enthusiastically, that his organization now had its own connection to the groups in Moscow and that the action could be carried out successfully and secretively." The same reports adds a little bit further that Weinberger even called the leader of the British organization, Professor Peter Reddaway, in London while still being in the presence of Otto and told him that "Giselle" was with him and that he was "enthusiastic about

241 Friedrich Weinberger himself; Weinberger refers to himself in the third person.

242 *Rundbrief* 1-1999, p. 9-10

her report and in particular because of the fact that he now had his own connection to Moscow." [243]

Indeed, Peter Reddaway continuously had people going to Moscow as couriers, and hence had access to a constant flow of fresh information. Our Dutch group also contributed our share, both through my own work as a courier and through a number of fellow Dutch couriers. By having his own "secret courier," Weinberger could compensate for this, create a greater importance for himself and boost his contribution to the cause. However, he never understood how secret his "secret courier" was in reality.

Liquidation

In 1980, Jaekel received information that the liquidation of the Working Commission had started, that some members had been arrested and that one member had died in a car accident. In the minutes of a high level meeting between the Stasi and the KGB on November 24-28, 1980 in Moscow, Colonel Shchadrin of the Fifth Department of the KGB is reported to have said that "the organized political underground in the USSR was beaten in the years 1979-1980 in preparation of the Olympic Games through a variety of political-operational measures. That concerns, in particular, also the Helsinki Group, which with its branches in Moscow, Ukraine, Lithuania and Georgia was completely uncovered and liquidated. In total, 150 persons were arrested. In connection with this in 1980 measures were implemented to liquidate the so-called "Working Commission to Investigate the Political Use of Psychiatry." The leaders of this group, Bakhmin, Ternovsky, Podrabinek [and] Grivnina were arrested. Irina Kaplun, who was connected with this group and who, according to the estimation of the KGB, agreed to immigrate to Israel under influence of IM Jutta, had a fatal car accident before her departure."[244]

Irina Kaplun, indeed, had been killed in a car accident on July 23, 1980, near the Lithuanian town of Panavezys under unclear circumstances.[245]

[243] HAXX 2941, p. 69-70

[244] HAXX 1386/1, p. 216. Irina Kaplun, whose father was shot in 1938, had become politically active in 1965, when with a couple of fellow students she distributed anti-Stalinist leaflets. She was arrested and excluded from the Komsomol. In 1969 she was arrested again, this time with Vyacheslav Bakhmin, with whom she had prepared a protest against the official commemoration of Stalin's 90th birthday. They were both charged with anti-Soviet agitation and propaganda, but the case was dropped for unknown reasons and both were released.

[245] *Chronicle of Current Events* No. 57; *Soviet Psychiatric Abuse in the Gor-*

According to the KGB, "Jutta" had made a crucial contribution to the liquidation of the Working Commission: "In connection with the liquidation of the Working Commission to Investigate the Use of Psychiatry, comrade Shchedrin praised the contribution of IM "Jutta." On the basis of the new operational situation, it is no longer necessary to employ the IM in the USSR, as through new deployment, new contacts would be established that are only in the interest of the enemy."[246] In February 1981, Gisela Otto was given the "Medal of Merit of the National People's Army in Silver" by MfS Director General Erich Mielke because of "special achievements, … initiatives and personal readiness in carrying out orders."[247]

Until 1983, Otto visited Weinberger several times in Munich, but "as ordered" didn't respond to his request to travel again to Moscow to meet with relatives of those incarcerated, or to be part of the work of the DVpMP.[248] The last visit recorded in the Stasi archives was in May 1983, when she was sent to Munich by Lieutenant Colonel Jaekel to get information on the decision of the Soviet psychiatric association to withdraw from the World Psychiatric Association.[249] Between 1983 and 1985, Dr. Otto was only used by the Stasi for the delivery of information as director of her policlinic, and a year later she didn't return from a business trip to France. Apparently the Stasi tried several times to win her back, but unsuccessfully.[250]

Interestingly, Weinberger knows many details about her subsequent fate that are not recorded in other documents. According to him, she met him again and told him that from now on she would not return but stay in the West.[251] This indicates clearly that at least until, 1986 contact with Weinberger was maintained, also after her defection to the West. The question is whether these meetings are part of the six mentioned by him earlier, or in addition. This also suggests, however, that the relationship was closer than Weinberger now prefers to admit.

---

bachev Era p. 25; communication with V. Bakhmin, July 2009.

246 HAXX 1386/1, p. 217. *Zielgruppe Ärzteschaft*, p. 134

247 *Politisch Missbraucht*, p. 647

248 *Zielgruppe Ärzteschaft*, p. 134

249 BstU, 10707/86, 2, p. 175

250 *Zielgruppe Ärzteschaft,* p.134. In the mean time Jaekel initiated a separate file on the DVpMP on June 20, 1982, but it seems this file was destroyed by the Stasi on December 19, 1989 in the months before the Stasi archives were taken under control by the new authorities.

251 *Rundbrief*, 1-1999, p. 10

Dr. Otto set up a gynecological practice in the *Schulstrasse* in Elmshorn, a town in the district of Pinneberg in Schleswig-Holstein in Germany, approximately 30 kilometers north of Hamburg.[252] In 1994, she had a fatal car accident on the Autobahn to Berlin.[253] The rumor is that she, realizing that her role in the Stasi became clear, took her car and drove it into a concrete pillar.[254] She was 60 years old.

For Weinberger, the revelation of Jutta's contribution to the liquidation of the Working Commission, and his role in this, must have been extremely painful. He wanted to impress others, by having his own "secret" ally. Yet his secrecy turned out to be not an asset, but a huge liability. He turned out to be entry point for infiltration by Eastern European secret services, and all the texts he wrote later to minimize his role and responsibility in this only indicate that he really suffers from the tarnish on his good name. Friedrich Weinberger visited Moscow in 1994 and asked the members of the Working Commission what they felt about the whole affair. They, of course, said that all was OK and that they would have been arrested anyway, which was probably the truth.[255] However, one can wonder whether this remark calmed the conscience of Friedrich Weinberger.

Pity

Having been there myself, I can only feel pity. Indeed, theses were confusing times, and many of the offered opportunities were fishy and raised many questions. We all made mistakes, and Weinberger's mistake could have been somebody else's. However, at the same time, one has to realize that Weinberger should have realized that keeping "Jutta" all to himself, without consulting any of the people around him who were much more familiar with these issues and could have issued a warning, was rather foolish. Perhaps he understood what their reaction would have been, and thus decided to keep it secret.

Keeping aside the deceit and the damage she caused, I can even understand the situation in which "Jutta" found herself having been coerced to work for the Stasi and then being trapped in an ever-deepening spiral of deceit.

---

252 Rundbrief 1-1999, p. 9. Letter Elmshorn Municipal Archive, June 22, 2009

253 Letter Elmshorn Municipal Archive, June 22, 2009. Rundbrief 2-1998, p. 29. In Rundbrief 1-1999, p. 9 the year 1995 is provided. The Rundbrief 1-2008 of the DVpMP confirms that she had a fatal car accident.

254 Interview Jochen Neumann, June 3, 2009.

255 *Rundbrief*, 1-1999, p. 11

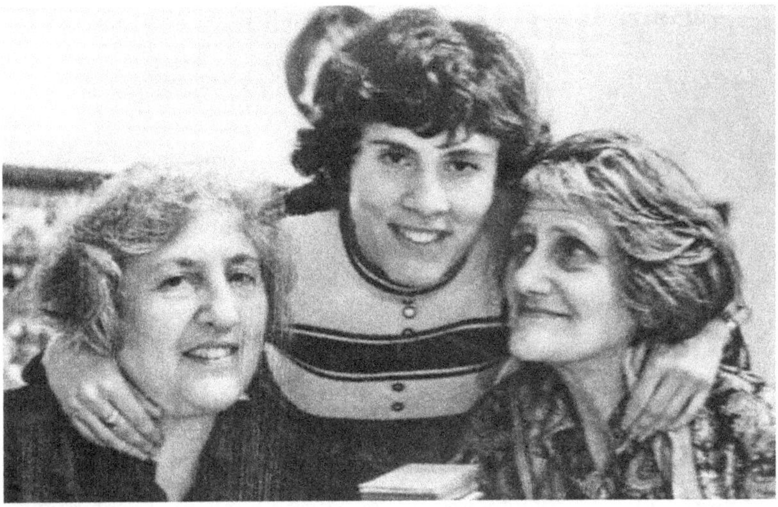

Irina Kaplun with her mother (left) and aunt (right)

Especially at a later date when real people were being hurt, it must have been a horrendous experience, like being sucked into a whirlpool, too much to digest. And when disclosure seemed inevitable, she apparently decided to end her own life. It is hard to imagine that this all happened without any psychological consequences. As Aleksandr Solzhenitsyn wrote: "The line that separates good and evil does not go through classes or groups, but right through every human heart. The line is movable, it fluctuates over the years. A bridgehead of good will remain even in a heart occupied by evil, and likewise even in the most merciful heart there will be an impregnable hiding place for evil".[256]

[256] Aleksandr Solzhenitsyn, in the 1999 Holocaust Lecture by Prof. Philip Zimbardo, Holocaust Studies Center, Sonoma State University

Chapter 14 – The End of the Working Commission

We shall sit together in the kitchen for a while.
The white kerosene smells sweet.

Osip Mandelshtam, 1931[257]

Of course, when looking back without having any possibility of access to the relevant KGB files, it is hard to establish what contribution "Jutta" had to the conviction of the members of the Working Commission. Undoubtedly, many of the materials she handed over to the KGB were already known to them, found during house searches among dissidents or intercepted while being smuggled out of the country. The reports on the conversations "Jutta" had with Working Commission members probably also contained very little news, as most if not all of the apartments were bugged and thus full records of the conversations were already available to them. And Jutta's testimony that the Working Commission members were hostile to the USSR and planned all kinds of "hostile activities" should also not have been much of a surprise.

Probably, the evidence collected by "Jutta" was only a limited part of the "evidence" that was used during the trials of the members of the Working Commission. Nowhere in the reports on their trials is such evidence mentioned, although relatives of the accused attended the trials and reference to such evidence would certainly have stood out.[258]

Vyacheslav Bakhmin, one of the persons mentioned repeatedly in the reports by "Jutta," was arrested on February 12, 1980, the third member to be arrested after the conviction of Feliks Serebrov in 1977 and Aleksandr Podrabinek in 1978.[259] In the same month, a consultant to the Working Commission, psychiatrist Aleksandr Voloshanovich, was told to emigrate from the USSR or face arrest as well.[260] By then it was clear that the KGB had decided to clean Moscow and the other "Olympic cities" of dissidents and other undesired elements in preparation for the Olympic Games of July

257 From Mandelstam, O., *Selected Poems*, Farrar, Strauss and Giroux, 1973

258 See the reports on the trials in the Information Bulletins of the Working Commission itself and the relevant issues of the Chronicle of Current Events

259 *Chronicle of Current Events* No. 47 (trial against Feliks Serebrov), No. 50 (trial against Aleksandr Podrabinek) and No. 56 (arrest of Bakhmin)

260 Aleksandr Voloshanovich, born 1941 in Kharkov, Ukraine, currently living in the United Kingdom. Voloshanovich is the author of forty psychiatric diagnoses of former or potential victims of political abuse of psychiatry in the USSR, and in all cases he concluded there was no evidence of mental illness.

1980. What was unknown, yet suspected, was the fact that KGB Chairman Yuri Andropov had decided to use the Olympic Games as a pretext to finish the dissident movement once and for all. The Working Commission was only one of the many dissident groups that would be liquidated in the course of this campaign.

I entered the orbit of the Working Commission when Jutta had already done most of her destructive work and the preparations for the arrest of Vyacheslav Bakhmin were in full swing. In fact, it was Bakhmin who advised me to come to Moscow if I still wanted to meet any of the dissidents at liberty, as one after the other was being arrested. His arrest took place on the day I booked my first trip to the Soviet Union.[261] By the time I got to Moscow, first in early March 1980 and - quickly after - during the first half of April 1980, the situation had become even more desperate. I visited the home of Irina Grivnina, a Moscow computer programmer who had been involved with the Working Commission from early on but who had joined the Commission officially only in March 1980, and heard the story of Bakhmin's arrest while in her apartment. Her two best friends – Aleksandr Podrabinek and Vyacheslav Bakhmin – were now behind bars and there was no doubt in her head that she would soon meet their fate. It was merely a question of how long she would still be able to continue her dissident activities.

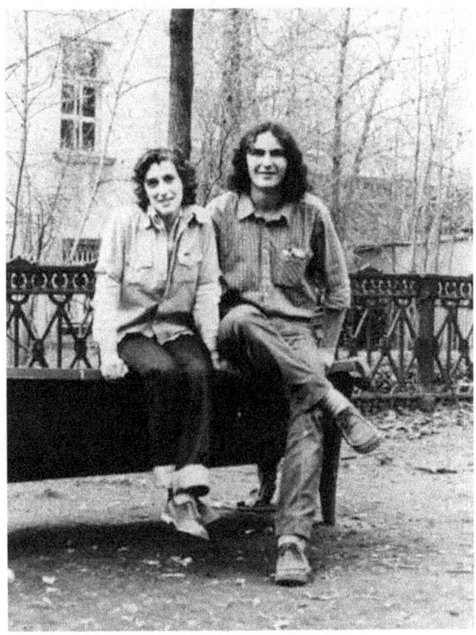

Irina Grivnina and Robert van Voren, 1980

Irina Grivnina was an impressive character, and had in her all the elements of a classic Soviet dissident. She was then 35 years of age, intelligent, with strong opinions, extremely loyal to her friends but harsh to those

261 *Dissidents and Madness*, p. 5-6. Incorrectly, I noted that the day of arrest of Vyacheslav Bakhmin was February 7, 1980; in fact it was February 12.

she disagreed with, courageous and as stubborn as can be. I was quite overpowered by her presence and her stories, and the unusual circumstances made the effect on me even stronger. Undeterred, she continued to do what had to be done. We visited one dissident after the other or, more often, the relatives of a dissident who had been arrested shortly before, and I carefully collected all the information in order to smuggle it out. Some documents were photographed, so I could smuggle them out on film.[262] Also, we would sometimes go to the post office, where Grivnina had ordered an international telephone call with Kronid Lubarsky in Munich. Because the telephone lines were pretty awful, she would be standing in the telephone booth shouting information on arrests, searches and other events into the receiver, so loudly that everybody in the post office could follow word for word. We also went around the city, trying to find ways to photograph places of detention, such as the Serbski Institute for Forensic Psychiatry at Kropotkin Street, where many dissidents were declared insane, or the Lefortovo prison of the KGB, where Grivnina soon would find herself as well. Also, one evening she took me out to the railroad tracks not far from her home on the northern edge of the city center, where at night convoys of prisoners were loaded in special train wagons to be taken out to the archipelago of camps in Siberia.

The rest of the time we would be sitting in the kitchen, listening to one dissident after the other dropping by and delivering more bad news. The days would almost unnoticeably change into evenings and then into nights, until the early birds would announce daybreak. Days without sleeping resulted in a permanent heightened state of alertness and sensitivity, with outside stimuli having a much stronger effect than usual, and the knowledge that those around you could or would soon be gone added an extra emotional layer to the whole affair. Being a fresh courier coming into the cold, still naïve and without any experience, this was the worst environment to start a "courier's career." Only two outcomes were possible: either I would be so shocked that I would never return, or I was hooked. The fact that I am still involved, after more than thirty years, proves that in my case it was the second option.

What was overwhelming, time and again, was the endless hospitality of the dissidents we visited. When moving around Moscow with Grivnina at least it was clear to our hosts that I was "one of them," but also before, when alone and just ringing the doorbell out of the blue, the treatment was no different: I was immediately pulled into the apartment and be seated at

262 *On Dissidents and Madness*, pp. 22-26

the kitchen table and fed. Only then the inevitable question would come: “What is it that brings you here?” At that time, we took this hospitality almost for granted, it was just part of it. Only later, in the late 1980s, when “glasnost” and “perestroika” had become the keywords of Soviet policy and the dissident movement was back in full force and hyperactive, we noticed the difference. Dissidents would tell us to come at a certain time, or told us they had no time at all. At first we were upset, even a bit angry, but soon we realized that this was the beginning of a new era, in which even dissidents had an agenda and appointments were inevitable: being a dissident was almost like having a job!

These days were still far away in 1980, an unimaginable distant future. During this first trip in 1980 I was directly confronted with the wave of arrests that hit the dissident movement: day in, day out, week in, week out. On April 10, a few days after I met him and while still in Moscow, Commission member Leonard Ternovsky was arrested, leaving only Grivnina and a second Commission member, Feliks Serebrov, at large.[263] Serebrov, a somewhat silent bearded man, was a self-educated worker and a poet. He had been in the Gulag several times before, the last time in 1977 having been the first member of the Working Commission to be arrested.[264] However, because of the publicity following the 1977 World Congress of the WPA in Honolulu, the authorities had been weary of evoking too much protest from the West and had meted out a sentence of only one year in camp. However, Serebrov was also a member of the Moscow Helsinki Group, and that made him an even more important target of the KGB.

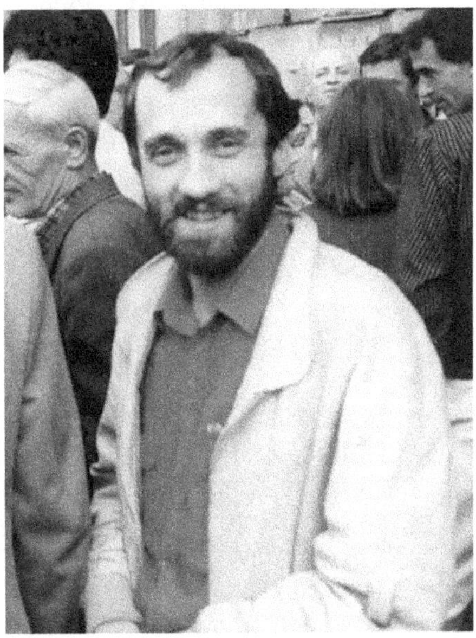

Aleksandr Podrabinek, 1989

During the summer of 1980, the pressure on the Working Commission continued unabated. In June, Aleksandr Podrabinek was re-arrested again in

263 Leonard Ternovsky (1933-2006), a radiologist by profession.

264 Feliks Serebrov, born 1930, spent four terms in the Gulag in 1947-1954, 1957-1958, 1977-1978, 1981-1987 (early release).

his place of exile in Ust-Nera, Yakutia. Life had been pretty harsh out there, in particular because of the climate. I will never forget the explanation a visiting friend gave upon his return on how to measure the temperature. If you spit and it reaches the floor and then freezes, it is warmer than minus 45 degrees Celsius; if it hits the ground with a tick and is immediately stuck to it, it must be between minus 45 and minus 55. However, when it hits the ground and bumps away, like a rubber ball, it is less than 55 degrees below Celsius. Podrabinek's re-arrest resulted in his wife and baby son Mark returning to Moscow, and he himself being sentenced to three years in camp, which he served in Yakutia.[265]

A month later, on July 23, 1980, Irina Kaplun died in a car accident in Lithuania, under unclear circumstances. She had left the Working Commission for personal reasons in 1978, and with her husband Vladimir Borisov (himself a victim of political abuse of psychiatry) she was mostly active in promoting the independent Free Trade Union that her husband and some others had set up.

In September 1980, I was back in Moscow again, my third trip that year. I spent most of my days going around Moscow with Irina Grivnina, and it was clear her days at liberty were numbered. She was tense, much more tense than before, and although this was my third trip, I was still partially oblivious of what was going on a round me. All I knew was that bad times were here. I knew rationally, but emotionally it was too much to handle for the young man from Holland that I was.

One evening, we went to the home of Leonard Ternovsky, who had his birthday but was awaiting trial in Butyrka prison. Repeatedly, a tape was played to those present at the party, and the room filled itself with the voice of Leonard Ternovsky reading poetry by his friend Feliks Serebrov. After a while I was introduced to an unknown man. "Realizing that I was a foreigner, he started up a conversation in German. His German, much better than my Russian at that time, was far from fluent. But we managed to carry on a conversation. The man was well built, with an open, handsome face. He wore a nicely cut, glossy grey suit and a wide tie. In some ways he resembled Pasternak. He was strikingly calm, and although very few knew him at the party, in a strange way he was a central figure. He radiated kindness and was self-assured yet unpretentious; a charismatic presence. After he allowed me to take his picture, the man left. Later that evening upon return to the city center, I was told that this was Anatoly

265 *The Story of the Opposition*, p. 7-9

Koryagin, a psychiatrist by profession, and a consultant to the Working Commission..."[266]

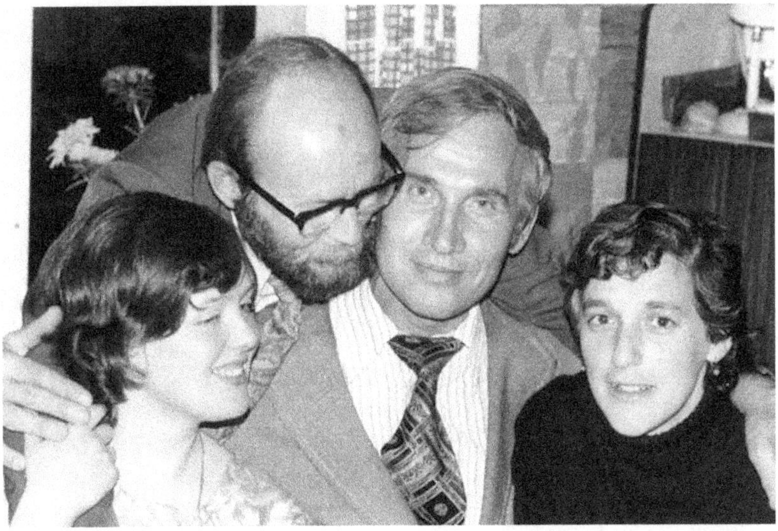

l.t.r. Olga Ternovskaya, Feliks Serebrov, Anatoly Koryagin, Irina Grivnina, September 1980

That night, Anatoly Koryagin had insisted to Grivnina and Serebrov be allowed to join the Working Commission. The reason was not that he saw any hope for its future; it was clear that an arrest of its members was merely a matter of time. Yet Koryagin wanted to share responsibility for the Commission's work. His contribution had been to examine former and potential victims of political abuse of psychiatry, writing psychiatric diagnoses in which he concluded that the person was not suffering from any mental illness. These reports were used as a means of defense: if the person was picked up again and sent to a psychiatric hospital, the Commission had proof that this was for non-medical purposes. These activities, as well as his essay, "Unwilling Patients," in which he exposed some of the mechanisms behind the political abuse of psychiatry, made Anatoly Koryagin a number one target for the KGB.[267]

A week after my departure, Irina Grivnina was arrested, and soon Koryagin officially joined the Commission. In January 1981, Feliks Serebrov was

266 *Koryagin*, p. 11. Koryagin (born 1938), emigrated to Switzerland in 1987, returned to Russia in 1995. According to the latest information he lives in the town of Pereyaslavl-Zalessky.

267 *Unwilling Patients*, in Koryagin, pp. 43-51

picked up by the KGB. Shortly after, on February 13, 1981, Koryagin met the same inevitable fate. He was arrested on the train from his hometown Kharkov to Moscow. The couple was on their way to the capital, where Koryagin wanted to introduce his wife Galina to some of his friends so she could turn to them for help after he was gone.[268] Koryagin's arrest ended the existence of the Working Commission.

In the course of 1980 and 1981, one member after the other was convicted. Bakhmin had already been tried in the summer of 1980 and sentenced to three years in camp for "slandering the Soviet state;" he would be re-arrested again in the beginning in 1983 while still in camp. This time he was sentenced to an additional year in camp, and was eventually released in February 1984.[269] Leonard Ternovsky's trial was in December 1980, resulting in a sentence of three years of camp.

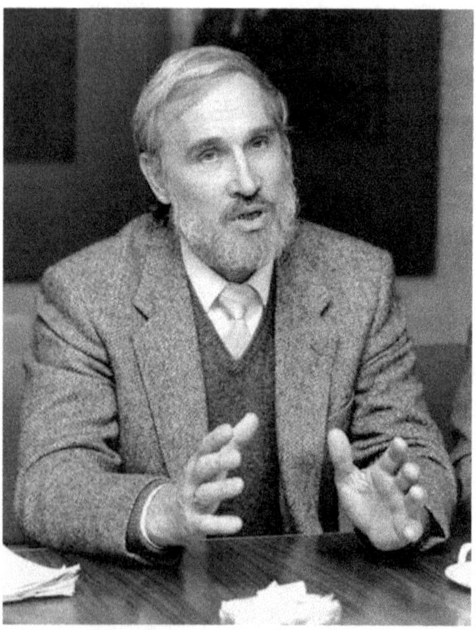

Anatoly Koryagin, Amsterdam , May 1987

Much later, in the summer of 1981, Irina Grivnina was tried, and sentenced to five years in exile. With her time in pre-trial detention deducted from the sentence, she was released in June 1983.[270] Following a long battle to avoid having her expelled from Moscow for not having a residence permit,[271] she was allowed to immigrate to Amsterdam in the fall of 1985, where she still lives today. Feliks Serebrov made a partial recantation, but somehow this didn't very much help him.[272] Instead of receiving a lighter sen-

268 *Koryagin*, p. 12. During the following years, Galina's main contact in Moscow would be Irina Yakir, a Moscow dissident and grand-daughter of Marshal Iona Yakir. See *On Dissidents and Madness*, pp 53-4.

269 *List of Political Prisoners*, 1983, p.61

270 One day in prison equals three days in exile.

271 Many dissidents were not allowed to live in cities like Moscow, Leningrad or Kiev after the completion of their sentence. For more information on the Grivnina case see *Schaakmatch tegen de KGB* (Chess match against the KGB), Amsterdam, 1986

272 *Chronicle of Current Events*, No. 63

tence the accusation was aggravated from "slandering the Soviet State" to "anti-Soviet agitation and propaganda," and he was sentenced to four years of camp and five years of exile.[273] He was released in 1987 together with many of the other political prisoners in the USSR.

The harshest sentence was meted out to Anatoly Koryagin. He was the main object of the authorities' wrath, being a psychiatrist who not only obstructed the authorities' systematic use of psychiatry as a tool of repression by writing independent psychiatric diagnoses, but also having been the author of a number of highly critical and damaging *samizdat* articles, such as *Unwilling Patients*, in which the system behind the abuse was explored. In June 1981 he was sentenced to seven years of camp and five years of exile, and in 1985 an additional sentence of two years of camp would be added in order to maximize the pressure on him. After an intense international campaign he was released in February 1987 and allowed to leave the USSR.[274]

---

273 *List of Political Prisoners*, p. 160

274 For more information on the campaign and Koryagin's lobbying in the West see *On Dissidents and Madness*, pp. 96-121.

Part III

Act One

Chapter 15 – The WPA Becomes Involved

They exchanged a hooligan
For good old Luis Corvalan
Where a creep can be found
To swap with Lyonya this time round[1]

"Bukovsky is after his expulsion politically used... in the fight against the USSR, even though he is a criminal."

Ivan Abramov, KGB[2]

The World Congress of the WPA in Honolulu was the first Melvin Sabshin attended in his new position of Medical Director of the American Psychiatric Association. He had obtained that position three years earlier, after a successful career in Chicago, Illinois.

As noted earlier, Melvin Sabshin started in Chicago in 1953, thanks to Roy Grinker, the Director of the Institute for Psychosomatic Research and Training at Michael Reese Hospital (the Psychosomatic and Psychiatric Institute – PPI).[3] Grinker had been one of the authors of the book *"Men Under Stress,"* that played a key role in understanding the psychiatric casualties of the Second World War. In the early 1950s, Grinker, along with several members of his staff, also published a study of paratroopers at Fort Benning (Georgia), in which the whole aspect of the soldiers' adaptation to the stressful conditions of parachute jumping was researched.

The PPI not only cared for a sizeable group of patients, it also ran a clinic and a package of advanced educational programs. Among these, the residency program was particularly notable and selected residents simultaneously went through psychoanalytic training at the Chicago Institute of Psychoanalysis.[4]

---

1 Saying in Moscow after Vladimir Bukovsky was exchanged for the Chilean Communist leader Luis Corvalan in December 1976. Lyonya stands for Soviet leader Leonid Brezhnev.

2 HAXX 1386/1, p. 81. Ivan Abramov was deputy of Filipp Bobkov, Director of the Fifth Directorate of the KGB, and his successor as head of the Fifth Directorate in 1985.

3 Roy R. Grinker, Sr. (1900-1993), is considered to be a pioneer in American psychiatry. He founded the psychiatry department at the University of Chicago, was the founding editor of the *Archives of General Psychiatry*, and was a prolific author.

4 Roy Grinker Sr. himself had been analyzed by Sigmund Freud, see *Sigmund*

Quite a few of the residents at Michael Reese later became psychoanalysts. Melvin Sabshin completed psychoanalytic training in 1962 and, although he did not intend to practice psychoanalysis, he treated some patients as part of the training process and, later, during his work at the PPI. One of the most important aspects of Sabshin's work at PPI concerned research, including participating in Grinker's multi-disciplinary projects on anxiety and depression.

During his stay in Chicago, Melvin Sabshin met Edith Goldfarb, "who was one of the psychiatric trainees who rotated through the three affiliated residency programs. She was enormously attractive and the most psychologically astute person that I'd ever met in my life."[5] As a young physicist, Edith had been selected to work on the Manhattan Project at the University of Chicago. After the war, she decided to become a physician and soon became interested in psychiatry and psychoanalysis. Upon completion of her residency, she continued her psychoanalytic training and began an appointment with the Chicago Institute for Psychoanalysis that continued until she left Chicago. She joined Melvin Sabshin in Washington, D.C., in 1976, two years after his appointment as Medical Director of the APA, and became active at the Washington Psychoanalytic Institute.[6]

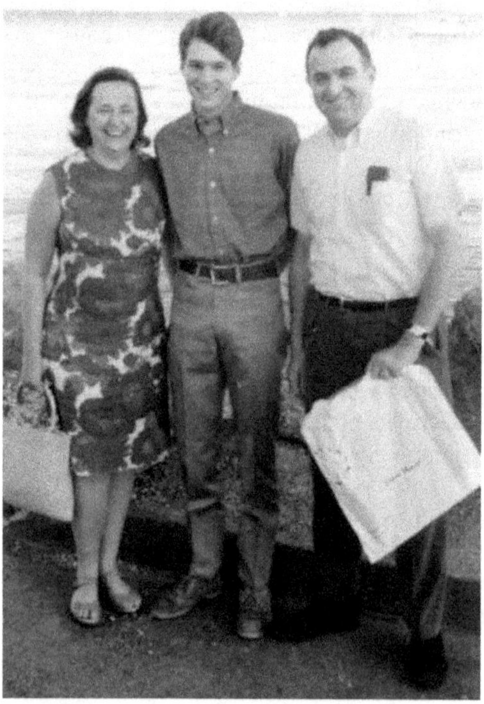

Edith, Jimmy and Mel Sabshin

Freud and his Impact on the Modern World (Annual of Psychoanalysis, vol. 29), edited by Jerome A. Winer and James William Anderson.

5 *Changing American Psychiatry – A personal perspective*, p. 32-3

6 Edith Sabshin remained a close companion of Melvin Sabshin throughout her life. She died in 1992, leaving Melvin Sabshin heartbroken. In 2000, he married his current wife Marion Bennathan.

The FBI is back

In 1955, Melvin Sabshin was deleted from the list of persons with a security risk, even though the document that led to this decision concluded that he had been a member of the Communist Party and various front organizations "within the past five years." However, "inasmuch the subject's activities do not now come within the revised criteria for inclusion in the Security Index, Sabshin's Security Index card is being cancelled."[7]

However, this does not mean that the FBI ceased to be interested in Sabshin as a source of information. Two years later, on May 5, 1957, two FBI agents were standing on his doorstep for a conversation. "Sabshin was cordial and indicated he had long been expecting a visit from the FBI."[8] The FBI made clear they came to visit him became he was in the "envious position to be of valuable assistance to the government" and that they wanted him to provide information on the Communist Party, even though they "did not desire to embarrass him or incriminate him nor have him make any statement which he deemed to be against his better interests."[9]

Even though Sabshin, according to the FBI, had expected their visit, he was apparently reluctant to provide them with the information they wanted. He "stated he felt a deep reluctance at furnishing information concerning other individuals since many of the individuals with whom he was associated in the movement are personal friends. He did state, however, that with additional interviews he might come to fully appreciate the government's position and, if so, he would then have no reluctance in furnishing the identities of those individuals with whom he was associated." As to his membership in the Communist Party, "he did admit that he was formally associated with the Communist Party but has now severed all relationships with the movement, both from a standpoint of membership and ideology."[10]

In the FBI report, the reasons that Sabshin gave for having been a member of – or having been associated with – the Communist Party are listed. In the first place, the influence of his parents, who had escaped from a Russia with a Tsar who condoned and stimulated anti-Semite repression and who had been toppled by the Communists. Secondly, Sabshin saw the Communist movement as the main opposition to the "Hitler movement"

7 Decision by Assistant Attorney General William F. Tomkins of June 13, 1955, communicated to the director of the FBI.

8 Report by FBI Chicago to the Director of the FBI, May 6, 1957, p. 1

9 Report by FBI Chicago to the Director of the FBI, May 6, 1957, p. 1

10 Report by FBI Chicago to the Director of the FBI, May 6, 1957, p. 1

and "he could see the Communist movement as only a means of salvation for members of the Jewish faith." Thirdly – and here the FBI combined the three remaining arguments into one – Sabshin had indicated that his membership was the result of "immaturity" and that he had been excited to "belong to an organization that was more or less a closed group and one which held surreptitious meetings." The fact that he had come 'out of the closet' was thanks to the fact that he now understood all this, as well as the fact that his new relationship (Edith Goldfarb) had "berated him for his former associations. He stated her feelings were also a contributing factor for his desire to furnish the FBI with information concerning his past activities."[11] On basis of the conversation, the agents concluded that "with additional contacts, Sabshin will be fully cooperative in this regard" (meaning furnishing the desired information) and advised that "interviews with Sabshin will continue until all information in his possession has been obtained and a determination made as to whether or not he possesses potential as a security informant."[12]

That follow-up meeting took place on May 8, 1957, and the FBI's earlier assessment had been correct. From the start, Sabshin made clear that he had decided to provide the FBI with "any information in his possession regarding his association with the Communist Party (CP) in the New Orleans, Louisiana area."[13] At the beginning of the meeting, the FBI agents asked Sabshin "in order to place in its proper perspective the information" to date his own CP membership. Sabshin indicated that he had been "near and around the Communist Political Association and the CP from October 1944 to some period in 1949. Sabshin stated he preferred not to make a definite statement of fact concerning CP membership since he felt the possibility exist that he was actually never a registered CP member. He could not recall ever having actually been registered. He stated he was treating the matter in a technical fashion but preferred it this way since upon entering the U.S. Army in 1944, he signed an oath that he was never a CP member. Sabshin, however, asserted he considered himself a CP member without ever having definite knowledge that he was. He stated that during the pertinent period, he was a believer in the Communist ideology and was active on behalf of the Party."[14]

---

11 Report by FBI Chicago to the Director of the FBI, May 6, 1957, pp. 2-3

12 Report by FBI Chicago to the Director of the FBI, May 6, 1957, p. 4

13 Office Memorandum of the FBI Chicago to the Director FBI, file 100-383716, May 20, 1957, p. 1

14 Office Memorandum of the FBI Chicago to the Director FBI, file 100-383716, May 20, 1957, p. 1

Subsequently, the FBI asked Sabshin to provide information on persons he knew to be members of, or associated with, the Communist Party. The document shows that he named two dozen individuals, and indicated whether they were CP members, ardent CP members, held any rank or position within the organization and what other information might be of use to the U.S. Government. Satisfied, the FBI agents conclude: "it appears that Sabshin has been fully cooperative in furnishing the information in his possession regarding his association with the Communist movement. The Agents believe he is sincere in his thought that he may never have actually been a registered CP member. He was given the opportunity to deny CP membership, which he would not do."[15] Sabshin indicated his willingness to meet again and furnish "information on any individual he recalls" and that considering his current position at the Michael Reese Hospital in Chicago, there was no chance he would re-associate himself with the Communist movement. "In addition, he stated he now has a very strong dislike for the Communist movement and further association with the movement would be repugnant."[16]

According to another FBI document, a further interview took place on June 28, 1957.[17] Apparently Sabshin provided no additional information during that meeting, as is reported in a FBI Office memorandum of July 24, 1957, and the document confirms that "his present feeling of repugnance towards the Communist Party precludes any possibility of his actively assisting the FBI in the role of an informant."[18]

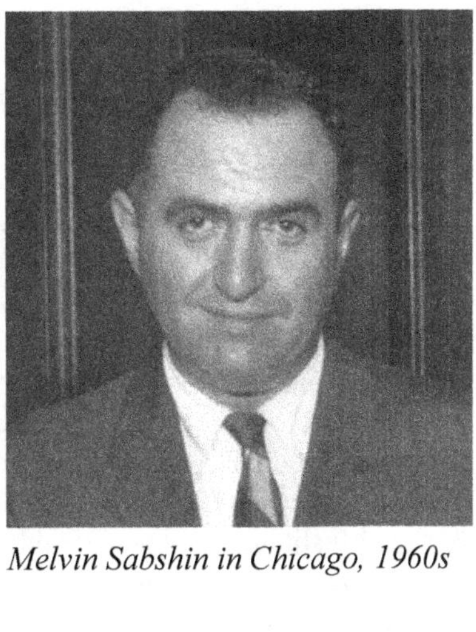

Melvin Sabshin in Chicago, 1960s

The case was, however, still not closed. Almost a year later, in May 1958, Sabshin was contacted by an investigator of the House Committee on Un-American Activities (HCUA) and asked whether he was willing to

15 Office Memorandum of the FBI Chicago to the Director FBI, file 100-383716, May 20, 1957, p. 5

16 Office Memorandum of the FBI Chicago to the Director FBI, May 20, 1957, p. 6

17 FBI report on the investigation into Sabshin, CG 100-28265

18 FBI Office Memorandum, FBI Chicago, dated July 24,1 957

testify. "Sabshin has consented to voluntarily appear and will reveal all he knows regarding CP activity in the New Orleans area. Sabshin was not advised of the hearing date but is to communicate with [name deleted] who will advise him."[19] However, Sabshin's appearance before the HCUA raised some concern, as his testimony might reveal the name or names of informants of the FBI within the Communist movement. The FBI investigated whether that would indeed be the case, and by the time they concluded that Sabshin could safely testify it was already summer. On July 30, 1958, Sabshin was informed that the "Committee was pressed for time and did not have time to hear Sabshin's testimony."[20] Sabshin left for a four-week holiday but contact was not resumed until late September;[21] however, for unclear reasons it never came to any public testimony. A FBI document of September 28, 1958, reports that Sabshin "openly appeared before the HCUA in Washington D.C. and testified as a Government witness," yet then adds: "The memo contains no further information regarding this matter. Review of Chicago indices disclosed no other statement that Sabshin had testified before HCUA."[22] Melvin Sabshin confirms that he never appeared before the HCUA and when asked why he thinks he was not called up, his answer shows to what extent the confrontation with his personal file has had an emotional effect on him: "your resume [of my FBI file] stirred many memories, some of which I still find quite painful, even with 60 years gone by. I always believed that I was not important enough to be called as a witness before the HCUA. If there was any other reason that I was not called I don't know what it would be..."[23]

More than a decade later, in March 1970, it is the White House that requested a name check of Melvin Sabshin. According to the files, during that investigation no new information came to light. A year later, in August-October 1971, another thorough investigation was carried out by the FBI at the request of the Department of Health, Education and Welfare, following his nomination to the Continuing Education Training Committee of the National Institute of Mental Health (NIMH). The investigation was again a full scale one, involving interviews with former colleagues and friends, a "neighborhood check" and conversations with neighbors, check of credit and arrest, etc. "No pertinent additional information was developed as a result of this investigation and our files do not reveal any action taken by the Department of Health, Education and Welfare concerning captioned

19 FBI Office Memorandum, FBI Chicago, May 6, 1958
20 FBI Office Memorandum, FBI Chicago, August 5, 1958
21 FBI Office Memorandum, FBI Chicago, September 22, 1958
22 FBI Chicago Airtel document to Director FBI, September 28, 1971
23 E-mail from Melvin Sabshin, February 12, 2010.

individual."[24] This information, however, was incorrect. A FBI document dated August 16, 1971, clearly states that "based on information received from the FBI in a memo dated March 25, 1970, to the White House, Sabshin was not offered a position with the above committee."[25] A further explanation adds that FBI investigation in 1952 "furnished derogatory information concerning the employee [M. Sabshin]."

The last name check, carried out at the request of the White House, is of November 1974. Melvin Sabshin is then already Medical Director of the American Psychiatric Association.

Global forum

The time in at Michael Reese Hospital and its Psychosomatic and Psychiatric Institute (PPI) in Chicago proved to be an excellent breeding ground for Sabshin's later career. His responsibilities at PPI increased over time and eventually he was promoted to the position of Associate Director. In the fall of 1961, Melvin Sabshin became Head of the Department of Psychiatry at the University of Illinois. As far as numbers of students concerned, the medical school at Illinois was the largest in the United States and it continued to grow even larger during the 1970s and 1980s. Gradually Sabshin also became involved in state and national activities in psychiatry. He became President of the Illinois Psychiatric Society, sat on several committees of the APA, was elected as Trustee on the APA's Board and, in 1972, he became the chair of the APA Program Committee, which had the responsibility of organizing APA's national annual conventions. In 1974, the Medical Director of the APA, Walter Barton, resigned from his position and a search committee selected Melvin Sabshin as his successor.[26]

Although his appointment as Medical Director of the American Psychiatric Association was a major step career-wise, for Melvin Sabshin it was particularly important intellectually. Here he had the chance of influencing American psychiatry as a whole and put his ideas to practice. From very early on it was clear to him that psychiatry needed a clear concept of diagnostics, one that would end the prevailing lack of clarity and in

---

24 Document of November 11, 1974, following a renewed name check request by the White House

25 FBI Airtel dated August 16, 1971, FBI Washington D.C., number WFO 121-26112

26 Walter Barton (1906-1999) was Medical Director of the APA from 1963 until 1974.

his view also led to abuses. Under his leadership the organization grew immensely, and from a small professional organization mainly active in organizing annual meetings and publishing two journals, it became an organization with 40,000 members and an annual budget of 28 million US dollars.[27] More importantly, the APA developed the Diagnostic and Statistical Manual of Mental Disorders (DSM), the American classification scheme used in psychiatry worldwide, which was one of the first attempts to compare diagnoses in different environments. Considering the enormous amount of time and energy he put in its development, it is not strange that the fourth edition of DSM was dedicated to him.[28]

The election to the Executive Committee of the WPA in 1983 was, in a sense, the next logical step in his career, as it enabled him to implement his ideas and concepts on an international level and to continue to promote clear diagnostic criteria as a means to curb improper use of his profession. In Sabshin's view, the political abuse in the Soviet Union had been made possible primarily because of the absence of clear diagnostic criteria and, thus, the main barrier against such abuse in future would be the development of an internationally accepted psychiatric nosology.[29]

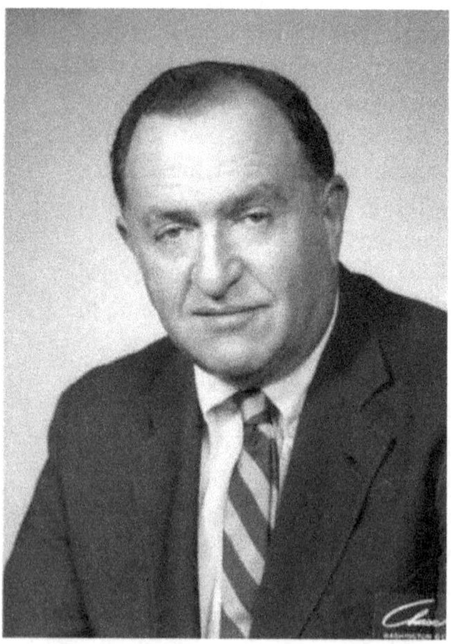

Melvin Sabshin, mid 1970s

With that in mind, the World Psychiatric Association (WPA) provided the right forum to Sabshin, as it was not only the organization on which the international campaign against Soviet psychiatric abuse concentrated itself, but it also constituted the international umbrella organization of psychiatric societies. It was, as such, probably one of the largest non-governmental

27 See the interview of Claus Einar Langen with Melvin Sabshin on the eve of his retirement, published in *Mental Health Reforms*, 4-1997, p. 15

28 *Changing American Psychiatry – A personal perspective*, p. 128. The dedication reads: *To Melvin Sabshin, a man for all seasons.*

29 For a much more extensive description of Melvin Sabshin's views and work regarding these issues see chapter 10 of Melvin Sabshin's memoirs *Changing American Psychiatry – A personal perspective*

organizations in the world. Originally created with the sole purpose of organizing world psychiatric congresses, it evolved into an international body that not only organized regional psychiatric meetings, but also promoted professional education and set ethical, scientific and treatment standards for psychiatry.

The organization had initially been set up in 1950 as an Association for the Organization of World Congresses of Psychiatry, with the Frenchmen Jean Delay as its President and Henry Ey as its Secretary General. The World Health Organization had just published the Sixth Revision of the International Classification of Diseases (ICD) that, for the first time, included a section devoted to mental, psychoneurotic and personality disorders. A few years later, the American Psychiatric Association produced the first edition of its DSM. After two World Congresses of Psychiatry, held in Paris in 1950 and Zurich in 1957, the organization was officially founded in 1961. By then, there was a generally accepted perception that empirical knowledge was more important than old or novel theories and that a mechanism was necessary to share the newly acquired knowledge with colleagues around the globe. At the same time, more and more psychiatrists recognized the need to agree on more precise and comprehensive definitions of mental disorders and to deepen the understanding of the socio-cultural settings in which the new knowledge was to be applied. The WPA united psychiatrists of different national and cultural origins and of different schools of thought, and thus provided a global forum to professionals united in the quest for increased knowledge in the field.[30]

Key events for the World Psychiatric Association remained the World Congresses of Psychiatry, which initially took place every six years but starting in 1989 were to take place every three years. The WPA also organized regular Regional Meetings. In order to ensure the continuous vitality and productivity in the WPA between World Congresses, Scientific Sections were established that carried out joint scientific work and also organized symposia and, when appropriate, position papers.

---

30 In the course of its existence, the WPA continued to grow, with ups and downs, and *anno 2009* the organization unites 135 national psychiatric societies representing more than 180,000 psychiatrists worldwide. The societies are clustered into 18 Zones and 5 Regions: the Americas, Europe, Africa, Asia, and the South Pacific. Representatives of the societies constitute the WPA General Assembly, the governing body of the organization. The WPA also has individual members and there are provisions for affiliation of other associations (e.g., those dealing with a particular topic in psychiatry).

From 1971 onwards, the agenda of the World Psychiatric Association was dominated by the issue of political abuse of psychiatry, initially with regard to such abuses in the Soviet Union (1971-1989) and later, in the beginning of the twenty-first century, in the People's Republic of China. As a result of the debates, WPA General Assemblies formulated ethical guidelines on psychiatric practice, including the Hawaii Declaration of 1977, its amendment in Vienna in 1983, and, more recently, the Madrid Declaration of 1996, expanded in 1999. In addition, the organization set up Committees on Ethics and on the Review of Abuse of Psychiatry.

Throughout the years, the organizational structure of WPA evolved in order to increase its efficacy. Until 1983, the organization was strongly dominated by the Executive Committee. The larger board, called the Committee, had very little influence over the actual running of the organization. Under Stefanis' chairmanship, the role of the Committee was enhanced.[31] Also, the 1983-1989 Executive Committee of the WPA and, in particular, its members Melvin Sabshin and Jochen Neumann, worked hard on a new organizational structure that would increase the democracy in the organization and result in a more balanced representation of the global psychiatric community. The goal was to decrease the domination of the large Western psychiatric societies but, due to the international political climate, these attempts were often seen in the light of the Cold War and, thus, interpreted as mainly attempts to strengthen the position of the socialist bloc and their subsidiaries in the Third World. The fact that Neumann and Sabshin managed to develop a compromise structure that was eventually adopted by the 1989 General Assembly must be seen as a major feat.

The Honolulu Congress

The request by the British and Americans to discuss the Soviet issue during the World Congress of the WPA in Honolulu had been supported by other societies as well and, thus, only a miracle could prevent the issue from being put on the agenda. This was also clear to the Soviets authorities, who received disturbing signals about the "anti-Soviet campaign with nasty fabrications regarding the alleged use of psychiatry in the USSR as an instrument in the political struggle with 'dissidents'."[32] According to the

---

31 For instance the election of Jochen Neumann as successor to the late Pal Juhasz in October 1984 was a decision of the Committee, on basis of a proposal by the Executive Committee.

32 Report by Yuri Andropov, Chairman of the KGB, to the Central Committee of the CPSU of September 10, 1976, p. 1

KGB, the campaign was a "carefully planned anti-Soviet action," in which a prominent role was played by the British Royal College "under influence of pro-Zionist elements. ... The KGB undertakes through operational channels measures to counter hostile attacks..."[33]

In October 1976, the Ministry of Health established a special working group under chairmanship of Deputy Minister of Health Dmitri Venediktov to work out a plan of action for a counter campaign. Among the members of the working group were leading Soviet psychiatrists Andrei Snezhnevsky, Georgi Morozov, Eduard Babayan and Marat Vartanyan. The plans they developed were, inter alia, the composition of documents with counter-arguments to be disseminated before and during the World Congress; active lobbying of the media to explain the humane nature of Soviet medicine; lobbying within the World Psychiatric Association to prevent the issue from being put on the agenda; lobbying the World Health Organization to put pressure on the WPA to not allow this unacceptable "anti-Soviet campaign;" and establishing closer working relations with positively-inclined Western colleagues. It was suggested to elect some of them to honorary membership of the Soviet All-Union Society.[34]

In February 1977, representatives of the secret services of the USSR, DDR, Bulgaria, Czechoslovakia, Hungary, Poland and even Cuba met in Moscow to discuss a common approach to the issue of political abuse of psychiatry and the upcoming World Congress in Honolulu.[35] The meeting was mostly led by Major General Ivan Pavlovich Abramov, deputy head of the Fifth Directorate of the KGB (which dealt among others... with dissidents), with the support of Colonel Romanov, deputy head of the First Division of the Fifth Directorate. It is interesting to note that according to the report, Colonel Romanov would travel with the Soviet delegation to Honolulu as "political advisor."[36] Eberhard Jaekel, then deputy head of Division XX/1 of the Stasi, had prepared a *Concept* particularly for this meeting, outlining how the Stasi could contribute to this joint operation.[37] Jaekel pointed out that the Stasi, at that moment, had no concrete evidence of planned anti-

33 Report by Yuri Andropov, to the Central Committee of September 10, 1976, pp. 2-3

34 Report of the Ministry of Health of the USSR to the Central Committee of the CPSU, signed by deputy Minister S. Burenkov, of October 22, 1976.

35 HAXX 1386/1, p. 61. The document is an announcement by the KGB that on February 8-10, 1977, a meeting will be held in Moscow of representatives of the various secret services.

36 Document HAXX 1386/1, p. 84

37 Document HAXX 1386/1, pp. 71-73

Soviet activity, but that in case it would discover anything, it would happily share it with the KGB. The minutes of the meeting clearly show not only the leading role of the Soviet KGB, but also the concern the Soviets had over Western preparations for the Honolulu World Congress.[38]

Shortly before the World Congress, a high-level conference took place in East Berlin, and the Soviet psychiatric leaders met with colleagues from Bulgaria, Hungary, the DDR, Poland and Czechoslovakia in order to coordinate their positions.[39] Much to the chagrin of Georgi Morozov, the Romanians didn't even appear at this meeting, while both the Poles and Hungarians openly criticized the Soviet position.[40]

However, all this Soviet activity could not prevent the issue from dominating the Congress from the very start. The first plenary session of the Congress saw the introduction of the Declaration of Hawaii. This statement of the ethical principles of psychiatry had been drawn up by the Ethical Sub-Committee of the Executive Committee set up in 1973 in response to the increasing number of protests against the use of psychiatry for non-medical purposes.[41] One of the principles stated in the Declaration was that a psychiatrist must not participate in compulsory psychiatric treatment in the absence of psychiatric illness, and also there were other clauses that could be seen as having a bearing on the political abuse of psychiatry. The Declaration of Hawaii was accepted by the General Assembly without difficulty, and without opposition by the Soviets delegation.[42] Also an Ethics Committee was established, chaired by Prof. Costas Stefanis from Greece; one of the members was Dr. Marat Vartanyan from the Soviet Union.[43]

The Soviet issue passed the General Assembly less easily. The Soviets did everything possible to make their point, and according to the Soviet delegation's report, Marat Vartanyan had successfully prevented former Soviet political prisoner Leonid Plyushch from being registered as a delegate at the Congress and "anti-Soviet materials" from being disseminated in the main congress hall.[44] Prior to the meeting, both sides held press-conferences and

---

38 Document HAXX 1386/1 pp. 78-93

39 *Report on the outcome of the VI World Congress of Psychiatry* by D.D. Venediktov, Eduard Babayan and Andrei Snezhnevsky, sent to the Central Committee on November 21, 1977, p.1.

40 Oltmanns, R., *Spurensuche auf Verbrannter Erde*, Norderstedt, 2009, p. 318.

41 See *The Issue of Abuse*, P. Berner and P. Pichot, p. A

42 *Report on the outcome of the VI World Congress of Psychiatry,* p. 4

43 See *Soviet Psychiatric Abuse - Shadow over World Psychiatry,* pp. 54-71

44 *Report on the outcome of the VI World Congress of Psychiatry,* p. 2

discussions continued during the Assembly. Two motions were put to the vote, a British one condemning the systematic political abuse of psychiatry in the Soviet Union, and an American one calling on the WPA to establish a Review Committee to examine the allegations of political abuse of psychiatry. The British resolution passed with 90 votes against 88, but only after a long debate not only about the issue itself but also about the allotment of votes and other procedural issues. The Soviets later claimed a moral victory, because only 19 societies had voted in favor of the resolution and 33 against. The Polish and Romanian delegates had been absent, who together had six votes.[45]

An American resolution asking for the establishment of a Review Committee received a larger majority of votes, 121 to 66 votes, but was also contested, not only by the Soviet delegation but also by the Greek delegate (and future WPA President) Professor Costas Stefanis, who said he could not see the point of such a committee and that, just as the All-Union Society had been condemned on what he considered inadequate evidence, so the Review Committee might act in the same way.[46]

The Review Committee would be one of the main focuses of attention in the coming six years. From the very first day, the Soviets refused to acknowledge its existence. Initially they tried to prevent its establishment, claiming that it would distract the WPA from its main function, namely the exchange of scientific ideas. When it was established in December 1978, however, in spite of all Soviet resistance, the Soviet society declared flatly that they would not cooperate with the Review Committee, and they confirmed this position in three letters, in which they maintained that the Review Committee was an "illegal formation," that it would continue not to recognize its existence and that no collaboration could be expected.[47] This position would remain unaltered over the coming years. Eventually, the Review Committee was largely made impotent when the WPA President and Secretary General decided to bypass it and started communicating with the Soviets directly. I will get to that point later.

---

45 *Report on the outcome of the VI World Congress of Psychiatry*, p. 5. In their report the Soviet delegation does not elaborate on the reasons why the Polish and Romanian delegates were absent, but they clearly must have been not amused.
According to Prof. Karl Seidel of the DDR the secretary of outgoing Secretary General of the WPA, Denis Leigh, remarked that the performance of Dr. Eduard Babayan had cost the Soviets ten votes. "The view of the Soviets that they can win voting with protests, is wrong." See: MfS 13788/83, p. 177

46 See *Soviet Psychiatric Abuse - Shadow over World Psychiatry*, p. 69

47 *The Issue of Abuse*, P. Berner and P. Pichot, p. 2

In April 1978, the Ministry of Health of the USSR presented a two-year plan to the Central Committee of the CPSU outlining the various activities it would undertake to counter the outcome of the Honolulu Congress. Among the decisions was to ignore the existence of the "illegal" Review Committee and to break off all relations with the British and American psychiatric associations "until they apologize to their Soviet colleagues.[48] In addition, decisions were made to actively lobby the media and friendly Western colleagues; increase the number of international scientific exchanges; publish brochures that explained the "exact" nature of Soviet psychiatry and countered the "lies" in, among others, the book by Bloch and Reddaway.[49] A joint task for the Ministry of Health and the KGB consisted of "organizing the collection of information on the fate of mentally ill persons and former Soviet citizens, who left the USSR, and to use this information while keeping in mind the demands of medical ethics, in order to expose the slanderous character of the accusations addressed to Soviet psychiatry (period: 1978)."[50]

Also, the links with fraternal psychiatric associations were strengthened. In August 1978, a meeting was held in Sofia between Georgi Morozov and Nikolai Zharikov on behalf of the All-Union Society, Ivan Temkov from Bulgaria,[51] and Dr. Rohland[52] and Karl Seidel on behalf of the DDR. During this meeting the improvement of collaboration and the exchange of information were discussed. The Soviets were told that it would have been better if they had kept their socialist colleagues better informed. One of the examples raised was the fact that one of Morozov's deputies, Dr. Yuri Novikov, had defected to West Germany. The DDR psychiatrists

48 *Report on the outcome of the VI World Congress of Psychiatry*, p. 8

49 Bloch, S., and Reddaway, P., *Russia's Political Hospitals*, Gollancz, 1977

50 *Plan of main activities in 1978-1979 to disclose the anti-Soviet slanderous campaign with regard to the so-called "political abuse" of psychiatry*, April 1978, p.2

51 The Stasi archives contain a report on a meeting of the Executive Committee of the WPA in Kyoto, Japan, on April 9-11, 1982, which is a German translation from Russian and Bulgarian and marked "top secret". Considering the fact that Prof. Ivan Temkov was, at that time, a member of the Executive Committee of the WPA, it is logical to assume that Temkov was the source of information and possibly fulfilled the same role as Jochen Neumann later. See HA XX 498 pp. 188-9. As we see later in this chapter (footnote 81), Temkov was not very positive about his Soviet colleagues and described Morozov and Professor Zharikov as functionaries of Soviet psychiatry who had not made any scientific progress.

52 Dr. Rohland was at that time Director of the General Secretariat of medical-Scientific Societies of the DDR.

found out only because a series of interviews that had been published in the journal *Stern*. "Also in this case we would have liked to have received direct information, because there is theoretically the possibility that one would meet this Novikov on the occasion of a congress. The reactions from the Soviet guests to both questions was indifference; we had the impression that they were embarrassed."[53]

Still the meeting had a positive follow-up. In November 1979, a symposium was organized, in which delegations from Bulgaria, Czechoslovakia, the DDR, Hungary and Poland as well as some 400 Soviet psychiatrists took part.[54] A special meeting was organized to discuss regional collaboration amongst psychiatrists from the socialist countries. Among others, a decision was reached to organize a yearly psychiatric conference for socialist countries. Also an attempt was made to develop a mechanism by which the socialist countries would coordinate their response to Western allegations of political abuse of psychiatry, an issue to which the Polish delegate Prof. Dabrowski protested, as the Poles "had not prepared themselves" for this item of the agenda. An attempt by the Soviets to convince the Poles to give up their resistance failed; they insisted that their disagreement would be noted in the minutes of the meeting, something that resulted in irritation among the delegates from the DDR (and possibly of others too). The East Germans were invited for a special meeting with the Soviet psychiatric leadership, where they were thanked for their ongoing support. According to Jochen Neumann, who was a member of the DDR delegation, the DDR psychiatrists were "the most reliable partners of the USSR."[55]

In the meantime, the Review Committee, chaired by Canadian psychiatrist Prof. Jean-Yves Gosselin,[56] started its work. In August 1979, it received the

---

53 Report by Dr. Rohland and Prof. K Seidel on a meeting in Sofia on May 26, 1978. HA XX 498 pp. 312-3

54 See the reports by Prof. H. Schulze and Prof. J. Neumann, HAXX 499 pp. 453-8

55 HAXX 499 p. 458. Interestingly, in February 1985 the same Jochen Neumann would write in a report on a visit to Moscow, where he and his colleague Bernd Nickel held meetings with among others Georgi Morozov, that according to Morozov "the collaboration with colleagues from our country is worse than with those from any other socialist country, and the chances to exert political and professional influence on Western colleagues through various research programs of the WHO is not enough used by us." See: *Bericht* by Jochen Neumann, February 1985, p. 2

56 Dr. J.Y. Gosselin has been Emeritus Professor of the Department of Psychiatry at the University of Ottawa since 1996. Dr. Gosselin was, among others, President of the Association des psychiatres du Québec (1968 – 1971), the

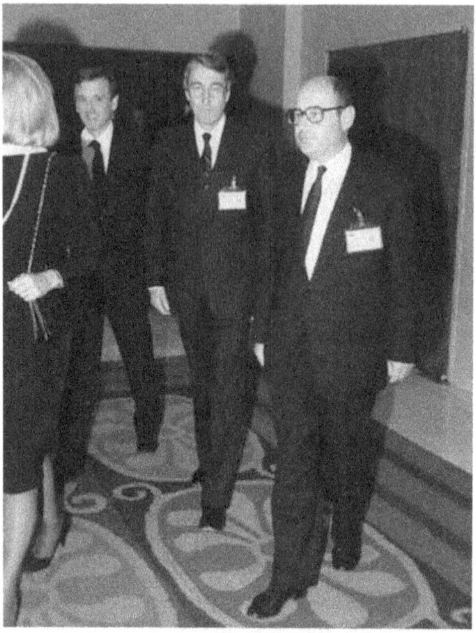

left Jean-Yves Gosselin, right Jochen Neumann, Athens, 1985

first complaints submitted by the British Royal College. By early 1983, 27 complaints had been made by nine member societies of the WPA. However, the Soviets remained mute and no response was received to any of the inquiries. Although not in line with procedures, the Executive Committee itself contacted the Soviets urging them to respond, initially also without success. By October 1981, when the Executive Committee received a report by Dr. Gosselin in which he expressed his frustration about the inability to move ahead, it became clear that patience with the Soviets was wearing thin. Even the Executive Committee agreed to increase pressure on the Soviets, but refused to consider suspension of membership.[57] A month later, the British College of Psychiatrists adopted a resolution calling on the General Assembly of the WPA to expel the Soviet society from its membership.

The final confrontation

More societies joined the campaign, either by adopting resolutions calling on the suspension or expulsion of the Soviet society, or in support of dissident psychiatrists such as Dr. Semyon Gluzman and Dr. Anatoly Koryagin who had both been sentenced to long terms of imprisonment because of their opposition to Soviet psychiatric abuse. In the course of 1982, it became clear that the General Assembly of the WPA would almost certainly vote for suspension or expulsion of the Soviet All-Union Society.

President of the Ontario Psychiatric Association (1986 -1987), and the President of the Canadian Psychiatric Association (1992 – 1993). He was Chairman of the Committee to Review the Abuse of Psychiatry for Political Reasons of the World Psychiatric Association from 1978 until 1985.

57 See Shaw, C., *The World Psychiatric Association and Soviet Psychiatry*, in Van Voren, R. (ed.), *Soviet Psychiatric Abuse in the Gorbachev Era*, Amsterdam, IAPUP, 1989, pp. 44-46

In preparing for the Vienna World Congress, the American Psychiatric Association sent out a memo to all member societies of the WPA on August 12, 1982, in which they announced their intention to organize a forum to discuss the issue prior to the General Assembly in Vienna. They invited other member societies to co-sponsor this event, and also suggested that member societies explore whether the foreign ministries in their countries would be interested in a discussion on the issue that was developing within the United Nations Human Rights Commission. During that session of the UN Human Rights Commission in Geneva in February 1983, the use of mental institutions to control dissent was to be discussed, and this discussion should either lead to a resolution condemning such use, or the adoption of an instrument to investigate such abuses.[58] The Soviets were livid when seeing the letter from the APA, realizing that the net was closing; they later used the letter as one of the main reasons for withdrawing from the WPA.

As mentioned earlier, in the course of 1982 the Soviets had actually started to respond to requests for information from the Executive Committee (deliberately bypassing the Review Committee that they still refused to acknowledge), albeit in a very limited form and in Russian, not one of the official languages of the WPA. In a report titled *The Issue of Abuse 1970-1983*, WPA President Prof. Pierre Pichot and General Secretary Prof. Peter Berner wrote that "The Executive Committee has been successful in obtaining from the member society assurance of imminent, active cooperation in any stipulated form, i.e., provision of medical records as well as on-site examination – and all possible avenues will be explored during the months still remaining until the Association's General Assembly convenes its next meetings, in order to employ the cooperation the Executive Committee has thus been assured of, in clarification of the circumstances that have occasioned the allegations of professional abuse in reference to the complaint cases submitted to the Association by several of its member societies."[59] Clearly, Professors Pierre Pichot and Peter Berner had tried to accommodate the Soviets as much as possible, even by providing an overly optimistic message to the WPA that the Soviets were willing to collaborate fully.

In a press release of February 15, 1983, issued after the Soviet's withdrawal from the Association, Pichot and Berner maintained this optimistic view, by stating that "the All Union Society began to react to enquiries forwarded to them by the Associations' Executive Committee and, also provided a number of case histories. In January 1983, the Chairman of the All Union

58 Memo from Dr. Keith Brodie, President of the American Psychiatric Association, to member societies of the WPA, August 12, 1982.

59 *The Issue of Abuse 1970-1983*. WPA, January 1983.

Society's Directorial Board [Dr. Georgi Morozov] visited the Vienna Secretariat of the World Psychiatric Association and personally handed over the medical data still missing on cases officially enquired upon by the WPA Executive Committee. The discussion carried through on that occasion, between the Soviet visitors and the undersigned, justified the hope that consent might yet be reached upon this controversial issue."[60] In a letter to the All-Union Society of February 15, they elaborated on this and added that "the WPA Executive Committee in their endeavor to resolve the differences… had expressed their desire to be permitted an on-site visit to the Special Psychiatric Hospitals in the Soviet Union" to which "Prof. Morozov and Prof. Saarma had consented to benevolently consider this possibility. This demand for cooperation was responded to by both Prof. Morozov and Prof. Saarma in the most amiable and conciliatory way, thereby justifying the hopeful expectation that this medical discipline might yet be spared the disastrous consequences of a world-wide rift."[61]

60 Press release by the WPA, February 15, 1983

61 Letter by Berner and Pichot to the AUSNP, February 15, 1983. Dr. Juri Martinovich Saarma (1921-2001) was a leading Estonian psychiatrists and member of the USSR Academy of Medical Sciences since 1974, closely related to the Moscow psychiatric nomenklatura. He was generally considered as a psychiatrist with close links to the KGB. He was fluent in German, which was a great asset in maintaining communication with foreign colleagues and not a regular feature among Soviet leading psychiatrists.

Chapter 16 - The Soviets Leave the WPA

"In the opinion of the KGB, there are secret services behind the leading [Western] psychiatrists..."[62]

The Soviet's "comparatively active cooperation in reference to the abuse issue" had been too little and too late.[63] On January 31, 1983, the All-Union Society officially resigned from the WPA.[64] The WPA leadership learned of this move only on February 8, 1983, during a trip of Professors Pichot and Berner to London. They had traveled there to convince the Royal College of Psychiatrists to take part in the inspection tour of psychiatric facilities in the USSR, which they had proposed to Georgi Morozov and Yuri Saarma during the Soviets' visit to Vienna a few weeks earlier. The news from Moscow left them stunned.

They would have been more stunned if they had known that the actual decision had been taken much earlier, not later than just one week after the visit of Georgi Morozov to the WPA Secretariat on January 8-11, 1983.[65] On January 18, the Ambassador of the USSR in the DDR, G. Gorinovich, delivered a message from the Central Committee of the Communist Party of the USSR to the Central Committee of the SED in which it said that "the abnormal situation that has developed within the World [Psychiatric] Association puts in fact the whole activity of the organization in question. For that reason, the All-Union Society... has taken the decision to withdraw from the World Association. About the date of the official withdrawal our friends will be informed (the same information has also been handed over to the other closely related fraternal Parties)."[66] On January 27, 1983, still several days before the official letter was sent, Eberhard Jaekel was

62 Colonel Romanov of the Fifth Directorate of the KGB, 1977. See: HAXX 1386/1, p. 84

63 Quote from the response of Profs. Berner and Pichot to the AUSNP of February 15, 1983, in reaction to their withdrawal from membership.

64 Interestingly, in December 1983 the WPA received 5,000 US dollars from the USSR Ministry of Health, apparently payment of the membership dues of the AUSNP – while usually the Soviets were notoriously bad in paying. The WPA had to write to the Soviets on January 25, 1984, with the request to order their bank to take the money back.

65 Dates mentioned in the minutes of the Executive Committee of the WPA, March 20, 1983, p. 3. According to a report by Prof. Szewozyk, found in the Stasi archives, a meeting was held on January 12, 1983, during the First Congress of the Hungarian Psychiatric Association, in which Morozov reported on his meeting with Berner and Pichot in Vienna. See HAXX 498 pp. 162-4

66 HAXX 41, p. 206

informed of the turn of events,[67] while the DDR Psychiatric Society learned about the decision only on February 11, more than two weeks later.[68] It seems that the decision was taken on the (highest) political level and then passed on for implementation to the AUSNP. . ."This decision was not discussed by psychiatrists and not adopted by Parliament; it was the result of a decree of the Supreme Soviet of the USSR on basis of a proposal from the Central Committee of the CPSU."[69]

In their letter of resignation, the Soviets complained of a "slanderous campaign, blatantly political in nature ... directed against Soviet psychiatry in the spirit of the 'cold war' against the Soviet Union. ... The leadership of the WPA, instead of taking the road of uniting psychiatrists, has embarked on the path of splitting them, and has turned into an obedient tool in the hands of the forces which are using psychiatry for their own political goals, aimed at fanning up contradictions and enmity among psychiatrists of different countries."[70] They were particularly angry about the memo of the American Psychiatric Association of August 1982, and accused the WPA leadership of complicity by not having spoken out against this mailing.

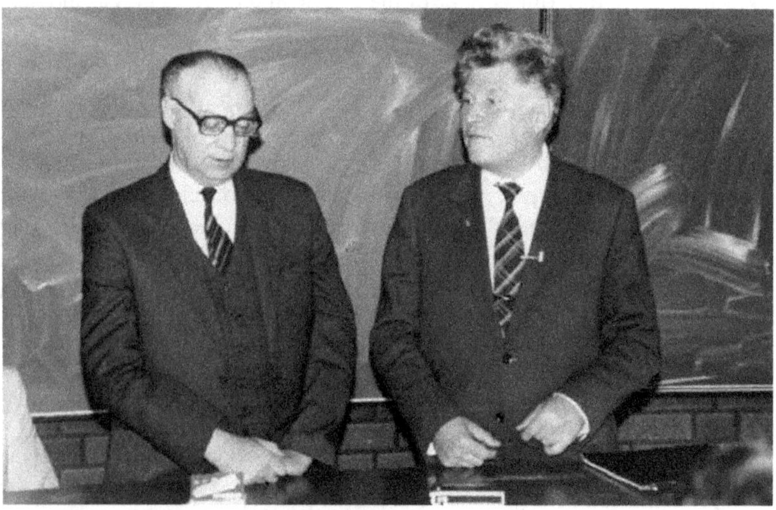

Finish psychiatrist Karl Achte and Georgi Morozov

[67] HAXX 41, p. 75. Jaekel found out during a conversation with Professor Karl Seidel; on Seidel see also note 91.

[68] *Politisch Missbraucht*, p. 629. Officially, the AUSNP informed the WPA and other societies on February 4; why their letter reached the addressees so late is unclear.

[69] *Psychiatry, psychiatrists and society*, p. 47

[70] *Soviet Psychiatric Abuse - Shadow over World Psychiatry*, pp 249-252.

In an article in the newspaper *Meditsinskaya Gazeta*, Georgi Morozov and Grigori Lukacher[71] explained why the AUSNP left the WPA and repeated that no political abuse of psychiatry occurred: "... Certain patients' outwardly behavior is not always an absolute index of their mental health, since it may be combined with delirious ideas of persecution and grandeur, messianism or delusions that they are great reformers and inventors. Such patients can sometimes act the role of so-called 'pathological prophets' and 'morbidly passionate idealists' and exert a certain influence on mentally healthy individuals who, not being specialists, cannot make a correct assessment of the mentally ill person's condition. From a clinical point of view, these patients are suffering primarily from exaggerated or delirious ideas that manifest themselves within the framework of psychopathic-like, paranoiac or hallucinatory-paranoiac syndrome. It is these patients, who once outside the Soviet Union, are widely used for political purposes by certain circles in Western countries."[72] Behind the scenes, however, the fact that the AUSNP had been forced to withdraw from the WPA had an impact, and some cracks started to appear in the unified position of Soviet psychiatrists. Some were not convinced by the arguments of the Soviet authorities and psychiatric leaders. "The weakness of the argumentation was evident. And we all understood something was wrong. (...) Softly, at first only in the corridors, talks started about the need to carry out changes..."[73]

In the months between the Soviet's resignation and the July 1983 World Congress of the WPA in Vienna, accusations regarding who and what had caused the crisis went back and forth. Professors Pichot and Berner angrily denied the Soviet accusation of 'misconduct' and claimed that they had only carried out the orders of the General Assembly.

The meeting of the WPA Executive Committee on March 20, 1983, in Buenos Aires, was attended by some twenty other invited guests and completely focused on the issue. In his opening remarks, Prof. Pichot pointed out that already during a meeting of the Executive Committee in Marrakech in October 1982, the Soviet member of the WPA Ethics Committee, Marat Vartanyan, had "raised massive objection to the WPA Report on "*The Issue of Abuse*" presented there in a draft form, as well as to the content of a letter circulated by the American Psychiatric Association

71 Grigori Lukacher, a neuropathologist and scientific secretary of the AUSNP. He was head of a department at the Serbski Institute. In 1988, when the neuropathologists left the AUSNP he decided to stay on and remained its scientific secretary. Peter Reddaway's travel notes, June 1990, p. 2

72 *Meditsinskaya Gazeta,* March 25, 1983

73 *Psychiatry, psychiatrists and society* p. 119

in August 1982... and containing information to the effect that the APA would vote... for a suspension of WPA membership."[74] He then continued by saying that he had told Vartanyan that it was "still possible ... to amend the draft of the WPA report on the "Issue of Abuse" by adding to it a preface which made mention of the cooperative manner in which the All Union Society had reacted to abuse inquiries ... Prof. Vartanyan had declared his readiness to recommend to the All Union Society a more effective manner of collaboration..."[75]

In the ensuing debate, Dr. Melvin Sabshin, representing the APA as its Medical Director, explained the nature of the letter of the APA and added that "it must be considered an absolute aberration and a distortion of the factual situation to adjudge circulation of the said letter as a major reason for the action taken by the all Union Society. Prof. Pichot replied by stating that Dr. Sabshin, in turn, seemed to misinterpret the situation. The APA letter certainly had not changed the basic position, but it had provided the All Union Society with an effective argumentation and with an overt reason for their resignation. Dr. Sabshin thereupon lodged an official objection to that argumentation."[76]

The Chairman of the WPA Ethics Committee, Prof. Costas Stefanis from Greece, said that the Soviet resignation had all been caused by the resolutions adopted in Honolulu and that establishing the Review Committee had been fundamentally wrong. He recommended "the abolishment of the Review Committee and a reversal of the development to the state prior to the [Honolulu] Congress. He stated further that the All Union Society had expected such an action from the Executive Committee, after it had declared its readiness to collaborate directly with the Association's officers."[77] His remarks were countered both by Prof. Pichot, who pointed out that it had not been the Executive Committee who had installed the Review Committee but had only carried out a resolution of the General Assembly. The same point was made by Jean-Yves Gosselin, the Chairman of the Review Committee himself. The latter also criticized the Executive Committee's readiness to communicate with the Soviets directly, thereby bypassing its own Review Committee and thus accepting its boycott by the Soviets.

From the minutes of the Buenos Aires Executive Committee meeting one gets the impression of an executive body at a loss: the departure of the

74 Minutes, Executive Committee Meeting, Buenos Aires, March 20, 1983, p. 2
75 Minutes, Executive Committee Meeting, Buenos Aires, March 20, 1983, p. 2
76 Minutes, Executive Committee Meeting, Buenos Aires, March 20, 1983, p. 3
77 Minutes, Executive Committee Meeting, Buenos Aires, March 20, 1983, p. 4

Soviets - in fact the only logical step they could have taken to avoid a public humiliating defeat - has taken them by a complete surprise. The "amiable and conciliatory" attitudes of Morozov and Saarma in mid January had put them on a completely wrong footing. Their main worry seems to be what the other societies are going to do, and whether this would mean a further disintegration of the WPA. Also in the official report of Prof. Berner to the General Assembly, this worry about the effect of the Soviets' withdrawal on the future of the WPA was highlighted: "The officers that have administered the WPA during the last election period have been obliged ... to countenance open confrontation between the national member societies, and have thus been unable to prevent the ultimate outcome of that confrontation, namely the withdrawal of psychiatric societies from membership of the Association. In consequence, the Association's influence has decreased. A most dangerous precedent has been set, which does not augur well for the future of the Association."[78]

The consequences of the Soviets' decision were far-reaching. According to Professor Laszlo Tringer, the WPA Congress had originally been planned in the Hungarian capital Budapest, and that suddenly had to change: "The WPA congress was moved to Vienna, because in the midst of the organizational work of the congress planned in Budapest, the Ministry of Health (under the pressure of the Communist Party) obliged us to cancel the congress in Budapest with the reasoning, that the city had no adequate facilities for such a huge congress ... The real reason was that the Soviet professional society has withdrawn from the WPA. ... Vienna "jumped in" half way thanks to Professor Peter Berner ... (I think no other country would have undertaken such a congress with the short time at disposal)."[79] Also, several other socialist psychiatric associations followed the Soviet example. On May 20, 1983, the Czechoslovak Psychiatric Society withdrew from the WPA by stating that "we refute, in particular, the offensive attitude of the World Psychiatric Association to the mystifying campaign of the American Society of Psychiatrists. As [the] WPA did not refuse this offensive attitude inspired by the State Department of the USA, it obviously lost its independence and by its lack of response manifests its consent."[80] Coincidentally (?) on the same day, the Bulgarian Society of Psychiatry wrote the WPA that it had decided to suspend its membership of the WPA because the association "had

78 *Report of the Secretary-General, 1983*. WPA, Vienna July 1983. Following the Soviet resignation, several other Eastern European societies withdrew from the WPA, as well as the Cuban Association.

79 Letter from Prof. Laszlo Tringer, September 16, 2009

80 Letter by Prof. Spacek on behalf of the Czechoslovak Psychiatric Society, May 20, 1983.

overstepped the limits" and got involved "in a campaign with a pronounced political [content]. ... Bulgarian psychiatrists are closely familiar with the organization and humaneness of Soviet psychiatric care."[81] Only on July 14, 1983, at the end of the session of the WPA General Assembly in Vienna, the Cuban Psychiatric Society followed suit, also referring to the actions "supported by the US Department of State."[82]

However, some other socialist societies refused to take similar action. The Poles and the Hungarians remained members of the WPA, even though the Poles did not receive an exit visa from their own government to attend the congress.[83] The East Germans only sent a letter to the WPA leadership protesting the turn of events and indicating that they might leave later. In its letter, the Society for Psychiatric and Neurology of the DDR expressed its regret that the Executive Committee of the WPA had "failed to undertake effective steps in order to counteract the anti-Soviet activities and the personal defamation which has been leveled against the Soviet colleagues." The Society wished to "reserve the right to any further steps in the matter."[84]

---

81 Letter by Prof. Milev on behalf of the Bulgarian Psychiatric Society, May 20, 1983. Not all Bulgarian psychiatrists were pro-Soviet in their attitude. In the Stasi files is a report on remarks by Professor Temkov from Bulgaria during a congress of the DDR psychiatric society in Karl Marx Stadt in October 1977. "He held the opinion that psychiatry in our countries was stagnated and that there was little hope for improvement. (...) According to the statements of Prof. Temkov is also in 'Russia' the level of psychiatry completely unsatisfactorily. Examples of that were the presentations by Prof. Morozov from Moscow in Sofia. Temkov described Morozov and Professor Zharikov, who was also present in Karl Marx Stadt, as functionaries of Soviet psychiatry who had not made any scientific progress. Prof. Temkov also voiced his opinion with regard to the so-called dissidents in the USSR. In his view there were clearly differences in opinion in psychiatry in the Soviet Union. The 'School' of Prof. Snezhnevsky from Moscow makes the schizophrenia criteria so wide that also people with a disturbed behavioral pattern can be hospitalized in psychiatric clinics with the diagnosis 'schizophrenia'. (...) The 'Russians' are very rigid with regard to their views and do not want to be helped." See MfS-HAXX, 2941, pp. 32-33

82 Statement dated July 14, 1983

83 *Report on the WPA Congress*, IAPUP, undated, p. 5. Additions in handwriting by Dr. Christine Shaw, who was then editor of the *Information Bulletin* of IAPUP. According to this document "the Polish psychiatrists have declared themselves ready to dissolve their association rather than resign from the WPA at the instigation of the USSR".

84 Letter by Prof. Heinz Schulze, President of the Society for Psychiatric and Neurology of the DDR, and Prof. Ehrig Lange, a member of the WPA Committee, March 15, 1983

World Congress in Vienna

The World Congress in Vienna was for me the first time that I attended such a large meeting. The IAPUP had sent a sizeable delegation to Vienna, partially as congress participants and journalists but also with some of our team members being delegates to the WPA General Assembly.[85] "As courier to the Soviet Union, I thought it would be best not to show my face too much, and in order to hide my true appearance a bit I had grown a beard. On top of that I decided to stay in the shadows. That was not so difficult, because although I was the only one who knew most of the members of the Working Commission personally, I was and remained a strange element in the team. I was not a psychiatrist, had no medical background, had just turned 24, with long hair and a beard, was an activist by nature and was inclined to take action and not waste too much time on discussions and diplomatic approaches. One of the members of our group would regularly remind me that I was not a psychiatrist and, therefore, should remain in the background."[86]

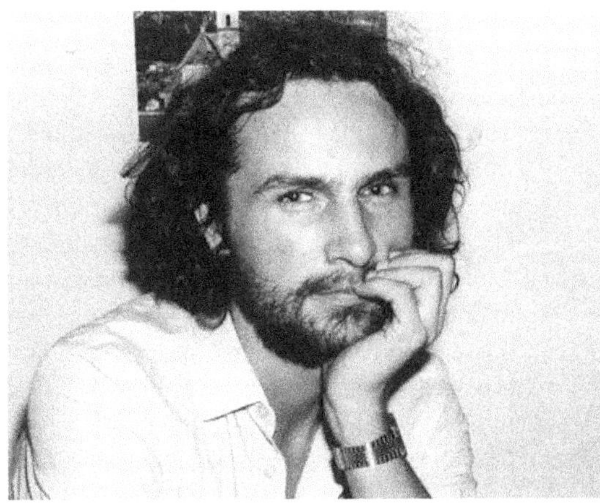

Robert van Voren, 1983

A much more prominent role was played by Ellen Mercer. Interestingly, everybody considered her to be an ally: the Soviets, the WPA and IAPUP as well. "What the others did not know, however, was that she was closely linked to us. As Director for International Affairs of the APA, she participated in most meetings, had direct access to internal documents of the WPA and knew exactly who was taking which position. Ellen participated in the meetings of our committee of representatives and helped develop our strategy. She was our secret weapon."[87]

---

85 E.g. Gérard Bles, at that time General Secretary of IAPUP and at the same time delegate of the Federation of French Psychiatric Associations., and Prof. Hugo Solms, delegate of the Swiss Psychiatric Association. Also Prof. W. von Baeyer from Germany was one of our team members.

86 *On Dissidents and Madness*, p. 64

87 *On Dissidents and Madness*, p. 64

Ellen played this role also in Vienna. When the Executive Committee forbade IAPUP to disseminate their literature during the congress, Ellen Mercer decided to allow us to put our public relations material on the table of the APA, together with announcements for a Forum on Psychiatric Abuse that the APA was organizing together with a number of other psychiatric associations. The WPA Secretariat had made it clear that the meeting was not to be advertised within the bounds of the Congress, even though other meetings outside the Congress could be advertised. A couple of posters, giving details of the venue of the meeting and its sponsors attracted the attention of Peter Berner. This resulted in an angry outburst of the WPA General Secretary. He "almost had a heart attack on the spot, swept the materials angrily off the table and ran off, fuming. Ellen was threatened with disciplinary action, but was supported by her immediate boss, Melvin Sabshin. ... It ended with a fizzle, but the atmosphere remained very tense."[88] At a press-conference later that day Berner explained that he had taken the posters down "not because he was trying to prevent a discussion of what he described as 'this important problem,' but because they had been put up in contravention of decisions previously taken by the organizing and executive committees, and recorded in the minutes of these committees."[89]

The activities of IAPUP were also noted by the East German delegation. In his *Sofortbericht* of July 27, 1983, Jochen Neumann writes: "...Small meetings were held by the International Association against the Political Use of Psychiatry and the West-German 'Association against the Political Abuse of Psychiatry. They disseminated their views through leaflets, which mainly concerned Soviet but also Czech psychiatry. These leaflets are in the possession of the leadership of the [DDR] delegation."[90] Later, during my research, I found these leaflets in the files of Professor Karl Seidel, who, like Jochen Neumann, worked as *Inoffizieller Mitarbeiter* for the Stasi until he became a full member of the Central Committee of the SED.[91]

---

88 *On Dissidents and Madness*, p. 65

89 *Report on the WPA Congress*, IAPUP, undated, p. 5

90 *Sofortbericht* Jochen Neumann on the Vienna Congress, July 2, 1983, p. 4

91 Prof. Seidel was recruited as an *Inoffizieller Mitarbeiter* of the Stasi in November 1967. His nickname was Fritz Steiner (MfS 13788/81 p. 41). According to one of the documents in his Stasi file he was a private physician of Party leader Erich Honecker (MfS 13788/83, p. 185). An interesting coincidence is, that during a visit to Romania in 1969 he met Dr. Ion Vianu, who at that time worked as a psychiatrist at the Marinescu psychiatric hospital in the Romanian capital and after his expulsion from Romania in 1977 would become the first Chairman of the board of IAPUP. (MfS 13788/83 pp. 79, 81).

The General Assembly of the WPA in Vienna was probably one of the most disorganized and tense meetings in its existence. The meeting was chaired by WPA President Prof. Pierre Pichot from France, who "occasionally allowed the proceedings to become extremely tangled. ... The atmosphere throughout was edge, fractious, uneasy and at some times belligerent."[92] Contrary to the session at the Honolulu World Congress, the press was not allowed to attend.

Some delegates, in particular those from East Germany, Cuba,[93] Egypt, Mexico and Israel, angrily called upon the WPA Executive Committee not to accept the Soviets' resignation, while others voiced the opinion that it was a fact of life one had to live with, a view supported by WPA President Prof. Pichot. The debate was followed by a discussion about various resolutions that had been submitted, but the situation was so confusing that some delegates didn't even know which resolution they were asked to vote upon. Eventually a resolution drafted by the British delegate Prof. Kenneth Rawnsley was adopted with a large majority of 174 votes in favor and 18 against, with 27 abstentions. The resolution was remarkably conciliatory in tone: "The World Psychiatric Association would welcome the return of the All-Union Society ... to membership of the Association, but would expect sincere cooperation and concrete evidence beforehand of amelioration of the

As noted before, there was one golden rule in the DDR, and that was that the highest Party echelons of the SED could not be infiltrated by the Stasi, and this included members of the Central Committee (See *Der Mielke Konzern*, p. 149). When Seidel was promoted to a top position within the Central Committee his work as IM was officially terminated on November on June 5, 1978 (MfS 13788/83, p. 196). As a farewell, he was given the Gold Medal of the *Nationale Volks Armee*. Reason for this award is "that [he] prepared valuable information on the political-ideological diversion and enemy contact-policy, in particular at international congresses. During the past years he has made a significant contribution to the exposure and suppression of hostile ideological attacks against the USSR because of the alleged abuse of psychiatry." (MfS 13788/83, p. 182). His file was closed in November 1983 (MfS 13788/83, p. 196).
However this did not necessarily mean that Seidel's political role in the psychiatric issue ended as well. In a letter dated October 12, 1982, to comrade Sieber of the division of International Relations of the Department for Health Policy, Prof. Seidel wonders whether the DDR-representation in Austria shouldn't contact the Austrian authorities to ask whether it is at all acceptable that in July 1983 Austrian territory will be used for a campaign against the Soviet Union. The letter was written after a visit to the Central Committee of the CPSU in Moscow. See MfS-HAXX 41, p. 37

92 Report by Prof. Kenneth Rawnsley, British delegate, to the Royal College of Psychiatrists of which he was then President, 26 July 1983.

93 Which withdrew from the WPA later during the session

political abuse of psychiatry in the Soviet Union."[94] Subsequently, Soviet dissident psychiatrist and political prisoner, Dr. Anatoly Koryagin, was elected Honorary Member of the WPA, with 119 votes for and 58 against.[95] A resolution calling on the WPA to take up the defense of opponents of political abuse of psychiatry was voted upon by a show of hands, 21 societies in favor and five against. And finally, the General Assembly agreed that the work of the Review Committee was important and should be continued, but also agreed that the mandate should be widened to include other forms of abuse of psychiatry. The latter decision effectively made the Review Committee impotent, and it would no longer play an effective role.

The General Assembly concluded with the election of the new Executive Committee. "As a first-time observer to such proceedings, I didn't know if regular procedures were followed, but I had the distinct impression that quite a number of delegates were completely unprepared. Names were mentioned and disappeared again off the table. In the meantime, every now and then a delegate friendly to our cause would step outside in order to report to us. We were sitting in the lobby outside the meeting hall, anxious for news, as if we were watching a soccer game."[96]

Kenneth Rawnsley, author of the resolution on the Soviet issue, later reported to his College: "The Executive Committee had provided two names for each office from the many submitted. However, the first office to be dealt with was that of Secretary General and in addition to the "official" slate the name of Professor Fini Schulsinger ... was proposed from the floor. He was duly elected by secret ballot. The Presidency was next and Professor Berner promptly withdrew his candidature on the grounds that he had had no opportunity to discuss future policy with Schulsinger. There followed a great deal of discussion with several recesses and eventually other candidates were proposed."[97]

Prof. Fini Schulsinger had been nominated by Dr. Neils Reisby from Copenhagen (who later was appointed as Treasurer of the WPA), and was not even present at the meeting, something to which another candidate for

---

94 Report by Prof. Kenneth Rawnsley, 26 July 1983; Bloch, S. and Reddaway, P., *Soviet Psychiatric Abuse*, p. 218.

95 The Society of Psychiatrists and Neurologists of the DDR officially protested against his nomination and subsequent election, "as an abuse of that honor in recognition of political activity." (minutes of the General Assembly, July 14, 1983, p. 17).

96 *On Dissidents and Madness*, p. 65

97 Report by Kenneth Rawnsley, 26 July 1983, p.2.

the position strongly protested.[98] However, Prof. Pichot pointed out that nowhere in the statutes it said that a candidate had to be bodily present, and Schulsinger was elected with a large majority. [99] Also the election of President caused some debate because of Professor Peter Berner's decision to withdraw his candidacy. According to Costas Stefanis, then present as Chair of the Ethics Committee, Berner might have suspected that Schulsinger's candidacy had been prepared by the groups opposing the political abuse of psychiatry, and thus saw some hidden "conspiracy" behind it, reason not to go ahead with his nomination.[100]

The second candidate happened to be a national from Iceland, and thus undesirable, as this would have meant that three members of the Executive Committee would be Scandinavian (the Treasurer was automatically from the same country as the General Secretary, Denmark). Confusion ensued. Kenneth Rawnsley suggested the Dutch Professor Bastiaans as candidate, a well-known expert on the treatment of concentration camp survivors and a member of the WPA Committee, while the Italian delegate suggested Prof. Stefanis from Greece, who immediately accepted his candidacy and stated "that he would accept the nomination in order to prevent an impasse in the

98 The person concerned was Prof. Juan Jose Lopez Ibor, who would become General Secretary of the WPA in 1989.

99 Prof. Schulsinger received 142 votes out of 232 available votes. Many delegates supported him because he was believed to be a member of Amnesty International and had previously spoken out against the political abuse of psychiatry in the Soviet Union. For instance, in an open letter to the paper *Politiken* on February 21, 1982, he wrote that "there have been multiple Soviet-psychiatric reports published in the West. Their content has never been disputed from the Soviet side. It is apparent from these reports that they operate with diagnoses like 'reformational paranoia' and 'sluggish symptom-poor schizophrenia'. (…) Some of the victims of these diagnoses are treated, against their will, with high doses of psychopharmaceuticals, which can only be characterized as torture. (…) Perhaps the fading socialist image of the Soviet Union could be improved if the incredible misuse could be brought to a halt."
According to Jochen Neumann, Schulsinger had at several times difficulties in his career because of his political views: "Some years ago he had not been selected as director of a large social research institute in Denmark because of his political views. And for the same reason he had not been given a much desired position with UNESCO in Paris three years ago, even though until now the position had not been filled." *Ergänzungen zum Bericht*, Jochen Neumann, October 1984, p. 15. Costas Stefanis added during an interview on November 18, 2009, that Schulsinger had told him that he was a Communist and had been active in the resistance during the German occupation of 1940-1945.

100 Interview Costas Stefanis, July 15, 2009. See also Chapter 18 – *Meeting Costas Stefanis*.

proceedings."[101] According to Stefanis himself he did not want this election and begged Berner to reverse his decision. Only when the latter declined he agreed to be nominated, thereby ending the sense of desperation among the delegates.[102] In the run-off between Bastiaans and Stefanis, the latter was elected President with a clear majority.[103] His election was met with approval by the DDR delegation: "[his election] can be seen as a positive step. … In his capacity as chairman of the Ethics Committee, he decided that this committee should not deal with complaints or individual cases, but with general principles of ethics in psychiatry. In his report, he praised he valuable work of the late American Professor Weinberger [sic!] and of professor Vartanyan (Moscow)."[104] However, the Stasi was less positive: "It is not possible to classify Stefanis exactly professionally and politically, but clearly he is not unwelcome to the Anglo-American lobby."[105]

Subsequently, the other members of the Executive Committee were elected. Vice-President became Prof. Pal Juhasz from Budapest, quite to the surprise of the remaining socialist member societies, as we will see later.[106] Other

---

101 Minutes of the General Assembly, July 14, 1983, p. 6. The Dutch candidate had been solicited by the author, see *On Dissidents and Madness*, p. 66

102 Interview Costas Stefanis, July 14, 2009.

103 Costas Stefanis received 162 votes, to 60 votes for Bastiaans. See *Minutes of the General Assembly*, July 14, 1983

104 HAXX 1386/2, pp. 79-80. The American professor referred to was Jack Weinberg (not Weinberger), a former President of the American Psychiatric Association. Interestingly, according to Prof. Karl Seidel it was Soviet psychiatrist and Ethics Committee member Marat Vartanyan who in 1978 tried to prevent the WPA from electing Weinberg as Honorary Member. According to Vartanyan, Weinberg was a "most reactionary, Zionist representative of the American Psychiatric Association". See: MfS 13788/83, p. 169

105 HA XX 498, p. 122

106 "Dr. Pál Juhász was born in Nagyenyed in 1916. He earned his diploma in medicine at the Medical Faculty of the University of Debrecen, and it was here he gained qualifications in neurology and psychiatry. Later, in recognition of his merits, he was awarded titles in forensic psychology, neuropathology, electroencephalography and psychology. During the war and for years afterwards, he was a student, and then an assistant, of Kálmán Sántha at the Debrecen Clinic of Neurology and Psychiatry. [He] founded the first EEG laboratory in the country. (…) Between 1950-1957, he was chief neurologist of the Hungarian People's Army, in the rank of colonel. He habilitated in 1957, at the age of 41, and became director of the Neurology and Psychiatry Clinic of the Debrecen University of Medicine. For four years, he was rector of the same university. In 1967 he was invited to head the … Clinic of Psychiatry … of the Semmelweis University of Medicine. (…) He was the president of the Hungarian Society of Psychiatry from 1980 until his death. He was an honorary member of the

elected members were Dr. Neils Reisby from Denmark as Treasurer (in those days the Treasurer was automatically from the same country as the General Secretary); Dr. Melvin Sabshin from the United Sates and Dr. Jorge Costa e Silva from Brasil were elected as Associate Secretaries.[107]

The meeting continued for some time, but very much in disarray and under severe time pressure. The Hungarian delegate, Prof. Pal Juhasz, asked the attention of the General Assembly for his complaint against the Swiss Professor Charles Durand, who had traveled to Budapest to meet an alleged victim of political abuse of psychiatry in Hungary and who had published a report in the Swiss press.[108] Juhasz considered this a violation of professional ethics, which in turn evoked a response from the Swiss delegate Hugo Solms who said Durand's trip had been entirely of a private nature and had nothing to do with the WPA. A Nigerian delegate tried to put forward a resolution concerning South Africa, but it was turned down because of insufficient time. The Mexican delegate lashed out at the Executive Committee, attacking them for not allowing sufficient time for discussion. Pichot subsequently read aloud a statement by several gay associations, calling on the WPA to petition the World Health Organization to have homosexuality removed from the list of mental diseases. And then the report by Rawnsley ended with a typical British understatement: "Proceedings terminated abruptly at 11.00 PM when the interpreters walked out."[109]

French psychiatry society and of the society of neurology and psychiatry of the DDR. The World Psychiatric Association also counted on his work, and gave him a vote of confidence." Quotes from an obituary by Dr. Ilona Huszar. See also an obituary in the WPA Newsletter 21, May 1984.

107 Juhasz received 164 out of 232 votes; Sabshin received 152 votes, Costa e Silva 115. See *Minutes of the General Assembly*, July 14, 1983. According to Costas Stefanis, Costa e Silva had been propelled to his candidacy by WPA President Pierre Pichot. Interview with Costas Stefanis, November 18, 2009.

108 This concerns the case of Tibor Pakh. In his statement to the General Assembly, Pal Juhasz explained that Mr. Pakh has been treated three times for short periods by psychiatrists who were present at the Vienna Congress, that the publication of his conclusions in a bulletin by Prof. Durand are not in line with the Hawaii Declaration and that at no time the opinions of the family and treating doctors have been taken into account, which in Juhasz' view was incorrect and not in line with international practice.

109 Report by Kenneth Rawnsley, 26 July 1983, p.2

Hungarian rebellion

The Hungarian delegate, Dr. Pal Juhasz, was elected to the Executive Committee very much against the wish of the Soviets and his own political bosses in Budapest.[110] Juhasz is described by many as a forceful figure, often characterized as "headstrong, but ...very friendly, polite. He was a very active, goal-oriented person, who tried – as he often said – to go up to the border of possibilities in changing things. In dynamic terms, he was always in 'antithesis,' trying to change the given circumstances."[111] Hungarian psychiatrist Dr. Janos Furedi, knew Pal Juhasz well: "Together with 71 others, we founded the Hungarian Psychiatric Association in 1980.[112] He was in a very good friendship with President Pichot and was nominated to be the Vice President. The KGB was much against having a high post in WPA from the Eastern Bloc, so there was pressure on Juhasz not to accept the nomination. I was there when it was told to him."[113] From the Stasi archives, it becomes clear that the socialist member associations had made an advance agreement not to agree to have one of them be a member of the Executive Committee: "The Hungarian delegate... has not kept to the agreements between the socialist countries and violated the issued instructions. Among others, he did not turn against the anti-Soviet attacks and has let himself be voted to the position of Vice-President."[114] In general, the East Germans were not very satisfied with the attitude of the Hungarians, including that of Pal Juhasz. In his travel report on the Vienna Congress, Jochen Neumann writes: "Remarkable and worrying is the fact that the Hungarian colleagues have not appeared at all as a

110 According to Prof. Laszlo Tringer, "Juhász was forbidden to accept the position of vice-president for the World Psychiatric Association, for which he became a serious nominee at the 1983 World Conference of the WPA, whose new venue was in Vienna. Despite the prohibition, he agreed to run for the position. There were about 100 Hungarian delegates at the conference, and the mood was festive when Juhász was elected, in effect unanimously, to be vice-president of the WPA. He accepted the nomination although he knew it would entail a disciplinary procedure from the Ministry of Health."

111 Letter from Prof. Laszlo Tringer, August 25, 2009.

112 Initially Hungary had a Hungarian Neuro-Psychiatric Society, and Juhasz was President of the Psychiatric Section. However, when the psychiatrists separated from the Neurologists, Juhasz was elected President of the newly formed society.

113 Letter Janos Furedi, April 27, 2009. According to Prof. Laszlo Tringer, who knew Pal Juhasz as well, the Minister of Health of Hungary had prohibited Juhasz to stand for a post on the WPA Executive Committee. Letter to the author, August 25, 2009.

114 BstU, ZA, HAXX 498, p. 83

representation of a socialist country and kept themselves even out of the political discussions."[115]

Apparently Juhasz knew already in Vienna that he would be in trouble. He said so to Costas Stefanis, the newly elected President, who did not fully understand what Juhasz meant with this remark. The latter explained that not everybody would like his decision and that trouble was awaiting him in Budapest. He indicated that he had received the first signs of that already.[116] And indeed, immediately following the World Congress, Juhasz was called in for questioning by his authorities. Stasi archives indicate that this happened on several occasions. "The Hungarian delegate has been called to responsibility by the relevant state institutions upon his return from abroad. The Minister of Health has started disciplinary action against him. Also the Party started proceedings against him. He was relieved from his position as President of the Hungarian Psychiatric Association. When the possibility is there, he should lay down his function as Vice-President of the World [Psychiatric] Association."[117] Janos Furedi remembers: "The meeting was held in the Ministry of Health, but the Ministries of Foreign and Internal Affairs, the Communist Party and many others were there. From our side, the General Secretary (Dr. Janos Szilard) and myself were there (I was then advisor in the Ministry and Vice President [of the Hungarian Psychiatric Association]). I do not know anymore what exactly happened, but as I remember he was expelled from the Party as well from the College (Advisory Board of the Minister)."[118] However, it seems that the report from the Stasi archives,

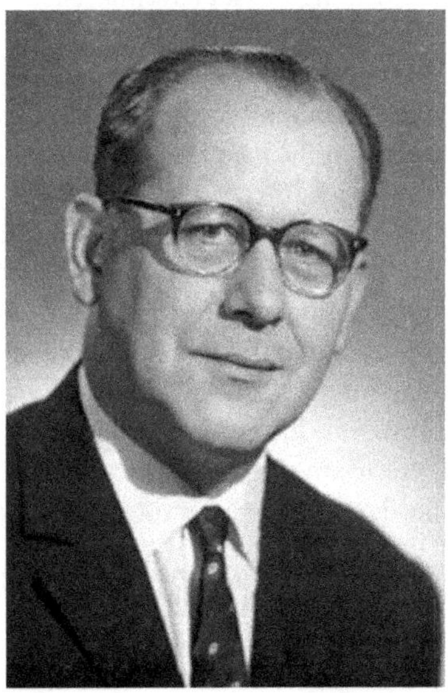

Pal Juhasz, 1982

115 *Sofortbericht* Jochen Neumann on the Vienna Congress, 8-14 July 1983, p. 3

116 Interview Costas Stefanis, July 15, 2009

117 BstU, ZA, HAXX 498, Bl. 83. Süss, p. 648. According to Dr. Tringer he did not lose his position as President of the Hungarian Psychiatric Association. Letter to the author, August 25, 2009

118 Letter Janos Furedi, May 1, 2009. Dr. Tringer confirms that a disciplinary process was started, but disputes that he was expelled from the Party. Letter to the author, August 25, 2009.

indicating that he was also relieved of his Presidency of the Hungarian Psychiatric Association, was incorrect.

Still, all was not lost for the Socialist bloc. Even Georgi Morozov, director of the Serbski Institute and generally seen as one of the main architects of Soviet political abuse, saw some use in having Juhasz on the Executive Committee. In his view, Juhasz' position should be used. The latter apparently told the East-German Professor Schulze in Berlin that Morozov had given him "moral backing."[119] His suggestion had been to view his position within the WPA positively and that because of this he could influence the positioning of the Executive Committee. The upcoming November 1983 meeting of the Executive Committee should be used to gather information on their position vis-à-vis the Soviets. One of his tasks should be to "influence the new President of the World Association, Professor Stefanis/Greece, to go to Moscow in order to have a meeting with the leading Soviet psychiatrists."[120]

It is unclear how much this affected Juhasz' health and whether the pressure was too much for him to bear. It was known that he was seriously ill with cancer of the pancreas, even though he himself seems to have been initially unaware of this.[121] On January 13, 1985, he wrote to Professor Peter Berner that "on December 10 [I] went through serious pancreas surgery, which, by the way, was completely successful. Fifteen days after this surgical intervention, I could leave the hospital. I have lost a lot of weight, and my abdominal pains have already diminished a lot. Little by little, I am regaining my working capability. I am preparing the trip to New York…"[122] However, Juhasz' health deteriorated again, and on January 23, he informed Peter Berner by telegram that he would not attend the handover meeting of the Executive Committee on February 2, 1984, in New York.[123] Instead,

119 *Politisch Missbraucht*, p. 649

120 BstU, ZA, AIM8249/87, Teill II, B. 1, p. 217.

121 According to Prof. Tringer (letter of August 25, 2009) Juhasz had undergone surgery before the World Congress yet believed he had been operated because of a gastric ulcer, and was unaware of the true nature of his disease. This is also confirmed by Jochen Neumann, who heard the same from a different source.

122 Letter to Peter Berner from Pal Juhasz, translation, no exact date marked. WPA archives.

123 Telegram from Pal Juhasz to Peter Berner, January 25, 1984, and Peter Berner's response of January 28, 1985. See also memorandum by Ellen Mercer on the Executive Committee Meeting, February 5, 1984, and minutes of the EC Meeting, February 1984. The fact that those present discussed the issue what to do when a member of the Executive Committee becomes incapacitated while in office indicates that those present knew Prof. Juhasz was seriously ill.

he sent his views on a variety of issues in a long letter to Peter Berner. Interestingly, his first remark concerned the election of Costa e Silva to the Executive Committee: "Particularly I find the abundance of his explanations alarming. … It has not been uttered in connection with his election that he would be a representative of either Latin America or the developing countries."[124] With regard to the Soviet issue, Juhasz explained that in his view "establishing contact with the Soviet Psychiatric Association would be a matter of major importance, and that the documentation presented by Profs. Morozov and Saarma personally in January 1983 in Vienna ought to be studied in the greatest detail. … Likewise I find it reasonable, if the EC will undertake to write a letter to the Bulgarian, Czechoslovak and the Cuban associations, before they themselves approach the WPA, in which letter the new EC – after having declared that it will abstain from political questions, and after having asked the mentioned associations to recognize this – ask these associations to take steps regarding a revision of their statement from last year…" [125] Clearly, Juhasz formulated a position that very well fit the Soviets, and it is surprising that the authorities still decided to act so strongly against him and put him under so much pressure.

Shortly after the New York EC meeting, on February 27, Juhasz died, merely seven months after the World Congress, 1984.[126] The Hungarian authorities informed the WPA Executive Committee that their presence at his funeral was undesirable. In none of the obituaries was his membership of the WPA Executive Committee mentioned, on strict orders from above.[127] A clearer sign that Juhasz had run into trouble with the authorities was not possible.

---

124 Letter of Pal Juhasz to Peter Berner, January 13, 1985.

125 Letter of Pal Juhasz to Peter Berner, January 13, 1985. See also the EC Minutes of Feb 2, 1984, p. 9.

126 Laszlo Tringer writes: "He died suddenly after getting up of his bed to go to the toilet, the cause of death was – as I remember – pulmonary emboli."

127 Letter Prof. Laszlo Tringer to the author, September 16, 2009. Half a dozen obituaries are in my possession and indeed nowhere his membership of the EC of the WPA is mentioned. The WPA instead asked the Danish Embassy to put a wreath on Juhasz' grave, with the sign "World Psychiatric Association" a move that was very much welcomed by Juhasz' colleagues: "I have gladly noticed at the funeral ceremony the last greeting of the World Psychiatric Association; the wreath of the President." Letter from Prof. Attila Liposey to Peter Berner, March 19, 1984.

Chapter 17 – Another Hidden Factor

> *"By taking on the position of Vice-President there are undoubtedly possibilities to fight the known anti-Soviet positions within the World [Psychiatric] Association determinedly and energetically and to expose those forces that try to abuse a big and influential international medical scientific association for the propaganda of a misanthropic ideology."*
>
> Dr. Ludwig Mecklinger, Minister of Health of the DDR[128]

The death of Pal Juhasz put the WPA in a difficult position. The position of Vice-President was now vacant, and had to be filled. Juhasz had, in spite of all objections within the Hungarian political leadership and that of the whole Eastern bloc, been a representative of the socialist countries, and now a new one had to be found. Only the Polish, East German and Hungarian psychiatric associations remained within the WPA (the Romanians were not considered part of that group, due to the independent political course of Party leader Nicolae Ceausescu), so the choice had to be made out of those three. The Hungarians had been invited to nominate a successor,[129] but they immediately indicated they could only nominate a candidate after a new President of the Hungarian Psychiatric Society had been elected (a position that was vacant following Juhasz' death); finally, on October 6, they would inform the Executive Committee by telegram that no candidate would be nominated by them.[130] The Polish association was deemed unreliable by the socialist bloc, because of the political situation in the country following the Solidarnosc period and the subsequent imposition of martial law.[131] A Polish psychiatrist, Dr. Stefan Leder, had been nominated by the time the Executive Committee convened in June 1984, but the nomination had come from a Turkish psychiatrist, Dr. Özek, and not from a psychiatric association.[132] Time was pressing to find a solution, and the WPA Executive was a bit in limbo.

---

128 Letter from DDR Minister of Health Ludwig Mecklinger to Kurt Hager, member of the Politburo of the SED, October 10, 1984. See HAXX 499, p. 418

129 Minutes of the WPA EC, June 1984, p. 2

130 Minutes of the WPA EC, October 1984, p. 5

131 Martial law in Poland refers to the period of time from December 13, 1981 to July 22, 1983, when the government of the People's Republic of Poland drastically restricted normal life by introducing martial law in an attempt to crush the political opposition against the Communist rule in Poland. Thousands of opposition activists were interned without charge and as many as 100 people were killed.

132 Minutes of the WPA EC, June 1984, p. 2

But not only the WPA had an issue to resolve: also the Soviets and their allies now had a problem. They lost a person on the inside of the Executive Committee, however unreliable Juhasz might have seemed to them. This called for action, and, interestingly, it was again the East Germans and not the Soviets who understood that something needed to be done.

Why the East Germans? One of the factors that played a role was probably the keen interest of Lieutenant Colonel Eberhard Jaekel in the issue of Soviet psychiatric abuse and the key role he saw for his service in the affair. Already on September 27, 1984, he sent a proposal to his boss in the Stasi "for the nomination of a representative of the DDR as Vice-President of the WPA."[133] Jochen Neumann, at that moment Director of the Hygiene Museum in Dresden and one of the top DDR psychiatrists,[134] thinks the first initiative came from Greece: "I think it was Stefanis who initiated the process that led to my election. He contacted Vartanyan and discussed with him the idea to have the position of Juhasz filled with a new representative from Eastern Europe."[135] Stefanis, however, strongly denies any involvement in the matter.[136]

According to Jaekel's document, the idea was that the Deputy Minister of Health of the DDR, Rudolf Müller, should contact Marat Vartanyan in Moscow with the request to contact Prof. Stefanis and inform him of

133 HAXX 499 p. 424. See also *Politisch Missbraucht*, p.650.

134 Jochen Neumann studied from 1954 until 1959 at the Universities of Leipzig, Greifswald and Humboldt University in Berlin, after which he spent his residency at the Charité hospital of the Humboldt University in Berlin and the Pathological Institute of the City Hospital Berlin-Friedrichshein. In 1961 he started his professional career in psychiatry as research assistant at the psychiatric clinic of the Charité, where he climbed up the ladder via the positions of chief doctor, head of a department to the position of deputy medical director. In 1971 Neumann received his PhD at the Humboldt University in Berlin. From 1972 until 1977 he was medical director and chief doctor of the neurological clinic of the Wilhelm Griesinger hospital in Berlin. In 1975 he became lecturer in psychiatry at the Academy for Continuous Medical Education in Berlin, where he was appointed professor in 1977, a position he held until 1990. In 1977 Neumann was also appointed Professor of Psychiatry at the University of Jena and director of the psychiatric department of the Clinic for Psychiatry and Neurology "Hans Berger" in the same city. In 1983 he moved to Dresden to become director of the German Hygiene Museum. A year later he was also appointed Honorary Professor at Dresden University. He held both positions until 1990. See a later chapter in this book.

135 Interview with Jochen Neumann, July 29, 2009.

136 Interview with Costas Stefanis, November 18, 2009.

the plan to have a DDR-psychiatrist nominated for the position of Vice-President. Stefanis should then contact the DDR Psychiatric Association, which would respond to this request with a nomination.[137] Rudolf Müller could be easily entrusted to do this. He worked for the Stasi as IM "Ernst Lache" and spoke Russian fluently, since he had studied in Leningrad in the 1950s.[138] "Prof. Müller ... had the necessary connections with the various services in Moscow and was a personal friend of Prof. Vartanyan."[139] Müller happened to be also a personal friend of Jochen Neumann, with whom he had studied medicine in 1957-1959, and several years later they worked together at the Charité clinic in Berlin. Neumann in turn knew Vartanyan from his work at Snezhnevsky's Institute in the second half of 1966. "It was [Vartanyan] who through his openly friendly relationships with Prof. Costas Stefanis catalyzed my candidacy and promoted it through tactical maneuvering."[140]

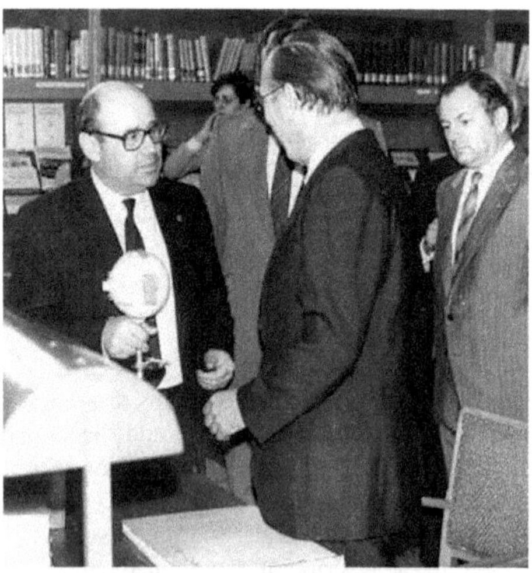
Deutsche Hygiene Museum, 1987. On the right Dr. R. Müller

Whoever took the first step is unclear. As indicated above, Neumann thinks it was Vartanyan who contacted Müller first, after discussions with Stefanis, and that is how the process was set in motion.[141] However, according to the Stasi files, it was the Stasi that was supposed to take the initiative and contact Vartanyan "through operational channels" (in other words: via the KGB) "with the instruction to inform Prof. Stefanis accordingly (as far as I know the KGB works with Prof. Vartanyan in relation to the World Associa-

[137] HAXX 499 p. 423, and 424.

[138] Dr. Rudolf Müller (born 1933), studied medicine in Leningrad in 1954-1957 and in Berlin in 1957-59, was deputy chief doctor of the sport medical service of the DDR in 1964-1969, studied psychiatry in 1969-1973 and was from 1980-1989 in charge of international relations of the Ministry of Health of the DDR. According to Jochen Neumann he also completed additional studies at the Party University in Moscow.

[139] Personal notes of Jochen Neumann, August 16, 2009.

[140] Personal notes of Jochen Neumann, August 16, 2009

[141] Interview Jochen Neumann, February 26, 2009

tion)."[142] It is clear, however, that the line Stefanis-Vartanyan-Müller was a crucial one, and that this line was known to the relevant institutions as being sufficiently strong to be used for such an operational enterprise.

The DDR leadership considered several persons for the vacant position. Until then the leading DDR-psychiatrist had been Prof. Schulze, who had also been head of the DDR-delegation to the WPA World Congress in Vienna. However, he had informed his *Führungsoffizier* on July 18, 1984, that he was no longer President of the DDR Psychiatric Association and that as a result his travel possibilities were much more limited.[143] Two other candidates were now brought forward: Professor Bernd Nickel, Director of the Wilhelm Griesinger Hospital and Professor Jochen Neumann. Both were considered to be politically reliable and were members of the board of the DDR Psychiatric Association. Of the two, Neumann was considered to be the best option, as he "has the experience in dealing with Western psychiatrists and in communicating with the bourgeois ideology and other hostile views. Prof. Neumann is an intellectual character, who is internationally also able to develop contacts and adapt himself."[144]

Success in Rome

And so it happened. "On a Friday, it was September 29, I received a phone call in my office at the Hygiene Museum from the General Secretariat for Scientific Societies in Berlin. The Deputy Director, Comrade Buhlert, asked me what plans I had for the weekend. I answered him that I planned to go with my family that evening or the next morning to Köthen (to my house on the edge of the Unterspree forest). Comrade Buhlert explained that that was impossible, because he would visit me on Saturday at 10:00 AM in the Museum in Dresden in order to discuss issues related to an important and short-term business trip. I also should not make any plans for the end of the following week. … Comrade Buhlert, who came especially for this meeting from Berlin, told me succinctly that I would travel to Rome on October 6."[145] Neumann was further informed that the relevant authorities had decided that the East-German Society for Neurology and Psychiatry, being one of the few remaining professional associations in the WPA

142 HAXX 499, p. 423

143 *Politisch Missbraucht*, p. 651

144 *Politisch Missbraucht*, p. 651. Undoubtedly, the theme of Neumann's dissertation in 1961 helped create this image of him as an intellectual: "*Mimical expressions as an essential component of the artist's expression in Ilya Yefimovich Repin*".

145 Personal notes of Jochen Neumann, August 16, 2009

from socialist countries, should try to exert influence on the developments within the WPA, preferably by obtaining a position within the Executive Committee or at least within the Committee. "With and through Prof. Vartanyan, the first arrangements had already been made."[146]

The operation was one with much haste, as very little time was left, yet it was organized with German *Gründlichkeit*.[147] "Comrade Prof. Neumann is to be sent to Rome on 7-8 October 1984 as a participant in the Regional Meeting, because during this Regional Meeting, a session of the Executive Committee will take place where among others the election of a Vice-President will be held. Prof. Neumann has agreed in taking this position and to travel. As a regular registration as participant in the Regional Meeting is at this moment not possible any more, Comrade Dr. Rohland asks the Stasi for support in connection with the following:

- To order the Embassy of the DDR in Italy to register Prof. Neumann for the Regional Meeting and to arrange his accommodation;
- In order to get an entry visa for Italy the Ministry of Foreign Affairs should put pressure on the Italian Embassy in Berlin;
- Quickly making available travel funds by the Ministry of Finance as well as an airline ticket for October 5, 1984, to Rome."[148]

And thus Neumann was nominated for the position and the trip to Rome was organized. "I received a VIP ticket in the name of Prof. Mecklinger (our Minister of Health) on which at the airport and at the last minute the name of the passenger was changed into mine. Because of the fact that, due to lack of foreign currency, whenever possible DDR-business trips should be carried out with Interflug, I had to travel with our own airline company to Milan and then change planes. All details of the trip were meticulously planned; in Milan I was to be shuttled in a car to the Alitalia plane as a VIP."[149] The DDR Embassy in Rome made the local arrangements for the trip.

The week before the actual departure was used for strategy planning. Neumann had two meetings with Prof. Karl Seidel, head of the department for health policy within the Central Committee of the Party and a friend of Jochen Neumann, during which strategy was discussed. An important element during the discussions was, according to Neumann, the assertion by Seidel that in the DDR no political abuse of psychiatry took place

146 Personal notes of Jochen Neumann, August 16, 2009

147 German *Gründlichkeit*, best translated with German thoroughness, is a character trait often used to describe German precision.

148 HAXX 499, p. 421

149 Personal notes of Jochen Neumann, August 16, 2009

or had taken place in the past, and that, in that sense, Neumann could function assertively without running the risk of having to deal with claims otherwise. "I remember that Prof. Seidel, already years before he became involved in high-level politics, both among colleagues and also in private strongly recommended absolute correctness when political factors played a role within the case of a patient. During one of the two meetings, Prof. Seidel pointed out that the DDR in no way should subject itself always to the wishes of the 'friends' (that is: the Soviets; RvV) and that at least with regard to health policy the country had its own independent view."[150]

A crucial role in the preparations was played by Deputy Minister of Health Rudolf Müller, "who coordinated all necessary logistical steps, as well as, behind the scenes, the necessary permissions in Berlin and Moscow and who had – at that time the most important element – a private hotline with Prof. Vartanyan, who discussed the tactical arrangements with his friend Costas Stefanis and provided feedback with regard to the actual situation. ... During those days the telephone lines between Rudolf Müller, Marat Vartanyan and Costas Stefanis, who was by then already in Rome, must have been red hot. According to information that I got, Prof. Vartanyan and Prof. Stefanis had agreed that I would be nominated..."[151] However, the nomination would be kept secret until the last moment, in order not to allow the opponents to prepare themselves. "In that sense, in planning my candidacy and my appearance in Rome, a surprise element was calculated with. As far as I know, only Prof. Stefanis knew this in advance (I do not know to what extent Prof. Stefanis had informed Prof. Schulsinger)."[152]

---

150 Personal notes of Jochen Neumann, August 16, 2009. In the Stasi file of Karl Seidel there are a number of interesting documents that show that he was much less a staunch believer in the socialist regime than one would assume. A document from 1964, for instance, which reports on a meeting between a Stasi officer and Seidel, mentions the fact that Seidel "said... that even officers of the NVA [*Nationale Volks Armee*] and the MfS (that he told the officer in passing, softly) are disappointed how socialism was being built in the DDR. They had something else in mind (freedom)." MfS 13788/83. p. 15. The same document indicates that through contacts with the Stasi Seidel had been able to obtain an apartment in Dresden. An extensive document that contains a transcript of a recording from 1968 expands on Seidel's convictions and positioning, and concludes that he is not so much a believer in the system but that he understands that he will live and have to make a career in the DDR and that in order to do so certain things are expected. He appears to be rather opportunistic in his behavior, adjusting himself to the opinions of the majority and avoiding anything that would rock the boat. See: MfS 13788/81, pp. 14-23

151 Personal notes of Jochen Neumann, August 16, 2009

152 Personal notes of Jochen Neumann, August 16, 2009. Schulsinger knew about

"In Rome, I was picked up by our Embassy, but nobody had actually any idea where the meeting was taking place. The next day – I slept near the Embassy in the guesthouse that probably belonged to the Embassy – we went around the city in a car, looking for the meeting place of the WPA symposium. Eventually somebody at the *Urban VIII* hospital knew of the symposium and thus we found the location. However, it turned out that the Executive Committee was actually staying and meeting at the hotel *Leonardo da Vinci*, in another part of town. The next day I went there on foot, as I had no money whatsoever. And that is where the election process took place."[153]

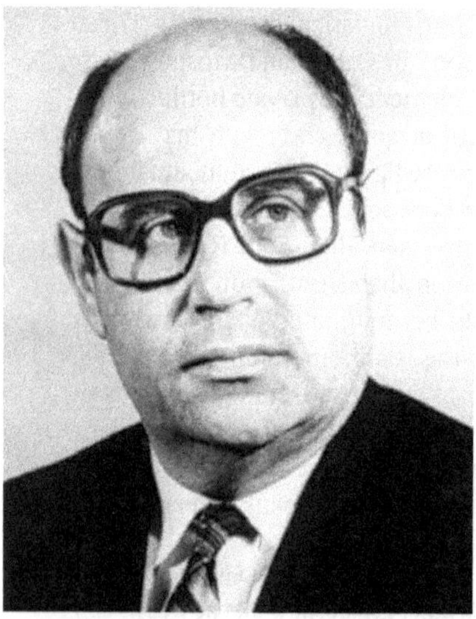

Jochen Neumann, 1984

The minutes of the Executive Committee give the impression that everything went relatively smoothly, and was prepared well in advance. In reality, the nomination of Jochen Neumann was tabled at the very last minute, and was a surprise for most of the people present. "He was suddenly there," recalls Costas Stefanis, but the question is whether Stefanis was not one of the few or even the only one who knew of Neumann's nomination from the very start. According to Neumann, Stefanis knew very well that he would be there: "In time – all persons involved were still asleep – I came to the hotel in the morning of October 8 and hid myself somewhere in a corner, waiting for things to happen. At a certain moment, Prof. Stefanis (whom I hadn't met before) appeared on the scene, and introduced himself. He was fully briefed and informed me of the planned agenda and time schedule and told me when I should be available in the lobby."[154]

The Executive Committee had discussed Neumann's nomination during an earlier afternoon session the day before, while Neumann himself was

the proposal and had even called Prof. Lange in Dresden to find out more. See later in this chapter and the report of Jochen Neumann on the Rome EC meeting, p. 6

153 Interview Jochen Neumann, February 26, 2009

154 Personal notes of Jochen Neumann, August 16, 2009; Interview Jochen Neumann, July 30, 2009

trying to find out where the Executive was actually meeting, and concluded that of the three candidates nominated (Dr. Leder from Poland, Dr. Robert Priest, nominated by the British Royal College of Psychiatrists, and Jochen Neumann) the latter was the best candidate. "The EC shared the opinion of the President, that the nomination from the GDR [DDR] was a signal to welcome, and it was decided that the President in his presentation of this item to the Committee, should express the EC's support of Dr. Neumann's candidature."[155]

The Committee of the WPA met the next Monday morning, initially with the members of the Executive Committee present, and was informed by WPA President Costas Stefanis that three nominations had been received, but that only two of them had been nominated by a member society, which the Executive preferred, and that the Executive was in favor of Neumann's candidature. It then reconvened without the Executive Committee, and a discussion ensued during which Neumann's candidature was seriously questioned. Several members wondered how they could vote for a person whose curriculum vitae was not made available in advance and whom they did not know; former General Secretary Peter Berner said he was not against a DDR candidate but that he knew other psychiatrists from there who would be more suitable as a Vice-President. One of the Committee members added Ahmed Okasha from Egypt to the list of candidates, which only strengthened the confusion. Eventually, the Committee decided to postpone the decision until the next session that afternoon, when more information could be received from the Executive Committee.[156]

After a two-hour lunch break, the Committee reconvened, this time again with the Executive Committee present. The meeting was chaired by an American psychiatrist, Alfred Freedman, member of the Committee. He had met Neumann earlier during the latter's visit to the United States in 1978 and was favorably disposed towards him. He informed the Committee that he had been informed by Fini Schulsinger that Neumann was actually present and suggested to invite him in, to which the others agreed. "…He invited Professor Neumann to the meeting introducing him to those present and asking him to introduce himself. Professor Neumann explained how he trained with Professor K. Leonhard at La [sic!] Charité in Berlin; how he had been Director at the Neurological-Psychiatric Clinic at the University of Jena and that his present appointment was Professor and Head of the Department of the University of Dresden and Director

155 Minutes of the WPA EC, October 1984, p. 3
156 Minutes of the WPA Committee, October 1984

of the Hygiene Museum of the Medical Academy of Dresden, a highly prestigious institution in his country. He also informed about his interest in biological psychiatry and psychopharmacology."[157]

Neumann remembers: "I was brought in, questioned, sent back, and that happened several times. Some of those present supported me, like Alfred Freedman, but others had strong objections. In particular, Peter Berner was very explicit about his reservations, repeating again that he was not against a Vice-President from East Germany but that he knew better candidates (e.g. Professor Leonhard).[158] Eventually when the election took place I was elected."[159] The election had been a major success: Neumann received 12 of the 16 votes, one person voted for Ahmed Okasha, one vote was void and two votes were blank. The Stasi was immediately informed of the successful outcome of the venture by urgent telegram.[160]

"After I was elected, Mel Sabshin suggested that the EC now needed to get to know the new "Acting Vice President"(Acting because I had been elected by the Committee and not the General Assembly and thus I was only Vice President ad interim). They decided to go out for dinner with their wives, but I had no money and had no idea how to pay for this. I feigned illness and said I would come along, but would not eat. They had an extensive dinner and the water was running through my teeth, but I couldn't pay so decided to pretend I was ill. One of them – I think it was Al Freedman - realized probably what was happening and said "Don't worry, we will pay" but I couldn't lose my honor and say: "Oh well, then I will eat as well" so I continued to pretend I was ill and had only a glass of mineral water and some mushrooms, while they were feasting next to me. Such were the times."[161]

---

157 Minutes of the WPA Committee, October 1984, p. 5

158 Professor K. Leonhard, an internationally renowned professor of psychiatry, taught at the University of Frankfurt/Main and later Director of the "*Psychiatrische und Nerven Klinik*" of the Charité, author of several important manuals in psychiatry.

159 Interview Jochen Neumann, February 26, 2009. In his report on the Rome EC meeting of October 17, 1984, he writes: "It is known that Berner, Austria, has tried with much effort to prevent the election of the DDR delegate. When all the arguments failed the main argument became that if somebody would be suggested from the DDR, it should be a well-known figure as Prof. Leonhard." *Ergänzungen zum Bericht*, Jochen Neumann, October 1984, p. 4

160 HAXX 499, p. 419. See also *Politisch Missbraucht*, p. 653

161 Interview Jochen Neumann, February 26, 2009

Mixed reactions at home

Upon his return from Rome, Neumann was met by Deputy Minister Rudolf Müller and a Major Koch of the MfS at the Airport Berlin-Schönefeld for a debriefing.[162] He reported, mistakenly, that he was elected with only one vote majority. Most of the opposition to his candidacy, he added, had been because, as a Director of the Hygiene Museum, he was not perceived as a good representative of psychiatry. However, he managed to counter these objections.[163] He promised to prepare a report for the Ministry of Health before October 17, after which a report would be prepared for the KGB in Moscow.[164]

The DDR Association of Psychiatrists did not automatically welcome the election of Neumann to the position of Vice President. The only person within the association who had known about the move was its President, Prof. Günter Rabending, who had been involved in organizing the selection and nomination and who himself worked as an "*Inoffizieller Mitarbeiter*" for the Stasi.[165] The others were surprised, to put it mildly, about the sudden way in which this all was organized. "Within the association there were fierce discussions about the way and method … in which the nomination and trip of Comrade Professor Neumann [had been arranged]…. The speed in which the trip had been organized was extraordinary even according to DDR standards."[166] Also Prof. Ehrig Lange from Dresden had expressed his surprise when called by WPA General Secretary Fini Schulsinger before the Rome EC meeting: "He had tried to clear his concerns during a personal telephone conversation with Prof. Lange from Dresden, whom he knew well, but the conversation was not very helpful because the latter had only voiced his surprise, according to Schulsinger, and could not really explain the DDR proposal."[167]

162 HA XX 499, p. 419

163 HA XX 499, pp. 412-3

164 HA XX 499, p. 413

165 Prof. Rabending, born in 1931 and at that time Director of the University Psychiatric Hospital Greifswald, functioned since 1971 under the nicknames "Rabe" and "Schäfer". See Süss, p. 652.

166 *Politisch Missbraucht*, p. 654

167 *Ergänzungen zum Bericht*, Jochen Neumann, October 1984, p. 6. See also HAXX 499, pp. 412-3. Prof. Ehrig Lange was also an *Inoffizieler Mitarbeiter* of the MfS with the cover name "Ehrenberg". He was recruited in February 1977 and became an official IM in September of that year. Personal circumstances, which are confidential yet known to the author, led to his agreement to work for the MfS. His personal Stasi file gives ample proof of this. In 1981 the Stasi concluded that he was not "honest" in his reporting an that his collabora-

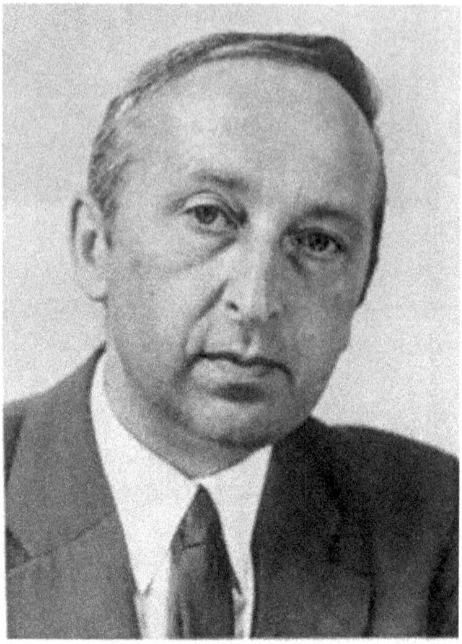

Prof. E. Lange, 1982

Possibly the reaction was also caused by Prof. Neumann's positioning within the Association. From conversations with him, I learned that no love was lost between most of the members of the Board of the Association and Neumann himself. He saw most of them as being mediocre opportunists with much less "intellectual baggage" and understanding of the outside world, and he knows that many of them considered him to be a bit arrogant, showing his intellectual superiority.[168] It is a combination that does not work and proved to be the main source of friction when Neumann is propelled into the Executive Committee of the WPA. Probably also jealousy played a role, because many had only limited travel possibilities.

In the West Neumann's election also resulted in surprise, partially because very few knew him or had heard his name before. Melvin Sabshin was curious about this new member of the Executive Committee and tried to gather information. "I met Mel [Sabshin] in 1984 in Washington on a study tour of our Social Psychiatric Center to places of psychiatric reforms in the US," remembers Dr. Helmut Bieber, at that time an active member of the German DVpMP. "In Washington, we visited, of course, the APA and Ellen Mercer. Knowing Mel [Sabshin] from his activity against the abuse, I tried to get to know him. ... It was during this *tour d'horizon* that he asked me my opinion about this East German, Dr. Neumann, who had become a member of the WPA Executive Committee. We had some friendly information in our group about him - I don't know from where - and that was all I could tell him."[169]

In an "Immediate Report" of October 15, 1984, Neumann outlines his tasks as he envisaged them.[170] According to this document, he saw it as

tion was based on fear, not on conviction. For that reason the collaboration was terminated in November 1981. BstU 4344/81.

168 Interview with Jochen Neumann, June 3, 2009

169 letter Helmut Bieber, April 25, 2009

170 The document is later followed up by a 27-page outline of Neumann's policy for the coming years, filed as BStU, ZA, HA XX 498, pp. 2-28.

his primary task to represent the socialist countries within the WPA and to make sure that "the socialist countries are informed about all developments either at all or in time. … The delegate finds himself as the only socialist under people who position themselves as either neutral, however in an unreliable manner, or as clearly pro-Western. … There will be a constant need for militant clashes until 1989, if we want to influence the positions in our advantage to a certain degree surely and reliably, even without the ability to make a positive prognosis when the time is there."[171]

The DDR leadership is jubilant. Politburo member Kurt Hager, Secretary of the Central Committee of the DDR Communist Party for Science, writes to "dear Professor Neumann: we consider the election of a representative of the DDR in this position in relation to the political conditions that exist in this context, as a big success. With accepting this position, you have taken upon yourself an important task. We wish you a lot of success in the interest of your profession and in strengthening the interests of the fraternal countries."[172] At the same time, having Neumann in the Executive Committee, the Stasi understands it is of pivotal importance that he functions in accordance with the wishes of the Soviet authorities, and in particular of the KGB. On October 24, as indicated earlier, a three-page document is produced for the KGB in which the East Germans express the view that "we consider it necessary that for a further targeted functioning of Prof. Neumann within the World Psychiatric Association in disclosing and countering the activities of anti-Socialist powers, a close collaboration and coordination of our operational interests and measures is implemented. We ask you, therefore, for instructions, information and tasks, that are suitable for the deployment and instruction of Professor Neumann."[173] In the Year Plan 1985 of the Directorate HA XX/1, the Stasi-division that was responsible for the deployment of Jochen Neumann, it is put equally clear: "In determining certain priorities in the deployment, a continuous fine-tuning with the KGB of the USSR is to be maintained."[174]

An interesting aspect of Neumann's work as *Inoffizieller Mitarbeiter* is the fact that although Eberhard Jaekel was chief of Chief Directorate (*Haupt Abteilung*) HA XX/1, which was responsible for surveillance of

171 BstU, ZA, HA 499, p.407

172 Letter from Hager to Neumann on October 25, 1984. See Süss p. 655. Interestingly, Hager addresses Neumann with "*Du,*" which suggests a friendly and relatively close relationship.

173 *Politisch Missbraucht*, p. 656

174 Arbeitsplan der HA XX/1 für das Jahr 1985, MfS GVS 741/84, BstU, ZA, HA XX, 421, p. 154. Süss, p. 656.

the churches, culture and illegal groups, Neumann was not recruited as agent for that directorate. Instead, he was working as IM 'Erhard' for HA II, which was responsible for counter-espionage. Still, many documents prepared by Neumann for HA II were found in the files of HA XX/1, and apparently they were forwarded for use by that department. Sonja Süss points out in her book, "*Politisch Missbraucht?,*" that in the files of HA XX/1, there are repeated references to "a reliable and checked source of Chief Directorate II/3," which clearly refers to Jochen Neumann. Also, in the collaboration plan of HA XX and the Fifth (Dissident) Directorate of the KGB for the period 1985-1990, one finds repeated references to an IM 'Lotos,' functioning as an agent in the "disclosure and prevention of anti-Soviet plans, intentions and activities" of organizations involved in the issue of the WPA and Soviet psychiatry. However, the personnel records of HA II do not produce an IM 'Lotos,' and Süss suggests this might have been a fictive creature by Jaekel in order to avoid the necessity of explaining to the KGB why information was coming from a different directorate than his.[175] Whatever the organizational position of Neumann within the Stasi structure, it was clear that all information eventually wound up on the desk of Eberhard Jaekel and subsequently found its way to the KGB in Moscow.

[175] See HA XX 499, p. 217. Also: *Politisch Missbraucht*, p. 656

Chapter 18 - Meeting Costas Stefanis

It had been twenty years since I had been there, in Athens, and I still remembered the drive from the airport to the city. Not so much the one after my own arrival, several weeks before the WPA World Congress started in October 1989. Rather, I remembered going with a colleague to the airport to meet Semyon Gluzman, the Soviet psychiatrist who served ten years in camp and exile for opposing the political abuse of psychiatry and was now part of our "team." Like me, he arrived around midnight, a few days before the Congress started, on an Aeroflot plane from Moscow (at that time there were no direct flights from Kiev, where he lived). Coincidentally, the same plane had brought the Soviet delegation to the World Congress, like a whale spitting out both opponents and proponents of a return of the Soviet All-Union Society to the WPA onto the Greek shore. Gluzman was sitting in the car next to me, mostly silent, looking out of the window. It was his first trip outside the Soviet Union. "Mmm," he said, "just like Tbilisi." With that he had given the city a place in his frame of reference, which until then only spanned the USSR. However, at that moment I didn't know what he meant; I had not yet had the chance to visit the Georgian capital myself.

On my visit twenty years later, while driving to the city, I understood. We now have an office in Tbilisi, which I visit regularly, and I immediately grasped what Gluzman meant back then. Especially in the evening when leaving the airport building, with the air still reverberating from the heat of the day, men standing in groups at the exit and around the taxi stand, talking agitatedly with short sleeved shirts and dark complexions, all very similar. Yet it was different, and not only because of the difference in the level of development. Athens has clearly grown, is much more modern than twenty years ago, thanks to its membership in the European Union. A more important difference is the smell of the sea nearby, the smell of the Mediterranean. It is mixed with car exhaust and pollution, but it is distinctly there. I opened the window and let the breeze circle through the taxi. This smell brought back the memories of the eventful days of October 1989.

I was in Athens again to meet with Costas Stefanis, the President of the World Psychiatric Association from 1983-1989. He is now in his early eighties, with failing health, but when I met him the next morning, in his office in the University Mental Health Research Institute that he established and built from scratch, he looked pretty vital. He actively moved around, with almost youth-like speed, and had prepared well for our meeting. All over of his office were photocopies of texts, minutes of WPA Executive

Committee sessions and a copy of one of my books from 1989, full of memory marks and notes scribbled on the side.

We had met a few times during the intermediate twenty years, but very brief meetings, not more than a handshake, a sign of recognition, that's all. Actually, we never really talked before, and nor did we talk during the 1983-1989 period when we were on opposite sides of the barricades. When I wrote him and asked for this meeting, more than half a year before, he immediately corrected this image that I had: "Personally, I never felt that I belonged to any camp," he answered my request, "and definitely, I never felt that we were opponents, because of some minor differences in assessing events or interpreting motives." But he gladly agrees to meet: "I have no objection at all to meet with you some time in the spring, ... I do not know how much I can contribute to your project, but I will try my best to recall events twenty years later." A sequence of illnesses and hospitalizations resulted in our meeting being postponed, but we had finally made it.

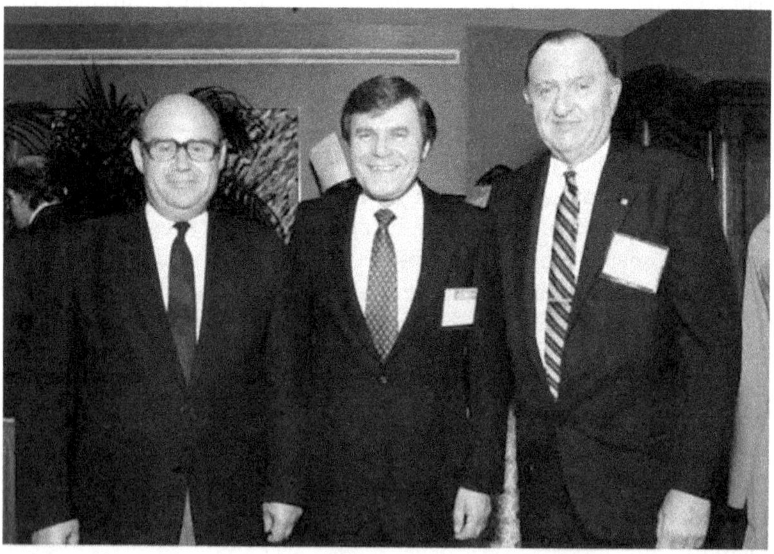

l.t.r. Jochen Neumann, Costas Stefanis, Melvin Sabshin, Washington, 1988

The meeting turned out to be a long one; many hours, and continued over dinner at night in a small tavern. Stefanis likes to talk, he admitted, "it is one of my vices. When Jochen Neumann was elected as Vice-President in Rome in 1984, his first move was to vote with Schulsinger to curb the length of the Executive Committee meetings. They were usually very long, seven to eight hours, very fatiguing. And so Schulsinger proposed to limit the length and there suddenly this guy from East Germany, just elected, yet unknown to us, seconds his proposal! I was quite surprised."

The conversation went back to 1983, the General Assembly of the WPA, where Stefanis was nominated from the floor. "It was a mess, there was total confusion; people were getting desperate. Schulsinger had just been elected as General Secretary, without being present himself; he had just given a written confirmation that he was willing to accept the position. Peter Berner had withdrawn his candidacy for Presidency. I don't know why. Maybe he thought that Schulsinger had been the choice of your people; that it had all been organized behind the scenes, and he refused to work with him. I pleaded with him, I told him 'I know Schulsinger; he is OK. Why don't you work with him, I don't understand. The organization needs you, it needs leadership.' But he refused, and people were upset, shouting, begging for a solution. There were people who proposed me from the floor, and others seconded them. Yet somehow this did not stop the confusion. And then the Italian delegate, Cazzullo[176] stood up and shouted loudly. "Stop this interminable discussion, I repeat let us vote for Stefanis…" I agreed, but I said that I wanted Berner to be President, not myself. But when Berner persisted, I agreed to my nomination." Stefanis was duly elected. "I didn't ask for it," he added. "Actually, I never asked for anything. All the time in my life I am proposed, asked, I never had to go for it myself. Elections, of course, followed the proposals, but I never felt as a career chaser. Neither, though, did I feel that anything was given to me without deserving it."

Born in 1928 to a lower class family, his father being a civil servant, Stefanis had an impressive career. He studied medicine, specialized in psychiatry and conducted post-graduate studies at Montreal's McGill University in

176 Professor Carlo Lorenzo Cazzullo, born in1915, graduated from the School of Medicine at the Institute Carlo Best in Milan (Italy). Cazzullo was in 1946 among the first Italians to cross the ocean to become a researcher at the Rockefeller Institute, where he studied electrophysiology with R. Lorente de No and with Nobel laureate Herbert Gasser. He was a member of the Committee of the WPA since 1966 and the Executive Committee from 1989 to 1993. In the 1980s Prof. Cazzullo was involved in developing and expanding relations between the Milan Institute of Psychiatry and psychiatrists from the People's Republic of China. Since 1959 Cazzullo was Professor of Psychiatry and Neurology at the University of Milan, Italy. In his *Ergänzungen zum Bericht*, Jochen Neumann writes in October 1984 that Cazzullo was known to be a friend of Georgi Morozov. *Ergänzungen zum Bericht*, Jochen Neumann, October 1984, p. 19. Later Neumann calls him a "bourgeois opportunist and a businessman with intelligence". *Reisebericht* of Jochen Neumann on the World Congress in Athens, October 1989, p. 3

Quebec, Canada. Back in Athens he became professor of psychiatry during the Colonel's Regime of 1967-1974,[177] built up the Mental Health Research Center at the University of Athens and was propelled into the position of WPA President in 1983. Five years after his WPA term of office ended, he was elected into the Athens Academy, and retired as professor of psychiatry in 1996. In the meantime, he became Minister of Health of Greece for the socialist PASOK Party. "The same post was proposed to me in the past ... and I declined, being more than hesitant to get involved in the political arena. I conceded in 2002 to Simitis government's proposal under special circumstances. My contribution to get out of impasses was mainly a citizen's obligation. I do not regret it. Several things were accomplished in less than two years."[178] And even now, at the age of 81, he continues to be professionally active, in spite of ill health. "I have been dead three times," he says, but somehow he manages to carry on in spite of an endless series of serious ailments. He just left the hospital after another serious surgery. "Let's see how long I manage to live."

The conversation continued, but then it gradually gained a bitter undertone. He remembered how he was accused of "clandestine communications" with the Soviets, and he targeted me as one of the main culprits. "There was nothing clandestine about it," he continues. "Everything I did was open and clear, never did I do anything secret. I was accused of having secret

[177] The Greek military junta of 1967-1974, alternatively "The Regime of the Colonels" are terms used to refer to a series of right-wing military governments that ruled Greece from 1967 to 1974. Rule by the military started in the morning of 21 April 1967 with a coup d'état led by a group of colonels of the Greek military, and ended in July 1974. According to Antonis Vgontzas, Stefanis' liberal views were not liked by the authorities. After the end of the junta regime he found documents of the Ministry of Health in which the complaint is voiced that Stefanis was made professor but that with his liberal or 'progressive' views he shows ingratitude to the military regime. Unfortunately, Vgontzas added, the documents were discarded during his moving from one house to another. Interview with Antonis Vgontzas, September 3, 2009.

[178] Letter to the author, July 28, 2009. During an interview Antonis Vgontzas confirms the story: "There were three professors: Andreas Papandreou and Konstantinos (Costas) Simitis were professors of economics, and Costas Stefanis was professor psychiatry. The relations between Stefanis and Simitis were much less strong than with Papandreou, and that is why people were very surprised that Stefanis, who always refused to become Minister of Health under Papandreou, agreed when Simitis asked him. Papandreou many times asked him before: 'please, become Minister of Public Health', but he always refused. He agreed when Simitis asked, because he saw it as something interesting, a sort of provocation."

meetings with Marat Vartanyan in Moscow, but I was there with a whole delegation. How could it have been clandestine? And why did you repeat these accusations, without any proof? Anything you said was immediately taken for granted, as the truth, and it was just nonsense."

All these years, rumors surrounded Stefanis, rumors that we also disseminated, it is true. It was said that he was a long-time friend with Marat Vartanyan, the main apologist of Soviet psychiatry, and allegedly even friends with Evgeni Chazov, the Minister of Health of the Soviet Union. Rumor had it that he was high up in PASOK, and the personal physician of the socialist leader Andreas Papandreou. "Nonsense," he says. I am politically unaligned, not a member of any party. I am independent, and don't belong to anyone. I vote PASOK, yes, so what? And yes, I was friends with Papandreou, but that had nothing to do with politics. And friends with Evgeni Chazov – how can you be friends with Evgeni Chazov? He was high up in the Soviet hierarchy and I met him only once in 1988!"

Antonis Vgontzas, a long time friend of Stefanis, later confirms the independence of Stefanis. "He was never a member of PASOK, but he is what in the United States you would call a liberal. Here in Greece you call it 'progressive.' He is a completely independent mind, not belonging to any party, but, of course, his political allegiance is clear. He was a close friend of Andreas Papandreou, for many years. He is also on friendly terms with the son, George Papandreou, and he is still an important figure in the Papandreou family, but it is different than the close personal relationship he had with the old Papandreou. And yes, he was sometimes also his personal physician, but that was part of the friendship."[179] That Stefanis and Andreas Papandreou were good friends is also apparent from one of Neumann's travel reports from 1985, in which he mentions a private party at Stefanis' home. "At this party was also the Prime Minister Papandreou, a friend of Stefanis, who was introduced to [me]. During our meeting, Prime Minister Papandreou referred to his talks with Erich Honecker."[180]

Marat Vartanyan is a different story. Stefanis met him the first time in 1971, at the WPA World Congress in Mexico where Vartanyan was elected as Associate Secretary of the WPA Executive Committee, and they met many times after. "I liked the man," says Stefanis. "Here was a Soviet guy you could talk to, relate to, who responded normally – a human being. Not

179 Interview with Antonis Vgontzas, September 3, 2009

180 *Sofortbericht*, 11-18 October 1985, on the WPA EC meeting in Athens, p. 2

like this Georgi Morozov, a stiff Soviet official, or this Nikolai Zharikov.[181] These were people that did not communicate; they remained stiff, like robots. Vartanyan was different: flamboyant, charming, and easy in communicating with people. He was a survivor. That is the best way to describe him: a survivor. He enjoyed life, but somehow there was always a sad undertone. When I asked Vartanyan about whether he believed in the system he immediately shrugged it off: 'I don't want to talk about that.' There was something there, a kind of underlying fear." But then, again, indignation takes the overtone: "I wasn't the only one who met him, who maintained contact with him. Take Ellen Mercer, she also met him regularly. So why pick on me?!"

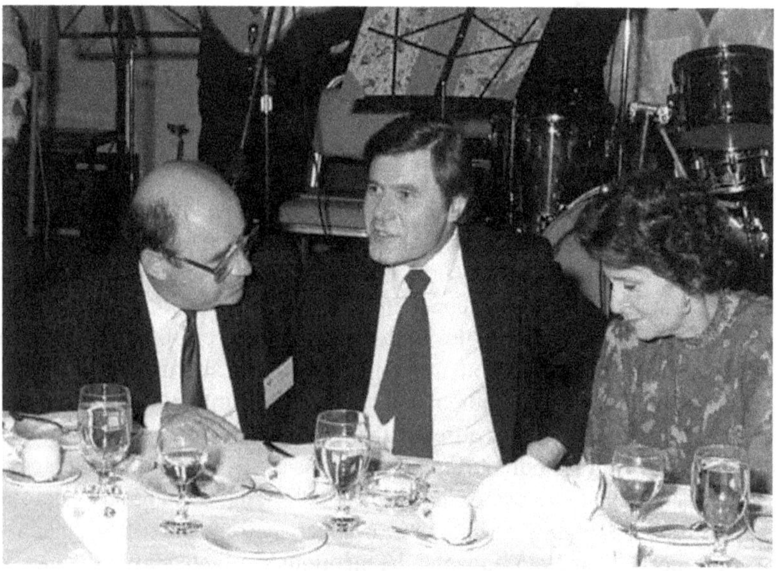

l.t.r. Jochen Neumann, Costas Stefanis, Adela Stefanis, Athens, 1989

Particularly painful is the fact that his wife Adela was accused of making disparaging remarks about Anatoly Koryagin, the dissident Soviet psychiatrist who was released from camp in February 1987 and gave a talk at an APA meeting in Chicago later that year, which both Stefanis and his wife attended. "In fact, she said that he looked like a saint, but also this was turned around and made into a negative remark." His wife confirms his

181 Nikolai Mikhailovich Zharikov, born 1920, finished the Military Medical Faculty in 1943, took active part in the Eastern front and was seriously wounded twice. After demobilization in 1946 specialized in psychiatry and became a psychiatrist in 1950. In 1999 he became professor of psychiatry.

story. "Yes," she says, "It is true. Koryagin was like a saint to me. He even looked like a saint. I felt his story was very moving."[182]

When talking about the past, about these attacks on his person, the bitterness became visible on Stefanis's face. Yet it is a sadness that prevails, not anger, at least not ostensibly. He never defended himself against the accusations. "Why didn't I defend myself?" he wonders. "I didn't, because it doesn't fit to my personality. I don't go out and tell people that it is all wrong, I just let it be." But clearly he was deeply hurt. "I never did anything illegal, and there is nothing I regret. I did what I had to do for the WPA, in spite of ill health. The organization was under imminent threat of falling apart. Latin American associations were angry with me for not allowing the Soviets back in. In the East, there were plans to set up a socialist WPA, which would unite the socialist countries and their supporters in the Third World and split the profession completely. The WHO was limiting their collaboration with us because we had forced the Soviets to withdraw. It was very serious, and it was my task to salvage the situation and try to make the WPA stronger."

Gradually, the conversation became more pleasant, amicable. We talked about totalitarianism, about the effect of Soviet rule on the population, the terror, the fear, how every family in the country was affected. Stefanis is well read, and very much aware of what was happening in the Soviet Union. He was also knowledgeable about the political abuse of psychiatry; actually, much more than I anticipated. And his opinions were clear, and not really different than mine. Somehow we found a common wavelength. When we went out for dinner in the evening, walking down the street, I tell him it is the first time I am back since those fateful days in 1989. "Ah," he says, "so you are full of memories. Can you imagine, then we were adversaries, we would walk past each other, not talking, sort of enemies. And look at us now!"

Indeed, this was a fateful meeting. More than anything it showed how destructive the political standoff was, how much it poisoned human

182 Indeed, there is a document that was published in the IAPUP *Documents*, titled "Why is Dr Stefanis Clandestinely Negotiating with the USSR about its Return to the WPA" and authored by Peter Reddaway, which states that "The same evening [of Koryagin's presentation at the APA Annual Meeting] Koryagin spoke briefly at an APA dinner for foreign visitors, spelling out the conditions on which, in his … view, the Soviet psychiatric society should be readmitted to the WPA. At this, Stefanis and his wife made disparaging remarks about Koryagin to the other guests at the table."

relations, and created fixed images of each other that made it impossible to see the person on the other side and understand his intentions. I feel so fortunate to be able to revisit those days, to digest them, together, and be able to close the book and put it to rest.

Yet the meeting also disturbed me. It caused me to look back, to my earlier activist days, and wonder whether I did everything right. His indignation towards me personally stayed on my mind, keeping me from falling asleep. I remembered the bitterness on his face, and with a feeling of sadness, I finally dozed off.

Chapter 19 – Soviet Actors

Already doctor Faust sold his soul to the devil; there were people before him, and after him.[183]

During the years between the Vienna Congress and the March-April 1989 WPA Regional Symposium in Granada, Spain, there were no official direct contacts between the Soviets and the WPA. The Soviet All-Union Society was not a member association, the conditions for their return were worded in the 1983 resolution of the WPA General Assembly, and the officers of the WPA had made it clear they would abide by the resolution: "The WPA Executive Committee… is bound by the resolutions voted upon by the General Assembly. We will honor the rules and will implement the resolutions of our governing body." [184] Yet this official position did not mean that there was no contact whatsoever, to the contrary. Representatives of the All-Union Society appeared at international meetings where WPA Executive Committee members were present, and they were bound to walk into each other, deliberately or coincidentally. Yet it is safe to assume that the unofficial relations between Soviet psychiatry and the WPA were mostly limited to four persons: on the side of the WPA, President Costas Stefanis and General Secretary Fini Schulsinger, and on the Soviet side since 1983 the President of the All-Union Society Georgi Morozov, and also Director of the infamous Serbski Institute in Moscow Since 1957), and Marat Vartanyan, first Deputy and since 1987 Director of the All-Union Center for Mental Health of the Academy of Medical Sciences. I say mostly, because as we will see in the next chapter, Jochen Neumann maintained contact with Georgi Morozov and Marat Vartanyan, out of his special position as an *Inoffizieller Mitarbeiter* of the Stasi.[185] We will return to those contacts in the next chapter.

Of the four persons mentioned, only Vartanyan and Stefanis maintained close personal relations. For Stefanis, Morozov was an almost inaccessible personality, a stiff Party bureaucrat, while Vartanyan with all his flair was a real person with whom one could connect.[186] This very well suited the Soviets, however, because Vartanyan was used exactly for that purpose: mellowing Western psychiatric leaders.

183 *Psychiatry, psychiatrists and society* p.97

184 WPA Newsletter 21, May 1984, p. 4

185 Interview Jochen Neumann, July 30, 2009

186 For more information on Stefanis' views regarding Vartanyan see the previous chapter.

Dark mournful eyes

Marat Enokhovich Vartanyan was maybe one of the internationally most successful and disputed representatives of Soviet psychiatry. Initially employed at the Institute of Psychiatry of the Academy of Medical Sciences, headed by Andrei Snezhnevsky, he became Director of the All-Union Research Center for Mental Health in 1987. A year earlier he had become Professor of Psychiatry. As noted before, he was a member of the WPA Executive Committee in 1971-1977 (as Assistant Secretary), and was a member of the Ethics Committee of the WPA (1977-1983). In 1985 he had also become a Corresponding Member of the USSR Academy of Medical Sciences.

Vartanyan was also a member of the Presidium of the International Physicians for the Prevention of Nuclear War (IPPNW), which was co-chaired by American Professor Bernard Lown and Soviet cardiologist Evgeni Chazov,[187] who happened to be a friend of Vartanyan. Chazov was an extremely influential doctor and politician in the Soviet Union, who professionally treated many of the top Party leaders including Leonid Brezhnev.[188] Andrei Kovalev, a diplomat working at the Ministry of Foreign Affairs during the late 1980s, remembers: "Many people in the West considered Chazov as a reformer, and he created that impression.

---

[187] Evgeni Chazov, born in 1928 and originally from Kiev, was in 1967 appointed head of the 4th Main Administration in the Ministry of Health at the age of 38. This department was in charge of the health care system for the nomenklatura, which consumed about half of the Ministry's budget. As a result, Chazov became the personal physician of many Soviet and Russian leaders, such as Leonid Brezhnev, Konstantin Chernenko, Yuri Andropov and Boris Yeltsin, as well as the leaders of several other countries. It seems that Chazov managed to develop a personal relationship with Leonid Brezhnev, who when dying made him a full member of the Central Committee of the CPSU. Apparently, Chazov had favored a different career and wished to succeed Aliyev as First Deputy Prime minister and head of the governmental bureau for Social Development. He was apparently blocked in this move by Yegor Ligachev, second in command to Mikhail Gorbachev and responsible for all appointments in the health field, and instead told to replace Burenkov as Health Minister, telling Chazov: "You have taken good care of the leaders' health, now take good care of the people's." See Peter Reddaway's travel report to the USSR, *Documents* 6, April 1988.

[188] For instance, in 1981 and 1985 Vartanyan traveled to the United States on behalf of the IPPNW. See David Lown, *Prescription for Survival*, and a letter from Harold Merskey, October 29, 1985, to Peter Reddaway. In 1983, Vartanyan co-authored with Chazov an IPPNW paper "The Psychological Effects of Nuclear War."

Actually, he was quite reactionary and behaved like royalty. I once brought him a document for the Central Committee that needed his signature, in the time of the preparations for the American psychiatric visit in 1988. It was a weekend day, Saturday or maybe even Sunday. He was sitting in his office with some other people, behind his desk. He didn't even look up, just made a move with his hand in the air, waving it backwards over his shoulder, indicating that I should just give him the document. He glanced through it, without ever looking up to me, put his signature and then with the same move over his shoulder handed it back to me. Not a word, no personal contact whatsoever."[189]

In December 1987, after the death of Andrei Snezhnevsky, Vartanyan managed to obtain a promotion to the position of Director of the All-Union Research Center for Mental Health, in spite of a nasty affair in 1985-1987, when the Disciplinary Committee of the Communist Party of the Soviet Union (CPSU) carried out an investigation against him on charges of corruption, to be discussed more later. He was finally let off with a Party rebuke, but his position was much weakened. However, in October 1987, Moscow Party Chief Boris Yeltsin was demoted, and as a result the political landscape changed. This allowed Vartanyan's friend Chazov, who had by then become Minister of Health of the USSR, to push through the latter's promotion.[190]

For those opposing the political abuse of psychiatry, Vartanyan was the epitome of how low Soviet psychiatry had sunk. He was on record multiple times as a liar and a cheater, yet, at the same time, people found him charming, hospitable, and entertaining. And not only within the psychiatric field: being on the Presidium of the IPPNW, he regularly met one of the Co-Chairs, Bernard Lown, who was very much impressed

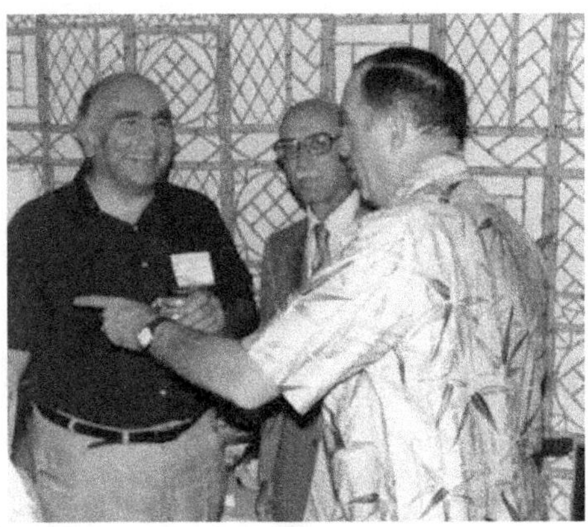

Melvin Sabshin and Marat Vartanyan, 1988

[189] Interview with Andrei Kovalev, October 12, 2009

[190] *Biographical Dictionary*, p. 50-51

by him. "Marat Vartanyan was a major spokesman of the Soviet delegation, and experimental psychophysiologist dealing with animal models.[191] He was highly cultured, reticent in speech and demeanor; his English was impeccable. I remember him as a brooding person with a ready laugh. I was attracted by his dark mournful eyes. Though he was in his early fifties, a fringe of white hair surrounding his bald head made him look a decade older. Marat's life was charged with tragedy. When he was still a young teenager, both his parents were caught up in the Stalinist terror and disappeared into a gulag.[192] He and his brother were street children, left to fend for themselves and hounded by their peers for being the offspring of counterrevolutionaries. I was awed by his ability to get an education, let alone a medical degree, and mount to the top of the profession."[193]

According to an obituary in the Korsakov Journal, Vartanyan was several times threatened with removal from the Yerevan Medical Institute as an "enemy of the people," but professors and students managed to prevent this. He was a very active sportsman, and at some stage, a member of the Armenian national basketball team.[194]

From all reports on him, it is clear that he managed to get the maximum out of life, albeit under Soviet circumstances. With his Armenian flair, he managed to get things his way, appearing at international congresses, winding people around his finger and always playing double games. Norman Sartorius, for many years Director of the Mental Health Division of the World Health Organization remembers that after the World Congress of the WPA in Honolulu and thanks to Marat Vartanyan "Soviet psychiatrists spoke ill about me. A story that was told at the time may explain this. I was in Honolulu at the World Congress of psychiatrists, and was present at the General Assembly as an observer. My wife came to the *antechamber* of the hall where the General Assembly took place and met there with Bert

191 Elsewhere in the book Lown calls him "a highly respected psychiatrist and experimental biologist." As we see later in this chapter, he also liked to present himself as a medical geneticist.

192 According to the obituary of Vartanyan, published in *the Korsakov Journal of Neuropathology and Psychiatry,* 1994, volume 94, issue 1, the father of Marat Vartanyan was arrested in 1939, after which the family moved to Yerevan. There is no mention of his mother's arrest.

193 *Prescription for Survival,* p. 282-3. This story sounds very unlikely. In the obituary in the *Korsakov Journal* it says that Vartanyan finished secondary school in Yerevan and the Yerevan State Medical Institute in 1955 at the age of 24. If he had been a street child this would hardly have been possible.

194 *Korsakov Journal of Neuropathology and Psychiatry* 1994, volume 94, issue 1, p. 109-110

Brown who was then Director of NIMH. I went out at the time when she said she would come, saw them sitting there, went over, gave my wife a kiss and shook the hand of Bert Brown. Right at that moment, Marat Vartanyan came out of the toilet, saw me shaking Brown's hand, and soon after that I heard that the reason I should not be trusted was that I was on the American side, against the USSR – since I had been seen shaking the hand of the American "chief psychiatrist" to congratulate him on the victory of Honolulu. The Soviets warned their people against me, they kept at a distance. However, Marat Vartanyan actually helped me on two occasions when I really needed his help, and he did this even though it was not at all to his own personal benefit.[195]

Ellen Mercer also had this somewhat dual attitude about him. "When reporters approached him with questions about the political abuse of psychiatry, he said, waving his arms, "come and visit us!" Yet when they then would ask how the trip could be arranged, he would make a sign in the direction of Ellen Mercer and say: 'Just talk to Ellen Mercer here, she will arrange it!' When we walked away, I asked him: 'what do you mean, just talk to Ellen Mercer?!' Yet that is how he was, he always turned things around and made sure he benefited from it. They probably must have thought – 'Gee, they are really close!"[196]

Marat Vartanyan knew Costas Stefanis from earlier times, when they collaborated on a joint WHO research project. Their relationship became friendlier during the years 1977-1983, when both served on the WPA Ethics Committee.[197] Following my interview with him in mid-July 2009, Costas Stefanis confirms their friendly relationship: "It is true that I met Vartanyan several times, mostly in the frame of international scientific meetings abroad or our common membership to several scientific organizations … I met him in Moscow a few times in various capacities (as WPA Ethics Com-

---

195 Interview Norman Sartorius, April 16, 2009. Norman Sartorius, born 1935, joined the World Health Organization (WHO) in 1967 and soon assumed charge of the program of epidemiology in social psychiatry. In 1977, he was appointed Director of the Division of Mental Health of WHO, a position that he held until mid-1993. In June 1993 Dr Sartorius was elected President of the World Psychiatric Association (WPA) and served as President-elect and then President until August 1999.

196 Interview Ellen Mercer, June 28, 2009

197 Marat Vartanyan was automatically excluded from that committee in January 1983 when the AUSNP left the WPA. See the EC Minutes of February 2, 1984.

mittee Chair, in the '87 "Forum,"[198] on two or three other occasions, almost all of them with several world known psychiatrists). … I do not hesitate to say that my acquaintance with him started as a strictly scientific and professional one and evolved into a friendly relationship. … He was open, not stiff, and knowledgeable of progress in our field worldwide (a rare exception among Soviet psychiatrists of that time). Moreover, he was very easy to communicate with, with an element of humor and he was clever enough either to be tolerant to the other's opposing views or to bypass them by saying: 'let's discuss it some other time.' I never discussed the All Union Society's withdrawal or potential reentry into the WPA; although, publicly he was the apologist of the Soviet view on abuse, he declined to discuss it in private, but in a humoristic way. Personally, I still think that he did not take part in this practice, but for reasons that he himself only knew, he was ordered to become the apologist. One factor that should be considered is under what political conditions - if ambitious enough - one had to function in order to retain his post and confront his inner enemies."[199] Later, during my second meeting with Stefanis in November 2009, we discuss Vartanyan more extensively, trying to understand the person behind the apologist. The picture that emerges is a complex one, and confirms much of the above: a man with a very painful past, who for reasons of his own, fulfilled a function for the Soviet authorities yet at the same time had no illusions about the Soviet system and its ruthlessness. And by not wanting to discuss these issues, he said more than if he had agreed to talk.

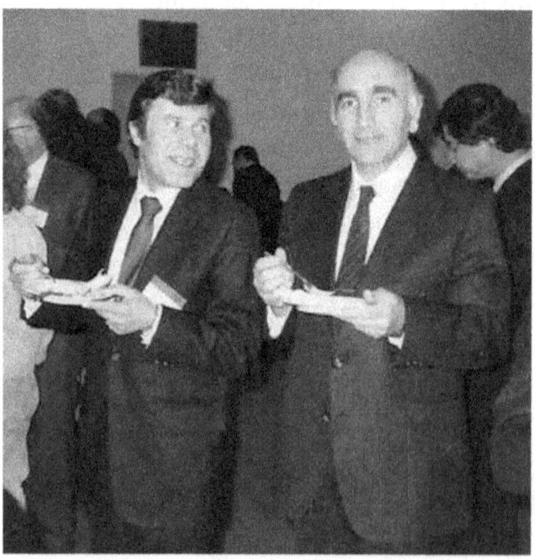

Costas Stefanis and Marat Vartanyan, 1988

Indeed, when looking at the fact that Vartanyan was allowed to travel abroad alone, mingle freely with Western psychiatric leaders and socialize with them, one can only conclude that he had an unusual position within the Soviet context. Usually, Soviet psychiatrists would never travel alone, always in groups of at least two or three, with at least one of them functioning as the ears and eyes of the secret service. If one traveled without others, it almost automat-

198 Stefanis refers to the Conference of the IPPNW, which was held in Moscow in 1987 and where Stefanis was one of the speakers.

199 Letter from Costas Stefanis, July 28, 2009

ically meant that the person concerned was ears and eyes of the secret service himself. In other words, there is ample circumstantial evidence to suggest that Marat Vartanyan was linked to the KGB. The aforementioned remarks about Vartanyan from the Stasi archives points exactly in that direction. Also Viktor Gindilis, a geneticist and colleague at the All-Union Institute for Mental Health, who was initially a friend but later turned against him, confirmed in his memoirs that "Marat has links with the [security] organs."[200]According to confidential sources, Vartanyan used to bring back medication from abroad for a family member of Evgeni Primakov, who was suffering from schizophrenia.[201] Primakov, who later became Foreign Minister and for a year also Prime Minister, was a General in the KGB.[202]

But there is also direct proof of Vartanyan's link to the KGB. In the *Mitrokhin Archive*, one document refers directly to KGB agent "Professor", and although the full name of the person concerned is not mentioned, there can be no doubt that "Professor" is in fact Marat Vartanyan. The document mentions the KGB's influence on the WPA as follows: "WPA Executive Committee – agent 'Professor', USSR; WPA Committee – professor Vencovsky, CSSR, professor Lange, DDR."[203] At the time the document was composed (1975), Marat Vartanyan was a member of the WPA Executive Committee; there can be no mistake in the identity here. Later, the document

200 Gindilis, p. 165

201 Yevgeny Maksimovich Primakov (born 1929) is a Russian politician, a former KGB general and a former Prime Minister of Russia. He was also the last Speaker of the Soviet of the Union of the Supreme Soviet of the Soviet Union, and the Russian Foreign Minister. Primakov is an academic and a member of the Presidium of the Russian Academy of Sciences. Primakov became involved in politics in 1989, as the Chairman of the Soviet of the Union, one of two houses of the Soviet parliament. From 1990 until 1991 he was a member of Soviet leader Mikhail Gorbachev's Presidential Council. After the failed August 1991 putsch attempt, Primakov was appointed First Deputy Chairman of the KGB. After the formation of the Russian Federation, Primakov was appointed Director of the Foreign Intelligence Service SVR, serving in that position from 1991 until 1996. Primakov served as foreign minister from January 1996 until September 1998, and as Prime Minister from 1998 until 1999.

202 The source of information is known to the author, but wishes to remain anonymous. According to the same source, former Serbski Institute director Tatyana Dmitrieva took over the psychiatric support after Marat Vartanyan died in 1993.

203 Mitrokhin Archive, Woodrow Wilson International Center for Scholars, Cold War International History Project, folder 28, *Practicing Psychiatry for Political Purposes*, document 4 (Plan 5/1-18230 of December 25, 1975, signed by KGB department heads Kryuchkov, Grigorenko and Bobkov, and confirmed the next day by KGB deputy chairman Chebrikov), p.4

indicates that "in preparation for the WPA World Congress in Honolulu, agent 'Professor' [should] strengthen and continue his contacts with WPA General Secretary Denis Leigh with the goal of receiving information on the state of affairs within the WPA leadership."[204] The same document also names three other KGB agents that were active in the psychiatric field ("Vaikin", "Krayevsky" and "Petrov") and lists a number of psychiatric leaders by their initials, who are considered to be "reliable" and having contacts with important foreign psychiatrists that are of use to the KGB. Among them are BEA (there is also mentioning of BAE, but probably the last two initials were wrongly swapped and both refer to Babayan, Eduard Armenakovich), LDR (Lunts, Daniil Romanovich), MGV (Morozov, Georgi Vladimirovich), MVV (Mikheyev, Vadim Vladimirovich), NRA (Nadzharov, Ruben Aleksandrovich) SAB (Smulevich, Anatoly Boleslavovich), SAV (Snezhnevsky, Andrei Vladimirovich), and SZN (Serebryakova, Zoya Nikolayevna).[205] Unfortunately there is not sufficient information in the document to establish whom the three agents named above actually were.[206]

It is also important to note that fellow EC-members Jochen Neumann and Melvin Sabshin do not agree with Stefanis' claim that he and Vartanyan were on friendly terms but had contact only occasionally. According to Neumann, these contacts were much more frequent, also by telephone, and there is no doubt in his mind that Stefanis and Vartanyan maintained intensive contact during Stefanis' tenure as President of the WPA.[207] The latter disagrees, sometimes angrily, and thus the issue will remain subject to debate.

In the USSR, not all shared the prevailing attitude among Western psychiatric leaders regarding Marat Vartanyan. Actually, he was feared by many and despised by others. In a handwritten travel report of Melvin Sabshin on his

204 *Practicing Psychiatry for Political Purposes*, document 4, p.5

205 *Practicing Psychiatry for Political Purposes*, document 4, p.2

206 When listing Soviet leading psychiatrists that were actively communicating with Western colleagues at that time, and then deducting those names by their initials in this document as well as agent "Professor" (Marat Vartanyan), less than a dozen names are left, and most probably the three agents are among them. Among those is Juri Saarma, who was widely suspected of being a KGB agent and who for many years was internationally quite active in the defense of Soviet psychiatry, but also Sergei Semyonov of the Serbski Institute, who was also widely considered to be linked to the KGB, Georgi Morozov's colleague and future AUSNP President Nikolai Zharikov and also Yuri Novikov, the Serbski psychiatrist who defected to the West in 1977.

207 Interview Jochen Neumann, July 28, 2009

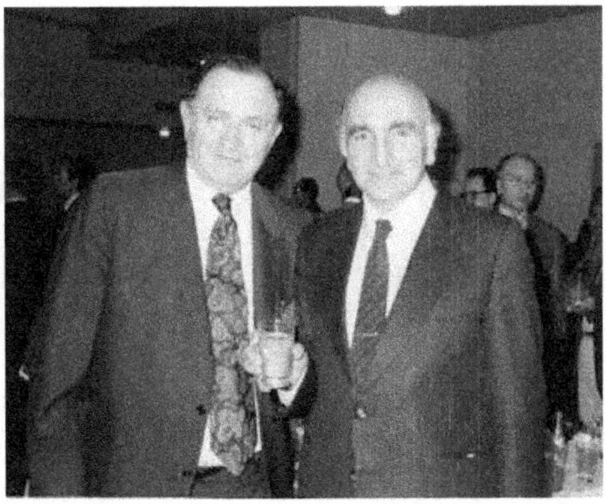
Melvin Sabshin and Marat Vartanyan, 1988

trip to the USSR in March 1990, he mentions that "Tiganov – he is afraid of Vartanyan."[208] Tiganov had his reasons, as we will see.

One person who fundamentally disliked Vartanyan was Dr. Viktor Gindilis, a Moscow based geneticist who worked with Marat Vartanyan for many years and was Head of the Genetics Laboratory of the All-Union Research Center for Mental Health.[209] He met Vartanyan for the first time in 1964 and joined him at the Institute in 1969. For many years, they were friends, and Gindilis often visited him at his home. However, according to Gindilis, Vartanyan's ambitions were uncontrollable and bad management led to the fact that he was twice turned down during elections as Candidate member of the Academy of Medical Sciences. "Marat ... still had an oriental mentality, within the framework of which failure during elections for the Academy was not only a painful matter, but looked like a serious defeat in the eyes of his ethnic group."[210]

According to Gindilis, Vartanyan tried in the beginning of 1985 to use all his tricks and networks to upgrade the All-Union Research Center to the level of a Scientific-Clinical Center of the Academy of Medical Sciences, of which there were at that time only two, the Oncology Center of N.N. Blokhin and the Cardiology Center of Evgeni Chazov. Apparently, both Blokhin and Chazov supported Marat in his plans. The idea was the Center would have three Institutes (Clinical Psychiatry, Biological Psychiatry and Social Psychiatry) and that initially Snezhnevsky would be the general director. However, he was then already more than eighty years old and "almost demented and quietly getting used to the nonsense that was happening around him."[211] It was clear that he had not long to live

---

208 Tiganov was at that time President of the Soviet Psychiatric Association AUSNP

209 Gindilis was also the author of the essay ridiculing the Moscow School and its ideas about schizophrenia, see chapter 9. The letter regarding Marat Vartanyan was given in translation to the author by Dr. Gindilis during a meeting at the home of Moscow dissident Larisa Bogoraz in late 1988 or very early in 1989, with the request to publish it as widely as possible. This was done in February 1989.

210 Gindilis, p. 154-5

211 Gindilis, p. 201

and Vartanyan was already maneuvering himself in place to take over. He decided that, for the time being, he would head the Center of Biological Psychiatry. He managed to get Snezhnevsky to sign a statement, prepared in advance by Vartanyan, that he recommended appointing Vartanyan as his successor. And in order to flatter his boss a bit further, the charmer Vartanyan had decided that after Snezhnevsky's death the Center would be named after him and a statue of Snezhnevsky would be placed in the entrance hall. He even had a sculptor come and take Snezhnevsky's measurements, but when the latter found out the purpose he threw the sculptor out and never forgave Marat for what he had done.[212] Apparently, Snezhnevsky was not yet that demented.

It all went terribly wrong for Marat, and instead of becoming head of a magnificent new Center he found himself in the center of an investigation by the Disciplinary Committee of the Communist Party. According to Gindilis, it was the "demented" Snezhnevsky himself who took the statement Vartanyan had made him sign and went to see Candidate Politburo Member Zimyanin, then responsible for science and medicine. Many of the people in the upper echelons of the Party knew Snezhnevsky well and regularly made use of his services. Unfortunately for Vartanyan, another Candidate Politburo Member, Boris Ponomaryov, counted Serbski Director Georgi Morozov among his entourage and Morozov and Vartanyan were already at war. For Morozov, this offered a unique opportunity to get rid of his opponent; and it was an opportunity he grabbed with both hands. Viktor Gindilis himself became involved, and with help of a colleague, he sent a letter to the Central Committee in which he leveled accusations against Vartanyan. Soon, he had Georgi Morozov on the telephone, who suggested meeting and discussing the issue.[213]

The accusations leveled against Vartanyan consisted of financial irregularities, plagiarism, administrative manipulation and involvement of corrupt actions by his associates. He was severely interrogated by the Disciplinary Committee of the CPSU, under chairmanship of Politburo member Mikhail Solomentsev. They even sent a delegation to the All-Union Research Center for an investigation on the spot. "Among them were well-known psychiatrists from outside, geneticists and bureaucrats of the Academy of Medical Sciences and the Ministry of Health. Marat knew them all, greeted them noisily and patted them on their backs."[214]

212 Gindilis, p. 201
213 Gindilis, p. 204
214 Gindilis, p. 207

Although it was clear this was a serious investigation, and Vartanyan was running around trying to use all his connections to stop the process, Gindilis also noticed that the inspectors came less and less regularly, and eventually stopped coming at all. It was clear that a different wind was blowing.[215] According to information from Moscow, it was Candidate Politburo Member Mikhail Zimyanin who intervened at the request of his daughter, as Vartanyan had helped her.[216] Three months later, the Communist Party officially reprimanded Vartanyan. "A Party meeting took place in our Center, during which Marat was reprimanded. I understood that for him it was terrible; as I was told, he left the meeting in tears."[217]

Three years passed, in the course of which Snezhnevsky died on July 12, 1987, at the age of 84, and, several months later, was succeeded by Vartanyan. By that time, November 1988, "glasnost" and "perestroika" were in full swing in the Soviet Union. Viktor Gindilis published an Open Letter to the Biological Medicine Department of the USSR Medical Science Academy in which he accused Marat Vartanyan and his wife of a whole series of irregularities, plagiarism and even pushing associates to suicide. The reason for the letter was Vartanyan's attempt to become a full member of the Academy. "It is clearly unjustified to 'reserve' for M.E. Vartanyan the Medical Science Academy's elective position for a 'geneticist specializing in mental illness.' Since his activity as an academic manipulator has long needed investigation by the State's Procurator's Office, I feel compelled to bring a number of important matters to the attention of yourselves, and of the leaders of the Academy, the Ministry of Health, and the Science Department of the Party Central Committee."[218]

In his letter, which was disseminated through *samizdat*,[219] he wrote that "I am the author of almost all the publications and research initiatives attributed to M. E. Vartanyan in the field of medical genetics, particularly with regard to the genetics of mental illness. ... *There is no immoral and unscrupulous act that Vartanyan would not commit for the sake of careerist goals* [italics by Gindilis] ... The real moral level of this would-be Academician has been revealed specially vividly by tragic recent events

215 Which was probably caused by the sacking of Boris Yeltsin, as noted earlier.

216 Travel report Peter Reddaway, *Documents* 6, April 1988

217 Gindilis, p. 208

218 Considering the content of his letter, it is not excluded that Gindilis was one of the sources of information on basis of which the investigation against Vartanyan was carried out in 1985-1987.

219 Samizdat is "self-publication", the unofficial way of disseminating forbidden literature in the Soviet Union.

involving the simultaneous deaths of two scientists at our Center, which resulted from the disorder in Vartanyan's own laboratory, and even more by subsequent cover-up attempts which included the forgery of documents and the spreading of slander about those who perished."

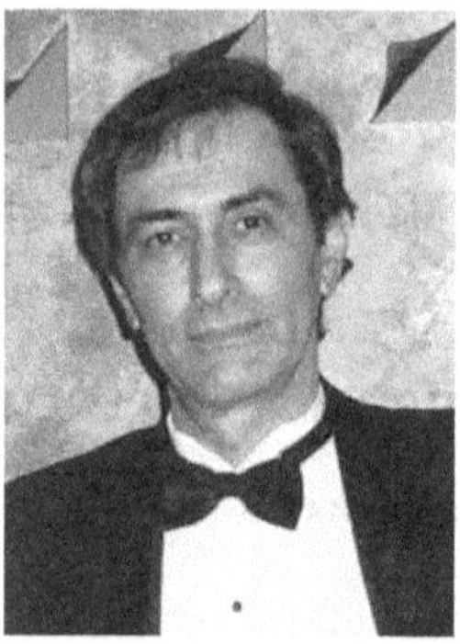

Dr. Viktor Gindilis

In his letter, Gindilis accused Vartanyan point by point of a whole range of misdoings. "Although Vartanyan presents himself, when it suits him, as a medical geneticist,[220] he has, in fact, not received or examined a single patient for the last thirty years... Vartanyan is simply illiterate even in the simple issues of medical genetics, and when it comes to complex aspects of the contemporary genetics of mental illness and molecular neurogenetics, he is completely incompetent. ... Everything he attributes to himself in official papers submitted to top bodies, e.g., in connection with the forthcoming Academy elections, is the fruit of the creative work of particular scientists. Most of these people have been cruelly done in by him as he has climbed the administrative ladder."

Gindilis then continued by giving several examples of plagiarism and stealing other scientists' work and publishing it under his own name. He also lashed out against Vartanyan's wife, D.D. Orlovskaya: "probably it is a unique situation for the Academy where neither of two spouses heading specialized labs in a single scientific institution should have the professional right to do so." According to Gindilis constant harassment by Orlovskaya ("without even knowing how a microscope is built, or how to use it...") and Vartanyan led to a number of people leaving the department or even committing suicide.

Several times Gindilis pointed out that opposing Vartanyan was impossible, because he had "constant protection ... by a certain group of people in the Science Department of the Central Committee, the Ministry of Health, and the Medical Science Academy." Most people decided not to resist, but, rather, to let Vartanyan get his way. "The view that Vartanyan is an adventurer, an academic manipulator, a fixer, an unprofessional administrator, etc., is shared by many people, including even former leaders of our Center like Academician A.V. Snezhnevsky..."

Interesting are Gindilis' remarks about Vartanyan's election as Director of

220 Interestingly, this is the third "profession" ascribed to Vartanyan, next to the two mentioned in Lown's book.

the All-Union Institute of Mental Health in December 1987. "The outcome was a behind the scenes pressure and autocratic decision. First, the decision went against the majority of the Center's staff, which was clearly expressed in a resolution of the staff union, and also against the wishes of a number of high bodies, including Party ones. Secondly, it ignored the fact that not long before, a special commission of the Central Committee's Party Disciplinary Committee had, in the face of powerful pressure from the forces protecting Vartanyan, nonetheless officially confirmed that he had grossly abused his official position and violated the norms of scientific ethics. To all appearances, however, the administrative reprimand imposed on him by the Party was viewed by him and his associates as merely a temporary hiccup…"[221]

And still the list was not complete. Accordingly among the other crimes committed by Vartanyan were that he "senselessly wasted foreign currency, illegally spent state funds for non-designed purposes, cooked [forged] the books, and committed scientific bluff. … The ethical corruption of subordinates by various means, and the ability to prove his usefulness to top nomenklatura officials – these are probably the only two things that Vartanyan does professionally...One can only express futile surprise that, at a time when perestroika has been proclaimed, the very title of Academician is being debased. The evidence for this is that such obvious careerists as M.E. Vartanyan, for whom scientific looting and administrative banditry are the ethical norm, have enjoyed such longstanding and sure protection within the Academy itself, the Health Ministry, the State Planning Committee, and the Science Department of the Central Committee."[222]

Interestingly, although Vartanyan's name is inseparably connected to that of political abuse of psychiatry in the Soviet Union, there is no evidence that he ever participated in these abuses himself. He was an apologist, a spokesperson for Soviet abusing psychiatry, and a very good one indeed, considering the widespread admiration he managed to evoke even among those who opposed that what he represented. "Vartanyan was quoted on the radio constantly together with Morozov and Snezhnevsky (and Marat was very happy with it, because he was of the opinion that it spread his fame and made him look better in the eyes of his [Armenian] community). Yet in fact he never had any direct involvement in dissident cases, because he was not a clinician, he did not make any official diagnoses and did not sign any such reports."[223]

---

221 It is worth considering which power in the Soviet Union was strong enough to have a Disciplinary Committee of the CPSU headed by a Politburo member back off.

222 Letter published in *Documents* 16, February 1989

223 Gindilis, p. 213

Dr. Georgi Morozov was in many ways the opposite of Marat Vartanyan, as Gindilis continues to write: "With G[eorgi] M[orozov] it was, of course, completely different. He sanctioned diagnostic reports on those dissidents that were put in his Institute, which means that he clearly took responsibility for it."[224]

Faithful Party psychiatrist

Some people, mainly foreigners, describe Georgi Vasilievich Morozov as a rather rigid person, morose, one that completely missed the flair of Marat Vartanyan. When Jochen Neumann tries to describe Morozov he frowns, pulls down the corners of his mouth and looks as if he has just heard something very disturbing. However, others (mainly people from his Russian environment) describe him as a rather easy-going character, absolutely not a hard worker, and some even refer to him as a womanizer. Dr. Yuri Novikov, the former department head of the Serbski Institute who defected to the West in 1977, describes Georgi Morozov as a "typical product of Soviet society… He too is a split personality, and, like with all the leading figures in the Soviet Union, it is hard to describe him because he has very polar character traits, a conglomerate of positive and negative ones. The positive ones are probably primary personal ones, the negative have developed in the course of his life. For instance, it is interesting that Morozov stays in the background during official gatherings, and doesn't defend the Soviet position during international meetings. In Honolulu, for example, it was [Dr. Eduard] Babayan who was the spokesperson of the Soviets. Morozov is always a bit in the shadow. Why? I know from my personal experience that Morozov doesn't like to participate in meetings where the issue of psychiatry and dissidents is being discussed. He comes too late; he cancels. That is interesting."[225] Others de-

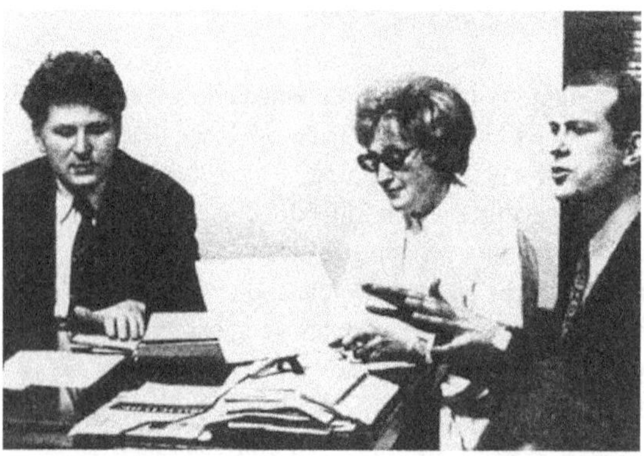

l.t.r. Georgi Morozov, Margaretha Taltse and Yuri Novikov, approx. 1976

[224] Gindilis, p. 213

[225] Interview of the author with Yuri Novikov, November 28, 1979, in Hamburg, p. 24. The quote is from the unpublished full record of the meeting, which lasted for three and a half hours and which is in the author's possession.

scribe him as an ascetic, not interested in titles and positions. "He didn't claim to be a thinker of international standing. 'Leading Soviet psychiatrist': apparently he considered this title for him as being sufficient."[226]

All agree, however, that Morozov was a typical example of a faithful follower of the Party line. Born in 1920, he completed his medical studies at the Moscow Medical Institute in 1942. He then joined the army, served at the front and resumed his studies after the war and finished his dissertation in 1950. A year before he joined the CPSU.[227] At first, he lectured at the First Moscow Medical Institute and at about the same time he married Galina Anatolyevna Strukova, who was ten years younger and daughter of Anatoly Strukov, a famous pathological anatomist.[228] According to the membership list of the Academy of Medical Sciences of 1977, the couple lived in the same Moscow apartment of her father, on Kutuzovsky prospect 43, an apartment block for the top party echelons.[229]

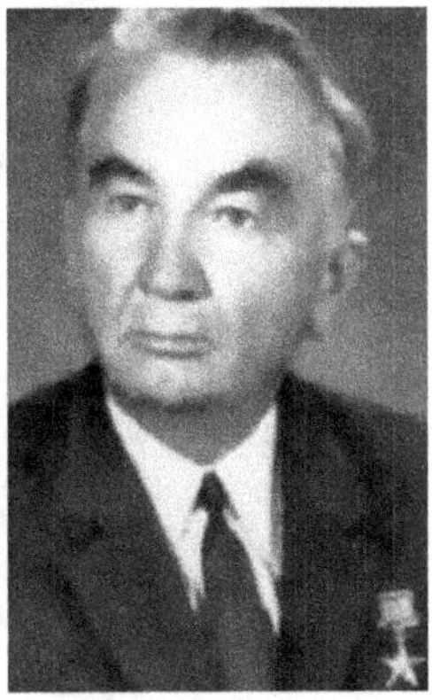

Anatoly Strukov

[226] Gindilis, p. 212

[227] *Korsakov Journal of Neuropathology and Psychiatry*, 1990, volume 90, issue 6, p. 156

[228] Galina Anatolievna Strukova, born in 1930. The couple has a son, Sergei Georgievich Morozov, born in 1967.
The father, Anatoly Ivanovich Strukov, born April 6, 1901in Spasskoje (Tula region), Soviet pathologist, member of the Academy of Medical Sciences (1966), Hero of Socialist Labour (1971). Member of the Communist Party of the Soviet Union since 1943. Graduate of the medical faculty of Voronezh University (1925). In 1938-1945 Chair of Anatomical Pathology in Kharkov Medical Institute (situated in Orenburg in 1941-1944). In 1945-1948 Chair of the Pathology of the Lungs in Moscow Institute of Anatomy and Pathology. In 1953-1972 Chair of Anatomical Pathology in Moscow 1st Medical University. Since 1961 also had of the laboratory of the Human Morphology Institute. Strukov wrote significant publications on tuberculosis, lung pathology, atherosclerosis, hypertensive heart disease, myocardial infarction, collagen diseases. Received the Lenin prize in 1974 for his research on pathomorphology of rheumatic diseases. Editor in chief of the medical literature publishing house (1948-1959) and the journal *Pathology Archives* (since 1968). Founder of the pathologists' school. Member of the German Academy of Natural Sciences (Leopoldina) since 1966. Awarded the Order of Lenin, three other orders as well as various medals. He died on March 13, 1988.

[229] Membership list of the Academy of Medical Sciences, look at http://www.dtic.mil/cgi-bin/GetTRDoc?AD=ADA376076&Location=U2&doc=GetTRDoc.pdf , p. 11 and 14.

Strukov had been head of the Medical Department of the Central Committee of the CPSU since 1949 and was one of the doctors who carried out the autopsy on the body of Soviet leader Iosif Stalin after his death in March 1953, the ultimate sign that he was fully trusted. For this, he was given the position as head of the Faculty for Pathological Anatomy of the First Medical Institute, a position he held until 1972. In 1966, he became a member of the Academy of Medical Sciences. It is clear that Anatoly Strukov was a very influential man within the highest possible Party circles. Confidential sources known to the author indicate that an aunt of Morozov was working at the Central Committee of the CPSU and through her position she helped Morozov further his career. According to Yuri Novikov, who appears to have been a protégé of Morozov until his defection to the West, Morozov was very close to KGB Chairman Yuri Andropov and had unlimited access to him. Also Konstantin Rusakov, Secretary of the Central Committee of the CPSU, was one of his friends, according to Novikov.[230] Other sources claim that he was also close to Candidate Politburo Member Boris Ponomaryov but it is unclear in what way they were related.

In 1957, Georgi Morozov was appointed Director of the Serbski Institute of General and Forensic Psychiatry in Moscow, a position he held until his official retirement in 1990. In that year he also retired as Professor of Psychiatry. Morozov became Corresponding Member of the Academy of Medical Sciences in 1973 and full member in 1988. During the same period, he held leadership positions of the All-Union Society: he became Vice-President in 1973, and in 1983 President, a position he gave up in October 1988, probably under pressure and as part of the Soviet efforts to mellow Western psychiatrists and to make a return to the WPA possible. However, he was quickly elected Honorary Chairman of the AUSNP, thereby retaining influence over the organization. Also, the Serbski Institute remained strongly in his orbit, being its "Honorary Director" and visiting the Institution daily for many years. Only several years ago, his successor, the late Tatyana Dmitrieva, took over his office; until then she had a much smaller office on the ground floor of the Institute, while Morozov's office was only used for meetings.

Apart from his psychiatric career, Morozov also had a political one. He was an active party member, and according to some, a General of the KGB (although concrete evidence was never provided). In 1988, he was elected to the executive of the Moscow City Committee, a position that he probably lost in August 1991 when the Soviet Union dissolved after the failed coup against

230 Interview with Yuri Novikov in *Stern* magazine, April 1978, reprinted in Oltmanns, R., *Spurensuche auf Verbrannter Erde*, Norderstedt, 2009, p. 318.

Party leader Mikhail Gorbachev.[231] How high Morozov ranked in the political elite in the Soviet Union can be seen from the car he rode: at his disposal was a chauffeured "*Chaika,*" the same car used by the top leadership of the country. Chazov also had a *Chaika* at his disposal, but Vartanyan not.[232]

Morozov is generally seen as one of the main architects of Soviet systematic political abuse of psychiatry. Clearly, under his directorship, the Serbski became the central institution where dissidents of any importance - be it international fame or seriousness of the "crime" – were diagnosed and sent off to be "treated' in one of the psychiatric hospitals of the vast Soviet Union. Morozov personally participated in these commissions as well, and repeatedly found dissidents to be "mentally ill." To his name well-known cases can be ascribed such as Vladimir Bukovsky, Viktor Fainberg, Natalya Gorbanevskaya, Pyotr Grigorenko, Leonid Plyushch, etc. etc.

How much he prioritized the political issues over the psychiatric ones is nicely worded in a report from Prof. Karl Seidel, Director of the Charité Psychiatric Hospital in Berlin and IM of the Stasi, to the MfS on his meeting with Georgi Morozov on January 13, 1977 in Berlin.[233] In this report, he informed the Stasi that during their meeting they discussed the World Congress of the WPA in Honolulu and that Morozov had expressed the view that "participation in the Congress and the choice of participants should be made on basis of political rather than professional points of view."[234]

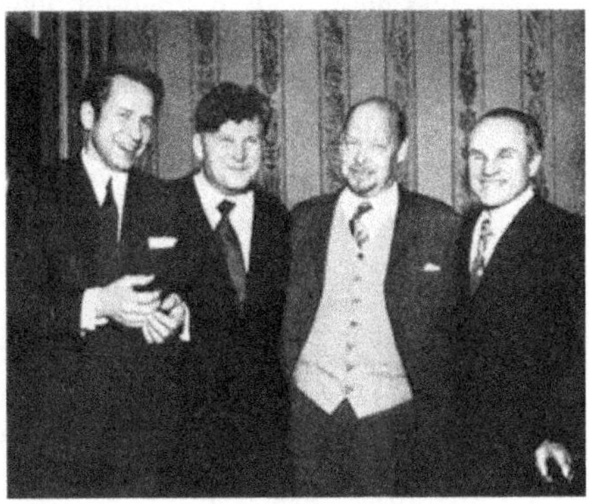

l.t.r. Kalle Achté, Georgi Morozov, Toivo Pikhanen, Nikolai Zharikov, 1973

[231] In May 1990 Peter Reddaway in a private travel report notes already that Morozov's position at the health department of the Moscow City Party Committee has been weakened, probably because Party officials do not want to be Associated openly with a man whose reputation is so much damaged as Morozov's. See Reddaway's travel report, May 21, 1990.

[232] Travel Report by Peter Reddaway, December 1988, published in *Documents* 15, January 1989.

[233] See Süss, p. 584.

[234] *Politisch Missbraucht*, p. 596.

Chapter 20 – Secret Negotiations?

You eat an elephant piece by piece
African saying

Indeed, from all information available, it is clear that Costas Stefanis saw it as his main task to turn the WPA again into a truly global organization. As he, himself, put it during a meeting of the Executive Committee in Rome in October 1984: "the association must be willing to deal with these problems if it were to stay alive and keep the **W** before the **PA**."[235] Also in his first address as President of the WPA, Costas Stefanis made his position every clear: "It was out of my deep concern for the Association's future and out of my desire to contribute toward a disentanglement from its internal disputes, that I accepted the challenge [of becoming President]. ... A number of societies encompassing thousands of psychiatrists, are no longer part of our association, others are apprehensive about its future and fortunately only few member societies fail to demonstrate concern. One may well ask how this situation came about. The opinion we are most frequently provided with asserts that it resulted from the intrusion of Cold War political antagonism into the Association's affairs and this might very well be true. ...It is both surprising and regrettable that such attempts ... succeeded in bringing about a rift in an organization of health professionals, a group least expected to succumb to outside pressures."[236]

For Stefanis it was clear that his primary task was to heal the rift in the organization and reunite the societies that left the association in 1983. For him, this was a goal that made all other issues of secondary importance. "In order to accomplish its goals, however, it has to be a truly global organization, representing psychiatrists from all countries, from all cultures and from all schools of thought. It has to develop within the framework of its founding principles and to become a meeting place where scientific knowledge is shared. ... Common sense only is required to apprehend that unless we all join forces in an effort to disentangle the association from the grip of political prejudice and restore its image as a truly scientific and professional organization, all our attempts are doomed to failure."[237] In fact, with this claim that the organization had become an arena for political conflict and Cold War politics, he inadvertently expressed a view very similar to that of the Soviet All-Union Society and their supporters. This very much angered the opponents of political abuse of psychiatry in the

[235] Minutes of the WPA EC, October 1984, p. 9
[236] *WPA Newsletter* 21, May 1984, p. 3
[237] *WPA Newsletter* 21, May 1984, p. 4

USSR, and was one of the factors that led to their suspicion of "clandestine negotiations" with the Soviets being carried out by Stefanis.

Stefanis further made clear that in his view it would take time, and patience was needed: "we should go steady and slow. The wounds need to be healed and must not be hastily covered up."[238] Yet at the same time, it was clear to him that the WPA should follow its own course, and not be influenced from outside: "We will firmly resist and we will not yield to the demands of any pressure group, regardless of its origin and intensions."[239] Yet he reiterated that he would try to bring the Soviets back into the WPA fold: "We will try to open new channels of communication and we will explore all legitimate ways of reopening the closed ones, an endeavor which is not easy and should not remain one-sided. ... I personally feel a moral obligation, neither to overlook obvious deficiencies in our organizational structure, nor to ignore minority voices which, as past experience has shown, monitor prevailing thinking more accurately than the majority vote..."[240]

Antonis Vgontzas, a long-time friend of Costas Stefanis, confirms that Stefanis' prime objective was to get the Soviets back: "Indeed ... he saw that as his primary task. He was totally against the abuse, against any abuse of psychiatry, but it was his conviction that the only way to change them was by bringing them in, to have them under some sort of control. He did this out of his own conviction; it was not an order of Papandreou, or of PASOK, or of any party. You have to understand that Greeks were anti-communist, but at the same time we had good relations with them. There were good relations with Tito, with Zhivkov in Bulgaria, with the Romanians. All disputes could be solved with them, no problem. And also with the Soviet Union we maintained good relations. We tried to be a bridge between East and West. Also the old Karamanlis of *Nea Demokratia* maintained excellent relations with the communist neighbors.[241] So you must also see his relations with the Soviets in that light. He had friendly relations with them, also with the Minister of Health as far as I remember, but that was quite normal and fit into his political thinking, which in turn was very much in line with general Greek political thought."[242]

---

238 *WPA Newsletter* 21, May 1984, p. 4

239 *WPA Newsletter* 21, May 1984, p. 4

240 *WPA Newsletter*, 21. May 1984, p. 4

241 See, for instance, *The Greek Socialist Experiment*, p. 131. Karamanlis was the first Greek prime minister who went on a state visit to Moscow and expanded Greek-Soviet trade relations. He also allowed Soviet vessels to be repaired at the Syros drydock.

242 Interview with Antonis Vgontzas, September 3, 2009

Indeed, PASOK's world view was based on the idea that the bipolar system of the Cold War was a matter of the past and that Greece should play the role of bridge between Western Europe and the Balkans, the Arab world, Africa and the Communist East. As Papandreou himself stated: "We are wrestling with the hawks in every part of the world. ... We are for peace, and only support Greece's interests." He added that Athens would become the 'crossroads' and 'meeting place' of world leaders. "Our policy has become the starting point of rapprochement among the nations."[243] PASOK's multi-dimensional policy of "national independence" was the result of the wish to free the country from Cold War commitments and to decrease the influence of both superpowers. However, in practice it mainly resulted in systematic criticism of the United States, which he called "the Mecca of imperialism," and avoiding criticism of the Soviet Union. He refused to condemn the imposition of martial law in Poland in 1981and later suggested himself as a mediator between the EU and the Jaruzelsky military regime.[244] Even when the Soviets shot down the Korean flight KAL 007 on August 31, 1983, killing all 269 passengers and crew on board, Papandreou avoided direct criticism and asserted that it had been on a spy mission and that "if such a plane came into Greece, we would have downed it."[245] A few months later, in February 1984, Papandreou participated in the funeral of Soviet leader Yuri Andropov, whom he called a "most capable" and "reasonable" man who had been "truly for peace."[246] In practice, however, Greece remained an integral part of NATO and the European Union and the Soviets' consideration of PASOK as the favorite socialist party that supported their policies and actively participated in their anti-nuclear campaigns changed into one of disillusionment. In the end, they just saw him as a "bourgeois nationalist" whose main goal was to have the Americans pay as much as possible for their military bases in the country.[247]

The Stasi reports of Jochen Neumann confirm Stefanis' favorable predisposition towards the Soviets. "Phenotypic is the fact that Professor Stefanis shows in general a neutral attitude which, however, is clearly

---

243 *The Greek Socialist Experiment*, p. 128

244 *The Greek Socialist Experiment*, p. 148

245 *The Greek Socialist Experiment*, p. 148. At that time Greece held the Presidency of the European Union and managed to prevent a strong condemnation of the Soviet Union. Instead, the statement didn't name any country specifically and only expressed the Community's "deep emotion", calling for a "thorough investigation."

246 *The Greek Socialist Experiment*, p. 151. Indeed, all sides agree that Yuri Andropov was a very intelligent man and one of the most cosmopolitan oriented members of the Politburo.

247 *The Greek Socialist Experiment*, p. 151

inclined towards the socialist concerns. This is supported by his friendly relations with our Soviet colleagues, his attitude in Helsinki and Rome and his reliability until now in keeping his agreements made before (for instance with Vartanyan). The collaboration with the DDR delegate was constructive from the very start and involved partially confidential discussions about the tactics to be used. He introduced the DDR delegate [that is, Neumann himself] to a few of his Greek friends, whose names I have forgotten, but who immediately asked me whether I as DDR-delegate also had known people like Prof. Kokkalis, Prof. Fotopulos and Dr. Kritzikis.[248] In all the three cases, although in the case of Dr. Kritzikis with the known limitations, they were communist emigrants, and because of the good familiarity of these Greek colleagues with these names, one can conclude that the circle around Stefanis consists of leftist oriented people."[249] Later he reports that Melvin Sabshin complained to a Polish psychiatrist about Stefanis, calling him a "sympathizer of the Soviets."[250]

Tension

From the very start, a competition developed between the WPA President and the General Secretary. The basis of the tension was not the Soviet issue, but a different view on their positions. Schulsinger intended to follow the line of Peter Berner, who as General Secretary had been the

---

248 Professor Kokkalis, Professor of Medicine at the University of Athens, was Minister of Health in the Cabinet of the Political Committee of National Liberation (PEEA) and a covert member of the Communist EAM movement. See Clogg, Richard: *A Concise History of Greece*, p. 132. According to Costas Stefanis, "following the defeat of the "Democratic Army" he emigrated to East Berlin. According to newspapers, he was appointed Director of Surgery at Charité Hospital.
Fotopoulos was in the past a Lecturer of Psychiatry at Athens University. He also worked in East Berlin, but came back to this country and worked in private practice before the fall of the Berlin Wall. He died after a few years. He was deeply disappointed about his experiences in East Germany.
Dr. Kritsikis also held an academic position in East Berlin in the field of Epidemiological Cardiology. He emigrated - before the fall of the Wall - to Paris and continued his career in Public Health and Cardiology - collaborating with WHO. (...) He came back to Greece and ... joined the University Cardiology Department." Dr. Kritsikis died in 2008. Letter from Costas Stefanis to the author, October 23, 2009.

249 *Ergänzungen zum Bericht*, Jochen Neumann, October 1984, p. 14. In a travel report of 11-18 October 1985 regarding a meeting of the Executive Committee in Athens Neumann reports that he met Kritzikis personally during this visit.

250 *Reisebericht Athen 11. bis 18. Oktober 1985*, p. 20

leading person within the Executive Committee, while President Pierre Pichot was more the ceremonial figurehead. Stefanis did not agree with this state of affairs at all. "Schulsinger followed the German example, where the Chancellor is the main person in charge and the President is a ceremonial leader, while Stefanis believed in the American model, where all the executive powers are vested with the President," Jochen Neumann later reflects. "Between the two men there was constant tension, because in no way did Stefanis want to yield any of his power. When I came into the Executive Committee for the first time in Rome, in October 1984, they had been shouting on each other. Fini had been angrily shouting at Stefanis that his leadership style was hopeless and that it was unbearable. Stefanis had been shouting back that Fini was merely the administrator of the organization, that he was the leader and that all content was his job, and that he would decide how to run the meetings. It was really emotions running high. [251] Between Schulsinger and Stefanis exists an insolubly deep conflict. From both sides, arguments are used that have some value and in a large degree correspond to reality. Schulsinger attacks Stefanis because of his lack of leadership qualities, but, in fact, criticizes his political position. Stefanis attacks Schulsinger, and says that it is his political positioning that causes the animosity, but does not see his own weakness as a leader."[252]

A letter by Costas Stefanis to Fini Schulsinger, written several months after the Rome meeting, clearly shows how high the emotions had run. In his letter, Stefanis offers two alternative descriptions of the proceedings to be included in the minutes. The first version was the most elaborate one, stating that "… the Secretary General … expressed his dissatisfaction with the rate of progress made by the EC with regard to the Agenda under the President's chairmanship and had stated his intention to bring for approval to the EC a proposal that would enable other EC members to alternate the chairmanship of the sessions… The President stated that he considers this move a violation of the constitutional principles and totally unjustified in view of the progress already made in vital areas for the future of WPA. All have agreed, including the Secretary General who expressed his regrets that his well-meant intentions to speed-up procedures met with such unforeseen reaction by the President whom he respects and in no way questions his policy making decisions."[253] The second version would be: "The Secretary General responded by expressing the view that by the proposed changes

---

[251] Interview Jochen Neumann, July 29, 2009

[252] *Ergänzungen zum Bericht*, Jochen Neumann, October 1984, p. 15. Stefanis referred here probably to Schulsinger's anti-American attitude.

[253] Letter from Costas Stefanis to Fini Schulsinger, January 21, 1985, p. 1

the EC would work more effectively and would cover in a shorter time a wider range of items. In the discussion that followed the President opposed this proposal by stating that is incompatible with the operational rules of the WPA and far from justified by past and current experience. Various comments were expressed by other EC members. All comments reflected a deep concern over the consequences that might arise if issues of this sort are not immediately dealt with and resolved."[254]

The letter ends with a recommendation by Stefanis: "The second version is less clear but may serve better WPA's policy, which definitely cannot be advanced with rifts within the EC. There is a third and preferable version, i.e. not to mention anything."[255] Yet Stefanis adds: "but it is too late for that." In the minutes, an abridged form of the first version was included, however only after Fini Schulsinger had consulted Jochen Neumann and some further modifications had been made. In a letter on March 6, 1985, Neumann writes to Schulsinger: "Recently I received the minutes of the meetings in Rome, and the papers concerning the 'cases.' In both papers is stated what's possible now and I agree. There are no comments."[256]

Neumann actually very much shared Schulsinger's views on Stefanis' leadership. In October 1984, right after his election to the Executive Committee, he writes: "The problem in the future will be the fact that Stefanis has certain incapacities as leader and is not capable of leading the EC firmly. He does not contain the discussions. He leads the talks with a certain Mediterranean generosity, spiced with emotional outbreaks. That already led to the situation in which the General Secretary proposed in every possible way to take away the chairmanship of the EC meetings. The emotions ran high."[257] But being of a different character and coming from the East (and thus less vocal in his indignation) Neumann took this in a different manner, as can be seen from his mediation in the case of the Rome minutes. He observed, and tried to steer the discussion in the direction he wanted whenever he saw the opportunity. He was supported in this by Melvin Sabshin, who also had his concerns about Stefanis' leadership style: "Sabshin's reservations about Stefanis were that he wished to have a President who gave directions in content, and not so much one that played the role of a dictator."[258] Retrospectively, both Melvin Sabshin and Jochen Neumann agree that in fact the real

254 Letter from Costas Stefanis to Fini Schulsinger, January 21, 1985, p. 1-2

255 Letter from Costas Stefanis to Fini Schulsinger, January 21, 1985, p. 2

256 Letter from Jochen Neumann to Fini Schulsinger, March 6, 1985.

257 *Ergänzungen zum Bericht*, Jochen Neumann, October 1984, p. 14

258 *Ergänzungen zum Bericht*, Jochen Neumann, October 1984, p. 17

driving force within the Executive Committee was not Stefanis but Fini Schulsinger and the two of them.[259]

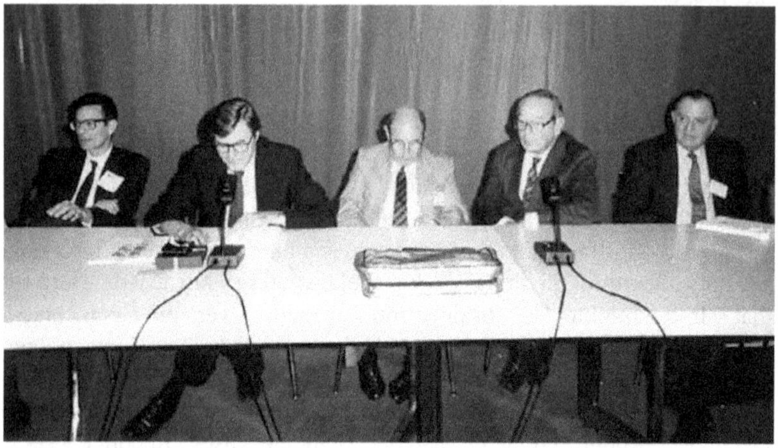

Washington 1988, l.t.r. Norman Sartorius, Costas Stefanis, Jochen Neumann, Fini Schulsinger, Melvin Sabshin

At the same time, Neumann developed a good working relationship with Costas Stefanis. In October 1985, a year after he was elected as Vice President of the WPA, Neumann reports to the DDR political leadership that "the collaboration between the President and the Vice-President can be considered to be excellent already from Rome, October 1984, onwards. Almost everything is discussed in advance and then together implemented. It was even possible to have the Executive Committee send a telegram of congratulations to the International Physicians for the Prevention of Nuclear War (IPPNW) on the occasion of them having been awarded the Nobel Peace Prize."[260] He reported another example of their good collaboration in April 1985 stating that he and Stefanis were able to weaken some formulations in the reports by the Review Committee on alleged cases of political abuse of psychiatry in the Soviet Union: "Of course the formulations are at moments not according to our taste, but still in none of the cases was it established that according to the Review Committee and the Executive Committee, a clear-cut case of [political] abuse [of psychiatry] took place. ... Neumann and Stefanis have positively influenced the proposed wording; otherwise, they would have been still a bit more negative."[261]

259 Interview with Ellen Mercer, Jochen Neumann and Melvin Sabshin, December 1-2, 2009

260 *Reisebericht Athen 11. bis 18. Oktober 1985*, p. 5

261 *Bericht* on the meeting of the WPA EC in Rio de Janeiro, 17-25 April 1985, p. 9

As far as Fini Schulsinger is concerned, Neumann initially viewed him with great suspicion, but after a year he concluded with satisfaction that since his own election as Vice-President, Schulsinger had become more neutral in his positioning. "Although it is assumed that Professor Schulsinger maintains, as before, close relations with Amnesty International, he said during his opening speech at the Congress in Athens [in October 1985] in his capacity of General Secretary that it is now more clear than ever '...that the World Psychiatric Association is no battlefield for Cold War.' On top of that he declared that all efforts should be concentrated on disarmament, the preservation of peace and the avoidance of a nuclear inferno. Prof. Schulsinger has found for himself a compromise position that makes it possible for him to come along in the Executive Committee without losing face: 'the World Psychiatric Association is no human rights organization. Activities in favor of allies that are forced upon us without justification would do more damage than help'."[262]

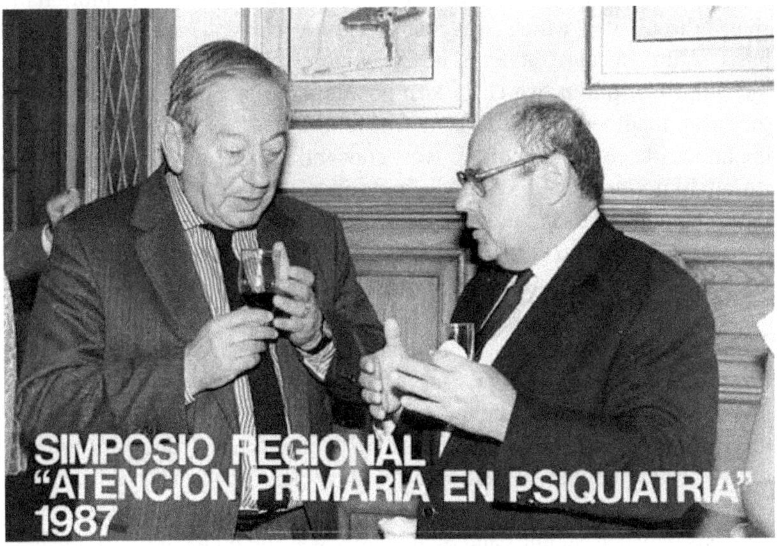

l.t.r. Fini Schulsinger and Jochen Neumann, 1987

For a while, things quieted down between the two chief executives, and a *modus vivendi* had been found by which the sessions would be shorter. However, when looking at the overview of the sessions of the Executive Committee throughout the period, one sees that the total number of hours spent in session actually did not change much over the years. The simple

262 *Reisebericht Athen 11. bis 18. Oktober 1985*, p. 11

calculation shows that the length of the sessions shortened, but that instead of two or three long sessions the Executive Committee met six – or sometimes even more – times, and that the total number of meeting hours was not much less. The tension between Schulsinger and Stefanis slowly subsided. In November 1984, Schulsinger writes to Melvin Sabshin: "Costas and I did a lot of useful work together, but his emotions from the Rome meeting flared up without any new reasons. It is nothing that will prevent the smooth running of the WPA, but it is a nuisance."[263] A year later, he wrote to Sabshin that "I talk to Costas on the phone once or twice a week, and I feel that all clouds disappeared some time ago."[264]

And then, towards the middle of the term of office of the Executive Committee, things worsened again. A new explosion within the Executive Committee came in November 1987, during which an angry Stefanis apparently threatened to resign. "He decompensated under pressure of the constant frustrations and attacks against him and started an emotionally sharp discussion, which was completely useless. That led to attacks by Sabshin. Because Stefanis in this concrete case was not right, it was difficult to help him, which in turn positioned him again in opposition to the other members of the Executive Committee. It is a fact, though, that the attacks from the side of the West concentrated on him and they tried to isolate him within the Executive Committee. He is certainly our best ally in fundamental issues, but his style of leadership is sometimes insufficient to such an extent that it becomes increasingly more difficult to support him without him losing face."[265]

Things quieted down again, but that did not change Stefanis' style of leadership. In a report to the Stasi of March-April 1989 Neumann wrote: "If Stefanis leads the General Assembly just as badly as the sessions of the Executive Committee and if the All-Union Society does not become more disciplined and prepare itself with a clear concept, it will become a disaster."[266] According to Neumann, one of the factors that led to new tensions between Stefanis and Schulsinger was the preparation for the next elections. In his report on the Executive Committee meeting in April 1988, Neumann wrote: "the atmosphere in Copenhagen was again a bit tense. The next World Congress and the next General Assembly cast their shadow, and a period is now starting in which everybody brings his own flock to dry land. … Stefanis would like to be re-elected as President and notices

263 Letter from Schulsinger to Sabshin, November 29, 1984.

264 Letter from Schulsinger to Sabshin, August 7, 1985

265 *Reisebericht,* Warsaw WPA EC Meeting, November 1987, pp. 6-7

266 Report Jochen Neumann on the WPA Executive Committee, April 1989, p. 4

that there is no chance for this and becomes embittered and unbusinesslike. Schulsinger is, at the moment, object of attacks in the press."[267] According to Neumann, Schulsinger wanted to be a candidate for the position of President, but Stefanis did not want to make clear whether he would go for a second term or not. In the mean time, the Brazilian Jorge Alberto Costa e Silva was also preparing himself for the position of President, and by the time the Executive Committee met in Granada in March 1989, his campaign was in full swing. Thus the competition between the men became a dominant factor during the meetings, which didn't really improve the productivity.[268]

With regard to the Soviet issue, the positions of Stefanis and Schulsinger initially differed. Not so much as far as the Soviets was concerned, because both were of the opinion that a return of the All-Union Society was necessary to preserve the unity of the organization. For Stefanis, this was just a matter of strategy, a way of reaching his goal of turning the WPA into a truly global psychiatric association; but for Schulsinger there was an underlying ideological issue. Schulsinger was strongly anti-American, and for him, Melvin Sabshin was the proponent of American dominance, or maybe even arrogance. He automatically took a position contrary to that of the American Psychiatric Association (APA) and, as the APA was against a return of the All-Union Society, he was in favor. Also, a return of the Soviets and the other societies that had left would reduce the American influence, and that was in line with Schulsinger's wishes. Basically from the very start, he made clear that in his mind the issue of abuse should be kept off the table in order to let the healing process do its work: "It is likely that the WPA which, inevitably, represents a target for various idealistic and/or political pressure groups, will for some time come to abstain from a pertinent involvement. However, our association remains committed to the promotion of psychiatric ethics and to combating the abuse of our discipline."[269]

Koryagin's Honorary Membership

A clear illustration of the rising tension between the two men and their different views can be seen in a discussion in February 1984 in New York, during the hand-over session of the Executive Committee. The issue on the table is the Honorary Membership bestowed by the General Assembly on

267 *Reisebericht* of Jochen Neumann, WPA EC Meeting Copenhagen, August 1988, pp. 3-4

268 Interview Jochen Neumann and Mel Sabshin, July 30, 2009

269 *WPA Newsletter* 21, p. 5

Anatoly Koryagin, the Soviet dissident psychiatrist serving twelve years in camp and prison in the Soviet Union for his opposition against the political abuse of psychiatry. The issue is a hot potato, which neither the outgoing President and General Secretary nor the incoming ones want to have on their plates.

Although the August 1983 issue of the WPA Newsletter announced that Koryagin "in accordance with a motion supported by several national member societies" had been conferred "Honorary Membership" (sic!) of the WPA,[270] later in the same report Koryagin was not listed as those upon whom Honorary Membership had been conferred (no quotation marks).[271] Clearly, Koryagin belonged to a separate category, which in such a way was sophisticatedly made clear.

Eventually, those present at the meeting in New York decided that outgoing President Pichot and outgoing General Secretary Berner should sign the Diploma of Honorary Membership, as his election took place while they were still in office. But they also decided that the "Vienna Secretariat prepare a letter – for signature by Profs. Stefanis and Schulsinger respectively – addressed to Mrs. Koryagin, giving notification of the conferment and enquiring into Dr. Koryagin's wishes concerning the Diploma's delivery into his hands."[272]

Even looking back twenty years later, or maybe especially so, this seems to be a strange situation. Not the decision that one team signed the Diploma and the other the letter, but the fact that seven months after the General Assembly, the Koryagins still had not been notified of the decision of the General Assembly, and that such a long discussion was needed as to how to handle the issue. The discussion was further intensified by the fact that the APA had decided to organize a press conference the day after the meeting of the Executive Committee to highlight the plight of Anatoly Koryagin, and that "the possibility of a WPA press-release to this conference, expressing the Association's concern at Dr. Koryagin's plight and solidarity with him as an honorary member of the Association, had been debated, and stood supported by Dr. Sabshin, Prof. Schulsinger and Prof. Reisby."[273]

Stefanis must have exploded. The minutes only record that "Prof. Stefanis thereupon strongly vetoed this proposal," but this formulation leaves no doubt that Costas Stefanis became extremely angry. He pointed out that he

270 *WPA Newsletter* 19, p. 3
271 *WPA Newsletter* 19, p. 8
272 Minutes of the WPA EC, February 1984, p. 13
273 Minutes of the WPA EC, February 1984, p. 14

saw it as his obligation to preserve the unity of the organization and recalled "that he had clearly declared his intention to support any action liable to promote the re-instatement of the, at present, endangered unity, and that he would do his utmost to prevent an escalation of dissent among the societies still holding WPA membership. He affirmed that solidarity with Dr. Koryagin had already been demonstrated by conferment of Honorary Membership and he considered the issue of a press release in special reference to Dr. Koryagin unnecessary and likely to aggravate an already difficult situation and thus a measure he did not wish to be associated with."[274] In a report written by Ellen Mercer, Director of International Affairs of the APA and present at the meeting, it is added that "Dr. Stefanis indicated that even though Dr. Koryagin's election to Honorary Membership didn't comply with the requirements of the WPA Statutes, that he is now a member and the election is past. He indicated that there were motivations other than scientific accomplishment and was yet another indication that the WPA had become a platform for political actions."[275]

A discussion took place, the minutes dryly report, followed by the probably somewhat cynical remark: "Prof. Schulsinger wished to know whether the Association intended to ignore Dr. Koryagin's situation," indicating that his irritation over what he considered Stefanis's dictatorial leadership style had reached a new peak. This cynical undertone is even clearer when reading Ellen Mercer's report, which says: "Dr. Schulsinger asked Dr. Stefanis if he wanted to pretend that Dr. Koryagin is not an Honorary Member and indicated that this could be interpreted from his comments. Dr. Stefanis stated that he could not pretend that Dr. Koryagin is not a member of the WPA, but that he did not want to focus on this."[276] Schulsinger added that not doing anything could be politically misinterpreted: "inaction and passivity all have consequences and that non-action is as political as action,"[277] to which Stefanis retorted that a press-release could also be misinterpreted and that many members of the WPA would be very upset by it. Schulsinger then added subtly that "although a general agreement seemed to exist on aims, it obviously did not extend to strategical means."[278] Ellen Mercer's report adds that Schulsinger "expressed his appreciation that Dr. Stefanis is able to express his views in a clear and strong way,"[279] again a subtle reference to the highly emotional interaction between him and Stefanis.

---

274 Minutes of the WPA EC, February 1984, p. 14
275 Memorandum by Ellen Mercer, February 5, 1984, p. 5
276 Memorandum by Ellen Mercer, February 5, 1984, p. 6
277 Memorandum by Ellen Mercer, February 5, 1984, p. 6
278 Minutes of the WPA EC, February 1984, p. 14
279 Memorandum by Ellen Mercer, February 5, 1984, p. 6

The discussion continued, now involving also the members of the outgoing Executive Committee, mostly agreeing with the fact that a press release could have political repercussions that should be avoided. Schulsinger then suggested mentioning Koryagin's Honorary Membership in the next *WPA Newsletter* with an addition including "an expression of regret and concern at Dr. Koryagin's situation." The discussion was closed with Stefanis' wish to be assured that all would answer questions from the press identically and, thus, the Executive Committee agreed "to abstain from any official public comment, apart from the reference that the next WPA Newsletter would contain a statement concerning Dr. Koryagin."[280]

Indeed, the *WPA Newsletter* contained a statement about Koryagin, but not in the May 1984 issue (21), nor in the September 1984 issue (22). Only in December 1984, eighteen months after Koryagin's election, did the *WPA Newsletter* contain the information that "as generally known, the Soviet psychiatrist Dr. Anatolij Koryagin was given honorary membership of the WPA at the General Assembly in Vienna, July 1983. When the present Executive Committee began the take-over procedures of the Vienna Secretariat on February 15, 1984, this honorary membership had not yet been announced to Dr. Koryagin (incarcerated in a prison camp) nor to his family. In March 1984, the new President and Secretary General wrote a letter to the wife of Dr. Koryagin… "Recently the WPA Secretariat learned that this letter was never received by Mrs. Koryagin, and a copy of it has now been sent to her via registered mail."[281]

While this last remark seems to be rather unimportant now, in those days, it either showed a complete lack of understanding of the situation or a deliberate carelessness. The Soviet Union was a closed society, a totalitarian state that controlled all internal and external communication. Anatoly Koryagin was serving twelve years of imprisonment and was considered a very dangerous enemy of the state and his wife was constantly watched by the KGB. No letter via ordinary mail would reach her, and certainly not from the WPA who had made the "political decision" to bestow a prize on this "enemy of the people." Yet the first letter was sent, after many months, by ordinary mail and it took the WPA a year and a half to send a letter via registered mail with at least a small chance of reaching its destination. And at no time, at least not according to the records, was consideration given to sending the Diploma and accompanying letter to

280 Minutes of the WPA EC, February 1984, p. 15. According to Jochen Neumann this tactical way out of the dispute was suggested by Melvin Sabshin. *Ergänzungen zum Bericht*, Jochen Neumann, October 1984, p. 16

281 *WPA Newsletter* 23, December 1984, p. 6

one of the Western embassies in Moscow with the request to make sure that they reached Galina Koryagina, Koryagin's wife. One can also note that no "expression of regret and concern at Dr. Koryagin's situation" was added to the statement in the *WPA Newsletter*.

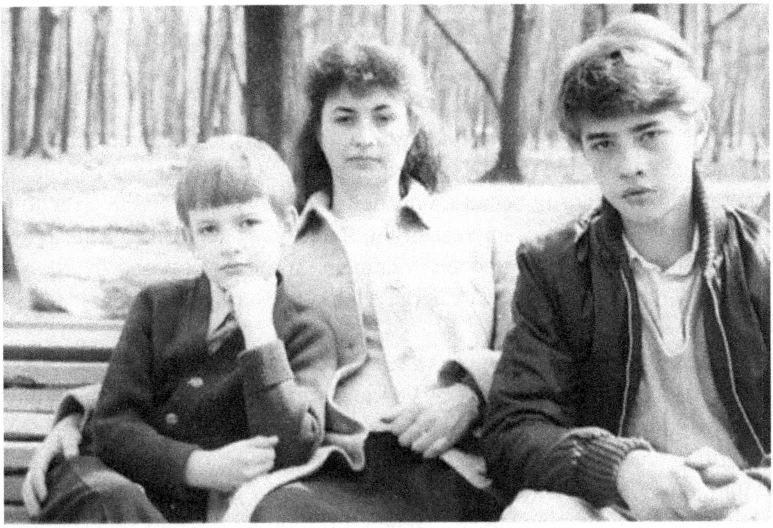

Galina Koryagina with two of her sons

More than a year later, in January 1986, the Koryagin issue reappears on the agenda of the WPA Executive Committee after the British Royal College urged the Executive Committee to take action in order to improve Koryagin's situation. The minutes record a negative response: "After an informed discussion on this issue, which is of immense importance to the future of the WPA, the EC agreed that any official action taken would lead to further difficulties for Dr. Koryagin, and that his prospects would be best served through diplomatic channels, in which the EC members would participate whenever possible."[282]

For those opposing the political abuse of psychiatry in the Soviet Union and campaigning against a possible return of the All-Union Society, the situation around Anatoly Koryagin's Honorary Membership was a clear sign of the disinterest of the WPA leadership and its predisposition to please the Soviets and lure them back into their fold.

282 Minutes of the WPA EC, Jaipur, January 1986, p. 16.Later in the same minutes it says: "The EC had agreed to act always in the interest of the WPA, and that in the present state of affairs, quiet diplomacy rather than open action would serve all parties best." See page 19 of the same minutes.

The issue would come back as a boomerang to the WPA leadership in early 1987, when Koryagin was released from prison after a long international campaign and allowed to immigrate to Switzerland. His interaction with Costas Stefanis would result in more emotions and misunderstandings, but I will come back to that later.

"Clandestine negotiations"

It is clear that from the very beginning of their tenure, contacts were maintained with the Soviets; Stefanis and Schulsinger were able to operate quite solitarily because only few other members on the Executive Committee showed any interest in the matter. In fact, in their endeavors, they were supported by Jochen Neumann, and only opposed by Melvin Sabshin and, rather weakly, by Jorge Alberto Costa e Silva.[283]

The first signs that the Soviets were actively preparing the grounds for a return to the WPA came in late 1984 and early 1985. Through the Soviet Embassy in Washington, the American Psychiatric Association (APA) was informed that the All-Union Society would be willing to resume relations with the APA if the latter would apologize for its "groundless criticisms of psychiatric abuse in the USSR." When this didn't work they reduced their demand to merely an apology.[284]

In the meantime, communications between the Soviets and part of the WPA leadership continued. In my interview with Costas Stefanis on July 15, 2009, he angrily refuted that "clandestine negotiations" took place[285] and, from

283 In his report on the EC meeting in Rome, Neumann writes that Costa e Silva expressed himself favorably to the Soviets in private ("You need to bring back the Russians. We in the Third World cannot do anything on world stage without the Russians and their enormous weight"), yet such expressions can also be a matter of friendliness and do not necessarily express real sentiments. In a travel report of April 1985 on the meeting of the WPA EC in Rio de Janeiro, Neumann is more critical of Costa e Silva, describing his wealth and also that other Brazilians refuse to consider him as their representative. *Bericht*, 17-25 April 1985, p. 5
A similar positioning Neumann ascribes to Jean-Yves Gosselin, Chairman of the Review Committee. *Ergänzungen zum Bericht*, Jochen Neumann, October 1984, p. 11 and 16; and *Ergänzungen zum Reisebericht Rio de Janeiro*, 18-23.4.1985: "Interesting is the fact that Gosselin always stresses his closeness to the Soviet Union and friendship with Vartanyan."

284 *Information Bulletin no. 11*, International Association on the Political Use of Psychiatry (IAPUP), April 1985.

285 See the chapter "Meeting Costas Stefanis."

his personal perspective, this might truly be so. This might also be an issue of semantics, because what is "clandestine" and what are "negotiations"? Indeed, one could say that discussing the prevailing situation during private conversations with Marat Vartanyan cannot be considered to be "negotiations" in the strict sense of the word, yet Stefanis's claim that they didn't discuss the membership issue seems fairly unlikely. Since a friendship between the two men existed, and communication between them continued as before, at least in the legal sense one could not say that these were "clandestine." Stefanis claims that these contacts were quite sporadic but, to Jochen Neumann's knowledge, were quite frequent.

Yet communication existed not only between Costas Stefanis and Marat Vartanyan as friends. Stefanis, Schulsinger, Morozov and Vartanyan met each other frequently, usually in the corridors of a conference or during other events. These meetings were informal, and you could say that they were not "clandestine negotiations," yet it is clear that a possible return of the All-Union Society was a subject of discussion.

"In July 1986, Prof. Stefanis was in Moscow for other business," Neumann writes, "and had unofficial contacts with Prof. Vartanyan, and explained to him the significantly changed situation in the WPA."[286] A bit further in the same report, Neumann writes that Stefanis confirmed to the other members of the Executive Committee that he maintained informal contacts, but that, at the moment, there was nothing to report to the public.[287]

Several months later, in November 1986, Stefanis informed the members of the Executive Committee of personal conversations with All-Union Society President Georgi Morozov and an exchange of letters. "After four personal conversations during a congress in Yugoslavia in September 1987, there was surprisingly full agreement about the necessity of the All-Union Society to return to the WPA. Prof. Morozov stressed that also within the All-Union Society, there was 'no resistance' against a new collaboration. It was clear that the split in the leadership of the All-Union Society had also left its traces and that Prof. Morozov did not know anything about the conversations that the Vice-President and the President had had with, among others, Vartanyan. In the mean time, Morozov had a letter delivered by Prof. Ivanets in a private envelope under the heading of 'Director of the Institute and Clinic,' in which

286 *Reisebericht* of Jochen Neumann on the WPA EC meeting in Copenhagen, August 1986, p. 1

287 *Reisebericht* of Jochen Neumann on the WPA EC meeting in Copenhagen, August 1986, p. 9

Morozov confirmed that 'he and his colleagues ... were in agreement with regard to their view on the current status quo in the WPA'.... In the Executive Committee, Morozov's letter to Stefanis was circulated along with some nice photographs made during the conversations between the two, showing a clearly relaxed atmosphere."[288]

In the same report, Jochen Neumann discussed the position of Melvin Sabshin, his fellow Executive Committee member. Reason is "Sabshin's unusual reluctance and demonstrative hesitation" with regard to the Soviet issue. According to Neumann, the President of the APA complained to him and Neumann about Sabshin's positioning; that the majority of American psychiatrists were in favor of a return of the Soviets, but also made clear that Sabshin is the real power figure within the APA against whom he can't do anything. "Both on Soviet and American sides, personal interests and sensitivities complicate the work enormously."[289] Apparently the decision was reached to expand the contacts with the Soviets and organize a meeting in Milan in 1987.

Thus the communications continued. According to the minutes of the WPA Executive Committee of April 1987, "The President [Costas Stefanis] had been to Moscow twice since the last EC-meeting [in November 1986] and had met with several Soviet psychiatrists. As a consequence of the latest developments, the President had been invited as an honorary guest to attend the 2nd Congress of Psychiatry for Socialist Countries in Varna."[290] The Minutes continue: "The EC agreed with the President that he had done well in showing that the WPA was open to discussions with non-member societies..."[291] In a report by Neumann on his trip to Moscow in February 1987, he expressly mentions the fact that Morozov had referred to "manifold conversations with the President of the WPA, the last time in mid-February [1987] in Moscow."[292] Shortly after, in July 1987, Stefanis sent a telegram to the Soviet Union following the death of Andrei Snezhnevsky, in which he wrote: "Soviet psychiatry has lost its father, and the scientists of the world one of their leading colleagues."[293] In a WPA Newsletter, Stefanis described

288 *Reisebericht* by Jochen Neumann, November 1986, p. 3

289 *Reisebericht* by Jochen Neumann, November 1986, p. 4

290 According to Neumann the costs of this trip were covered by the Bulgarians. See Neumann's *Reisebericht* on the WPA EC Meeting in Amman, April 1987, p. 4

291 Minutes of the WPA EC, April 1987, p. 2

292 *Reisebericht* by Jochen Neumann on his trip to Moscow, February 24-25, 1987, Haxx499, pp. 243-4

293 *Korsakov Journal of Neuropathology and Psychiatry*, 1987, no. 10, p. 1444

the late Snezhnevsky as a "great clinician" and he stated that Snezhnevsky "advocated international cooperation among psychiatrists."[294]

Between April and September 1987, Stefanis was again back in Moscow, and this time he also had a meeting with Evgeni Chazov, the Minister of Health of the USSR and, as we know, a friend of Marat Vartanyan.[295] In his report to the DDR leadership, Jochen Neumann writes: "Prof. Stefanis reported on a personal meeting with Soviet Minister of Health Chazov, whom he has known personally for a long time.[296] Chazov assured Prof. Stefanis of the interest of the Soviet Union in a renewed collaboration [with the WPA] and stressed that the issue should be resolved soon. Prof. Vartanyan joined the conversation and pressed Minister Chazov to be more cautious and less rushed."[297]

In October 1987, Costas Stefanis and Fini Schulsinger met again with Georgi Morozov. This time the meeting took place in Milan (Italy), as planned a year earlier, during an international psychiatric conference that Morozov attended together with Juri Saarma[298] and Nikolai Zharikov, the future President of the All-Union Society. The meeting was "informal," but Morozov left no doubt who took the initiative: "We ourselves did not raise the issue, but officials of the Association brought up the question with us, asking how we felt about returning."[299] Morozov said he told the WPA officials that the Soviet Union was interested in cooperating with the WPA but had to be sure before returning that a "businesslike atmosphere" prevailed "without prejudice and unfounded attacks." Morozov continued by praising the present officers of the WPA Executive Committee. He said: "We have a very positive attitude toward the new officers because they want a businesslike, scientific, clinical

294 WPA Newsletter No. 34, Autumn issue, October-November 1987. The remarks by Stefanis evoked a very angry reaction from Rick Scarnati, President of the Ohio Department of Mental Health, who pointed out that Snezhnevsky's name was closely related to the political abuse of psychiatry.

295 One of the occasions is the Seventh Congress of the International Physicians for the Prevention of Nuclear War (IPPNW), of which Chazov was co-chair and Marat Vartanyan a member of the board, on May 27-June 1, 1987, an occasion where Stefanis was one of the speakers. See *Psychiatric News*, August 7, 1987

296 Which Costas Stefanis denied in our interview on July 15, 2009

297 *Reisebericht* of Jochen Neumann on the WPA EC meeting in Buenos Aires, pp. 2-3. According to the same report Stefanis also had a "very constructive" meeting with the Soviet Ambassador in Geneva, Sofinski.

298 see chapter 15, footnote on Juri Saarma.

299 RL/FRE interview with Georgi Morozov, October 24, 1987, 23.37 h.

approach and we are for that."[300] Less than two hours earlier, WPA General Secretary Fini Schulsinger denied that the WPA had raised the possibility of a return of the Soviet All-Union Society to the organization.[301] However, he confirmed that he had met Georgi Morozov and Juri Saarma in Budapest in November 1986 at the Annual Meeting of the Hungarian Psychiatric Society and that both sides had then agreed "to continue mutually explorative contacts without obligations." He added, when asked, that at this stage he was negative about a possible Soviet return, but added "if political utterings and religious beliefs are no longer criminal … I would of course, be very positive because we try to be a world association." [302]

However, the travel report by Neumann shows that the meetings in Milan were far from harmonious. According to him, quite a few more people were involved in the discussions: Morozov and Zharikov on the Soviet side (Saarma is not mentioned), Stefanis, Sabshin and Schulsinger on the part of the WPA (and, interestingly, not Jochen Neumann himself) and the host, the Italian Dr. Cazzullo, who in an earlier report of Neumann had been marked "friend of Morozov" and in whose villa the meetings took place. "It came to a confrontation between Schulsinger and Sabshin and also between Sabshin and Stefanis, which led to Sabshin withdrawing from the meeting. As far as is known to me, Sabshin insisted that only the APA supports or declines initiatives for rapprochement with the Soviet All-Union Society and reports … to the WPA. Stefanis and Schulsinger angrily refused. On the other hand, Stefanis and Schulsinger were disappointed about the Soviet representatives, who were not only completely uninformed and unfit in their argumentation, but also allowed themselves to be misused by Sabshin and did not recognize that the latter tried to drive a wedge into the WPA. Apparently in Milan, it had come to a grouping of Sabshin/Morozov against the WPA, represented by Schulsinger and Stefanis."[303] During an interview in November 2009, Stefanis confirmed that Mel Sabshin had been on Morozov's side: "They were repeatedly together. I saw them even going to the opera together."[304]

As indicated, the push of Costas Stefanis and Fini Schulsinger to get the Soviets back to the WPA was actually very intense. On the basis of the available data, one can only conclude that, for instance, during the twelve

300 RL/FRE interview with Georgi Morozov, October 24, 1987, 23.37 h.
301 RL/FRE interview with Georgi Morozov, October 24, 1987, 21.51 h.
302 RL/FRE interview with Georgi Morozov, October 24, 1987, 21.51 h.
303 *Reisebericht* Jochen Neumann on the WPA EC in Warsaw, 20-26 November 1987, p. 2
304 Interview with Costas Stefanis, November 19, 2009

months between November 1986 and November 1987, the Soviets met with either Costas Stefanis or Fini Schulsinger, or both, at least six times.[305] This intense communication was no different in 1986, and would also continue throughout 1988.

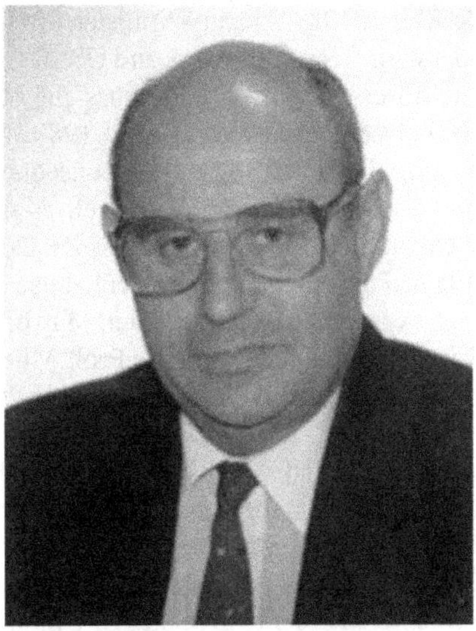
Jochen Neumann, 1985

We will return to those contacts later, but we should not forget that in addition to the above, contact was maintained between the Soviet psychiatric leadership and Jochen Neumann in East Berlin. For instance, in March 1988, Georgi Morozov traveled to the DDR to meet with Neumann.[306] Also, Jochen Neumann traveled to Moscow after almost every meeting of the Executive Committee of the WPA in order to meet with the Soviet psychiatric leadership and inform them of what was happening, of which, according to Neumann at least, Stefanis must have been well aware.[307] These contacts were maintained from the very start, and the reports of Jochen Neumann repeatedly record such communication. In February 1985, Neumann writes: "The discussions are held with Academy member Morozov, Academy member Snezhnevsky and corresponding Academy member Vartanyan. Academician Morozov is at the same time Chairman of the All-Union Society. The talks were very detailed and extensive and concerned mostly the preparations of the EC meeting of the WPA in April 1985."[308] In a separate report on the discussions with Georgi Morozov, Neumann

305 Nov 1986: Schulsinger meets Morozov/Saarma in Budapest; Nov 1986 – Apr 1987 Stefanis meets the Soviets twice; between Apr and Sep 1987 Stefanis is in Moscow and meets with Chazov; Aug 1987 Stefanis at meeting in Varna; Oct 1987 Stefanis and Schulsinger meet Morozov c.s. in Milan.

306 HA XX 499, p. 107

307 Interview with Jochen Neumann, July 30, 2009. Stefanis denies any knowledge of this and appeared sincerely stupefied when I told him during our meeting on November 19, 2009.

308 Report by Jochen Neumann on a visit to the All-Union Society and the Serbski Institute on February 3-6, 1985, Report dated February 14, 1985, p. 3

writes: ".... It is clear to them, and that has also been stressed by Prof. Stefanis, that the tendency to reconcile and find common interests, started by Prof. Stefanis, would not have been possible without the support of the DDR-Vice President in the Executive Committee."[309]

In March 1989, Deputy Minister of Health of the DDR, Dr. Rolf Müller, met with Georgi Morozov and USSR Chief Psychiatrist Aleksandr Churkin in Moscow in order to discuss the situation with regards to the WPA. Müller suggested that in May 1989, Neumann should come to Moscow to explain to the Soviets the consequences of the proposed new Statutes and Bylaws of the WPA, as well as the content of the report by the US Delegation to the USSR.[310] This US Delegation visited the USSR in March 1989 to investigate the political abuse of psychiatry; the report of the visit was expected to be published in May of that year. "Comrade Prof. Morozov very much thanked comrade Prof. Müller that he had found the possibility to discuss the above-mentioned issues with the Soviet side."[311]

Whether Stefanis really knew about these contacts between East Berlin and Moscow is not clear from the Neumann reports; but, in January 1988, both men agree that "independent from each other [they should] inform the leading comrades of the All-Union Society as extensively and precisely as possible, in order to give the All-Union Society the chance to act a bit more maneuverably and elegantly."[312]

Meeting Stefanis again

What do you do when a man whom you always considered to be an opponent turns out to not be that, but, in fact, increasingly shows character traits you can adhere to and understand? What do you do when you start developing a bond with a man thirty years your senior, who was, for you, the epitome of a fellow traveler but who turns out to be a free mind, a free spirit, and not the type of person to be put into a "box"? What do you do when your "enemy" increasingly shows signs of being a friend?

It is a strange question, which for many persons will remain unreal and

309 *Reisebericht* by Jochen Neumann on his trip to Moscow, 24-25 February 1987, p. 2. See: HA XX 499, p. 243-4

310 See chapter 27

311 HA XX 499, pp. 60-1

312 Report on a private meeting with Stefanis, by Jochen Neumann, January 1988, p. 4

unnecessary to answer, but, for me, it is a pressing one, especially after meeting Costas Stefanis for a second time at his home in Athens. During that visit, we lost all sense of time because of the intimate conversations, the revelations (the "confession time," as we started to call it during the meeting), and the growing sense that here we had a meeting of minds that refused to be caged and put into a set framework.

The meeting was supposed to conclude our discussions; at least that was my starting point. I thought I had a clear picture; all I needed to do was tell Costas Stefanis what I found and what will eventually appear in this book. Stefanis, on his part, had been seriously ill, again on the verge of death, and until the day before it was unclear whether we would actually meet. At first, he looked fragile, much more so than during our previous meeting, but gradually he gathered strength, as if the power of the mind empowered the body, and took over the physical forces that were lacking. We had lunch; the hours passed almost unnoticeably. We went deeper and deeper, both sharing "secrets" but, at the same time, understanding that something unusual was happening: we share an understanding of the world around us, we share an understanding of history and the role of the human factor, and above all, we refused to allow ourselves to give up our freedom of mind and accept the infringement of a system, whether capitalist or socialist or whatever. Step by step, more similarities appeared, amazing on one hand but gratifying on the other – even though it was twenty years later, we still were able to close the chapter and accept what happened.

The fundamental discussion centers on the issue of perception: how did we perceive each other, what did we think the other's intentions were? "You know," he says, "come to think of it. You were all focusing on me, and my 'clandestine negotiations' with the Soviets. Do you realize I was probably the least communist on the Executive Committee?" And indeed, considering the fact that Neumann was Communist, Sabshin and Schulsinger (ex) communist, Costa e Silva the son of a leftist politician and Reisby a clone of Schulsinger, it leaves Stefanis possibly as the only "unaligned person." "You know, they accused me first of being CIA, and then of being KGB," he adds. I smile, because I know the story, I have been accused of the same. "Really?" he said, "so you see, there is a similarity here."

We discussed his trips to Moscow, his interaction with Georgi Morozov and Marat Vartanyan. He listened attentively to Neumann's reports to the Stasi, which I ad-hoc translated from German to him and which deal with his connections with Moscow as well as his chairmanship. It was visible that he was hurt by the descriptions about his leadership style, about his

"Mediterranean flair." But he remained calm, no emotional outbursts, just tried to explain that this was not so much a lack of leadership but a desire to find consensus, to let all sides have their say. And this is what we accomplished, he adds, "We turned the WPA from something weak and floundering into a strong global building, into a true World Psychiatric Association. Before it was a travel agency; then, it became much more of a prestigious world organization." Several times he expressed his gratitude to the other members of the Executive Committee. "It is amazing, you know. We came from completely different backgrounds, with different agendas, but somehow we managed to achieve a lot." We then discussed various sessions of the Executive Committee, and laugh about the fact that having worked on this book I know some of the dates better, add names, situations… It was as if I had been there, the advantage of a younger mind over an older and more tired one.

When I leave, it is not a final goodbye. Costas is ill, even though you sometimes tend to forget, due to his indomitable energy. He is actually seriously ill and any small infection could mean the end of his life. Several times during our meeting, he reflects on this, as well as on the quality of life in the present, when he is confined to his home and his mind wants to go where his body is not able to take him. Yet our story is unfinished; apart from the obvious, the family, there is an additional reason to go on with life. He asks when the book will be finished, when it will it all be written down. I ask him jokingly "until when do you want to live?" indicating that it can be prolonged, as long as it keeps him going. He laughs, but our positions are different, it is clear: he is about to leave this earth, sooner rather than later, life is coming to an end; while I normally should be around for quite some time. It is all relative.

Chapter 21 – A Professional Career with Political Hurdles

"[Neumann] is marked by a high personal commitment, impatience with the implementation of innovations and directions into the future as well as by high professional ethics and morality."
Professor G. Wessel[313]

From 1954 until 1959, Jochen Neumann studied medicine at the Universities of Leipzig and of Greifswald, in the northeastern part of East Germany, and at Humboldt University in Berlin, after which he spent his psychiatric residency at the Charité Hospital of the Humboldt University in Berlin as well as at the Pathological Institute of the City Hospital in Berlin-Friedrichshein.

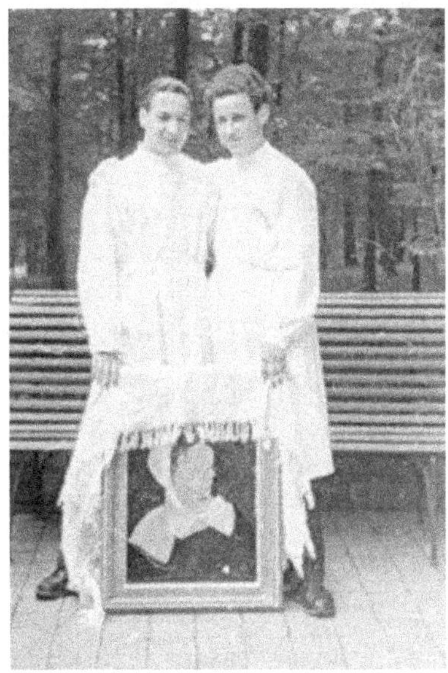

Neumann and a fellow student in University

In 1961, he finished his thesis, received his doctor's degree, and started his professional career in psychiatry as an assistant at the psychiatric clinic of the Charité.[314] Here he climbed up the hierarchical ladder and became eventually a senior lecturer and head of the department of neuro-radiology and assistant medical director. In the meantime, he spent months abroad,

---

[313] Deputy Rector of the University of Jena, in his assessment, see later in this chapter.

[314] In 1961-1969 Professor K. Leonhard, an internationally renowned professor of psychiatry who before had taught at the University of Frankfurt/Main in West-Germany and author of several important manuals in psychiatry was one of his teachers. Leonhard was Director of the "*Psychiatrische und Nerven Klinik*" of the Charité until 1969. In 1970 he was succeeded by Prof. Karl Seidel. In 1965 Neumann became a board certified neurologist and psychiatrist.
The title of his 1961 thesis was "*Mimics as an important component in the artistic expression of Ilya Yefimovich Repin*" (Mimischer Ausdruck als wesentlicher Bestandteil des künstlerischen Ausdrucks bei Ilja Jefimowitsch Repin), a title that clearly indicates the wide scope of cultural interests of Jochen Neumann.

working and studying at various psychiatric institutes and clinics.[315] At the Charité Hospital, he also met one of the men who would have a profound influence on his way of thinking, both professionally and politically, and one of the few people with whom he maintain contacts to this very day. Professor Karl Seidel became Director of the *Psychiatrische und Nervenklinik* (psychiatric and neurological clinic) of the Charité Hospital in Berlin in 1970, where Neumann worked as a department head. In addition, as member of the Central Committee of the SED, he was the top health politician in the country, and "was the one who was able to connect and later deepen my ... biological views of psychiatry with psychodynamic and social factors into a dialectic unity (also during conversations when he already had climbed the political ladder to the top and had turned psychiatry into a hobby. [He was] ostensibly a clever man with an open mind, in science he did not allow himself to be induced into speculative thinking and steered and formed noticeably and unnoticeably his psychiatric and political followers. On top of that, he established cross-connections with representatives from other disciplines that were of interest to our [psychiatric] profession and coordinated the exchanges. Not less important was the influence of Karl Seidel on my professional career that was the result of his political establishment in the top levels of the Party."[316]

315 In 1965 in Prague, in 1966 at the Serbski Institute in Moscow, in 1967 in Vienna and in Paris, where he had a close friend, a Jewish former Communist resistance fighter who had spent 4 ½ years in Auschwitz and Mauthausen and was also related to several top DDR politicians, with whom he had been imprisoned in the Auschwitz concentration camp, and was thus deemed politically reliable.

316 Bruckstücke *Narratives, Personales*, September 2009, p. 2. Karl Seidel, born in 1930, son of a physician, studied medicine in Leipzig in 1950-1956, specialized in psychiatry/neurology in 1957-1961, was chief physician in the university psychiatric clinic in Leipzig in 1961-196. In 1963-1971 he was director of the Academic Psychiatric Clinic in Dresden, from 1971 until 1978 Director of the psychiatric clinic of Charité in Berlin. Member of the SED since 1947. From 1967 until 1978 he worked as *IM* Fritz Steiner for the *MfS*, in 1978-1981 he was deputy head and during the period 1981-1989 head of the department for health policy of the Central Committee of the SED. Interestingly, Seidel himself was since 1986 under Stasi surveillance because of illegal trade in computer equipment from the West. He allegedly traded for 320,000 German Deutsch Mark (DM) worth of equipment, with a gain of some 130,000 DM (approximately 65,000 euro). In addition he illegally imported a Volkswagen Passat worth 40,000 DM. The case reached the highest echelons of the Party, including Party chief Erich Honecker and Stasi chief Erich Mielke, but somehow never led to criminal charges until the very end of the existence of the DDR. Seidel was arrested in December 1989 and spent three months in prison under pre-trail investigation. It never came to a trial, but the case was closed only in April 1991. See *Politisch Missbraucht*, pp. 239-242.

It was also Seidel's political protection that several times saved Neumann in a conflict situation with lower or middle-range Party officials, which happened repeatedly during Neumann's career. In fact, their friendship actually started as a result of such a conflict. When in 1970 Seidel became Director of the *Psychiatrische und Nervenklinik* of the Charité, the heads of the various departments that now fell under Seidel's authority were very independent minded and not inclined to subordinate themselves to their new boss. Neumann, then combining the positions of chief doctor and head of the neuro-radiological department became involuntarily involved in the skirmish with Karl Seidel. In fact, in the resulting conflict, he wrote a letter of resignation, as a "protest against the style of leadership of Karl Seidel." A few days later, he was asked to come to the director's office. "At his table was the chief of personnel of the Charité Hospital, comrade Dube, and on the table was my letter of resignation, with my reason for resigning underlined in red," remembers Neumann. "Karl Seidel asked me 'what is the meaning of this all?' and whether I was aware of the fact that I would walk straight into an open knife." The chief of personnel was asked to leave the room, and told she would later hear the outcome of the discussion. And with a cup of coffee on the table, a discussion ensued.

"KS: 'What do you actually think?'

JN: 'I think I clearly formulated myself.'

KS: 'And did you consider what consequences this can have for you?'

JN: 'Yeeees.'

The discussion goes back and forth.

KS: 'If you leave the Charité with a big leap because of a conflict with me, your academic career has ended… Probably you will wind up in a state practice somewhere in the province, in the middle of nowhere. Is that what you want?'

JN, proudly: 'I will stay in Berlin…'

KS: 'But not as a physician.'

JN: 'Also OK, then I will take over the management of a car wash in Mahlsdorf, for emergency sake I already investigated and I would have a better income there anyway…'

KS: 'It would fit you.'

Again back and forth, explaining our viewpoints.

Pause. Coffee…

KS: 'I suggest you take your protest back, we rip up your notice and you stay in the clinic. I will inform comrade Dube. So: you will stay?'

JN: hawking, undefined mumbling, thoughts back and forth without a word said, deep frowning.

Pause, vacuum.

KS, starting a suggestive monologue: 'In some way I like you. You are original, productive, you know what you want and you voice your opinion... But to a certain extent you are a clown.... To fight is good, but not at any price, just out of stubbornness or principle. A combative behavior makes only sense when it is coupled with the appropriate intelligence, when the chances of success are considerably bigger than of a failure. Only a stupid person would persist when it is clear it will end with an emergency landing. Your whole intelligence is useless when it is not used to assess correctly the existing circumstances.... Irrespective of the fact whether you are right or wrong, you stand no chance against me, because *those* who put me in this position *do not make mistakes.* With a jump from the television tower with a banner around your belly saying 'out of protest against Prof. Seidel,' you don't achieve anything, you only break your neck and you make a fool of yourself up there... When you want to continue working here, we could very well work together and we forget this story...'

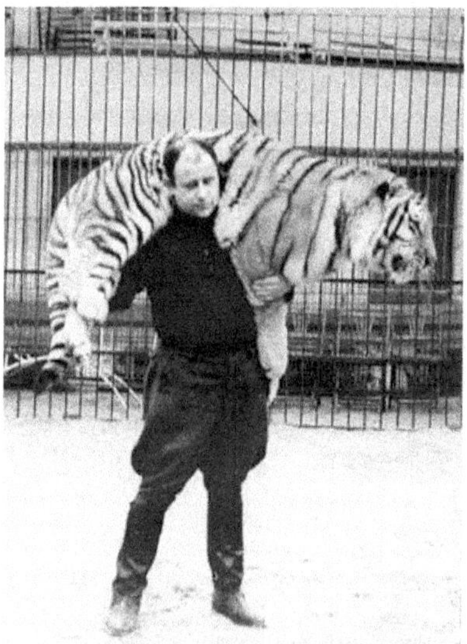

Jochen Neumann with a Siberian tiger, 1969

KS: 'So you stay?'
JN, with a small voice: 'Yes.'[317]

In 1971, Neumann received his PhD at the Humboldt University in Berlin.[318] A year later he was appointed medical director of the Wilhelm Griesinger Hospital in Berlin.[319] This appointment was

317 Bruckstücke *Narratives, Personales*, September 2009, p.3

318 The title of his dissertation was *Die Entwicklung des Hirnstammes und die topographischen Beziehungen zwischen Hirnstamm und Schädelbasis im Pneumencephalogramm bei Kindern* (The development of the brain stem and the spatial relationship between the brainstem and the cranial base in pneumoencephalograms of children)

319 Interestingly, this hospital was named after Wilhelm Griesinger, Wilhelm Griesinger, a 19th-century German physician, one of the founders of the concept of community-based care for mentally ill patients. In a time when such patients spent most of their lives in asylums in remote rural areas, he recommended their integration into society and proposed that short-term treatment of acutely ill patients could be carried out in clinics that were located in cities and linked to general hospitals. In his view short-term hospitalization could be effective only if professional and natural support systems cooperated closely.

cause for another serious clash in Neumann's career that could have had far-reaching professional and political repercussions.

Provocateur

Initially, Neumann was told that he had been hired and should start during the fall of 1971, and then, suddenly, his employment was cancelled for reasons that were not immediately clear. Later it turned out that Prof. Peter Hagemann,[320] the medical director of the hospital Herzberge in the same district, had been behind the politicking to keep Neumann out of this position. "Hagemann, a combination of a clever and educated man but with confusing personal relationships, was a devious schemer.... He tried with all possible means and still unknown reasons to prevent my getting the director's post in Griesinger. ... After I took office in October 1972, I found in the director's desk the entire correspondence of Professor Hagemann with all sorts of departments, colleague directors of other institutions and some leaders of university hospitals, in which he perfidiously tried to thwart my appointment."[321]

The Wilhelm-Griesinger Hospital was a municipal facility in Berlin-Lichtenberg and thus the appointment of Jochen Neumann as medical director had to be confirmed by the municipal council. "It is easy to guess that after these disputes, the relationship with my supervisor, the district medical officer, was not an easy one. A certain tension existed from the beginning."[322]

During his time at the Wilhelm Griesinger Hospital, Neumann managed to set a process in motion to restructure the hospital fundamentally. "The fundamental restructuring of a 1600-bed clinical hospital, that in a physical, moral and professional sense was still suffering from the after-effects of the Nazi period, demanded all my energy and the use of all my clinical-practical

---

He believed that most patients should be discharged from long-term treatment in remote asylums. For those unable to live without support in the community, he suggested setting up sheltered living conditions. His ideas were rejected by his contemporaries, but are implemented worldwide today.

320 Professor Peter Hagemann, who was chief doctor of the Charité at this time, worked for the Stasi since 1965 as psychiatrist. When after two years this work for the MfS became too difficult to combine with his job as medical director of the psychiatric clinic at Berlin-Lichtenberg (Herzberge), he suggested a successor to the Stasi. See *Politisch Missbraucht*, p. 690-1

321 Bruckstücke *Narratives, Personales*, September 2009, p. 5

322 Bruckstücke *Narratives, Personales*, September 2009, p. 5

skills. In spite of much resistance, financial barriers and fights, I managed, in a period of five years, to change a traditional psychiatric institution of the asylum type into a structured clinic with modern specialized diagnostic, therapeutic and social units, either fully operational or under development. After my departure, this formed the basis for a further development into a central research institution."[323]

This tension continued, however, and came to an explosion in the autumn of 1976 during a meeting at the office of the district medical officer of Berlin-Lichtenberg, Dr. Edgar Dusold.[324] The meeting irritated Neumann to such an extent that back in his hospital he voiced his irritation in the sharpest possible way. The same evening, he was called in by Dusold, who in carefully chosen but nonetheless threatening words expressed his deep anger. "It became dangerous when he accused me of the fact that my sole purpose was the damage the State and the DDR when I attacked my State superior, its authorized representative. By doing so, he concluded, I attacked the total health system of the DDR, subvert the influence and authority of the Party, and, as district medical officer, he could not allow his subordinates to go against managers in senior positions and turn against the State."

Dusold ordered Neumann to come back within twenty-four hours with an essay of at least one and maximally two pages on the theme: "How do I see my relation with my State employed superior." Neumann refused, which further angered Dusold, who made a direct connection between Neumann's behavior and the political protests that had developed in connection with the exile of the popular singer Wolf Biermann to West Berlin.[325] He

323 Bruckstücke *Narratives, Personales*, September 2009, p. 5

324 According to Jochen Neumann Dusold was an *OibE* (officer in special service) of the Stasi. "He was in charge of the Lichtenberg health care system, which he ruled with an iron fist and dictatorial gestures." See: Bruckstücke *Narratives, Personales*, September 2009, p. 5

325 Wolf Biermann (born 15 November 1936 in Hamburg), son of a German Communist resistance fighter who was killed in Auschwitz, was one of the few children of workers who attended the Heinrich-Hertz-Gymnasium in Hamburg. In 1953 he became a member of the Freie Deutsche Jugend (FDJ) and several times he represented West-Germany at the FDJ's first national meeting. In 1961 Biermann formed the Arbeiter- und Studententheater (Workers' and Students' Theater). It produced a show called Berliner Brautgang documenting the building of the Berlin wall that was shut down by the authorities in 1963. Although a committed communist, Biermann's nonconformist views soon alarmed the East German establishment. In 1963 he was refused membership of the SED. Two years later, publicly denounced as a 'class traitor', he was

announced that the next day an official "job interview" would be held to assess Neumann's performance.

During the next three-four days, several interviews and meetings took place, but increasingly the affair turned into a completely political one, "even though no political intention whatsoever had been behind my behavior and it basically concerned an authority problem with the district medical officer that I had handled unwisely. ... Quickly, within half a week, the conflict, which had originally been a personal one, spun out of control. In connection with the accusations, which were now purely political and put in relation to the exile of Biermann, followed by unrest among intellectual circles, I was dubbed to be a provocateur who questioned the integrity of the DDR and the authority of the State and Party officials, and whose personality and person needed to be scrutinized. I found myself fighting a losing battle."[326] Neumann became even more frightened by Dusold's remark that Neumann's wife also could be affected by this (she was in her last year of specialist medical training and working in the same district). Then, adding even more fuel to the fire, Neumann said to Dusold that, considering the situation and the effect of this on the future of his professional career, he might as well immediately apply for an exit visa to leave the country. The same evening, an official liaison officer of the Stasi visited Neumann at home to have a long conversation with him about the situation, most probably in order to assess whether Neumann had become politically untrustworthy.

The next day, Dusold gave Neumann only two options: "Either you are just a very bad type, and then we will proceed with you accordingly, or you are mentally ill. In the latter case, we leave you in peace, but you must agree to be examined psychiatrically, by a neutral colleague, and get a corresponding certificate." The latter was totally unacceptable to Neumann, and thus he chose the first option, and the case followed its own course, out of control, higher and higher up the political ladder. Eventually, Neumann was informed that on December 16, 1976, a meeting would take place where he would be relieved from his position as medical director of the Wilhelm Griesinger Hospital.

---

forbidden to publish his music or perform in public. In 1976 the SED Politbüro decided to strip Biermann of his citizenship while he was on an officially authorized tour in West Germany. It later turned out that the Politbüro had decided to do so before the first concert in Cologne, even though this concert was used as the official justification afterwards. Biermann's exile provoked protests by leading East German intellectuals.

326 Bruckstücke *Narratives, Personales*, September 2009, p. 7

However, it never came to this ultimate decision. A few days before December 16, Neumann received a phone call that the meeting has been postponed and that a new date would be set. The case was never discussed again. Only much later Neumann found out that a Prof. Kurt Winter, whom he had known during his student days and who was then Director of the Institute of Social Hygiene of the Medical Faculty of Humboldt University and now Rector of the Academy for Continuing Medical Education of the DDR in Berlin-Lichtenberg, had intervened.[327] "Kurt Winter had heard of the bickering and my impending dismissal and was interested in what really had happened. Among the leading staff of the Academy, he expressed his lack of understanding of what happened, saying that if comrade Neumann, whom I have known for two decades, has in fact made inappropriate remarks, then something special must have happened. ... He went to see his old fellow Spanish Civil War veteran Paul Verner,[328] a member of the Politburo, and voiced the opinion that my behavior as well as the behavior of Edgar Dusold should be weighed equally before any conclusions were drawn from my transgressions. From then on, events took an unexpected favorable outcome for me."[329]

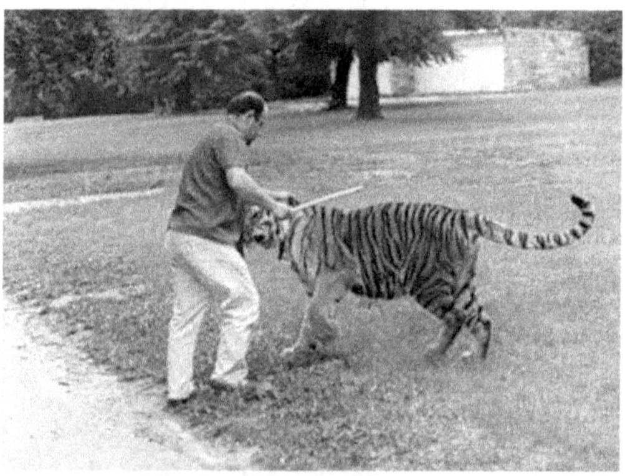

Neumann with a Siberian tiger in Volkspark Friedrichshain, Berlin, 1970

In September 1977, Neumann was appointed professor at the Academy for Medical Education of the DDR, where he had been lecturer since 1975, and simultaneously he became Professor of Psychiatry and Neurology at the Friedrich

[327] Kurt Winter, former combatant in the Spanish Civil War, German Communist of Jewish descent, Director of the Institute of Social Hygiene of the Medical Faculty of Humboldt University and later Rector of the Academy for Continuing Medical Education of the DDR.

[328] Paul Verner (1911-1986) was a German communist politician. He joined the communist movement at a young age, and went into exile during Hitler's rule. After the end of the Second World War, he returned to Germany. He became a leading figure in the FDJ. In 1958 Verner became a candidate member of the SED Politburo. He was also one of the secretaries of the party Central Committee. In March 1959 Verner became First Secretary of the Berlin district organization of SED, a powerful institution in the DDR. At the time the party district included West Berlin. Verner became a full Politburo member in 1963.

[329] Bruckstücke *Narratives, Personales*, September 2009, p. 8

Schiller University in Jena.[330] He also became director of the psychiatric department of the Clinic for Psychiatry and Neurology "Hans Berger" in the same city. Career-wise, he had now reached the highest step on the academic ladder.

However, his time in Jena was not altogether a happy one. After spending many years in Berlin, Jena lacked the cultural life he had gotten used to. In Berlin, he had full access to the theatre and museums. "A considerable part of my spare time I passed with artists (visual artists, writers, actors), and with some of them I was - and still am - friends, among them some circus people as well. For a long time, I felt myself partially at home in the studios of the Academy of Art, in the College of *Weissensee*, in the German Theatre and in the Winter Quarters of the Central Circus in the *Hoppegarten*."[331] One of Neumann's hobbies, and a rather unusual one, was taming tigers. In Jena, it was quite different; it was a provincial town, with all its consequences. "In this environment, there was no drive for deep ideological, political and philosophical digging. This concerned both religious cadres as well as the hard-boiled Party cadres. Exceptions could be found among the students who were still not integrated into the community, and among some artistic and socially sensitive intellectuals who were an exception to the rule, but they didn't really get into my orbit and I also didn't try to get in touch with them."[332] In addition, the academic environment was much less open to the outside world, and Neumann was surprised to find out that there were even colleagues in leading positions who did not speak any foreign language. Quite a few of them had actually never left Jena. They had started their careers there as students, slowly climbing up the ladder to the position of professors. For Neumann, whose eyes by then already reached well beyond the borders of the DDR, this was quite unbelievable, and in a way also unacceptable.[333]

Clearly, Neumann did not feel at home in Jena, but the discomfort was mutual. Also for the academic establishment, Neumann remained an outsider, a difficult person to deal with and even more difficult to satisfy. The Stasi file on Jochen Neumann of this period very much confirms the position of

330 He would hold this position until 1982. *Abschlussbeurteilung*, December 23, 1983, signed by Prof. G. Wessel.

331 Bruckstücke *Hygiene Museum I*, January 7, 2010, p. 3

332 Bruckstücke *Hygiene Museum I*, January 7, 2010, p. 3

333 One should not forget that Neumann by then had not only worked and studied in Moscow, Vienna and Paris, but had also participated in a tour of psychiatric institutions in ten States of the USA in 1978 as a member of an international delegation, which very much opened his eyes to Western psychiatric practice.

Neumann as an outsider. In a report, his *Führungsoffizier* is explicit about the fact that Neumann is not feeling well in Jena: "…he feels himself provincially constrained in Jena… and is looking for ways to keep himself busy elsewhere." He also adds that Neumann is very critical: "He complains about the poor Party work in the field of medicine… (…) He assessed that the current economic situation was not rosy. In the times of W[alter] Ulbricht[334] we supposedly had a better economic situation. (…) Such moments characterize his inconsistency, predisposition and sense of superiority. He has an outspoken tendency to wish to be instructive and likes to hear himself. (…) He was of the opinion that having the Intershops[335] were ideologically harmful and it was difficult to convince him of the economic value of these institutions (maybe he is angry that he himself cannot go shopping there in style)."[336]

This tension is diplomatically worded in an assessment by the Deputy Rector of the University of Jena, Professor G. Wessel, written at the end of Neumann's tenure in Jena. It is a combination of praise and criticism: "He is marked by a high personal commitment, impatience with the implementation of innovations and directions into the future as well as by high professional ethics and morality." According to Prof. Wessel, Neumann was a "difficult negotiating partner, who pushed his ideas through" [337] but at the same time he described him as "one of the scientists who has a wide overview in his professional field and who, as a leader, considers everything easy as something strange and everything inaccessible and every backlog as a challenge that needs to be met." Yet in spite of the fact that the relationship had been a difficult one, Wessel was full of praise for what Neumann had been able to accomplish during his stay in Jena: "…He has undertaken intensive efforts to give this institution again a clear profile in research and medical care. He carried out thorough reforms and gradually built up scientific collaboration with foreign institutions. That concerns particularly the link with an Institute of the Academy of Sciences of the USSR. …

334 Walter Ulbricht (1893-1973) was a German communist politician. As General Secretary of the SED from 1950 to 1971 he played a leading role in the early development and establishment of the DDR.

335 Intershop was a chain of government-run retail stores in the DDR in which only hard currencies could be used to purchase high-quality goods. The East German mark was not accepted as payment. Intershop was originally oriented towards visitors from Western countries, and later as an outlet where East Germans could purchase goods they could not otherwise obtain.

336 MfS/BV Gera, 780/80 Band 2, p. 69

337 "He is often a difficult negotiating partner, pushes his ideas through and uses in that context also a very temperamental and not usual path. Things that are considered by him to be defects or weaknesses are mentioned by him bluntly and openly, which is not always in his advantage."

During his work in Jena, Prof. Neumann has made special contributions to the introduction of work therapy, psychological diagnostics and addiction care for alcoholics and drug addicts."[338]

When in 1982, Neumann was offered a position as Director General of the German Hygiene Museum in the DDR, he immediately accepted the offer, even though it was much less of an academic position and seemingly a step down the career ladder.[339] It was a challenge and, at the same time, a possibility to get out of Jena. "Later a colleague reminded me of a quote that was ascribed to me (rightly or wrongly, both is possible): 'The best in Jena is the Saalbahnhof (train station), because from here late in the evening it is still possible to catch a train to Berlin'."[340]

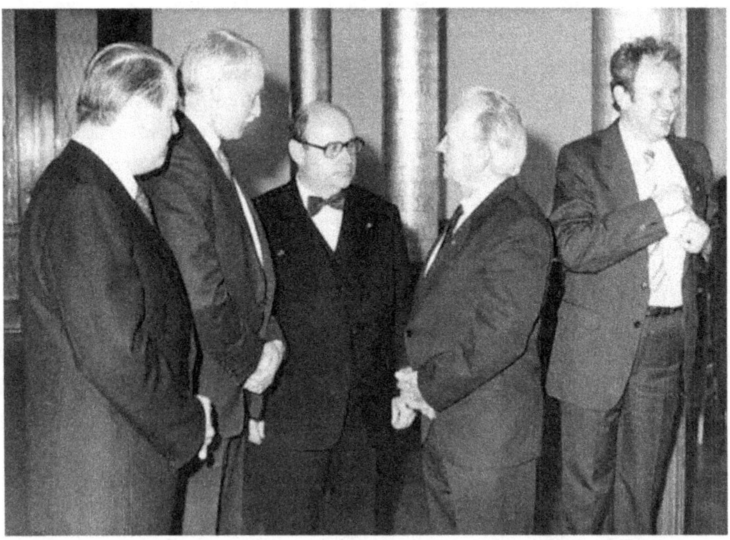

In the center Jochen Neumann with DDR Minister of Health Ludwig Mecklinger, 1987

338 Final assessment by Prof. Dr. G. Wessel, Deputy Rector of Jena, December 23, 1983.

339 A year later he was also appointed Honorary Professor at Dresden University. He held both positions until 1990.

340 Bruckstücke *Hygiene Museum I*, January 7, 2010, p. 3

Unacceptable behavior

The *Deutsches Hygiene Museum*, where Neumann started as Director General in early 1983, was indeed a totally different type of institution than he had known before. It was not a purely academic setting, yet, at the same time, the position was an opportunity to use all his skills and his broad view on his profession and on life in general. The Museum, with its manifold tasks of very different nature, had health as its only common denominator in the broadest sense. Its main task was to promote nationwide health-improvements on motivations and behavior patterns, with rather different institutions and sectors united under one roof each headed by a Director.[341] At the top, stood the position of "Director General," which was then occupied by Neumann. He represented the Hygiene Museum to the outside world and was solely responsible for work concepts and plans, as well as the coordination and facilitation of production processes. His position was directly subordinate to the Ministry of Public Health, who was, thus, his employer and a personal supervisor. As Director General, he frequently traveled abroad to trade fairs in order to represent the Hygiene Museum and conduct business on its behalf. For Neumann this period, which lasted until 1990, was "the best, most beautiful, interesting and exciting in my working life."[342]

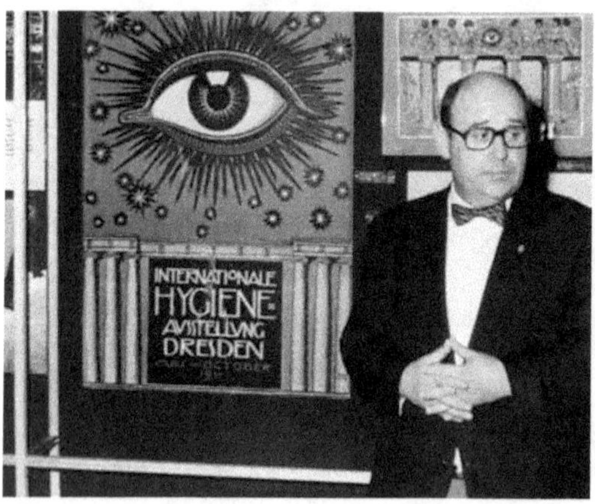

Jochen Neumann as Director of the Deutsche Hygiene Museum, 1986

The Hygiene Museum was not only a museum, although it also functioned as such and un-

[341] The Deutsches Hygiene-Museum was founded for mass education in hygiene, health, human biology and medicine. It stood in context of the Dresden industry of medicine and hygiene products. Karl August Lingner (1861-1916), the Odol mouthwash manufacturer, initiated the foundation of the Deutsches Hygiene-Museum in 1912. In 1911, Lingner was the driving force behind the First International Hygiene Exhibition that drew over 5 million visitors to Dresden. The museum building designed by Wilhelm Kreis (1873 - 1955) served as the venue for the Second International Hygiene Exhibition in 1930, and is still in current use by the museum today. The museum's Transparent Woman, showing the organs of human beings as a see-through sculpture, became world famous.

[342] Bruckstücke *Narratives, Personales*, September 2009, p. 9

der Neumann's leadership saw a constant increase in the numbers of visitors.[343] It was also one of the most important medical institutions of the DDR. It had a high international reputation, especially after it became a Collaborating Center of WHO in 1987. During his tenure as Director General, Neumann concentrated his own scientific work on the issue of mental health, his main slogan being "mental health is the central component of human health." High-ranking foreign visitors, mostly with public health or health pedagogic interests, would visit the institution. The position of Director-General was, thus, well endowed and prestigious. De facto, he was an important person at the intersection of health, health propaganda, domestic and foreign policy and even foreign trade (export-oriented production). In that sense, the name "Museum" was a rather misleading one, which undoubtedly also contributed to the hesitation in October 1984 to elect Neumann as Vice-President of the WPA. What contribution to the WPA could be expected from a museum director? In November 2009, during one of our meetings, former WPA President Costas Stefanis admitted he never actually knew the importance of Neumann's position: "I realize now that it was actually the most important export firm of the country with a huge cluster of operations that he directed."[344]

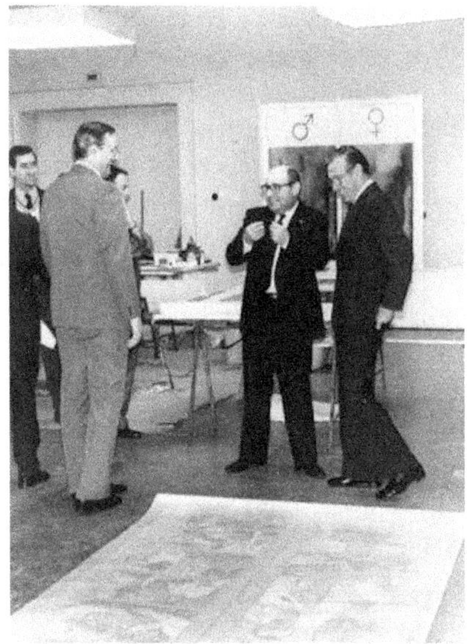

Jochen Neumann giving explanation in the Deutsche Hygiene Museum, 1987

The relationship with his direct superior, Health Minister Prof. Ludwig Mecklinger,[345] was a good and productive one, and became even closer

343 In an assessment of Jochen Neumann, written on the eve of his departure as Director General, it reads: "The number of visitors increased over the past years to a level not seen before. Up to several thousands of visitors had to be taken care of each day, which was almost impossible to handle with the number of personnel available." *Beurteilung*, October 30, 1989

344 Interview with Costas Stefanis, November 15, 2009

345 Ludwig Mecklinger (1919-1994) studied in 1939-1944 medicine in Leipzig, Hamburg and Berlin. In 1944 he was drafted into the army and was later in an American prisoner of war camp in Traunstein. In 1945 he joined the SED and during the years 1945-1947 he was in the provincial government of Saxony-Anhalt in charge of disease control, and later, from 1948 to 1952, he was

because of an incident in 1987. "On the occasion of the 1st May 1987 I received from my superiors a premium of 500 East-German Marks, in those days a respectable amount. Dr. Harig, one of the Deputy Ministers of Health, and others responsible for health education and the Hygiene Museum, appeared unexpectedly at the Museum and called a staff meeting at which he handed me this gift, garnished with an appropriate eulogy. I was duly impressed, and in thanking them, I vowed to contribute in the future even more remarkable, larger, and more significant benefits, etc.... Behind closed doors, I was furious."

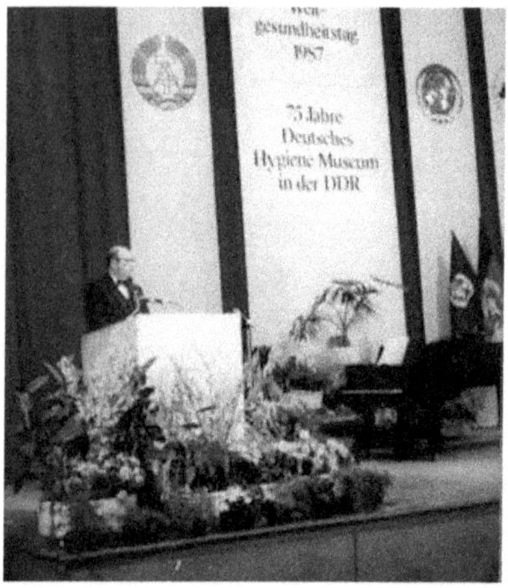

Neumann speaking at the World Health Day 1987

The reason for Neumann's anger was the difficult position in which the Hygiene Museum found itself, and for which nobody seemed to have any attention or understanding. The demands were increasing every day, from all sides, including the Ministries of Education and Foreign Trade, but nobody was able to explain to Neumann how this all should be realistically made possible. The only support came from personal contacts at the Department of Health Policy of the Central Committee, Professor Karl Seidel. Neumann felt betrayed and sold. "I told Dr. Harig over a coffee in my office that I experience this premium as a snub, and

Minister of Labor and Health of the Land Saxony-Anhalt. In 1954 he obtained a law degree from the German Academy for State and Law in Potsdam. In 1952-1954 he was deputy chairman of the Central Committee of the German Red Cross, 1954-1957 deputy chief of the medical service of the *Kasernierten Volkspolizei* and subsequently the *Volksarmee* (People's Army), and 1957-1964 head of the Military Medical Section at the University of Greifswald. In 1964 he became a professor and deputy Dean for Military Medicine as well as Deputy Minister of Health, 1969 Secretary of State and First Vice-Minister and from 1971 until 1988 Minister of Health. In 1981-1988 he was a member of the *Volkskammer* (Parliament) and in 1986-1988 a member of the Central Committee of the SED. Mecklinger worked for many years and at least since 1962 with the MfS, and when he celebrated his 65th birthday in 1984 the MfS had a problem deciding what medal to award him with, as he already received the Bronze, Silver and Gold Medals of the National People's Army (Nationale Volks Armee – NVA) as well as the *Kampforden für Verdienste um Volk und Vaterland in Gold* in 1974. Eventually he was given the Scharnhorst Orden. See *Politisch Missbraucht*, p. 179

that I was not prepared to accept, that he could take it back to Berlin to the Ministry."[346] A long discussion with Harig followed, without Neumann changing his mind.

A week later, Neumann went to see the Minister, who was clearly irritated and didn't understand Neumann's attitude. He first tried to convince Neumann to change his mind and take the premium. "During his long career, first as state secretary and then as Minister, he had never experienced somebody daring to refuse to accept an award or bonus from him, and to return it to him. Obviously, it was not quite clear to me what the issue was and whom I have before me."[347] A discussion ensued, which led nowhere and ended with the Minister summing up the situation: there was financially no technical possibility to take the premium back and they could have spared themselves all the discussions because Neumann had to keep the money anyway. He ended by saying: "And now let's put an end to these fruitless debates. You accept the money, won't you?" "No," was the answer of Neumann.[348]

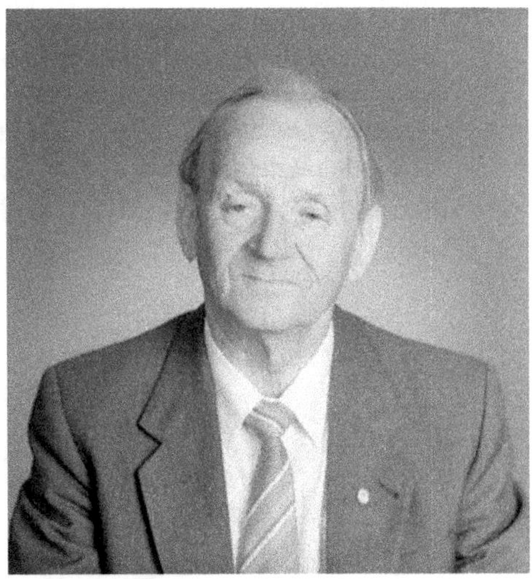
Ludwig Mecklinger in 1986

A week later, Neumann was again summoned to the Ministry. In a short conversation, the Minister asked him first whether he had changed his mind and would accept the premium, to which Neumann again refused. What followed was a sharp lecture by the Minister, who explained to Neumann that this was unacceptable behavior and that his patience was coming to an end. "Because of your productivity, we have, in the past, sometimes tolerated your behavior that we otherwise consider unacceptable by others. But at some point we have reached the limit with you. You have a few more days to think about your decision. My secretary will call upon you now and then I'll leave you for the last time, without putting further discussion, the question of whether you give up and take the money or not.

346 Bruckstücke *Narratives, Personales*, September 2009, p. 10

347 Bruckstücke *Narratives, Personales*, September 2009, p. 11

348 Bruckstücke *Narratives, Personales*, September 2009, p. 11

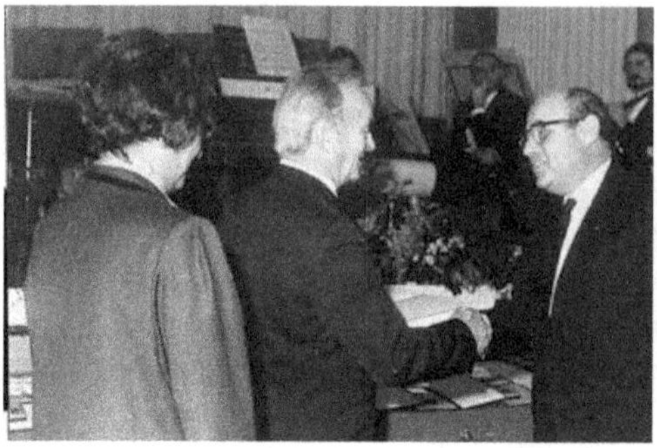

Prof. Ludwig Mecklinger with Jochen Neumann, 1987

You can then answer 'yes' or 'no,' and then that's your own thing. Meanwhile, the affair had reached higher circles, and wound up as a "special event" on the table of the Health Policy Department of the Central Committee."[349]

For a third time, Neumann was summoned to the Ministry. "The minister stood behind his desk and greeted me politely and coolly; without offering me a seat, he started the encounter with rolling pathos and with the following words: 'Comrade Neumann, I will ask you the key question. You can answer it with a yes or no. Nothing more. You had time to reflect on your attitude. Remember, and before you speak, you stand in front of a member of the Council of Ministers of the German Democratic Republic and a member of the Central Committee of the Socialist Unity Party of Germany… 'Do you accept the premium?' – 'Yes'."[350] The Minister came over to Neumann and embraced him. From that moment onwards, they addressed each other with the familiar "you" (*Du*) and the first name.

349 Bruckstücke *Narratives, Personales*, September 2009, p. 12
350 Bruckstücke *Narratives, Personales*, September 2009, p. 12

Chapter 22 - Reporting for the DDR Leadership

Before turning a page you need to read it.
Zheliu Zhelev [351]

It is a typical Jochen Neumann situation. During one of our interviews in the summer of 2009, we discussed his reports on the meetings of the Executive Committee, and inadvertently I referred to his "reports to the Stasi." "Robert," he says, "I have to correct you on this. I never addressed my reports to the Stasi. I wrote my reports for a number of governmental institutions. Of course, the Stasi obtained a copy, but it was not addressed to them." And he shows me the copy of a report he found at home, a few days prior to our meeting. Attached to it is a small note from his secretary, reading:
"2x Prof. Seidel, C[entral] C[ommittee];
3 x G[eneral] S[ecretariat] Medical Scientific Societies, Buhlert;
1 x Ministry of Health, Deputy Minister Prof. [Rudolf] Müller
2 x Prof. Neumann"[352]

"Of course," he continues, "one of the reports wound up on the desk of the Stasi, probably one of the three copies that went to the General Secretariat. I know that, because my *Führungsoffizier* referred to them, so they must have gotten it. But I never reported to them directly. The only time I did so was at the airport upon my return from Rome, after I had been elected in October 1984. Then two men, Deputy Minister Rudolf Müller and a Stasi major, met me on the plane and I was immediately taken to the government reception building at the airport and questioned for two hours about what had happened. That was the only direct reporting I ever did. With my *Führungsoffizier,* it was different, he just was making sure I was staying on track and not a security risk. Intellectually, he was not up to par, what interested me was too much for him, this psychiatric business went beyond his field of interest and understanding."[353]

---

351 Zheliu Zhelev, quoted in Tzvetan Todorov, *Hope and Memory*, p. 6

352 Report on the Executive Committee of the WPA, New York/Washington, November 1988. Original.

353 Interview Jochen Neumann, July 30, 2009. Probably at least two of the copies were forwarded to the Stasi, and on basis of the other documents with which it was stored in the various files one was probably sent by Seidel (himself an IM) and the other by Buhlert of the General Secretariat of Medical Scientific Societies. Among the papers received from Jochen Neumann is a document containing instructions for "the preparation and implementation of visits to

Yet also his *Führungsoffizier* sometimes received separate reports, written for him. They were usually small additions, such as the one to the travel report on the trip to New York, Washington and Mexico City. It is called an "*Ergänzungsbericht,*" a supplementary report, providing information on issues not directly related to the WPA. "I mostly wrote these to inform him whom else I had met," Neumann recalls, "to keep them informed of my contacts in the West."[354]

Jochen Neumann was adamant that he never fulfilled any orders while being a member of the Executive Committee, and merely kept the DDR leadership and, both directly and indirectly, the Soviets informed of what was happening within the WPA. In the document sent to me prior to an interview in June 2009, he wrote that "with regard to the influence [of the Stasi] on the Executive Committee and the WPA, I would like to make the following specification. *At no time did I receive any instructions* with regard to the WPA from the *MfS*. They were only interested in knowing in detail what was happening within the WPA. In my reports, I have tried to the best of my (subjective) ability to create an image as realistic as possible of what was happening in world psychiatry and the WPA, also with regard to individuals involved. In doing so, I have not taken into consideration any possible wishful thinking on the side of the recipient of the reports and have in these reports never answered any expectations involuntarily in order to stabilize my own position. My reports were (subjectively) uncompromising, honest, and reflected my knowledge and views of that time."[355]

In a way it is again a semantic discourse, a bit like in the case of Stefanis's "clandestine negotiations." Yet, for Neumann, it is of essential importance: he was not the regular spy, he didn't inform on people, he defended his country and kept the leadership informed, as instructed. That the

medical-scientific events abroad." The document indicates that of travel reports four copies need to be submitted, consisting of a "political part" (to be submitted within ten days) and a "professional part." The reports need to be marked "*Nur für Dienstgebrauch*" (only for official use; all of Neumann's reports are marked as such) and among the instructions for the "political part" is to report on political conversations, report on activities of representatives of West Germany and on unusual events. *Hinweise zur Vorebreitung und Auswertung des Besuches von Medizinisch-Wissenschaftlichen Veranstaltungen im Ausland*, no date. Jochen Neumann made of most reports more than four copies, and of some I have even three in my possession.

354 Interview Jochen Neumann, July 30, 2009. In September 2009, the author received the full file of all Neumann's travel reports, both the main ones and the additions, as well as his official requests for permission to travel.

355 Situation MfS/ WPA, June 1, 2009

Stasi would get his reports was clear to him from the very start, and his impression was that the Soviets were informed of what he was writing, hence their increasingly distant attitude. In his reports, Neumann was not overly friendly to the Soviets, increasingly critical actually and eventually outright hostile, as we will see later. It certainly didn't help him to obtain the trust of the Soviets, yet there is no evidence that he really cared. And, as noted before, after virtually each Executive Committee meeting he would travel to Moscow to report on what happened. Usually the meeting would be with Georgi Morozov and Marat Vartanyan, sometimes in the presence of Gennady Milyokhin, then in charge of international relations at the Serbski Institute, and often he would fly back the same evening. If he would stay over, he usually spent the evening with Milyokhin, who was doing his job but at the same time tried to take distance from the current leadership. And, by the way, Neumann is convinced that Stefanis was fully aware of Neumann's trips to Moscow.[356]

First Stasi contacts

Jochen Neumann's first contacts with the Stasi date back to long before his WPA period, and had nothing to do with the World Psychiatric Association. In fact, he was for a while subject to surveillance himself, which ended when the Stasi concluded there was nothing to find. What happened?

Sometime, toward the end of 1977 or at the start of 1978, Neumann was informed via the DDR Ministry of Health that he had been invited to the USA for a scientific exchange trip with regard to the issues of addiction and substance abuse, together with an internationally composed group of people active in the field. All costs would be covered by the US State Department, but there was only a very short time span left for the organization of the necessary trip formalities. The trip should begin the first part of February 1978. Neumann would receive the flight tickets from the US Embassy, as well as the dates of the start of the trip in Washington and an arranged meeting place. In Washington, he would learn all other information where he would go, etc.

Immediately there was a complication: after submitting the necessary registration forms for the trip via the relevant authorities of the Ministry of Health, Neumann received a call from Mr. Alexander, the cultural attaché of the US Embassy in East-Berlin, who invited him for a personal conversation. As a precaution, Neumann informed the Health Ministry,

356 Interview Jochen Neumann, July 30, 2009

who immediately replied that a visit to the US Embassy was impossible under any circumstances. The Ministry of Health was interested in the trip, they said, but he could not go to the Embassy, that could not be changed. When passing that message to Mr. Alexander, the latter's reaction was unambiguous: without a conversation, there would be no participation in the trip. The interview would serve first of all as an examination of Neumann's knowledge of English; either come to the Embassy or refrain from participation. The Ministry, however, stuck to its decision.

"The senior physician of the neurological department of our Jena university clinic, Dr. G. M., looked after a patient who had come to him with neurological complications as a result of another illness and who had come to him for professional consultation, in which I had also been involved. This patient, known under the name K. H., was an associate of the district administration Gera of the MfS (his service rank and tasks are unknown to me). Because I appreciated him as a humanly sociable, rather modest patient, I dared to turn to him with the request for advice how I should behave in the delicate situation," remembers Jochen Neumann.[357] "Comrade H. showed understanding for the situation and gave me the following advice: you go to the US Embassy without informing the Ministry of Health. I take that responsibility.... however, I expect a detailed report from you afterwards on the details of the visit and the conversation."

Mr. Alexander tested Neumann and came to the conclusion that his language ability was sufficient for his participation in the trip. "Moreover he gave me instructions and references how to complete the questionnaires (a membership in a Communist Party was normally a hindrance in the acquisition of a US entry visa), on the side saying that they knew anyway who I was but that the consular section worked under strict rules and, therefore, I should not mention my Party membership."

Two days later, Neumann was invited to a second conversation with Mr. Alexander and was informed that in a few days he would depart for the USA. "Also about this I gave a precise (oral) report, with which comrade H. was satisfied. He asked me on this occasion whether, in the future, I would be willing to collaborate with the MfS in a more or less similar form in comparable situations and within the framework of my travels. I confirmed my agreement to cooperate without hesitation (based on my Communist conviction, I felt that I was called upon to protect my country), on the condition that this work would concern international

357 Report by Neumann written and sent to the author on August 6, 2009

issues, especially regarding the defense against hostile activities damaging to the DDR. I further stipulated that I would **not** be ready to undertake activities linked to the collection of data and information on citizens of our country, patients and colleagues in particular."[358] Neumann is given the cover name "Hans."[359] Upon his return from the United States, where he coincidentally met Mel Sabshin for the first time during a visit to the offices of the American Psychiatric Association, he delivered a 27-page detailed report on his experiences. The report has an addition of 29 pages listing all the persons he met, institutions he visited and information on the other participants in the trip.[360]

---

358 The bold is Neumann's. In his report he adds that in the book of Sonja Süss these circumstances are not represented fully correctly: "All the subsequent events were described by Ms. Süss *in principle correct, in the detail occasionally somewhat distorted.*"
The Stasi archive includes a detailed report by the Stasi officer who met with Neumann on May 10, 1979, in which Neumann's personality is described in detail. The report confirms that Neumann refused to provide any personal information on others, including his friendship with a French communist and former Nazi-camp inmate: "because the person in question has been close to him for many years. He would act differently, when it would concern a person who would not be so close to him." (MfS/BV Gera, AOPk 780/80 Band 2, p. 71) However, this can also be seen as a tactical way of saying "no".
During the above-mentioned meeting, Neumann also explained how he otherwise could be useful to the MfS. According to the author of the report, Neumann behaved sometimes in an unusual way, putting questions to trigger answers and by doing so apparently trying to assess how much the Stasi knew about him. For instance, the Stasi officer reports, Neumann wanted to know what during a next meeting they would like to know from him about his private life, and whether he should report any connections to women. According to his report the Stasi officer answered that it would only be of interest if it had any operational significance, and concludes at a certain point: "…one can conclude, that 'Hans' underestimates us and overestimates himself. (…) In general terms, I am not convinced of the honesty and reliability of the person and it would be advisable not to make use of the operational possibilities suggested by him."BstU, MfS/BV Gera AOPk 780/80, pp. 72-3

359 *Politisch Missbraucht*, p. 621; BstU, MfS/BV Gera AOPk 780/80, p. 68-74

360 BstU, MfS/BV Gera AOPk 780/80, pp. 128-186. This report on his trip to the USA is the only document that contains personal information on his fellow travelers and the persons he met, including information on their "personality structure". However, in his reporting he limited himself to factual information, their positioning with regard to Eastern European countries and socialism and refrains from allegations that could be of operational assistance to the Stasi, e.g. to blackmail them. In addition, the file contains a six page record of a debriefing upon Neumann's return, written by his MfS *Führungsoffizier*.

The contacts with K. H. were soon abandoned and Neumann was handed over to colleague with the first name of W. "With W. I met several times in Weimar in a secret meeting place. This W. was an arrogant ass with a distinct ambition; he was psychologically unfit, somewhat clumsy and dull. He tried to make all of my personal acquaintances and friends into potential suspects, as a result of which distance between us grew, up to the point of more or less sharp discussions in which I referred to the clear boundaries that I had set regarding my readiness to cooperate." Neumann refused to continue the meetings and broke off contact with the Stasi.

The Stasi archives confirm that the relationship between W. and Neumann was certainly not optimal, but for them it is actually an indication that Neumann was not reliable and honest: "During the collaboration, the *Führungsoffizier* got the impression that, in the case of the person concerned [Neumann], one deals with a person whose reliability and honesty is not a given fact. … N. is, for instance, not prepared to give the MfS information on persons that are of interest – in particular DDR citizens. Work for the MfS he described in front of our associate in a degrading and impudent way as 'sniffing around'… In conclusion, there is a paradox in the initial declaration of willingness [to collaborate] and the current refusal to provide information, as a result of which the associate was not able to judge the motives of N. with regard to his collaboration with the MfS. Every now and then, he expressed only his willingness to report on his contact with the US Embassy and demands in that respect also clear instructions how to behave."[361]

In order to understand his motives and to assess his reliability, the Stasi puts Neumann himself under surveillance, and his mail and telephone is checked. For Neumann, the outcome is not unimportant, because with a negative outcome his permission to travel abroad and to work in higher State functions would be under direct threat. It could kill his career. To his benefit, the surveillance by the Stasi ended after nine months, when it was concluded that it was impossible to clarify his motives beyond doubt and that therefore further collaboration was undesirable.[362] His career continued undisturbed. In 1982, he became General Director of the Hygiene Museum in Dresden, and was appointed as Professor of Psychiatry at the University in Dresden. The same year, Neumann was registered again as an *Inoffizieller Mitarbeiter*, this time under the cover name "Erhard."[363] He reported on

361 *Politisch Missbraucht*, p. 622; BstU, MfS/BV Gera AOPk 780/80, p. 216

362 *Politisch Missbraucht*, p. 622

363 *Politisch Missbraucht*, p. 623. Neumann is registered as "Erhard" on August 26, 1982, under number 6048/82. His *Führungsoffizier* is Harry Sattler, who is known to Neumann as Harry Kupfer, see for instance in chapter 4, "Meeting

his foreign trips (e.g. his report on the WPA Congress in Vienna, July 1983)[364] but did not engage himself in spying on his colleagues, as most of his compatriot psychiatric leaders did. Two years later, in 1984, "Erhard" became active as a member of the Executive Committee of the World Psychiatric Association.

Subjective yet fascinating

The reports by Jochen Neumann are fascinating reading, without doubt. They are of high literary quality, clearly show his intelligence and his ability to analyze situations, at certain moments are humorous and unbelievably frank. The recipients must have taken a deep breath when reading Neumann's open criticism of the Soviets, his growing admiration of the Americans and, finally, his criticism of what is happening in his own country. Yet, at the same time, they also show his loyalty to the DDR, his desire to help build a Communist society in spite of the fact that he became increasingly disenchanted, and his principled behavior. He agreed to serve his country, and he did it, in spite of everything.

His criticism of the Soviets and admiration of the Americans is certainly not there from the very start. Clearly, during his five years on the Executive Committee, Neumann goes through a process of a changing his worldview, and develops a more balanced understanding of the political reality, which is also reflected in his use of wording. In his report on the Vienna Congress of 1983, he still very much uses all the obligatory political slogans and formulations. For instance, he writes that "a circle of Zionist agitators dominate the Royal College and this is in its turn in England in agreement with official circles the leading view. Exactly these Zionist connections led to the systematically prepared anti-Soviet attitude and the abuse of the voting machinery and open manipulation."[365] It is, as far as I could establish, the only report in which the term "Zionist" is used. In his 1984 report on the Executive Committee of the WPA, he has changed his wording already to "the Royal College group."[366]

Jochen Neumann". According to Neumann, his recruitment mainly concerned his foreign trips, and probably was an attempt to test his reliability and have him ready for a later assignment – which turned out to be the WPA. E-mail Jochen Neumann, August 30, 2009.

364 *Sofortbericht* Jochen Neumann, Vienna World Congress, 21 July 1983. 6 pages.

365 *Sofortbericht* Jochen Neumann on the Vienna Congress, July 27, 1983, p. 3

366 "The influence of the Royal College groups is extraordinarily big, as before, but less important than in Vienna." Report on the Rome EC meeting, October 19, 1984, p. 2

Surely, his reports are subjective, and when reading them I come to elements where I clearly see where his interpretation is not in line with what I perceive as the truth. For instance, in a report on the trip to New York, Washington and Mexico in October 1988, he reports on a reception at the American Psychiatric Association which Koryagin attended and where I, coincidentally, was his interpreter. Neumann writes: "I was able to observe, for instance, how at an evening reception Koryagin with Van Voren, who interpreted for him into Russian, were walking around alone for many hours and were not engaged by anybody in a conversation or recognized. Simply not any person was interested in them."[367] I raked my brains after reading this, and slowly the images of the meeting came back to me. Indeed, part of the time Koryagin and I had separated ourselves from the participants, discussing tactics and reviewing the day, as we often did. In addition, many of the professionals around weren't sure about how or when to interact and were cautious in doing so without being sure that it was OK to do so. In reality, I functioned as interpreter but, in fact, Koryagin and I formed a team, and these discussions were ongoing.[368] But reality is that Koryagin was considered a hero, and many people wanted to talk to him, even just meet him and feel his presence. He made an enormous impression, including on Stefanis's wife,[369] and his intransigence on the Soviet issue made this appeal to the wider public even stronger. Here you had a man who survived six years in the Gulag, who had been on hunger strike for two years almost consecutively, who had never given in and always showed the Soviets his contempt. Koryagin was, for them, the image of a real hero.

I very well remember several occasions, both in Europe and the United States, where Koryagin was welcomed as a pop-star. His first appearance in Amsterdam was in May 1987 at the Sakharov Congress held there, of which I was one of the organizers. He was not only welcomed with a standing ovation, the photography session after the meeting turned into a fist-fight among journalists who wanted to have the best photo opportunity. I was shocked at the journalists' behavior, but Koryagin accepted it more or less stoically, or maybe it all passed him as if in a dream, still trying to cope with the sudden change from endless isolation in Chistopol prison to being a star in the West.

This difference in interpretation makes documents sometimes a bit difficult to use, because they are subjective – as Neumann time and again stressed in our conversations – or hide the emotional connotation, such as in the

367 Report on the WPA EC, October 1988, p. 6

368 See, for instance, *On Dissidents and Madness*, pp. 119-120

369 See chapter 18, Meeting Costas Stefanis

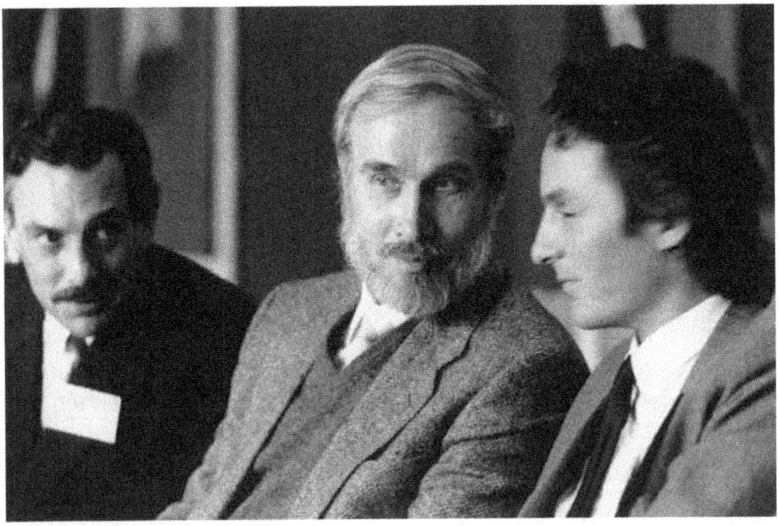

Koryagin in Amsterdam, May 1987

minutes of the WPA Executive Committee meetings where one has to really read between the lines in order to see what actually went on. A great help in retrieving at least part of this are the frequent interviews with those who were there; in particular, the double interviews with Melvin Sabshin and Jochen Neumann, where one stimulates the other and the factual knowledge of one is combined with the analytical knowledge of the other. Gradually, step by step, a picture of what really happened emerges, but it remains a limited reflection of what really took place.

Stasi files

The building is like any other office building in Berlin, a new structure on Karl Liebnecht Strasse in what used to be East Berlin, of which the traces are gradually fading away, either torn down to be replaced with modern high rises, or hidden behind an ever increasing amount of overpowering advertisements and other symbols of the "decadent West." Inside it is all well organized, almost sterile, with friendly staff taking you from one office to the next, like a patient in a clinic being prepared for surgery. One room is a sort of dressing room, but instead of taking off your clothes, you are told to leave your personal belongings behind, except pen, paper, laptop and your silenced mobile phone. Then, the door swings open, and you enter the reading room, where silence reigns and people are diligently working away. It brings back memories from university, the auditorium where exams took place, people sitting behind separated little tables with a chair, standing in long rows, and a supervisor sitting in front, making sure that you do not do something illegal. My table was in the far end, and the mountains of files were staring at me, inviting me to come over and explore. My fingers itch; this is real heaven for historians, files that hide their secrets that, by the end of the day will be yours.

Everything was meticulously prepared with unbelievable diligence and care. Little notes already indicate where and in which folder I probably could find what I was looking for, all the files have already been checked by my case manager, my *Führungsoffizier* as I almost automatically start to call her. Until recently the files were made anonymous in advance, with all the references to outside individuals blackened. This practice has since ended; it was too time consuming, so I now get to see the files in their full glory.

I started reading and soon any glorious feeling disappears. The first file contained personal information, referring to the way a person was recruited, operational information, agents' requests for surveillance of a potential suspect or references provided by others. But it also contains materials on why the person agreed to collaborate, and my first file was immediately a hit. For a long time, I had wondered why the person concerned agreed to collaborate; somehow, I couldn't fit the story into my head. And here it was: adultery. The person had a love affair with somebody who ran into serious trouble, trouble that threatened to spill over to her and her marriage, and only by agreeing to collaborate was she was let off the hook: no consequences, no information to her husband, but for a price, and a very high one indeed. The person reported on everything, from adultery by others, to alcoholism, homosexuality, political indiscretions and attempts to leave the country. It was a nasty sequence of petty spying, indicators of a person losing her moral dignity as a result of an earlier infidelity. And in the files her own story was filled with information on other love affairs, on warnings by others about the couple's alleged desire to flee the country, resulting in more investigations and surveillance, all concluding that she could still be considered "reliable." That is, until she actually flees, leaving her husband behind, and leaving the Stasi bewildered because of the unexpected turn of events.

I screened other files, on other *Inoffizieller Mitarbeiter*, and also there I found evidence of petty spying, of reporting on others in their private or work environments, either out of political conviction, defending the fatherland against traitors from inside, or just out of careerist opportunism. I had a bitter taste in my mouth, nausea caused by seeing so much dirt, mixed with a sense of disbelief because of the systematic and detailed control machinery that was in place, checking and double checking even the most ridiculous detail (like sending a pair of glasses to the "technical department" to have it checked as to whether there were any hidden compartments. Answer: "it looks like it is in its original state, nothing found," a document signed by two engineers). And I started to understand that Jochen Neumann really is an exception to the rule. He was almost a moral island in this sea of indiscretion, this gross violation of basic trust and normal human interaction, a person who, in spite of his agreement to work with the MfS, never lowered himself to their level. More than ever, I understand his remarks in a letter to Ellen Mercer in November 2008, before our communication was established: "I have been some kind of a hybrid between a deeply convinced communist on the one hand and a cosmopolitan on the other. I also was (culturally considered) a cross between a bourgeois of the XIX century and an engaged communist.... You may imagine how fragile my position within the country was: a mixture of an insider and an outsider at the same time. Higher levels of my party appreciated and made use of my capacity to create and to maintain international contacts on a more interpersonal and less official level. The majority of my East-German psychiatric colleagues, mediocre, poorly educated and small minded through and through, didn't know the world beyond the frontiers and had no confidence in my … intentions."[370]

I left the building with a full head, after a seven-hour plunge into the Stasi past. I walked into a changed East Berlin, which now more than ever seems to be a strange mix of two layers, two worlds – communism and capitalism. That same evening, I met Jochen Neumann, we had a drink. To my surprise, he brought me a pile of his reports, found in his home while preparing to move to a smaller apartment. They are the same that I found that afternoon in the Stasi files, but better preserved and with small notes attached, instructions to his secretary to whom to send copies. We talked and I tell him what I found that day. But I was not able to tell him to what extent one of the people he still respects was spying on his colleagues, and was certainly no better than the rest. I don't want to take away that last illusion from him; it is already too much.

[370] Letter Jochen Neumann to Ellen Mercer, November 11, 2008

Part IV

Act Two

Chapter 23 – Power Struggle in Moscow

No one is a villain gratis; there is always a determining motive, and that motive is always an interested one.[1]

Good and evil flow from the same spring.[2]

The relations between Georgi Morozov and Marat Vartanyan never recovered from the 1985 investigation by the Disciplinary Committee of the CPSU. To the contrary, they continued to worsen when the power struggle became more and more intense, further fired by the issue of a possible return of the Soviets into the WPA, by foreign influence and by the political changes in the country itself.

Georgi Morozov had a strong power base in the political elite, as noted before, being the son-in-law of Anatoly Strukov, a very influential Party official, and said to having close to a number of high level Soviet political leaders, including KGB Chairman Yuri Andropov. He knew many people high up in the political establishment and, thus, had strong political clout within the Party himself (as illustrated by riding a *Chaika* as his personal car). He reached the top of the scientific level by becoming first a candidate member of the Academy of Medical Sciences and later a full member, and was honored with the whole possible range of Soviet medals and awards. His relationship with the KGB will probably always remain unclear, but is, in fact, not of such great importance. As Viktor Gindilis points out in his memoirs, "the orders came from the party or the [security] organs. A Communist of whatever rank had to implement these demands, just like thousands of other rank-and-file and not-rank-and-file communist-psychiatrists in the whole country."[3] At the same time, however, he had not been able to push through the investigation against Vartanyan in 1985-1987, partially because of Zimyanin switching sides, and partially because of the sacking of Boris Yeltsin as party leader in Moscow.

Marat Vartanyan, as we saw in a previous chapter, was linked to a different political faction and his closest relationship was probably Evgeni Chazov, the cardiologist who treated many political leaders and who eventually managed to climb to the position of Minister of Health of the USSR and member of the Central Committee of the CPSU. He was severely threatened

1 Montesquieu, as quoted in Tzvetan Todorov, *Hope and Memory*, p. 79

2 Rousseau in *Letrte sur la vertu*, p. 325

3 Gindilis, p. 213

by the investigation of 1985-1987, but managed to escape with a Party reprimand, and continued his scheming to get to the top. He managed to become a candidate member of the Academy in 1985, and a full member in 1988, and in spite of Snezhnevsky's attempt to block his ambitions in 1985, he succeeded Snezhnevsky as Director after the latter died on July 12, 1987.

At the same time, Morozov lacked an international network. Not only is it very difficult to find anybody who really liked him (the most positive remark is Gindilis' that he was "ascetic"), but his name was also invariably linked to the political abuse of psychiatry. The same counted for Vartanyan, but Morozov was Director of the Institution that internationally was considered to be the Lion's Den. On top of that, he had diagnosed many dissidents himself, signing psychiatric diagnoses that sent them away for many years of psychiatric "treatment" in special and ordinary psychiatric hospitals. In other words, he was personally seen as a "hangman."

Vartanyan was, on the other hand, an international wiz-kid, who managed to win people over even though they may have been disgusted by what he represented, but who, at the same time, fell for his charm and nice stories. He skillfully used these international relations to impress the political bosses in Moscow, and show that, by betting on him, they could recover the lost political reputation within the international psychiatric community. That which got him in trouble in the Soviet Union – the wheeling and dealing – turned out to be his major asset internationally.

How much this clash between two psychiatric dinosaurs in the Soviet Union hurt Soviet interests vis-à-vis the WPA can be seen from the reports of Jochen Neumann. Time and again the members of the WPA Executive Committee noticed that communication was obstructed by either side, purely for reasons of personal interest. In November 1986, Neumann writes: "In the Executive Committee, there was a unanimous feeling that for quite some time, Prof. Morozov obstructed the resumption of contact because the conversations until now and also the support from the WPA Vice-President [Neumann] were linked to Prof. Vartanyan. They speak openly about the fact that everything that does not originate from Prof. Morozov directly is torpedoed by him, and that, vice versa, everything that is handled by him personally succeeds."[4]

---

4 *Reisebericht* Jochen Neumann on the WPA EC Meeting in Rio de Janeiro, November 1986, p. 3

In the course of 1988, the battle for power intensified. Morozov held the important position of President of the All-Union Society, through which he exerted enormous control over the psychiatric elite, but it was exactly this position that got him in trouble. It was clear that the All-Union Society had very little chance to return to the World Psychiatric Association if Morozov was still in place, and, thus, it became politically expedient for him to leave that position. A battle for power ensued.

The favored candidate for the position of President of the AUSNP among the political elite seems to have been Yuri Aleksandrovsky, at that moment Deputy Director of the Serbski Institute. However, Morozov managed to block his promotion to that position by exposing some minor misdemeanors from the past. Because of the uncertainty of Aleksandrovsky's candidacy, the Annual Congress of the AUSNP was postponed until October 27-28, 1988. Vartanyan, on the other hand, favored his deputy Aleksandr Tiganov as the future President of the AUSNP. Tiganov, who originally succeeded Snezhnevsky in the 1950s as Director of the Institute for Post-Graduate Medical Training, had recently been promoted to the position of Deputy Director of Vartanyan's Research Institute for Clinical Psychiatry of the Center for Mental Health of the Academy of Medical Sciences.[5] In the summer of 1988, he had also been promised by Vartanyan to be made a Corresponding Member of the Academy of Medical Sciences, a proposal that was apparently supported by Chazov. In other words, Vartanyan was moving him step-by-step in the direction of being a faithful replacement when necessary.

According to unconfirmed information from Moscow, collected by Peter Reddaway from reliable sources during one of his trips to the Soviet Union, Vartanyan made use of his friendship with Costas Stefanis to maneuver his candidate into a better position. During the meeting with Evgeni Chazov in October 1988, which according to Jochen Neumann lasted for about an hour,[6] and which took place just before the start of the Congress of the AUSNP, Stefanis is said to have lobbied for Vartanyan's candidate, while discrediting Georgi Morozov by saying that if the latter remained President of the AUSNP, the chances of a return of the All-Union Society were very small indeed.[7]

5 His predecessor as Deputy Director, Ruben Nadzharov, who was also heavily implicated in the political abuse of psychiatry, had suddenly retired in the summer of 1988 and thus the position had become vacant.

6 Report on the EC of the WPA by Jochen Neumann, October 1988, p. 4

7 Travel report by Peter Reddaway, *Documents* 15, January 1989. The meeting is confirmed by Jochen Neumann in Jochen Neumann's report on the WPA EC

However, Vartanyan's plan failed. Probably Morozov's clout among the political leadership was still stronger and thus, unexpectedly, his protégé Nikolai Zharikov was pushed forward and elected as President of the All-Union Society, after having been selected in advance by key Central Committee figures.[8]

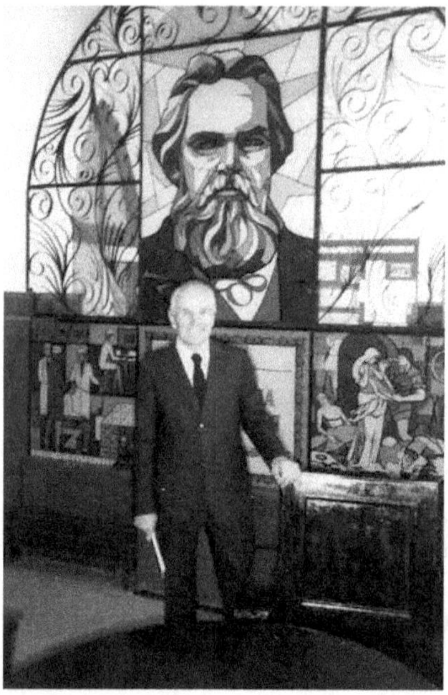

Nikolai Zharikov, 1989

The choice could not have been worse. Nikolai Zharikov, a psychiatrist working at the Serbski Institute and Deputy Editor of the Korsakov Journal of Neuropathology and Psychiatry, then the main psychiatric journal in the Soviet Union, was not only personally involved in the political abuse of psychiatry but also a person with the same inability as Morozov to communicate with Western psychiatry.[9] As we will later see, his clumsiness drove others to madness, not only the Western psychiatrists he was supposed to convince, but also Jochen Neumann, who was trying to defend the Soviet cause within the WPA leadership but saw his attempts constantly undermined by Zharikov's unsophisticated behavior. However, the choice was also a good illustration of the lack of understanding of the new political reality on the part of the old Party establishment that, in spite of the enormous changes in the country itself, stuck to old mechanisms and reactions.

The election of Nikolai Zharikov to the position of President of the All-Union Society was not the only major change voted upon at the Congress of

meeting, October 1988, p. 4. However, the details of the conversations are not mentioned there.

8 Travel report by Peter Reddaway, *Documents* 15, January 1989

9 Nikolai Zharikov, also a Corresponding Member of the Academy of Medical Sciences, had been personally involved in well-known cases such as Vladimir Bukovsky and Yuri Shikhanovich. See the *Biographical Dictionary on the Political Abuse of Psychiatry in the USSR.*

the AUSNP. The neuropathologists, fed up with being constantly associated with the political abuse of psychiatry and the resulting international isolation, left the association and joined the neurosurgeons in a new organization. Instead, the narcologists joined the All-Union Society, and thus it was renamed into "All-Union Society of Psychiatrists and Narcologists."

In addition, the decision was reached to re-apply for membership of the WPA.[10] But actually, the decision to apply had been taken earlier, and considering the way the AUSNP left the WPA in 1983, it would be safe to assume that also this decision was taken or at least endorsed by the political leadership of the country.[11] The AUSNP was still supposed to endorse it at their Congress, which was to take place after the meeting of the WPA Executive Committee had taken place.[12] A telegram informing the WPA that the Soviets were ready to rejoin reached the WPA leadership in mid-October, well ahead of the AUSNP Congress and just in time for applications as set by the WPA Statutes. The message reached the WPA Executive on the eve of a WPA Regional Symposium in Washington D.C, where the WPA Executive Committee would meet to discuss the situation.[13]

---

10 *Vremya*, October 28, 1988, 18.00 GMT. See *Documents* 12, November 1988

11 In 1983 the decision was clearly a political one taken at the highest possible level, and was for instance known to the DDR leadership and the Stasi before the WPA was informed. See chapter 16.

12 See Jochen Neumann's report on the WPA EC meeting, October 1988, p. 3

13 Jochen Neumann's report on the WPA EC meeting, October 1988, p. 3. See also *Documents* 12, November 1988

Chapter 24: Political Changes at Home

"Yesterday they gave me freedom...
What should I do with it?"
Vladimir Vysotsky

While leading Soviet psychiatrists remained intransigent and continued to deny that anything was wrong in Soviet psychiatry, attributing outside actions to being part of a Cold War slander campaign, Soviet society started to change with an ever-increasing speed and eventually found itself on a rollercoaster out of control.

In April 1985, Mikhail Gorbachev had been appointed General Secretary of the CPSU, following a long period of ailing and almost invisible Soviet leadership. Gorbachev was of a younger generation that had not participated in the Great Patriotic War (as the Second World War was called in the Soviet Union) and had seen Stalin's terror from the other side: his maternal grandfather had been subject to repression.[14] Initially very little changed and, in particular, the political repression of dissidents continued and even worsened, but by the end of 1986 a fundamental shift took place. The catalyst was the death of the well-known writer and dissident Anatoly Marchenko, who had served most of his life in prisons and camps and had been on hunger strike for three months in Chistopol prison.[15] The

---

14 Mikhail Sergeyevich Gorbachev (born 1931) was the last General Secretary of the Communist Party of the Soviet Union, serving from 1985 until 1991, and also the last head of state of the USSR, serving from 1988 until its collapse in 1991. He was the only Soviet leader to have been born after the October Revolution of 1917. Gorbachev was born in Stavropol Krai into a peasant family, and operated combine harvesters on collective farms. His maternal grandfather, a veteran Communist, narrowly escaped execution after having been branded a Trotskyite. He graduated from Moscow State University in 1955 with a degree in law. While in college, he joined the Communist party of the Soviet Union, and soon became very active within it. In 1970, he was appointed the First Party Secretary of the Committee of the CPSU of the Stavropol Krai (Kraikom), First Secretary to the Supreme Soviet in 1974, and appointed a member of Politburo in 1979. After the deaths of Soviet Leaders Leonid Brezhnev, Yuri Andropov, and Konstantin Chernenko, Gorbachev was elected General Secretary by Politburo in 1985. Gorbachev's attempts at reform as well as summit conferences with United States President Ronald Reagan contributed to the end of the Cold War, ended the political supremacy of the Communist Party of the Soviet Union (CPSU) and led to the dissolution of the Soviet Union. He was awarded the Nobel Peace Prize in 1990.

15 Anatoly Tikhonovich Marchenko (1938-1986) was an influential and well-known Soviet dissident, author, and human rights campaigner. Initially a

Soviets' decision to let him emigrate came too late: while his wife was preparing the emigration documents, he succumbed to a variety of ailments and malnutrition. At that moment, the CSCE was having one of its major conferences in Vienna, and the death of Marchenko caused uproar. The Americans threatened to walk out and freeze the process of détente, and Gorbachev understood that something fundamental had to be done. He called Andrei Sakharov, the dissident leader and Nobel Peace Prize laureate who had been exiled to Gorki in late 1979 after criticizing the invasion of Afghanistan, and asked him to come back to Moscow "to serve his country." Sakharov agreed.

Release of political prisoners

Less than two months later the first political prisoners were released, and one of them was Anatoly Koryagin, the imprisoned psychiatrist and Honorary Member of the WPA. "At the beginning of February 1987, the situation changed dramatically for Koryagin. Galina [Koryagina] on the phone, completely beyond herself of excitement: "He is home!" she shouted, "Tolya (her name for Anatoly) is at home! He is sitting in the bath scrubbing off the dirt and is unbroken. He is only talking about how he is going to continue his fight with the authorities!" A few hours before, she and her sister met him on the street by sheer coincidence, when they were on their way to the post office to call me. He was just coming from the train station. They had released him from Chistopol prison, where he had been

worker on a drilling gang, and not of intellectual background or upbringing, he became radicalized, and turned to writing and politics, after being imprisoned as a young man on trumped-up charges. During his time in the labor camps and prisons he studied, and began to associate with dissidents. He first became widely known through his book *My Testimony*, an autobiographical account of his then-recent sentence in Soviet labor camps and prison, which caused a sensation when it was released in the West in 1969. It brought home to readers around the world, including the USSR itself that the Soviet gulag had not ended with Stalin. He also became active in the Soviet human rights movement and was one of the founder members of the influential and much-emulated Moscow Helsinki Group. He was continually harassed by the authorities, and was imprisoned for several different terms, spending about 20 years in prison and internal exile. He died in Chistopol prison hospital at the age of 48 on December 8, 1986, as a result of a three month long hunger strike he was conducting, the goal of which was the release of all Soviet prisoners of conscience. The widespread international outcry over his death was a major factor in finally pushing then-General Secretary Mikhail Gorbachev to authorize the large-scale release of political prisoners in 1987.

incarcerated just like the deceased Anatoly Marchenko. He had taken a train home. Nobody was waiting for him, of course, because nobody knew he had been released. But suddenly he was there, standing in front of his wife. He was very emaciated, looking years older, but unbroken and in a very good mood. It was a complete miracle."[16]

Immediately following his release, Anatoly Koryagin started issuing his first official statements, in which he called upon the Soviet authorities to release all political prisoners and indicated that he was going to continue his struggle. He did not have to wait very long. Soon after, a wave of releases started, as a result of which hundreds of political prisoners were told to go home. "The main address to collect information was Larisa Bogoraz, the widow of Anatoly Marchenko. The reason was that everyone understood that his fatal hunger strike had forced the authorities to initiate the release of all prisoners, and so they first reported to her, first of all to offer their condolences, and, secondly, as a sign of respect to her late husband."[17]

The way in which they were released differed from case to case. Some were released unconditionally. Others had a conversation and were warned not to get involved in politics. There were also those who were asked to sign a statement in which they promised not to become politically active again. Even at that point there was a split: some refused and were released anyway, others refused and went back to their cells, only to be released much later.

The wave of releases lasted two years. Many political prisoners were released already in the course of 1987, yet the political prisoners from psychiatric hospitals had to wait longer.[18] Most of them were only released in 1988 and 1989, as part of the pressure on the Soviets to show that they mend their ways and the Soviet attempt to show that they were ready to return to the WPA. Possibly, their reluctance to release dissidents from psychiatric hospitals was related to their denial that anything had been wrong in Soviet psychiatry: if you release them, you indirectly admit that their hospitalization had been unfounded. How effective their resistance was is shown from the memoirs of Andrei Kovalev, who during those years

16 *On Dissidents and Madness*, p. 98

17 *On Dissidents and Madness*, p. 99

18 "This category of offenders appears to have moved very slowly in comparison to others. Sixty-four political prisoners were released from psychiatric hospitals this year and permitted to return home, compared to 19 released in 1986 and virtually none in previous years." *Soviet Abuse of Psychiatry for Political Purposes*, A Helsinki Watch Report, 1988, p. 3

worked at the Ministry of Foreign Affairs in Moscow and was involved in the negotiations on human rights with the US State Department, with a special interest in Soviet psychiatric abuse. When, in the spring of 1988, Gorbachev was about to embark on his first visit to the United States, orders were given to release a number of political prisoners form psychiatric hospitals. "It was unacceptable not to use this unique possibility of putting strong pressure on the psychiatrists, judicial authorities and courts that, unfortunately, happily prolonged the periods of compulsory treatment and only with reluctance ended them. ... At the last moment ... somebody somewhere decided to put a stick in the wheel. The mechanism to release dissidents from psychiatric incarceration was blocked. It turned out to be necessary to use strong methods of conviction and explain to the psychiatrists that not informing the General Secretary of the Central Committee of the CPSU could have severe consequences."[19]

Soviet press

Until 1987, the Soviet media had supported leaders of Soviet psychiatry almost unconditionally; virtually the only exception was an article in 1985 accusing psychiatrist Eduard Babayan, head of the department for addiction problems of the Ministry of Health, of "lack of principle" and other failings, which led to his removal from his position.[20]

However, psychiatry did not remain untouched by "glasnost." In the beginning of 1987, the first articles severely criticizing Soviet psychiatry appeared in the newspapers *Meditsinskaya Gazeta* and *Sochialisticheskaya Industriya*.[21] In these articles a number of leading psychiatrists were accused of taking bribes for issuing false psychiatric reports so that the person who paid for such a report could avoid military service.[22] The articles were restricted to this form of malpractice, however. What was remarkable was that the articles admitted that false reports had been drawn up and that two psychiatrists named were closely involved in the political abuse of psychiatry. One of them, Professor Margarita Taltse, was at that time head of the Fourth Department of the

---

19 *Page from the Book of Condolences*, p. 9

20 *Pravda*, October 30, 1985, and *Sovetskaya Rossiya*, November 24, 1985. Eduard Babayan had been one of the spokespersons of the Soviet delegation to the WPA World Congress in Honolulu, 1977, and was one of the apologists of Soviet psychiatric abuse.

21 May 20, 22 and 27, 1987 in *Meditsinskaya Gazeta* and January 31, February 1, March 24 and May 20 and 30, 1987, in *Sochialisticheskaya Industriya.*

22 *Sochialisticheskaya Industriya,* January 31 and February 1, 1987

Serbski Institute in Moscow, exactly the place where political cases were being assessed.[23]

In two further articles, published four months later, and in particular in the three articles published in *Meditsinskaya Gazeta*, this was explored further. Although there was no question of reports on political abuse of psychiatry in these articles, it could not be coincidental that of the twenty psychiatrists mentioned by name, five were closely involved in the political abuse and that of the eight clinics mentioned, five were places where dissidents had been held. Two of the psychiatric institutions named were even directed by key architects of the political abuse of psychiatry.

The reason for this sudden anti-corruption campaign was summarized by the Minister of Health of the Russian Republic Dr Anatoly Potapov as follows: "The acceptance of bribes and the practice of extortion in a number of clinics has become customary… it is time the truth was told… For sums of money, healthy people are changed into sick people. Evidently anything can be bought in the psychiatric hospitals in the Moscow area."[24] The author of the series of articles in *Meditsinskaya Gazeta* did not doubt who the guilty persons were: "Again and again the same group of psychiatric specialists have 'manufactured' schizophrenics out of normal persons."[25]

---

23 The Fourth Department was headed by the notorious Daniil Lunts until his death in 1977, after which Taltse took over. Prior to this she had been Lunts' deputy. She herself was involved in quite a few political cases, such as of Vyacheslav Igrunov, Yuri Shikhanovich, Iosip Terelya and Ivan Yakhimovich. See Koppers: *Biographical Dictionary*, p. 48

24 *Sotsialisticheskaya Industriya*, January 31, 1987

25 *Sotsialisticheskaya Industriya*, January 31, 1987.
Anatoly Potapov, a psychiatrist by profession, was from 1965 to 1983 director of the psychiatric hospital in Tomsk. He was closely related to Yegor Ligachev, leader of the more 'conservative' faction in the Soviet Politburo, who was party-secretary in Tomsk at more or less the same time. Potapov and Ligachev were said to be friends and went out hunting together, and it was Ligachev who brought Potapov to Moscow. Coincidentally, also Chief Psychiatrist of the USSR Ministry of Health Aleksandr Churkin was also from Tomsk and probably belonged to the same group. Also USSR Health Minister Evgeni Chazov thanked his position as Minister of Health to Ligachev.
In 1990 it was revealed in the Soviet press that Anatoly Potapov himself had been involved in the political abuse of psychiatry. "At a ceremonial meeting of the hospital staff in 1971 [in Tomsk], which I attended, Potapov said literally the following: 'We expect to register a great number of patients on November 4-7. There'll be a special mark on their papers. They are suffering from 'paranoid schizophrenia'. We are to accept them all no matter how many there are…". *Moscow News* no. 37, 1990, reprinted in *Documents* 38, September 1990.

According to *Meditsinskaya Gazeta,* the acceptance of bribes led to a "whole system by means of which criminals are enabled to escape punishment by being sent to a psychiatric hospitals. This system can lead to the release of very dangerous criminals after two or three years."[26] Among the psychiatrists responsible for these practices were two specialists who also played a part in the political abuse of psychiatry. Tamara Pechernikova, a head doctor on the staff of the Serbski Institute, was for a long time involved in declaring dissidents mentally ill.[27] In the case reported in the *Meditsinskaya Gazeta,* she recommended that a double murderer be discharged as 'cured' after a three-year confinement. The author of the article later found out that the man was not mentally ill, but had paid a large sum of money to have himself declared mentally ill, thereby escaping the death penalty. After his release, he committed two more murders.

A second psychiatrist, closely involved in the issue of political abuse of psychiatry, Dr. Aleksandr Churkin, at that time chief psychiatrist of the Ministry of Health of the USSR, sent a dangerous criminal to the Kashchenko psychiatric hospital for compulsory treatment. However, the clinic was not at all equipped for dangerous criminals and the man even got permission to go on vacation. During such an excursion, he carried out a large-scale robbery.[28]

From *Meditsinskaya Gazeta,* it also became clear that in the spring of 1985, a criminal investigation had been started against the corrupt psychiatrists. The head of the investigation reported to the newspaper that "the affair unexpectedly produced other cases, and new suspects came to the attention of the investigators. Some of them have already been sentenced."[29] As a result one of them, Dr. Yuri Massover of the Kashchenko Psychiatric Hospital, was sentenced to nine years of hard labor for accepting bribes.[30]

---

26 *Meditsinskaya Gazeta*, May 27, 1987. Since 2001 the Global Initiative on Psychiatry, of which the author is Chief Executive, has carried out a whole range of projects in the field of forensic psychiatry and prison mental health in former Soviet republics, notably Lithuania, Russia and Georgia. In all of these countries the same practice still prevailed.

27 Among her victims are the poetess Natalya Gorbanevskaya, Vyacheslav Igrunov and Yuri Yakhimovich.

28 *Meditsinskaya Gazeta*, May 27, 1987

29 *Meditsinskaya Gazeta*, May 27, 1987, and *Argumenty i Fakty*, no. 5, January 30, 1988, p. 7

30 It is not clear, whether this investigation is the same as against Marat Vartanyan, or a separate one. According to a travel report by Peter Reddaway of June 1990, Massover was strongly defended by his colleagues and asserted his innocence. Also well-known dissidents believed he might have been framed. The

Since the Kashchenko Psychiatric Hospital constantly reappeared during the criminal investigation process, a special commission was formed to study that particular hospital. The conclusion left no doubt: "The current procedures regarding the organization and execution of forensic psychiatric examinations in the Kashchenko Psychiatric Hospital are not in accordance with the directives of the Ministry of Health; the professional standard of the specialists is low; new personnel is not trained; the committees of specialists have not been revised for a long time, and almost half of the specialists have been inadequately trained."[31]

A long article in the government newspaper *Izvestiya* in July 1987 went even further.[32] The paper acknowledged that authorities had been sending troublesome Soviet citizens to psychiatric hospitals, where they had been declared to be mentally ill. *Izvestiya* discussed two of such cases in detail. The first concerned a woman who had complained about faulty treatment for cancer. She was taken from her bed in the middle of the night in order to be sent to a psychiatric hospital. The resistance by family and neighbors and the fact that she barricaded herself in a room made the attempt fail. In answer to questions by *Izvestiya,* the judicial authorities answered: "The sick person was visited at home in order to make a diagnosis. The medical committee [consisting of a psychiatrist, a doctor and a bench worker] concluded that she showed signs of paranoid schizophrenia.... She is insane, she inundates everyone with statements." Although the attempt to have the woman forcibly committed failed, she was put on the list of psychiatric out-patients, and only after four years of struggle and the intervention by *Izvestiya* her name was taken off the list.[33]

---

suspicion centred on Vartanyan, who might have framed Massover in order to take the attention away from himself.

31 *Sochialisticheskaya Industriya*, May 30, 1987

32 *Izvestiya*, July 11, 1987

33 The psychiatric register was a matter of serious criticism. In early 1988, Chief Psychiatrist Aleksandr Churkin claimed in an interview with *Corriere della Sera* (April 5, 1988) that 5,5 million Soviet citizens were on the register and that 30 percent would be removed from that list within two years. However, a year later the journal *Ogonek* (no. 16, 15-22 April, 1989, p.24) gave a figure of 10,2 million, that it had received from the state statistics committee. People on the psychiatric register were registered with a dispensary and had some of their civil rights taken away. On top of them, it was hard for them to find a job, housing etc., as a result of which they were outcasts in society. Severe criticism was also voiced in 1979 by Dr. Etely Kazanets in his article in *Archives of General Psychiatry*: "It was exceptional for a diagnosis to be revised in favour of an exogenous diagnosis or vice versa. This resulted in long and unfounded retention of patients on the dispensary list... Keeping these people on dispen-

The second case in *Izvestiya* concerned a woman who continuously complained about noisy neighbors. "When a letter addressed to the Ministry of Interior Affairs (MVD) was again received by the Petrovka [the popular name of the MVD in Moscow], the police reached the end of their patience." The woman was taken away by the police and, by means of a trick, hospitalized and compulsorily treated for a period of three months. When the police was asked why, the answer was quite simple: "She wrote, and wrote, it was clear that she was not normal." Also in this case *Izvestiya* intervened. An investigation carried out by the Ministry of Health revealed that the woman was quite normal and certainly did not need any psychiatric treatment."[34]

The authors of the article in *Izvestiya* quoted a directive of the Ministry of Health, which stated that "persons who disrupt work of institutions by numerous letters with a senseless content" were liable to be confined to a psychiatric hospital. The authors pointed out that in most cases commitment to a psychiatric hospital for compulsory treatment occurred without a court order and that no possibility existed to contest the decision. Apparently a law had been prepared in 1977 that made a court order for compulsory hospitalization obligatory, but the law had been held up by a highly placed official in the health care system. The authors argued that new legal measures should be taken that would guarantee the rights of the patient, including the right to appeal such decisions.[35]

---

sary lists for long periods constitutes a real threat to their individual rights. (…) [It] infringes on rights and influences a great many things, such as fitness for military service." See: Kazanets, E., *Differentiating exogenous psychiatric illness from schizophrenia*, p. 740-746

34 *Izvestiya*, July 11, 1987

35 On January 5, 1988, the Presidium of the Supreme Soviet adopted such legal measures. However, the law was severely criticized both inside and outside the USSR as being insufficient. Reason for this appears to have been the strong resistance within the medical establishment that led to a watering down of the proposed text. According to Andrei Kovalev, "that [draft] document was provided to Shevardnadze, who fully understood the overriding effect it would have on Soviet psychiatric inquisition. Work continued on getting a decision by the Politburo concerning the need to adopt a law that would regulate all aspects of psychiatric help. Unfortunately the Ministry of Health together with the repressive organs managed to win n the battle with the Foreign Ministry. (…) Although [the law] was worked out at the initiative of Shevardnadze, whose key parameters were written down in the minutes of the Central Committee, we managed to work on the text only in the course of the written voting within the Politburo." *Page from the Book of Condolences*, p. 11

After the visit of the US State Department delegation in March 1989 and the Athens World Congress in October that year, a new law was drafted. However,

At the same time, *Izvestiya,* for the first time, openly criticized the prevailing psychiatric theories is the USSR, and in particular Snezhnevsky's theories with regard to (sluggish) schizophrenia.[36] In November 1987, the newspaper *Komsomolskaya Pravda* added its voice, and quoted a number of Snezhnevsky's psychiatric symptoms, including "an exceptional interest in philosophical systems, religion and art." The paper quoted from a 1985 *Manual of Psychiatry* published by Snezhnevsky's Moscow School of Psychiatry:" We managed to find ten different kinds of this illness [schizophrenia] with all manner of forms and variations. The symptoms which may be found in different cases were astonishing. They include, for example, withdrawal, eccentricity, affectation, slovenliness, gluttony, hyperactiveness, and exaggerated opinion of oneself, exaltation, or conversely lethargy, absent-mindedness, undue sensitivity, capriciousness, a sense of inadequacy, irritability, vulgarity, argumentativeness, or the manifestation of a particular interest in philosophical systems, religion, art." The authors subsequently concluded: "In that way the diagnosis of 'sluggish schizophrenia' can be applied to virtually anyone who, in any conventional sense, is sane."[37]

Until then it seemed that the days of the leaders of Soviet psychiatry that were heavily involved in the political abuse of psychiatry were numbered, but immediately after the article in *Komsomolskaya Pravda* the tone in the Soviet press started to change. On November 20, 1987, a week after the *Komsomolskaya Pravda* article, *Sovietskaya Rossiya* published an interview by the extremely conservative journalist Eleonora Gorbunova with Anatoly Potapov, the Minister of Health of the Russian Republic, who had been so critical earlier that year. In the interview, Potapov confirmed that compulsory hospitalization occurred far too often and that patients were labeled schizophrenic too frequently, but he added that Soviet journalists should show more restraint. "We must use publicity in a responsible way, otherwise lawmen will get the impression that they can be locked up in a clinic without reason."[38] Potapov directly attacked *Komsomolskaya Pravda* for publishing their article. The change in atmosphere was undoubtedly linked to the dismissal of Boris Yeltsin, exactly on the day

buy the time it was ready to be introduced the Soviet Union collapsed; the law was subsequently adopted by the Russian Federation. One of the authors, Svetlana Polubinskaya, subsequently assisted many other former Soviet republics to draft their new legislation.

36 See chapter 9: The origins of Soviet political psychiatry

37 *Komsomolskaya Pravda,* November 11, 1987. The same day Boris Yeltsin was sacked as Party leader of Moscow.

38 *Sovietskaya Rossiya,* November 30, 1987

that *Komsomolskaya Pravda* published its article, which had also resulted in a discontinuation of the investigations against Marat Vartanyan.[39]

A different wind was now blowing in the Kremlin. Potapov's critical remarks were followed two days later by those of Evgeni Chazov, the Soviet Minister of Health. During a televised press conference he repeated earlier claims that alleged victims of political abuse of psychiatry had turned out to be mental patients upon arrival in the West. He also added another argument that would be used many times in the coming months, namely that the critical articles on psychiatry in the Soviet press had resulted in attacks against psychiatrists with deadly consequences: "One sad piece of news I can give you, for example, is that yesterday in Moscow a psychiatric doctor was killed, and another is in grave condition in the intensive care unit at Botkin Hospital. I believe the Soviet press must be aware of these situations."[40] Shortly after, the same Chazov managed to have Marat Vartanyan appointed by the Moscow City Party Committee, now headed by Yeltsin's successor Lev Zaikov, as successor of Andrei Snezhnevsky as Director of the All-Union Research Center for Mental Health.[41]

In February 1988, the newspaper *Trud* published an article by the same Eleanora Gorbunova, who repeated that the critical articles had led to attacks on psychiatrists, and also mentioned that in November 1987 a psychiatrist had been killed in Moscow. Since February 1987, sixty-five aggressive actions against psychiatric officials had been reported in the Moscow area alone. The article in *Izvestiya*, Gorbunova wrote, had "provoked an explosion of aggression from mentally ill people. ... Being sick people unable to answer for their actions, they are demanding of psychiatrists that

39 See chapter 20. On 21 October 1987 at a plenary meeting of the Central Committee of the Communist Party, Yeltsin, without prior approval from Gorbachev, lashed out at the Politburo and expressed his discontent with both the slow pace of reform in society and the servility shown to the General Secretary. In his reply, Gorbachev accused Yeltsin of "political immaturity" and "absolute irresponsibility," and at the plenary meeting of the Moscow City Party Committee proposed relieving Yeltsin of his post of first secretary. Nobody backed Yeltsin. Criticism of Yeltsin continued on 11 November 1987 at the meeting of the Moscow City Party Committee. After Yeltsin admitted that his speech had been a mistake, he was fired from the post of first secretary of the Moscow City Committee and demoted to the position of first deputy commissioner for the State Committee for Construction.

40 Moscow Television Service, November 22, 1987, 11.00 GMT

41 For more on this see Chapter 20. Lev Zaikov, a full member of the Politburo, was according to Moscow journalist Mikhail Poltoranin closely affiliated to Yegor Ligachev. See *Corriere della Sera*, May 12, 1988

they open the hospital doors, accusing them of treating them incorrectly and to no effect."[42] Quite possibly these claims were based on real facts, and it is no surprise that persons turned against their psychiatrists when finally, after many years of maltreatment and inhumane living circumstances, it seemed that the outside world now finally acknowledged that something had been wrong. However, the authors of these claims, among them Marat Vartanyan,[43] were not interested in the cause of the aggression towards psychiatrists; they used it as an argument to silence the press.

Only in the spring of 1988 did the climate change again, but much of the momentum was lost. One of the persons who managed to get a number of articles published in the Soviet press in 1988 was Semyon Gluzman, the dissident psychiatrist who had served seven years in camp and three years in exile for his "diagnosis in absentia" of General Pyotr Grigorenko. Gluzman had been one of the authors of the *Manual on Psychiatry for Dissenters*, together with Moscow dissident Vladimir Bukovsky, in which they gave guidelines to potential future victims of political psychiatry how to behave during investigation in order to avoid being diagnosed as being mentally ill.[44]

"During one of my travels to Moscow I visited, as usual, Irina Yakir. It was spring 1988, morning and time for a cup of coffee, and at Irina's you could always find out the latest news and gossips. ... When I entered her flat, somebody was already sitting in the kitchen. It appeared to be a slightly reserved and shy man, with a small beard, a somewhat nasal voice and with "ants in his pants," because he was about to visit a number of editorial offices to get his articles published. We were increasingly curious about each other, in particular because according to Irina we had a lot in common and because we shared the interest in the political abuse of psychiatry. He introduced himself: "Semyon Fishelevich." Bells started to ring, because I knew only

---

42 *Trud*, February 16, 1988. Eleanora Gorbunova had earlier published articles with the same message, such as a report for Novosti press agency on August 4, 1987, based on an interview with Marat Vartanyan, Vladimir Tikhonenko, Ruben Nadzharov and Vyacheslav Kotov.

43 Made during the Novosti interview, see the reference above.

44 See chapter 9. Some of the diagnoses they quoted in this *Manual* were from psychiatric diagnoses of Tamara Pechernikoca, earlier mentioned in this chapter: "ideas of fighting for the truth and justice most frequently arise in personalities with a paranoid structure" and "the ligious-paranoid state develops following psycho- traumatizing circumstances which affects the interests of the person concerned, and is typified by accusations of encroachment upon the legal status of the individual."

one Semyon Fishelevich and that was Gluzman. Indeed, it was Semyon Gluzman himself sitting in Yakir's kitchen across the table from me."[45]

The meeting in Yakir's kitchen was to be the beginning of a long process of rapprochement. Gluzman was a careful man, different than most of the dissidents I knew. He took a philosophical approach, putting things in perspective. His articles were careful analyses of the systematic abuse of psychiatry for political purposes, not attacks and listings of human rights violations. In spite of what had been done to him, and in spite of the fact that he had lost many of his friends and acquaintances in the camps, Gluzman had found the strength to put all the events in perspective. The reserved attitude of Gluzman changed only slightly during the following meetings. "He observed me, looked from a corner in the kitchen to the interaction between me and Yakir and, a certain sense of trust developed. At the same time, however, the difference in approach formed as big a barrier. I was an activist; I led a campaign to keep the Soviets out of the WPA unless they would admit their guilt. For me, everything was pretty much black and white, and that was a position that was fully shared by Anatoly Koryagin and other dissidents. For Gluzman, things were much more fluid, for him black and white didn't exist and the answer to who was good and who was bad was much less clear. For him, all were victims of the Soviet system, both prisoners and guards. So, for him it was not that all Soviet psychiatrists were wrong and all dissidents were right."[46] His articles were published in several Soviet journals and newspapers.[47]

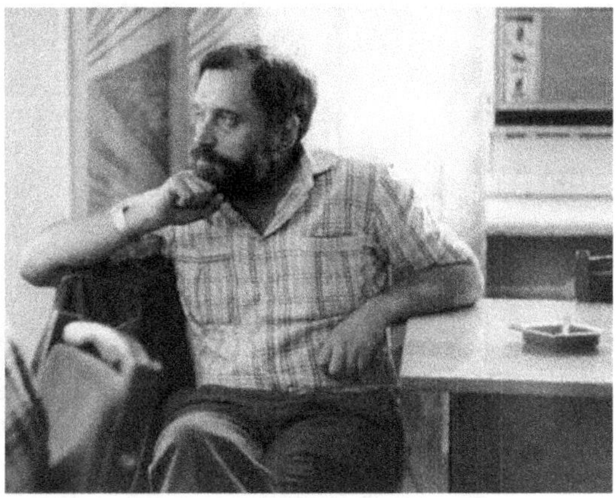

Semyon Gluzman 1989

---

45 *On Dissidents and Madness*, pp. 112-3

46 *On Dissidents and Madness*, p. 114

47 *Selskaya Molodezh*, No. 8, 1989, pp. 32-36; *Raduga*, October 1989, No. 10, pp. 56-67. A collection of the articles was published by IAPUP on the eve of the WPA World Congress in Athens in October 1989 under the title "*On Soviet Totalitarian Psychiatry*". The collection also contained other works by Semyon Gluzman.

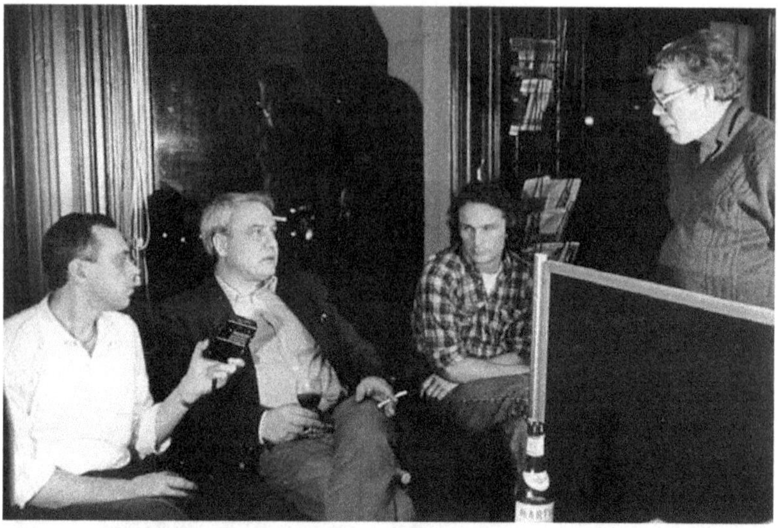

Vladimir Bukovsky is interviewed by the Sverdlovsk film studio crew. Right from him Robert van Voren

The interest in the issue did not wane, and also attracted other media. The television studios in Sverdlovsk (now Ekaterinburg) decided to make a film on the subject and producer Boris Kustov contacted Semyon Gluzman. Through him, they came to me and in the spring of 1989, the film crew stood on our doorstep in Amsterdam. A long list of former victims of political abuse of psychiatry had agreed to be interviewed and traveled to Amsterdam. This list included the well-known Ukrainian dissident, Leonid Plyushch, who had been released in 1975; the poetess Natalya Gorbanevskaya from Paris and, from Hamburg, the Bashkir poet Nitzametdin Akhmetov. The crew also did a large number of interviews in the Soviet Union, not only with well-known victims of political psychiatry but also with the leaders of Soviet psychiatry. They appeared on film in a good mood, sure of their cause and also of their eventual success in Athens: they were already celebrating their victory.[48]

[48] The film was eventually shown to the Soviet public in the spring of 1990 during a public viewing at the cinema "Strelya" in Moscow. See *Documents* 36, June 1990.

Chapter 25 – Irritation, Admiration and Disenchantment

The best political jokes were told within the Central Committee [of the SED]; the higher the joke-teller was ranked, the sharper the joke.

Jochen Neumann

From the very beginning, it was clear that the Soviets were not going to build their future on Jochen Neumann. This had not only to do with the person himself, even though it seems quite likely that the Soviet psychiatric leadership received copies of Neumann's reports to the Stasi and therefore knew his opinion of them.[49] If that was the case, they might have seen him as a "Trojan Horse," a peon who turned out to be a liability and not an asset. Equally important was probably the typical combination of Soviet imperial arrogance and Russian negligence that often played a factor in Soviet politics. And, to make things worse, the views on how a return of the All-Union Society should be brought about differed fundamentally. As Neumann states, "I had the 'class order' to find myself a position in the highest echelons of the WPA. The unspoken main goal was to represent the policy of the socialist bloc within the WPA. In what way this should be attained, that was clearly subject to differences between the comrades from the DDR and the Soviets. According to the DDR-view I should obtain respect through *fruitful professional collaboration* and then by building upon this success exert *political* influence. The leaders of the All-Union Society were, in majority, blockheads without any vision, they believed that only by showing their muscles could they recover the lost positions."[50]

Also the starting point was quite different between that of the Soviet All-Union Society and the new (Acting) Vice-President. Whereas the Soviets maintained that nothing was wrong with Soviet psychiatry and that they were deeply insulted by the unjust allegations leveled against them, Neumann's view on the situation was much more realistic: "One thing was absolutely clear: between Hawaii and Vienna, the Soviets (and with them all other socialists) lost one battle after the other and were eventually

49 There are several possible "tracks" along which the Soviet psychiatric leadership knew the content of Neumann's reports. It is quite likely that the Stasi forwarded the content to their colleagues at the KGB, who shared at least part of the content with people like Morozov and Vartanyan. At the same time, Vartanyan probably retained contact with his friend Rolf Müller, who was deputy Minister of Health of the DDR and himself an IM of the Stasi, and who received copies of all of Neumann's reports.

50 Personal notes of Jochen Neumann, August 16, 2009. Italics by Neumann.

forced to retreat. Even though the socialist professional societies presented themselves under Soviet leadership as militant and optimistic and grouped together in a bloc of protesters, the situation was a catastrophe: in the third biggest NGO in the world, the representatives of the Eastern Bloc had no longer a say, even worse, they were out of it."[51] This was a view that no Soviet psychiatrist would have ever ascribed to.

And thus the relationship was cool from the very start, and grew increasingly tense. In a report on his participation in a Congress of Psychiatrists of Socialist Countries held in Moscow in September 1985, Neumann does not try to contain his disdain: "The scientific level of the Congress was close to banal. … The language of the congress was only Russian, which did not facilitate communication."[52] The congress also results in the first conflict between the Soviets and Neumann. An interview is arranged with the Soviet press agency TASS, and Neumann is asked his opinion. "The interview was given in a way that clearly expresses our class position as is expected from a representative of the friendly DDR delegation." However, Neumann was not presented as a DDR psychiatrist, but as Vice-President of the WPA: "It was mentioned three times that it concerned the position of the Vice-President of the World Psychiatric Association, as a result of which there certainly will be problems with the WPA, as the DDR-representative is not allowed to make such statements and present it as the position of the Executive Committee. In a way there had been a bit of manipulation. … It is not good when the DDR-representative in the WPA is pushed in a corner in such a way."[53]

With time, Neumann became increasingly irritated by the way the Soviets dealt with the situation, an irritation that was very much shared by Stefanis. In June 1986, Stefanis expressed his frustration to Neumann, as quoted in the latter's travel report: "The Soviets did not know before Hawaii [Honolulu Congress 1977] what was going on in the WPA, and came to inadequate conclusions and measures. Before Vienna they were inadequately informed and lost a lot of time, and reacted not always with the right steps and decisions, and now again they do not know exactly what the atmosphere is, and will do again irreparable harm. It seems it eludes them completely that the world is counting on a renewed collaboration and that the majority of colleagues react to their extreme reluctance with lack of understanding. The WPA will exist like this also in the future, if necessary without the Soviet Union, which would be detrimental to the WPA and in

51 Personal notes of Jochen Neumann, August 16, 2009

52 *Ergänzungsbericht zur Reise Moskau 24-27.9.1985*, p. 2

53 *Ergänzungsbericht zur Reise Moskau 24-27.9.1985*, p. 3

particular to the socialist countries; this would leave the field, to a large degree, to two or three Western countries. The influence on the colleagues in the Third World cannot be underestimated."[54]

A year later, in November 1987, the situation was no different. Neumann angrily reports to the DDR leadership that "as before, the leading comrades of the All-Union Society are evidently completely uninformed about structures, persons and backgrounds, and function in international affairs extraordinarily rude and unprepared. In Warsaw, Prof. Kovalev ... was present as an official observer of the All-Union Society. ... He was not informed about anything, neither about the history of the issue nor about the statutes and [the organization's] bodies, and even less about persons and their backgrounds. He was not even informed as to who was a member of the Executive Committee and who has which opinion. He was completely unaware of the Committee, its tasks and its membership."[55]

Also, Neumann must have felt quite embarrassed when the Soviets were on the scientific program, as they usually presented something outdated or, by international standards, rather odd. For instance, on October 24, 1987, a press report on the scientific meeting in Milan points out that "before [Soviet psychiatrist Juri] Saarma took the podium, most of the speakers had outlined their research into schizophrenia with elaborate slides, which often showed results of extensive cooperation with leading researchers in various parts of the world. Saarma's speech on 'certain aspects of neurophysiological studies' seemed to confuse doctors in the audience when he did not use the usual international terms. He talked about measuring 'internal inhibition' in schizophrenics and demonstrated his remarks with brief handwritten notes flashed on a screen at the front of the auditorium. Some of the participants looked around in bewilderment, especially after Zharikov took the floor to talk about Pavlov's influence on Soviet psychiatry. ... The president of the meeting, Professor Carlo Cazzullo of Milan University, interrupted to provide an international term. He explained that Saarma was talking about 'psychometric tests.' Cazzullo said that Saarma had done extensive research into this field."[56] Cazzullo's intervention did not take away the doubts about the Soviets' scientific level.

During the same meeting, Georgi Morozov showed his 'negotiating skills' by putting three conditions on a Soviet return to the WPA, as if the ball

54 *Reisebericht Basel* by Jochen Neumann, June 1986, p. 10

55 *Reisebericht Basel* by Jochen Neumann on the WPA EC meeting in Warsaw, November 1987, p. 3

56 RL/RFE report, October 24, 1987, 01.56 AM

was in their court and they could afford to set the terms: "First, he said, the Soviet Union wanted the WPA's voting system changed. He said it was undemocratic that countries like Britain and France had 25 to 27 votes, while countries like India had three votes. Second, Morozov said, the Soviet Union wanted the WPA to reply to Soviet explanations of Western accusations that the USSR was abusing psychiatry. He said the Soviet Union had once supplied the explanations at the WPA's request, but the organization had never commented on them. Third, Morozov said, the Soviet Union wanted a guarantee that the WPA would not be used for political attacks on the USSR if the Soviet Union rejoined. He suggested asking WPA President Costas Stefanis of Greece, who was also in Milan, about the reaction from WPA officials."[57] Stefanis declined to comment, the report continues, but one does not have to be a clairvoyant to understand that his blood must have been boiling, and the same undoubtedly counted for Neumann, who was not present in Milan at the time but was informed later.

Neumann's irritation was further heightened by the fact that the Soviets continued to meet his attempts to represent the socialist bloc with disinterest and even suspicion. For instance in October 1988, when the AUSNP had informed the WPA by telegram of its intention to rejoin the WPA, Jochen Neumann met several times with Marat Vartanyan in New York at a symposium on "Steps that will Revolutionize Psychiatry in the 21st Century." Vartanyan had been invited to that meeting by a number of psychiatrists who were favorably inclined to the Soviets and he participated actively in the program. Later, Vartanyan was also in Washington D.C. at the time of the Regional Symposium, but only few people knew of his presence in the capital.[58] Also in this case, the Soviets did not make much use of the services of Neumann, as he somewhat bitterly remarked in his report to the DDR-leadership: "As before the Soviets (Prof. Vartanyan) are not very clever and psychologically sensitive in their choice of means and methods; as a result, because of their inconsideration with regard to clear psychological issues, already existing conflicts are strengthened and not brought to an acceptable solution. (…) The reporter [that is, Neumann] had repeated contact with [Vartanyan] in New York. However, it was like in the past, where they do not need any suggestions or situational descriptions from the DDR-representative; they are apparently of the opinion that they have an overview of the situation and are able to get things under control through personal relations and contacts with a number of individual - indeed respectable and important - personalities of American psychiatry."[59]

57 RL/RFE Report, October 25, 1987, 03.58 AM

58 See Jochen Neumann's report on the WPA EC meeting, October 1988, p. 4

59 Jochen Neumann's report on the WPA EC meeting, October 1988, p. 4

The October 1988 report by Neumann also shows that Morozov's attitude towards Neumann differed a bit from Vartanyan's: "Already during my stay in the USA, Prof. Morozov tried to inform the DDR-representative [Neumann] of what had happened. As far as I know the President of the WPA suggested inviting the Vice-President and DDR-Representative to the meetings in Moscow, but this was turned down by Prof. Vartanyan as being "not appropriate." [60]

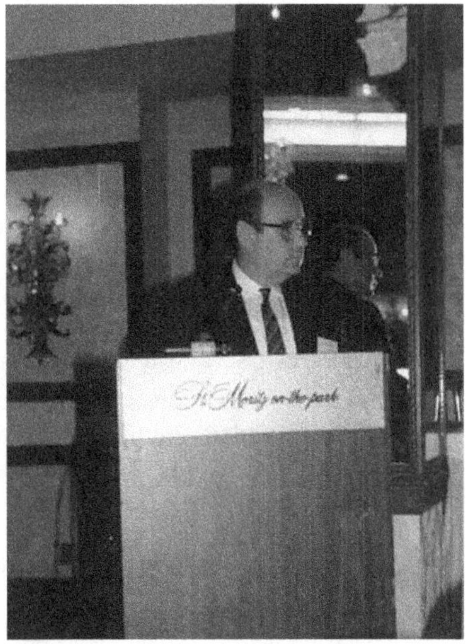

Neumann speaking in New York, October 1988

The relationship with Zharikov also was, from the very beginning, not really optimal, to put it mildly. In March-April 1989, Neumann's irritation level reached a new peak, and he wrote: "ACHTUNG [beware]: The All-Union Society is not even one bit more diplomatic, flexible and engaged than in the past."[61] But this is not all. Neumann continues: "Prof. Zharikov was present in Granada (via which line is not clear) and during a discussion on the changes in Soviet psychiatry, he behaved in a way that was close to pure stupidity. Because of his not answering concrete questions and by repeating boring long platitudes, the participants in the meeting were completely frustrated and irritated. Pyotr Morozov, who was also present, let me know that he belonged to a 'different Moscow School' as Prof. Zharikov and showed me more or less clearly that he was keeping a certain distance from him.[62] He told me personally that because of perestroika at this moment in Moscow one doesn't know who has to say what, but that this is perestroika. Comrade [Pyotr] Morozov is in his behavior of course much more flexible and clever and actively seeks contact with influential American psychiatrists."[63] And Neumann adds one final

60 Jochen Neumann's report on the WPA EC meeting, October 1988, p. 5

61 Report Jochen Neumann on the WPA Executive Committee, April 1989, p. 3

62 Pyotr Morozov, a relatively young Moscow psychiatrist and son of the late Professor V.M. Morozov (and not a relative of Georgi Morozov), probably referred to his belonging to the Vartanyan camp, while Zharikov clearly belonged to the Morozov faction.

63 Report Jochen Neumann on the WPA Executive Committee, April 1989, p. 3

remark on Zharikov, which doesn't need any comment: "The disregard of form and lack of being informed has not changed on the Soviet side. Prof. Zharikov asked the reporter [Neumann] at a certain moment the number of members of the Executive Committee and whether Schulsinger was one of them."[64]

From admiration to friendship

The reports by Jochen Neumann for the DDR authorities form a very valuable indicator of his changing perspective through his years of WPA service. Several years of continuous communication with Western psychiatry and exposure to life outside the DDR undoubtedly influenced his views and positioning, even though he maintained that he was a faithful Communist and representative of his country. One of the organizations that clearly impressed Neumann was the American Psychiatric Association, of which his fellow EC-member Melvin Sabshin was Medical Director. In May 1987, he reported on the sessions of the Executive Committee in Chicago[65] and makes use of the situation to write quite an extensive exposé on American psychiatry and the APA, in which he stresses the pluralist atmosphere within the organization and the fact that within the APA a wide variety of interests are being represented: "for instance in Chicago the Congress was supported by some very diverse psychiatric associations, of which the 'Gay and Lesbian Psychiatrists' were far from being the most obscure."[66] Interestingly, he also remarks that "according to leading representatives of the USA, the issue of psychiatric human rights is the number 1 problem for the survival of psychiatry in the USA; and that in spite of the misuse of these issues for political purposes by certain circles within psychiatry and in particular outside psychiatry, anti-socialist and anti-Soviet goals do not play a prominent role among the psychiatrists."[67]

In his report on the Executive Committee meeting in Warsaw in November 1987 Neumann is even more positive about the American Psychiatric Association: "The APA is a magnificently organized and functioning organization, without which nothing happens in American psychiatry, in addition to the fact that the APA in an equally magnificent manner organizes scientific life and is unusually rich. … A direct state influence on American psychiatry is absent. It is rather such that the APA, which is organized

---

64 Report Jochen Neumann on the WPA Executive Committee, April 1989, p. 3

65 May 10-12, 1987

66 Report by Neumann of May 26, 1987, on the sessions of the EC in Chicago

67 Report by Neumann of May 26, 1987, on the sessions of the EC in Chicago

according to purely capitalist principles, exerts influence that reaches into the lobby of the White House and in Congress. The APA possesses its own high-rise building and functions with an annual profit of millions.[68] The APA follows carefully political life in the USA and has direct influence on it."[69]

Initially his relationship with other members of the Executive Committee remained formal, with a hesitance to be more open and relaxed. Considering the fact that he initially considered himself to be among people who were "either neutral… or clearly pro-Western"[70] this attitude is not so strange: Neumann was not just a regular member of the Executive Committee, but also had the task to represent the interests of the socialist countries and on top of that lived a double life as IM of the Stasi – all factors that did not really stimulate the development of close friendships. Also he felt himself dropped into a lion's den, with Stefanis and Schulsinger openly and sometimes very vocally fighting over leadership of the WPA, Neils Reisby being invisible and Jorge Alberto Costa e Silva hiding behind Sabshin's back. For someone who had never functioned within the leadership of an international organization, this was a rather uncomfortable situation that needed time for adjustment.

From the very first moment, Neumann felt that, with Melvin Sabshin, he touched common ground: they shared the desire to do business and get the necessary work done. As far as the Soviet issue was concerned, they were clearly on either side of the barricades, but on most other issues they agreed. In his report on the Rome meeting, Neumann writes: "Sabshin is an extremely clever man and tends towards compromises and elegant formulations, which enable collaboration and a constructive attitude even in conflict situations. He seems to combine clear pro-Western ideological attitudes with a tactically shrewd, neutral positioning, during which he himself separates his position as a representative of the American Psychiatric Association and as member of the EC. … The formulation found in order to end [the discussion on] Koryagin's issue also comes from Sabshin."[71] Later that year, Neumann even reports that Sabshin "contributes constructively to the solution of the problem in which he often goes against the Royal College and even the APA."[72]

---

68 Actually the APA didn't own the building in which it had its offices.

69 Report by Neumann of November 1987 on the sessions of the EC in Warsaw; *Politisch Missbraucht*, p. 664

70 *Ergänzungen zum Bericht*, Jochen Neumann, October 1984, p. 2

71 *Ergänzungen zum Bericht*, Jochen Neumann, October 1984, p. 16

72 *Reisebericht Athen 11. bis 18. Oktober 1985*, p. 12

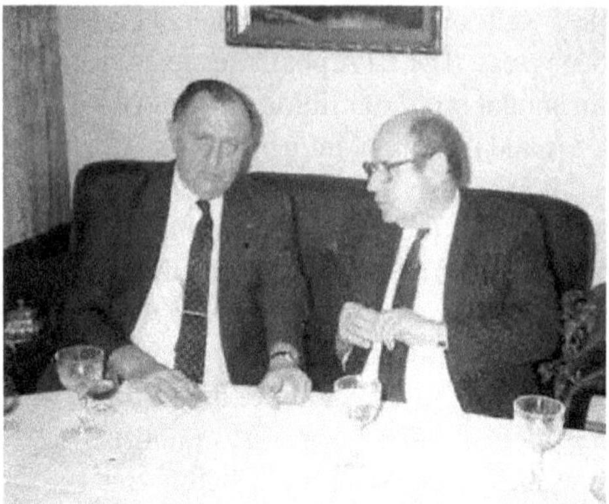

Melvin Sabshin and Jochen Neumann, 1988

During the first years, their relationship was businesslike, without any personal connotation, although Melvin Sabshin remembers that Jochen Neumann was quite ill during an Executive Committee meeting in Jaipur, India, in January 1986 and that he spent much time at his bedside, caring for him and at the same time discussing many issues. The real turnaround came during a session of the Executive Committee in Sydney in April 1988, almost three-and-a-half years after his inauguration as member of the Executive Committee. Unfortunately the minutes of these Executive Committee meetings have not been found, but according to both Jochen Neumann and Melvin Sabshin there was an item on the agenda with regard to the Soviet issue that was highly contentious. So contentious that for Neumann it was reason enough to put his EC-membership at stake. He went to Melvin Sabshin and said: "You need to be with me on this. You understand that if this passes, I will have to resign from the Executive Committee. Help me to avoid this from being adopted." Melvin Sabshin agreed, by answering: "I will support you, but I also have something important for me. If you vote with me on this, then I will support you." And thus it happened.[73]

After concluding this secret "deal," a relationship of trust started to develop between the two men, which then gradually turned into friendship. And such friendship also developed with Ellen Mercer, who usually accompanied Melvin Sabshin on his travels and met Neumann regularly. "With Ellen things were easier," Neumann recalls. "She was not a member of the Executive Committee, had no official position within the WPA and was therefore more accessible and easier to communicate with."[74] A big impact

73 Interview with Jochen Neumann and Melvin Sabshin, July 30, 2009. The deal concerned a symposium on Soviet political abuse of psychiatry, organized by IAPUP, which was part of the program of the WPA Regional Symposium organized by the APA in Washington D.C. in October 1988. Intense negotiations followed, in which Melvin Sabshin played a key role. The symposium became eventually an allied event, not under the responsibility of the WPA. I return to that issue in a later chapter.

74 Interview with Jochen Neumann, June 4, 2009

on their relationship was the aftermath of the WPA Regional Symposium in Granada, in March-April 1989. Because of bad weather, the flights were canceled to Madrid, and many of the congress participants and WPA leaders we stranded at Granada airport. Each and everyone went his way to make alternative arrangements, but for Neumann this was an impossible situation: without credit cards, without the necessary currency, he had no alternative than to sleep at Granada airport on a couple of chairs and wait for the next plane out. Ellen Mercer quickly understood the predicament and took Neumann under her wings. She cut a deal: if Neumann agreed to drive, she would rent a car, so that they could find their way to Madrid. Neumann agreed.

The trip to Madrid took quite a few hours, a perfect opportunity to get to know each other and to talk about issues. First general interests were covered, then their life stories, and eventually politically more sensitive issues, such as the issue of Soviet psychiatric abuse. By then, Neumann's irritation over the Soviets' position had reached a new peak thanks to Zharikov's behavior, as mentioned above, and gradually the acknowledgement that indeed something was fundamentally wrong with Soviet psychiatry had settled in his mind. The trip with Ellen Mercer and their long discussions strengthened this position.[75]

During the last year of his term as Vice President, Neumann developed a relationship with both Mel Sabshin and Ellen Mercer that would not only survive Athens and the subsequent fall of the Berlin Wall, but that would also help him through the most difficult period of his life and last until this very day. In fact, without this friendship this book would never have been written.[76]

Disenchantment

Even though twenty years after the collapse of socialism in Eastern Europe, Jochen Neumann still maintains affectionate feelings for the country he served loyally and at much personal expense, it does not mean he remained blind to the failures of the system he helped build. The period 1984-1989 very much helped him open his eyes, to see the world in a different

75 Interview with Jochen Neumann, June 4, 2009; interview with Ellen Mercer, June 28, 2009.

76 It was Ellen Mercer who informed Jochen Neumann on November 30, 2008 of my interest in meeting with him and encouraged him along the way. After initial hesitation, Neumann agreed. Our first meeting took place in February 2009.

perspective, and also to see how the system he faithfully represented had strayed far away from the ideal he had envisaged in his youth and which the Communist leaders of his country still proclaimed as a reality.

Throughout his travel reports, and from the very start, Neumann expressed dissatisfaction with the way his own country dealt with the situation. In his report on the Executive Committee meeting in Rome in October 1984, during which he was elected, he complained about the fact that the DDR authorities had provided him only with "an ancient copy of the statutes of the early 1970s, although statutes and regulations play an unbelievably important role in any organization. In fact, the Polish candidate was sidetracked because his nomination had not been in accordance with the statutes. Also the membership fee of the DDR was too late because a transfer had not yet been received; by chance, the General Secretary's assistant noticed this and the delegate [Neumann] could show proof of the paid amount."[77]

In a later report, Neumann complained about the fact that the East German society every year paid for the same number of members (225), which became a bit suspicious: "Maybe one should, for reasons of cosmetics, vary the numbers."[78] In addition, the fact that the DDR society did not answer questionnaires sent around by the WPA caused irritation: "Also the DDR Society has not used the chance to express its views."[79] Another point of contention was the fact that Neumann was not included as a member of DDR delegations to Congresses of Psychiatrists of Socialist Countries and thus "cannot be of assistance to the WPA President… This situation is not completely understandable; in particular, because DDR delegation of ten people did include some who neither politically nor professionally or organization-wise had anything to offer in any way."[80]

Also the constant problems obtaining visas and getting travel documents at the last minute were a constant reason for anger. In April 1985, Neumann complained angrily about the late provision of the necessary papers and the subsequent treatment by German customs officers: "This caused … an enormous hectic rush for a large group of associates and comrades and the unjustified involvement of high diplomatic channels under an extraordinary pressure of time. In the end, a whole day of the meeting of the Executive

77 Report by Neumann on his participation in the EC meeting in Rome, October 19, 1984, p. 5

78 *Reisebericht* of Jochen Neumann, WPA EC Meeting in Basel, June 1986, p. 5

79 *Reisebericht* Jochen Neumann, WPA EC meeting Amman, April 1987, p. 2

80 *Reisebericht* Jochen Neumann, WPA EC meeting Amman, April 1987, p. 4

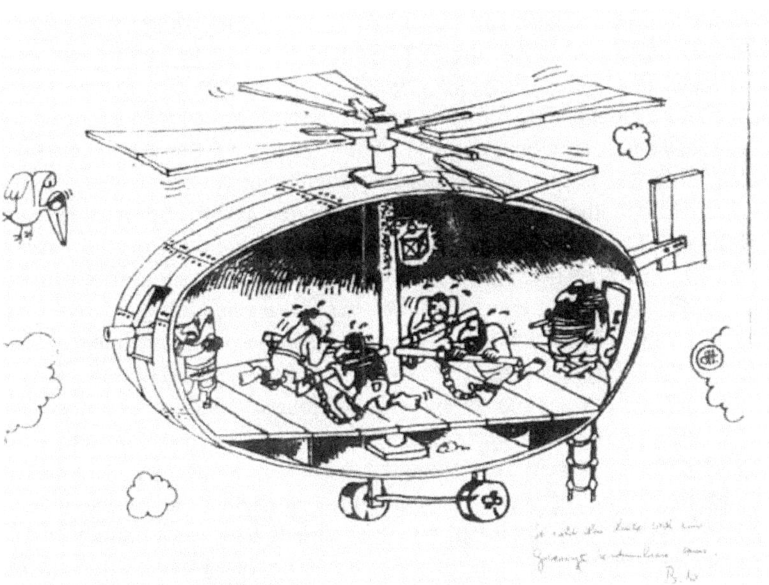

A drawing that for years hang on the wall of Neumann's office, symbolizing for him the economy of the DDR

Committee was lost, and as far as I know also 2,500 [West German] valuta-Marks were spent for an un-planned flight. During the last hustle and bustle, they forgot to give the delegate the yellow exit-card, which led to a quasi arrest of the DDR delegate at the border crossing at *Friedrichstrasse* without the possibility of making a supervised phone call. As a result, the booked flight from Tegel to Frankfurt was missed. The treatment by the border agencies went from unpleasant to disrespectful and one needed a long-time membership in the Party and ideological staunchness to deal with it."[81]

Yet Neumann's feelings of disenchantment went deeper, and well beyond relatively petty things such as lack of currency and the feeling of being from a second-rate country. These were issues that could still be dealt with through ideological conviction and the belief it was all the result of the encirclement by the Western world and the Cold War. The lack of support from the Soviets and the inactivity of other socialist countries also caused him frustrations. The Soviets ignored him, even insulted him by refusing to make use of his services, and seeing people like Zharikov making a fools of themselves must have been very upsetting. A particularly striking

81 *Ergänzungen zum Reisebericht Rio de Janeiro 18-23.4.1985*, pp. 4-5

document in this respect is his travel report on meetings of the WPA Executive Committee and the APA Annual Meeting in Chicago in May 1987. The fact that Anatoly Koryagin was received in Chicago as a hero seems to be manageable for some reason. He was anti-Soviet and used by the Americans for political purposes. Worse, however, was the fact that the Soviet side was unpredictable and that Neumann was blindsided. "I was confronted with the fact," Neumann writes, "that also the Soviet side itself speaks about political abuse of psychiatry and in this context gives names of people who are said to have been guilty of this, as a result of which my own positions and statements of the past three years are getting a very peculiar view. I was shown two press articles that were relevant but that I had not read myself. One was supposed to have appeared in the Soviet journal *Moscow News* and the other in the journal *Socialist Industry*. The contribution to *Socialist Industry* was in the hands of Prof. Stefanis who had it translated into Greek. He told me in broad terms about the content of the article."[82] The big issue for Neumann was whether the Soviets indeed abused psychiatry for political purposes and if it was continuing, albeit in a different form. For him, the main question was whether "the current board of the All-Union Society which must be considered partially guilty or knowledgeable of these events, can still be seen as a negotiating partner, or if one needed to wait 'until new people were in power'."[83]

At the same time, although in favor of a more democratic voting structure within the WPA that would give more power to smaller countries (and inevitably lead to a limitation on the influence of the Anglo-Saxon societies), he fully acknowledged that without them – and in particular without the APA – it would be impossible to run a WPA. "It is an illusion to try to lead the WPA without the influential USA… Outside the socialist countries there is almost invariably the view that the Soviet Union and the other socialist countries at this moment cannot give any valuable contribution (intellectually, culturally, technologically, regarding education and continuing education, research, finance, well functioning organizational structures)… For that reason, it is hard to assume that there are third countries willing to question the WPA in favor of the socialist countries."[84]

Neumann's disenchantment with socialist reality in the Eastern bloc did not go unnoticed. Having gotten to know Neumann during the process of writing this book, I realize that this would have been quite impossible,

82 *Reisebericht* by Jochen Neumann, May 6-15, 1987. See: HA XX 499, p. 240
83 *Reisebericht* by Jochen Neumann, May 6-15, 1987. See: HA XX 499, p. 240
84 *Politisch Missbraucht*, p. 665

actually, because throughout his life and career he never kept his mouth shut and voiced his criticism in front of his superiors whenever he felt the urge to do so. This time it was no different, and being on friendly terms with people like Seidel and Müller certainly helped him feel free to do so. "You know, when you were at a higher political level you were quite free to say what you thought. There were no repercussions and the conversations were sometimes quite frank."[85] Or, as he writes in a note in June 2007, "the best political jokes were told within the Central Committee; the higher the joke-teller, the sharper the joke."[86]

Still, this did not mean that his increasingly open criticism of the socialist system was not a matter of discussion by his (political) environment. The issue, for instance, was discussed in October 1988 during a meeting between Lieutenant Colonel Eberhard Jaekel, head of MfS Chief Directorate XX/1, and Deputy Minister Rolf Müller, as we know, a friend of Neumann's. Jaekel reported that Neumann "held the opinion that he and his generation felt betrayed by socialism. For many honorable people socialism has become an empty word. They think differently, hide their disenchantment and adapt. Neumann said that he had understanding for those doctors who left socialism… because they had a societal and human future under capitalism. The socialist social system is in urgent need of reform, in particular… to give the youth again a political future and motivation... Prof. Müller considers the remarks by Neumann to be confidential expressions of the questions he is facing. Prof. Neumann also expressed the view that for him leaving the DDR was not an issue. Prof. Müller has good relations with Neumann over many years and knows he needs concrete political guidance."[87]

The process of disenchantment continued until the very end of his membership on the Executive Committee. In his final report to the Stasi, after the Athens conference, he added that he never had the support from the DDR and the DDR Ministry of Health that he needed in carrying out his task. "Well-defined lobbying is part of the business."[88] Two weeks later the Wall came down, and Neumann's disenchantment with the system he served reached an all-time high.

---

85 Interview with Jochen Neumann, July 30, 2009

86 Note by Jochen Neumann, June 29, 2007

87 HA XX 499, pp. 176-8

88 *Zusatzbemerkungen* Jochen Neumann, 26 October 1989; *Politisch Missbraucht*, p. 669

Chapter 26 – Psychiatric Abuse and East-West Politics

It doesn't matter what color the cat it; it's more important whether it catches mice.

Deng Xiaoping[89]

There is no point in making too sharp a distinction between good and bad people... The distinction should rather be made between people's understanding of their own actions: between bad and good conscience, between memories of successes and of failures. Nothing is gained once and for all.

Tzvetan Todorov[90]

In the course of 1988-1989, the number of exchanges between Western psychiatrists and psychiatric bodies, political and non-governmental organizations and Soviet psychiatry multiplied; it is virtually impossible to provide a full record of all the exchanges, meetings and discussions. Clearly, the political changes in the USSR had their impact, and made the Soviet Union a very attractive object of interest. "This totalitarian state, closed for 70 years while serving as a superpower co-determining the agenda of international politics, changed at the end of the 1980s into an "Eldorado" for pioneers and adventurers. … Gorbachev had acquired enormous international respect. He was immensely popular in the West, often more popular than politicians in those countries. During his travels, he was often welcomed as a mix between a national hero and a film star. … The reduced tension between East and West and the new policy of openness increasingly led to a hype in the West. Key words of this policy were "glasnost" (openness) and "perestroika" (reform), and soon these terms were used in the West as well. Everywhere these key notions of Gorbachev's policy were repeated. Especially after Gorbachev published his book, *My Vision on the World*, it was an unstoppable process. In reality, it was a terrible book, long-winded and full of empty phrases, but after the Collected Works of Lenin and Stalin and the Memoirs of Leonid Brezhnev, the book was an enormous relief. Finally, we had a Soviet leader who was three-dimensional and not a retouched state portrait."[91]

89 *Human Rights, Perestroika and the End of the Cold War*, p. 267

90 Tzvetan Todorov, *Hope and Memory*, p.73

91 *On Dissidents and Madness*, p. 135

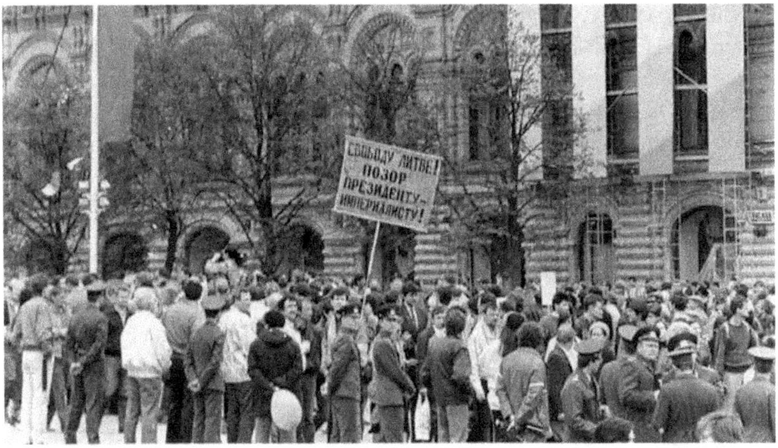

Demonstration in Moscow, 1990

Although under severe criticism at home, with a Soviet press exposing one case of abuse after the next case of corruption, naming psychiatrists and cases by name, the Soviet psychiatric leadership managed to cling on to power and even ride the high waves of Western attention. And as before, the attitude remained defiant, the denials that something had been wrong remained unaltered and until the very last moment, the Soviets thought that they could put demands on a return to the WPA. It was the game of flexing muscles that Neumann referred to in his memoirs: "the leaders of the All-Union Society were in majority blockheads without a vision, who thought that only by flexing muscles the lost positions could be recovered."[92]

How right Neumann was in his assessment is again shown in a report on a meeting on January 26, 1988 of the Serbski leadership (consisting of Georgi Morozov, Ruben Nadzharov and Gennady Milyokhin) with a delegation of the International Helsinki Federation. During the meeting Morozov claimed that "the Soviet Union… had voluntarily withdrawn because the situation created in relation to Soviet psychiatrists was unfounded and discriminatory. He said that Soviet psychiatrists would not return unless a 'more democratic' system of voting within the WPA was guaranteed. He implied that the WPA leadership had indicated that they would like the Soviet Union to join the association again, but he said he found the attitude of WPA towards Soviet psychiatry to be as unsatisfactorily as before."[93]

---

92 Private notes by Jochen Neumann, August 16, 2009

93 Minutes of the meeting, *Documents* 4, February 1988

In the meantime, Stefanis and Schulsinger continued their efforts to bring the AUSNP back into the fold. How often they met with the Soviet psychiatric establishment is hard to retrace, but it probably was not less than in 1986-1987 and it is clear that they did everything possible to stay out of the limelight. In a letter to Comrade Buhlert of the General Secretariat of Medical Scientific Associations in East Berlin, Neumann wrote in early October 1988 that "about two weeks ago consultations took place in Moscow, in which Prof. Stefanis and Prof. Schulsinger took part on behalf of the WPA. In these discussions, the Royal College was represented by the President, Prof. Birley, and its Registrar, Prof. Priest, and Melvin Sabshin represented the APA. I was informed by Prof. Schulsinger by telephone immediately upon his return."[94] Shortly after, in the beginning of 1989, Stefanis and Schulsinger were found by a German television crew in one of the psychiatric hospitals of Moscow. Again, both vehemently denied they were there for "secret negotiations."[95] Three months later, in April 1989, a Symposium was held in Moscow on Mental Health and Law, co-sponsored by the International Academy on Law and Mental Health and the Serbski Institute. Also the Institute of State and Law participated in the event. During that meeting, "relations between most foreign participants and Soviet psychiatrists remain distant, formal and mutually suspicious. Schulsinger was much closer, and obviously respected by senior Serbski psychiatrists."[96] It seems obvious that the earlier regularity of at least one meeting per two months was maintained throughout 1988-1989.

The wooing back into the WPA fold did not only focus on the Soviets, although, of course, they remained the prize target throughout the period. Three other associations had left the WPA, namely the Czechoslovak, Bulgarian and Cuban associations, and also they should be reintegrated into the WPA. Sometime before the summer of 1987, the WPA sent out letters to these non-member societies, and not unsuccessfully. As reported at the Executive Committee meeting in Buenos Aires in August 1987, "the President… received favorable reactions to his communication… among them letters from Bulgaria and Cuba. He was in full agreement with the EC, when stating that the result of the initiative had been satisfactory, and that, for the time being, the WPA need not take further steps in this direction."[97] On November 15, 1988, Neumann reported that the WPA has received

94 Letter to Buhlert by Jochen Neumann, October 6, 1988. The letter is attached to a travel request of Jochen Neumann to go to Copenhagen in November 1988 for a meeting with Schulsinger.

95 *The Times*, March 16, 1989

96 Report by Dr. Timothy Harding on the conference, *Documents* 22, June 1989

97 Minutes WPA EC, August 1987, p. 2

applications for reentry into the WPA from the Bulgarian and Czechoslovak psychiatric societies and contacts with Cuba were continuing.[98]

Koryagin on the scene

A complicating factor for both Stefanis and Schulsinger was the release of Anatoly Koryagin from Chistopol prison, and his subsequent emigration to Switzerland. With his release, the Soviets had put one of their worse adversaries onto the chessboard, and it was Koryagin's intention to make maximum use of it. Soon after his arrival in Switzerland, he resumed his political activity, as he had promised in the bathtub at home in Kharkov right after his release.[99] And waging a war was exactly what he was good at – his endless hunger strikes in camp and, subsequently, in Chistopol prison had shown his perseverance and determination.

Being his private interpreter, guide, travel companion and, eventually, friend I witnessed him from very close and during a protracted period of time. Koryagin was a real Russian from Kansk, Siberia, proud to be "Siberian" rather than "Russian" ("you know, in Siberia you find the real Russians, not those weaklings in Moscow that have been spoiled")[100] and

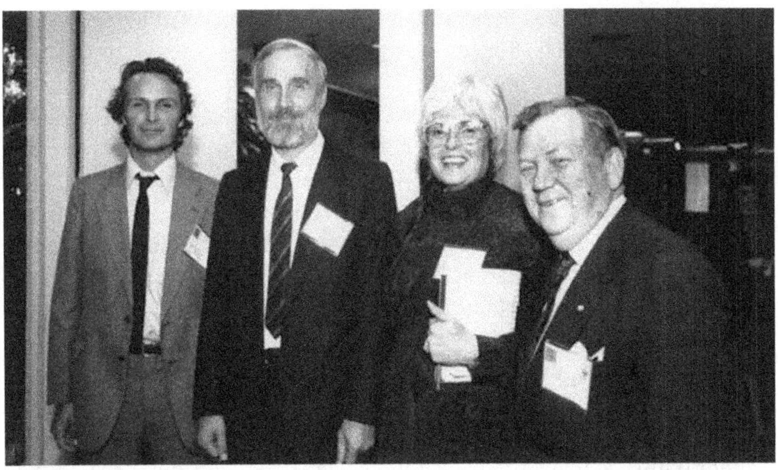

APA Regional Symposium, Washington October 1988. L.t.r. Robert van Voren, Anatoly Koryagin, Ellen Mercer, Harold Vysotsky

[98] *Reisebericht* of Jochen Neumann on his meetings with Fini Schulsinger, 6-11 November 1988, p. 2

[99] *On Dissidents and Madness*, p. 98

[100] This view Koryagin voiced many times during our joint travels.

fiercely anti-Communist. He had a great sense of humor, a zest for life and an indomitable spirit. He was pretty old-fashioned and traditional in his views, e.g. his wife Galya, was supposed to take care of the children and household and nothing else; but there was nothing bad in his character – he was kind, straightforward and, having never been outside the USSR, he had not been exposed to other cultures, perceptions, or approaches.[101]

The first encounter between Stefanis and Koryagin took place in Chicago, in May 1987. Koryagin was honorary guest at a dinner for foreign visitors to the APA Annual Meeting in Chicago, and gave a speech, outlining his conditions for a Soviet return. According to one report, they met very briefly afterwards, through an intervention by an American psychiatrist, shook hands and exchanged but a few words.[102] The atmosphere was very tense, and no constructive talks followed for almost a year. In March 1988, more than a year after his release, Koryagin met Stefanis in Switzerland on March 11, 1988 for a private meeting of six hours. A report, written by Koryagin immediately following the meeting, shows clearly the fundamental distrust. Whether this was mutual is hard to say, but it clearly existed on the part of Koryagin. Stefanis might have seen Koryagin as an imminent threat to his attempts to bring back the Soviets, but I also cannot exclude the possibility that deep down he might have actually admired the man – an independent spirit, who went against the grain and did what he believed in; exactly the position Stefanis felt he himself was taking.

Stefanis tried to explain his position to Koryagin. He said that the WPA was under immense pressure and that Third World countries were threatening to leave the organization; that the World Health Organization (WHO) had increased the pressure because it could not collaborate with an organization that excluded such an important country as the USSR; that he was stuck with a war he had not started himself, and, as WPA President, he could not prevent scientific contacts between Soviet and Western psychiatrists. He added that he himself maintained such contacts, with Marat Vartanyan-probably not the best name to mention during such a conversation.[103]

All in all, the conversation led to nothing, and neither side was willing to seek a compromise. Stefanis tried, even if not wholeheartedly, but the attempt to

---

101 For more personal reminiscences of Koryagin by the author see *On Dissidents and Madness*, pp. 96-98 and 119-121.

102 Report by Peter Reddaway, *Why is Dr Stefanis clandestinely negotiating with the USSR about its return to the WPA*, no date, probably spring 1987

103 See Koryagin's notes on his meeting with Stefanis, published in IAPUP *Documents* 8, June 1988

win over Koryagin had bitterly failed. For Koryagin, his arguments didn't count; he was a proponent of the black-and-white picture: either you are with us or against us. The delicate balance Stefanis was seeking, the Greek background of his political thinking, his policy of brinkmanship between East and West was, for Koryagin, all a matter of intellectual nonsense, a way of avoiding one's responsibility. The WPA should stand for medical ethics and defend those who were victims of political misuse of psychiatric practice; here no subtleties counted, either they did or they didn't, thereby betraying the Hippocratic Oath.

The two men would never come to speaking terms.

Regional Symposium in Washington

In a report of May 1988, following the meeting of the Executive Committee in Sydney, Jochen Neumann mentioned a "renewed sharpening of the Cold War full of attacks and aggression against psychiatry in the Soviet Union and (although less) also in other countries."[104] The explanation for his claim was not immediately clear. He pointed at the "institutionalized representatives of anti-Soviet positions," such as the Royal College and the American Psychiatric Association, represented in Sydney by Harold Visotsky, who, in earlier travel reports, was branded as an "anti-Soviet agitator." "It seems that the political détente at higher levels do not fit into the concept of certain circles. There are good reasons to assume that the anti-Soviet activities within the APA should disturb the course of détente and are steered by the secret service."[105]

Then the reason for Neumann's agitation later becomes clear. It turned out that at the Sydney meeting, the program of the WPA Regional Symposium in Washington D.C. was discussed, a meeting that was planned for October 1988 and organized by the APA.[106] Among the submissions was symposium submitted by IAPUP, "Soviet Psychiatry in the Gorbachev Era," and this submission caused a major discussion within the Executive Committee. For Neumann acceptance of this symposium would have far-

104 *Reisebericht* of Jochen Neumann on the WPA EC in Sydney, April 24 – May 9, 1988, p. 5

105 *Reisebericht* of Jochen Neumann on the WPA EC in Sydney, April 24 – May 9, 1988, p. 5

106 In the minutes of the meeting of the Executive Committee, it reads "Some of the EC members felt that a few of the submitted papers had titles which might indicate that they did not fully meet the goals of the WPA." See the WPA EC Minutes, Sydney, April 1988, p. 3. There is no reference to any heated debate.

reaching consequences. "I have announced that I will probably at least not take part in the meeting of the Executive Committee in Washington, if this sub-symposium takes place in its planned format, irrespective of what other steps might follow."[107] It is clear: Neumann might resign from the Executive Committee if this symposium takes place under the aegis of the WPA. This is the moment, mentioned earlier, that Neumann approached Sabshin and asked for his support. Sabshin agreed: "The point of view of the reporter [Neumann] was met with understanding by Sabshin, and was also immediately supported by the other four members of the Executive Committee. ... M. Sabshin will try to either have this symposium taken off the program or to reschedule it as a parallel meeting next to the official program."[108]

For Jochen Neumann, this situation must have caused a lot of anxiety. Another similar situation happened in October 1984, when he had to remain absent during an audience with the Pope in order to avoid having photographs taken with him; it would have been a problem for a representative of the socialist DDR to meet with the fiercely anti-communist Polish Pope Karol Wojtyla. It reminds one of how he could not afford the political risk of being seen in the same place as Anatoly Koryagin, let alone be photographed together. The extent of this issue was seen from his travel report in May 1987 when he attended the meeting of the Executive Committee in Chicago: "On top of that there were underlying tensions, because the *Corpus delicti* of Psychiatry, Anatoly Koryagin, recently released from the Soviet Union, was participating in the APA event as honored guest. The EC-members succeeded in keeping the WPA completely out of the affair. We were supported in this by some American colleagues."[109]

The symposium that caused the tension dealt with a range of issues related to Soviet political abuse of psychiatry and had among its speakers the same Anatoly Koryagin, at that time one of the most vocal opponents of a return of the All-Union Society to the WPA. Other participants included Aleksandr Podrabinek, one of the founders of the Moscow Working Commission and now editor of the unofficial newspaper "*Express Khronika,*" via a video message; Peter Reddaway, Paul Chodoff, the British psychiatrist Sidney Levine and the author, Robert van Voren. While the symposium

[107] *Reisebericht* of Jochen Neumann on the WPA EC in Sydney, April 24 – May 9, 1988, p. 6

[108] *Reisebericht* of Jochen Neumann on the WPA EC in Sydney, April 24 – May 9, 1988, p. 6

[109] *Sofortbericht* of Jochen Neumann on the WPA EC meeting in Chicago, May 6-15, 1987, p. 2.

was organized by IAPUP, it was at the request of the APA Committee on Abuse with full support from the APA Organizing Committee and, in all likelihood, also with Melvin Sabshin knowing about it.[110] On May 16, 1988, Costas Stefanis and Fini Schulsinger sent a message to Melvin Sabshin, in which they offered themselves as speakers on the program, but suggested removing a few proposed sessions, including the above-mentioned one, as "this symposium has a content which is well-known by everybody. The content is hardly scientific, and it will not serve to promote international collaboration."[111]

The response from Sabshin was probably not what they expected. In a message of June 1, 1988, he wrote: "after careful review, the Program Committee believes that you should assume the responsibility of expressing this point of view directly to the individuals involved [in this session]. In the absence of your memorandum, the Program Committee would have been inclined to accept almost all of these submissions and, in effect, your recommendations would overrule these decisions. The Program Committee agrees to abide by your decision ... if you take the responsibility of notification of the appropriate individuals who made these submissions."[112] The same day, Robert Hales, Chairman of the Scientific and Organizing Committee, sends a memo to the WPA Executive Committee with the same message.[113]

Schulsinger and Stefanis reacted by asking all Executive Committee members to put their personal opinions on paper and send their statement "as soon as possible."[114] In a separate letter to Melvin Sabshin, they explained: "we want you to understand that this request is not made to embarrass you... We understand very well possible difficulties on your side, but be assured that we do not wish to escalate any tensions. We are absolutely aware that you have done the best to promote the interests of the WPA."[115]

110 Letter from Ellen Mercer to Robert van Voren, February 5, 1988. The letter also has the following interesting remark: "I really think the WPA Executive Committee (with exception of Dr. Sabshin) really underestimate our 'network'! It will be great fun to watch them gradually realize all of this."

111 fax from Fini Schulsinger, May 16, 1988. Five symposia were questioned, apart from the one organized by IAPUP three of them concerned Soviet political abuse and one "anti-Americanism".

112 Memorandum to Costas Stefanis and Fini Schulsinger from Melvin Sabshin, June 1, 1988

113 Memorandum by Robert Hales, June 1, 1988

114 Letter from Fini Schulsinger to each of the Executive Committee members, June 3, 1988

115 Letter marked "Personal" from Stefanis and Schulsinger to Melvin Sabshin,

Two weeks after the mailing to the Executive Committee members, Jochen Neumann wrote to Schulsinger. He was clearly not happy with the way things were going, and put more pressure on the General Secretary by writing that "I would like to encourage you to do whatever you can to avoid a minor disaster. In case the anti-Soviet session would take place under the auspices of the WPA, at least I could not take part in the EC meetings in October. And maybe there could be bigger problems in so far as I would have to inform the board of our member society and this could mean further steps, which would not be supportive for WPA. Do what is possible, cautious and polite but with consequence."[116]

That same day, Stefanis and Schulsinger wrote to the APA Organizing Committee. The issue clearly had become almost too hot to handle. In a letter to Dr. Robert Hales, they explained that "five of [the EC members] endorse and adhere to the self-evident and traditionally established principle of close collaboration between the Organizing Committee and the WPA EC and Secretariat in the organization of the WPA Regional Symposia. This principle was not even questioned by the sixth member, Dr. Sabshin, who promptly offered his proposals regarding the issues raised in our memo of May 16, 1988. Four of the six members reaffirm the opinion they voiced in our discussions … while Dr. Costa e Silva, agreeing with Dr. Sabshin and with you, suggest that the EC should write directly to the contributors, and Dr. Sabshin himself is inclined to disapprove of only one of the five contributions listed in our memo."[117] However, Stefanis and Schulsinger offered a compromise solution. "In order to free the Organizers from any restrictions in applying their own judgment in the construction of the Scientific Program while the WPA's policy of promoting rather than restricting fruitful collaboration among its membership is preserved and in order to avoid embarrassing abstentions of EC members and of other segments of the WPA and thus trigger off chain reactions that will inevitably threaten the very existence of the WPA even before it's General Assembly, we submit as a compromising gesture the following proposal. An arrangement should be sought by which the contributions in question should appear in the Program in a way that would clearly indicate that it is the APA and the Organizers alone who have the sole responsibility for their inclusion … and that the WPA is not co-sharing the responsibility for their presentation."[118]

June 3, 1988

116 Letter from Jochen Neumann to Fini Schulsinger, June 21, 1988. The letter was also faxed the same day.

117 Letter of Schulsinger and Stefanis to Robert Hales, June 21, 1988

118 Letter of Schulsinger and Stefanis to Robert Hales, June 21, 1988

In 1988, being organizer of one of the disputed symposia, I read this letter carefully, as well as the letter Schulsinger and Stefanis sent to the organizers of the five symposia in question, explaining their position. However, I never paid attention to the remarks "to avoid embarrassing abstentions of EC members." Only now, after reading Jochen Neumann's reports, I realize that this is what they refer to: Neumann has threatened not to appear in Washington, and maybe even withdraw from the Executive Committee altogether. Stefanis and Schulsinger's warning in their letter is therefore not empty: "We trust that the Organizing and Scientific Committee... will respond positively to our compromise proposals. If, however, other considerations prevail and the Organizing Committee and the APA do not or cannot accept our proposals, then it is certain that we are heading towards a serious crisis and major decisions will have to follow."[119]

The compromise that Schulsinger and Stefanis offered was clearly to Sabshin's liking. In a memo to the other members of the Executive Committee, sent on July 8, he made clear that "the symposium proposed by Mr. Robert van Voren and the papers proposed by Drs. Paul Chodoff and Rita Newman will not be part of the official WPA Regional Scientific Program."[120] Some time later, in a letter of July 20, Stefanis and Schulsinger express their appreciation for Sabshin's efforts to "mitigate, and eventually remove the potentially serious problems which, due to minor, but still important, gaps in communication – threatened the smooth course of the... WPA Regional Symposium..."[121]

Jochen Neumann traveled to Washington D.C. but stayed away from the disputed session. "At this symposium, people like Koryagin, van Voren, Reddaway and another 1 to 2 persons of the same *couleur* spoke. The DDR-representative was purposely not present at his meeting. The representatives of the press, among whom there is also a Mr. Langen of the Frankfurter Allgemeine Zeitung (a former DDR citizen who is said to have been imprisoned for many years in DDR prisons), are well informed and have copies of letters that have gone back and forth between the WPA and the APA. It is an open secret that they receive detailed information and also support from Ellen Mercer of the Office of International Affairs of the APA, with support from Visotsky, the Chairman of the Council of International Affairs, and others."[122]

119 Letter of Schulsinger and Stefanis to Robert Hales, June 21, 1988

120 Memo by Melvin Sabshin to the WPA EC members, July 8, 1988

121 Letter from Stefanis and Schulsinger to Sabshin, July 20, 1988

122 *Reisesbericht* of Jochen Neumann on the WPA EC meeting in Washington D.C., October 1988, p. 5

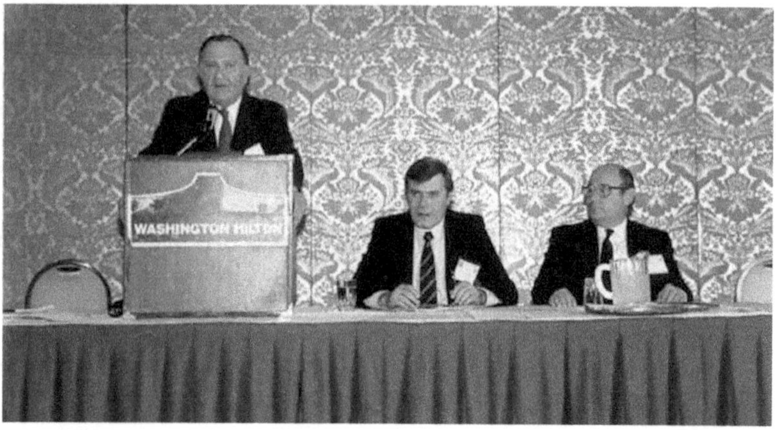

l.t.r. Melvin Sabshin, Costas Stefanis and Jochen Neumann, Washington, 1988

However, in spite of his avoidance of this symposium, a short confrontation with dissident psychiatrist Anatoly Koryagin could not be avoided, as noted in an earlier chapter, and Neumann also had his first encounter with the author of this book.

Chapter 27: the US Visit to the USSR

The KGB knew everything that was happening in the Central Committee, but the Central Committee didn't know what was happening in the KGB.
Aleksandr Yakovlev[123]

The first substantial discussion within the WPA leadership with regard to a possible return of the All-Union Society into the organization took place almost a year earlier, in November 1987, during a meeting of the Executive Committee in Warsaw, held on the occasion of a WPA Regional Symposium on alcohol and drug addiction. The WPA General Assembly in Athens was less than two years away and the critical articles in the Soviet press had raised hopes among the opponents of political abuse of psychiatry that changes were indeed forthcoming. Maybe the dismissal of Morozov and Vartanyan were a possibility, they thought, and although only few of the political prisoners in psychiatric hospitals had yet been released, the general political climate gave hope that this was just a matter of time.

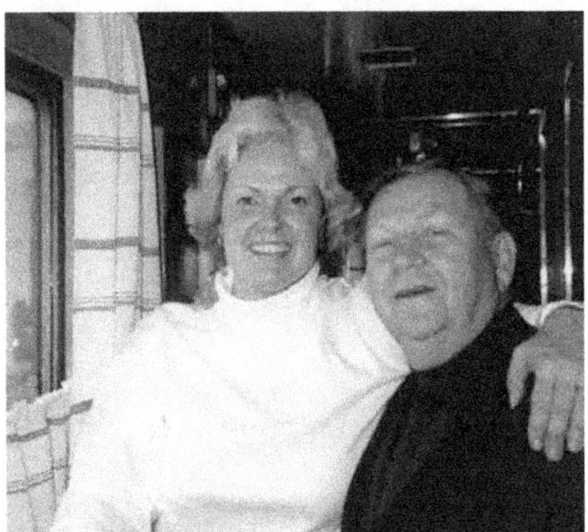
Harold Visotsky and Ellen Mercer in the USSR, March 1989

Also, new actors had appeared on the scene. The American Psychiatric Association's foreign policy was mainly represented by Melvin Sabshin, who, as a member of the WPA Executive Committee, had to meander carefully between the two organizations in order to avoid a conflict of interest. Ellen Mercer was Director of the Office of International Affairs of the APA, and Dr. Harold Visotsky, Chairman of the APA Council on International Affairs. In particular, the latter was, in the eyes of Jochen Neumann, one of the main agitators against a return of the All-Union Society and there clearly was no love lost between them. The British Royal College of Psychiatrists had a new President, Dr. Jim Birley, an internationally respected British psychiatrist who had been Director of the Maudsley Institute for more than two decades. Jim Birley was clear in

123 Adamishin, p. 270

his positioning, and although "British polite" in his behavior, he was also at times unusually direct and, for the Soviets, a hard nut to crack.

At the Warsaw meeting of the WPA Executive Committee, the Soviet issue was raised both by the Royal College and the APA. "At the moment, there are attempts by the London-based Royal College, the Australian Royal College and the APA, to delay the rapprochement of the All-Union Society. The Royal College and its new President Birley has sent letters to that effect, which try to commit the WPA in an almost neo-colonialist fashion. Their interests are not fully equal to those of the APA: Sabshin stresses that the APA is willing to bring the All-Union Society back into the WPA, under certain conditions. Only the hegemonic demands of the APA determine that they want to decide when and under what conditions this rapprochement will take place."[124]

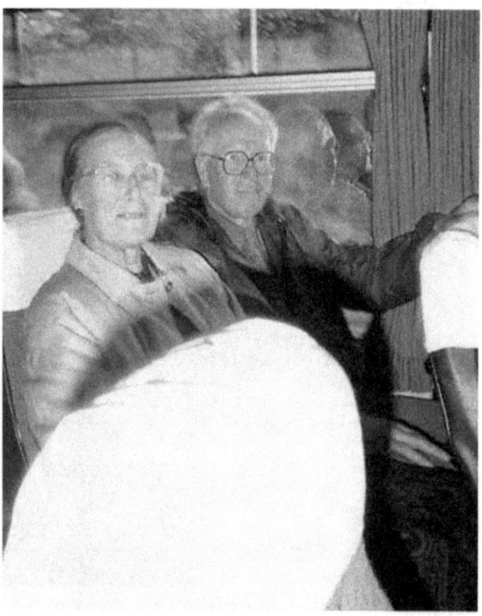

Jim and Julia Birley

During a combined meeting of the Executive Committee and the Committee of the WPA, the British psychiatrist Robert Priest tried to have a statement adopted by the larger WPA Committee, in which hope was expressed that changes under 'glasnost' and 'perestroika' would lead to a situation that the All-Union Society could return to the WPA, but that this moment had not yet come. A discussion followed which, according to Jochen Neumann, "in principle supported a rapprochement with the All-Union Society as soon as possible, which in this open form had not been expressed at the highest level within the WPA since 1982."[125] Neumann continues: "The discussion became a bit controversial because Stefanis, frustrated by the personal attacks, brought in a certain confrontational sharpness,

[124] *Reisebericht* of Jochen Neumann on the WPA EC meeting in Warsaw, November 1987, p. 2

[125] *Reisebericht* of Jochen Neumann on the WPA EC meeting in Warsaw, November 1987, p. 3

which was neither necessary nor helpful."[126] And also Schulsinger shows his feathers; Neumann refers to a "small mock battle with Stefanis."[127] The tension within the WPA Executive Committees was clearly rising.

Neumann was satisfied with the developments. In his report he wrote: "One cannot overestimate the importance of these developments. It gives room to further careful activity, with the precondition that the Soviet comrades in the future adapt themselves well to the existing situation and prepare themselves properly, and do not cluelessly and with banal arguments blab around a bit without clear strategic goals and tactical maneuvers."[128] At this moment, in spite of an obvious disdain for the Soviets' way of operating, his loyalty was still with them and he apparently still believed that the allegations of Soviet political abuse were part of the East-West confrontation. The revelations in the Soviet press had not yet altered his position, at least not to such an extent that he wavered in his task to help to bring about the return of the All-Union Society.

The campaign intensifies

In the meantime, IAPUP had become a more permanent entity with a permanent office in Amsterdam and three staff members. After Gérard Bles had stepped down as General Secretary in 1984, Catherine Kuhn from Geneva assumed this role temporarily. Catherine had been one of the founders of one of the first committees against the political abuse of psychiatry, set up in 1974 in Geneva.[129] The call for a more permanent secretariat became louder, in particular because the campaign in connection with the World Congress of the WPA in 1989 in Athens had to be started and the delays in releasing Soviet political prisoners from psychiatric hospitals demanded an intensification of IAPUP's international lobbying. In December 1986, after completing my studies at Amsterdam University, I was urged to assume the role of General Secretary, and, as a result, the seat of the organization moved in early 1987 to The Netherlands.

126 *Reisebericht* of Jochen Neumann on the WPA EC meeting in Warsaw, November 1987, p. 3

127 *Reisebericht* of Jochen Neumann on the WPA EC meeting in Warsaw, November 1987, p. 4

128 *Reisebericht* of Jochen Neumann on the WPA EC meeting in Warsaw, November 1987, p. 4

129 The first committee to be established was the British Working Committee on the Internment of Dissenters in Mental Hospitals, in 1971.

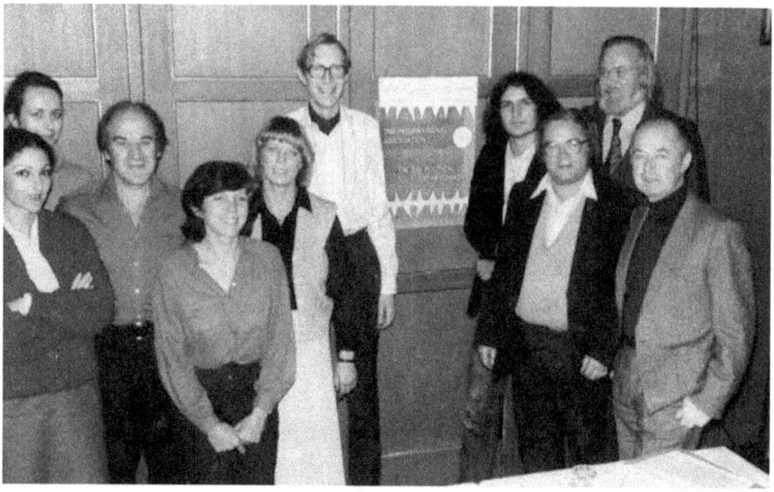

IAPUP, 1981

IAPUP had at that moment actually none of the tools that a permanent organization demanded: no official statutes, no registration as a legal entity, no formal board and not even a bank account. In order to be able to develop the campaign more professionally this had to change. At the same time, we wanted to leave the very horizontal "confederate" structure as a representation of national committees and groups as it was, so our notary set about the task of developing official statutes that, on the one hand, fulfilled all the requirements of Dutch legislation and, on the other hand, met all our wishes and demands. The result was draft statutes discussed during exhaustive meetings, commented upon by our lawyer, Professor Charles André Junod of Geneva, and eventually finalized by our Dutch notary and incorporated in November 1988. Shortly after registration, we received our first official subsidy, $40,000 from an American foundation, enough to finance our campaign.[130]

Our plans with regard to the World Congress in October 1989 in Athens were much more extensive than ever before. While the preparations for

130 The grant came from the Smith Richardson Foundation in New York, a private foundation that funded many initiatives in support of the democratic movement in the Soviet Union. We were much liked by the founder and President of the foundation, Ralph Richardson, because he had earned part of his wealth in selling mussel cleaning machines to Dutch customers, and he had fond memories of them. In addition, we managed to secure funding from a variety of private donors and small private foundations, totalling approximately 85,000 euro, for those days not a small amount.

Vienna in 1983 had been relatively amateurish, with very limited funds available, we now had the chance to move our campaign to a more professional level and make sure that the Soviet issue remained high on the psychiatric agenda, both within the WPA and outside. Our goals were to keep the Soviet All-Union Society out of the WPA as long as the political abuse of psychiatry continued. Considering the changing political climate in the USSR and the relaxation of relationships with the West, this was a complex task that called for strategic maneuvering. We also wanted the newly founded Soviet Independent Psychiatric Association be admitted to the WPA. And finally we wanted to do everything possible to facilitate the election of a new WPA Executive Committee that would prioritize medical ethics and would support our campaign against the political abuse of psychiatry. We had the feeling that we had failed to do this in Vienna, and the result had been a leadership with, as we saw it, a pro-Soviet Greek as President and an anti-American Dane as General Secretary. This mistake should not be repeated.

In order to be able to lobby successfully, we made sure that we were represented at all the important psychiatric congresses, and that included all the WPA Regional Symposia, but also meetings of the International Academy of Law and Mental Health (IALMH) and meetings of the CSCE. Usually our delegation consisted of four or five persons, supported by a number of influential psychiatrists and invariably by Ellen Mercer as our "secret weapon." She introduced us to leading psychiatrists and potential candidates for the future Executive Committee of the WPA and on the basis of these meetings we would consider whether to support their candidacy or not. Gradually an image was formed in our heads of a future Executive Committee that would be steadfast and continue to consider medical ethics as a priority. "That we were being used to further personal careers was something we did not even consider. At the same time, we were surprised as to how our influence had actually grown. It was the story of the mouse and the elephant that walk across a bridge, during which the mouse looks up to the elephant and says proudly: "Are we nicely marching or what?" Only in our situation it didn't only turn out that we nicely marched along, but it also seemed that we decided on the rhythm. It was a very strange realization."[131]

One of the standard members of our delegation was Anatoly Koryagin, who because of his strong personality and clear opinions, was widely admired and made an impact wherever he went. Here you had a man who had been

131 *On Dissidents and Madness*, p. 118-9

sentenced to twelve years of camp and exile because of his resistance against the political abuse of psychiatry, who came out of camp unbroken and who personally had examined a lot of victims of political psychiatry and had declared them mentally healthy. On top of that, Koryagin was an honorary member of the WPA, and also of a number of other Western psychiatric associations. In the fall of 1988, he was awarded an honorary doctorate from the Free University in Amsterdam, in the context of a conference in which Fini Schulsinger attended.[132]

As Koryagin's personal guide, I traveled with him from country to country, from congress to congress, from meeting to meeting. He was frequently invited to speak at meetings and, where possible, we would do that together. I would focus on the context and the debate as to whether the Soviets should be allowed to return or not, followed by Koryagin's personal testimony that almost invariably resulted in standing ovations. It was clear that the man had an enormous charisma.

In 1988, we were invited to give a lecture tour in Greece. The invitation came from a young parliamentarian, Kostas Karamanlis, a cousin of the "old" Konstantinos Karamanlis who, with Andreas Papandreou, dominated political life in Greece for a long time.[133] The young Karamanlis was building his political career,[134] elections were around the corner and thus a lecture tour with the internationally renowned and respected Koryagin was an excellent way of promoting himself. For us, it was a nice way to get the support of public opinion in Greece and to develop a network of contacts with the Greek press, so we could make use of that during the upcoming World Congress. It was a fight in the back garden of Costas Stefanis, one that we relished at the time but also one that made the fight between the WPA and IAPUP more of a personal one: several of Stefanis' colleagues participated in the organization of the tour, something he felt to be a sort of betrayal.[135] Looking back, I think we unwittingly allowed ourselves to be used in a national election campaign, even though we were convinced our cause was just and we did not voice any political preference. However, it surely didn't help to create an open dialogue with Costas Stefanis and, in fact, deepened the personal confrontation.

---

132 *Documents* 11, October 1988

133 See chapter 18: Meeting Costas Stefanis

134 In 2004 he would become Prime Minister of Greece, winning a second term in 2007.

135 Interview with Costas Stefanis, July 15, 2009

Meeting Shevardnadze

It is a rather affluent neighborhood of Tbilisi, and increasingly popular among the local *nouveaux riche*. The European Union Monitoring Mission had its headquarters there, 'modestly' occupying a huge compound surrounded by what is said to be a beautiful park. A little bit further up the road is Shevardnadze's residence, behind a high wall with a black gate. A group of elderly men and women are sitting on the opposite side of the street, hiding from the sun. Their purpose becomes clear when our car stops and I get out. They jump to their feet and start demonstrating. "Shevardnadze, die!" and "Shevardnadze in prison!" are the most popular slogans, and when we enter the gate their shouts follow us, amplified with a bullhorn. They are there three days a week, said to be paid 5 lari per day, orchestrating popular outrage against the man they see as the murderer of his predecessor, Zviad Gamsakhurdia. Inside the compound, our passports and bags are checked. A few guards hover around, a caged dog barks occasionally, probably seriously irritated by the mantra of slogans coming from behind the wall. After listening for ten minutes to the shouts, I can very well understand his irritation. The buildings are dilapidated, the garden badly maintained, quite different than the park of the EU Monitoring Mission a bit further down the hill. In the corner, a monument marks the grave of Shevardnadze's wife who died in 2004, a year after he was forced to step down as President of Georgia.

With a colleague I enter a building on the other side of the compound, and are asked to wait a few minutes in the corridor. I observe the paintings, an interesting combination of Moscow's Red Square and of mountain ranges. Then we are asked in, and we enter history: a large room, decorated with pictures of Shevardnadze at various stages in his turbulent life, rows of photos of the same man with leaders of the world, a wall full of books and, in the corner, a huge desk with a big black leather chair. The air is that of the working area of an elderly statesman, but also of a man living in isolation, only surrounded by the souvenirs of his years in power. And by his faithful secretary, who has stayed with him during all these years and who has a much smaller desk in front of the wall of books, and who assists where necessary, also by helping him to remember names and situations.

Being 81 years old, he has grown much older since he was ousted by an angry crowd from Parliament six years ago, images that were broadcasted around the world. The waves of white hair that were so characteristic of him have thinned considerably. But it is Shevardnadze, no doubt about it and, in the course of the conversation, he becomes more and more talkative, telling stories from the past about his favorite interlocutors on the international scene, of whom Ronald Reagan is clearly one of his top favorites. He tells the story how of visiting Reagan in California, unannounced, since he was in the neighborhood. He found that Reagan didn't recognize him anymore because of progressing Alzheimer's disease. His own memory of the issues I want to discuss is less clear, although at certain moments his mind suddenly flares up and he answers my questions in detail, and with a certainty that leaves no doubt that he very well knows what he is talking about. No dementia here, so much is clear, and when I show him the pack of photos of the 1988 Politburo, lifted from the GIP archives, he goes from one to the other, explaining the person's good and bad sides, and with whom he was friends. It is a strange feeling, cozily chatting away with the man who, with Gorbachev and Aleksandr Yakovlev, belonged to the main driving forces of 'glasnost' and 'perestroika,' while discussing the character traits of Politburo members who, for most of us, were one-dimensional retouched photos or whose names only evoked feelings of revulsion. "Chebrikov," he remembers, "he was an orthodox hardliner, very strict to the Party rule. His successor, Kryuchkov, was much more pleasant, already the younger generation and much more intelligent." Chebrikov, who had been KGB chief, was in 1988 Secretary of the Administrative Organs of the Central Committee of the CPSU, a crucial position within the Party apparatus.[136] Shevardnadze singles Chebrikov out as one of the people who opposed the ending of the political abuse of psychiatry and the liberalization in general.

Whatever he did as Minister of the Interior of Soviet Georgia and as General Secretary of the Georgian Communist Party (and certainly not all reports are positive)[137] and after the collapse of the Soviet Union as President of

---

136 Viktor Mikhailovich Chebrikov (1923 - 1999) was a Soviet Union spy and head of the KGB from 1982 to 1988. Born in Dnepropetrovsk in Eastern Ukraine, he served in the Red Army during World War II. Turned down for the military academy after the war, he earned an engineering degree in 1950 and began work at the city's metallurgical plant. That year he joined the Communist Party, and rose through the local ranks until 1967, when he was brought to Moscow as deputy chairman of the KGB under Yuri Andropov. Due to differing views regarding reforms, in October 1988, Gorbachev replaced Chebrikov with General Vladimir Kryuchkov (who in 1991 attempted a coup against Gorbachev). He remained a member of the Politburo and became Secretary of the Central Committee of the Administrative Department of the Central Committee of the CPSU, also a very powerful position.

137 Many Georgians describe Shevardnadze as a particularly zealous Party leader, who imposed a strict rule in order to show Moscow that he was capable of maintaining order in his own country. "For the liberal and anti-Soviet Tbilisi youth of the time, Eduard Shevardnadze was a completely unacceptable figure, regarded as just another power-crazy communist" writes David Turashvili in

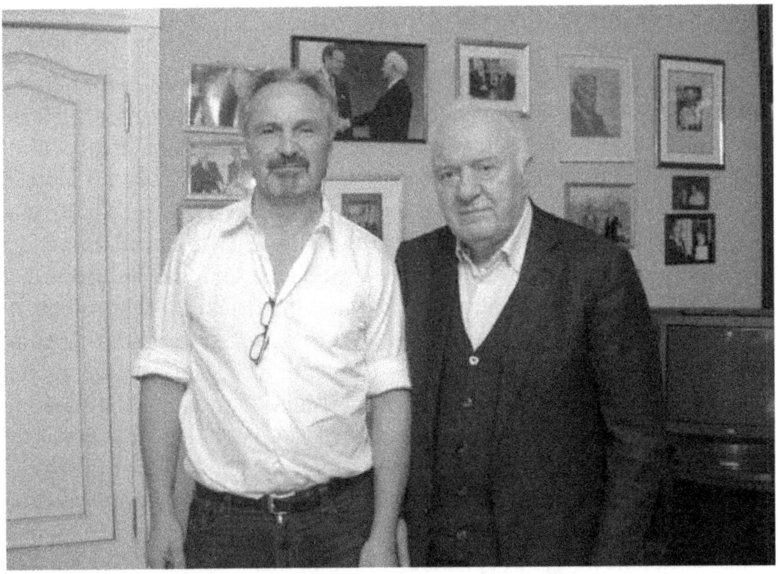

Van Voren with Eduard Shevardnadze, October 2009

Georgia, there is one thing that cannot be denied: Shevardnadze played a crucial role in opening the Soviet Union, moving it from totalitarianism to a growing adherence to international standards of human rights and the rule of law. As former US Secretary of State George Schultz writes in his memoirs: "I was well aware and appreciative of how much easier it was to deal with Shevardnadze than with Gromyko. The difference was absolutely dramatic. We could have a real conversation, argue, and actually make headway in resolving contentious issues."[138] In the case of the political abuse of psychiatry, Shevardnadze probably had a decisive voice in curbing the influence of the psychiatric establishment and of the KGB and making sure the practice ended, at least as a systematic government policy of repression. The value of that contribution to the cause of human rights cannot be underestimated. However, for many Georgians who know the other face of Shevardnadze, this is little consolation.

---

his book *Flight from USSR* (p. 23), referring to one of the most painful events during Shevardnadze's rule in Georgia, when a group of young Tbilisi students and actors tried to hijack a plane to escape from the USSR and failed. Together with a totally innocent priest the hijackers were sentenced to death and executed; only a 19-year old girl was spared, and was sentenced to 14 years after having undergone a forced abortion while being in prison. See Turashvili, David: *Flight from the USSR*, Tbilisi 2008

138 *Turmoil and Triumph*, pp. 744-745

High-level political involvement

It was in April 1987 that Shevardnadze's direct involvement in the issue began. A delegation under the leadership of US Secretary of State George Shultz was visiting Moscow in order to deal with arms control and Richard Schifter, then the US Assistant Secretary of State for Human Rights and Humanitarian Affairs, had suggested to Secretary Shultz that he would come along to discuss human rights. Shultz agreed and when the American delegation got to Moscow, Schultz told Shevardnadze that he brought the Assistant Secretary of State for Human Rights along as a member of the delegation. He suggested that Shevardnadze appoint someone to discuss human rights issues with him. Shevardnadze agreed and appointed his deputy Anatoly Adamishin. "I had my first meeting with Anatoly [Adamishin] on April 14, 1987. Anatoly had been involved in African affairs and was brand new to human rights. When I raised the issue of abuse of psychiatry with him, he told me he had no information on that subject. But the U.S. concern was obviously noted and at another arms control meeting, in September 1987, in Washington, we had another human rights meeting, this time with Yuri Reshetov, who conceded that the practice had existed but had been abandoned."[139]

Shevardnadze himself had only recently been alerted to the issue of political abuse of psychiatry, although he seems to have known about the issue before.[140] "In the winter of 1986-1987, on one of the Western information

139 Letter from Richard Schifter to the author, September 28, 2009

140 In our interview on October 15, 2009, Shevardnadze said that he had known of political abuse of psychiatry before he became Foreign Minister, when he was Minister of Internal Affairs in Georgia, "but I did not interfere with the work of judicial organs. It was an issue of the KGB". When checking documentation on political abuse of psychiatry in the Soviet Union, it is noteworthy that virtually no documentation exists on such abuses in Georgia, although some cases seem to have taken place. For instance, in the *Biographical Dictionary of the Political Abuse of Psychiatry in the Soviet Union*, no cases from Georgia are reported, and no Georgian psychiatrists or Georgian psychiatric hospitals mentioned.
The idea that top leaders of the country were not aware of some of the human rights violations is not so outlandish as it might seem. Anatoly Adamishin remembers that sometimes Western politicians would provide the Soviets with data they did not have themselves. "Gorbachev exclaimed once, with reference to Hans-Dieter Genscher's claim that there were 300,000 Germans in the Soviet Union who would like to move to Germany: 'In the West they know it better than we ourselves know it from our internal information!'" *Human Rights, Perestroika and the End of the Cold War*, p. 83

materials in which there was talk of political abuse of psychiatry in the USSR, [Foreign Minister Eduard] Shevardnadze wrote the instruction to inform him urgently of the real state of affairs in this area," remembers Andrei Kovalev, then working at the Foreign Ministry. "That evening, work started seriously on the preparation of reforms in Soviet psychiatry."[141]

The invitation was followed by many months of discussion on this issue at international gatherings, such as the Convention on Security and Cooperation in Europe (CSCE) and also at human rights roundtables between Schifter and his counterparts in the Soviet Ministry of Foreign Affairs.[142] One of the key officials at the Soviet Foreign Ministry was Anatoly Kovalev, First Deputy Minister of Foreign Affairs. According to his son, Andrei Kovalev, who worked in the Ministry's Department of Human Rights and Humanitarian Affairs, "moving in the necessary direction demanded a private conversation between my father ... with Prime Minister N.I. Ryzhkov, who was surprised and upset when he learned abut the political abuse of psychiatry. During one of the next meetings of the Politburo, he angrily spoke out on this issue. However, the network of those involved in psychiatric repression was so strong that a clear and strong position of the General Secretary [Mikhail Gorbachev], the Prime-Minister and the Minister of Foreign Affairs, was only enough to provide a legal basis to the work that was undertaken. This legal basis was only relative since on basis of the then-existing rules, everything that happened within the Politburo was kept strictly secret and I was not supposed to know, let alone refer to it."[143]

---

141 *Page from the book of condolences*, memoirs by Andrei Kovalev, p. 1.

142 The CSCE has its roots in the 1973 Conference on Security and Cooperation in Europe (CSCE). Talks had been mooted about a European security grouping since the 1950s but the Cold War prevented any substantial progress until the talks in Helsinki began in November 1972. The recommendations of the talks, "The Blue Book", gave the practical foundations for a three-stage conference, the Helsinki process. The CSCE opened in Helsinki on July 3, 1973 with 35 states sending representatives. Stage I only took five days to agree to follow the Blue Book. Stage II was the main working phase and was conducted in Geneva from September 18, 1973 until July 21, 1975. The result of Stage II was the Helsinki Final Act which was signed by the 35 participating States during Stage III, which took place from July 30 to August 1, 1975. The concepts of improving relations and implementing the Act were developed over a series of follow-up meeting, with major gatherings in Belgrade (October 4, 1977 - March 8, 1978), Madrid (November 11, 1980 - September 9, 1983), and Vienna (November 4, 1986 - January 19, 1989). THE CSCE is now called OSCE – Organization on Security and Cooperation in Europe.

143 *Page from the book of Condolences*, p. 4

Soon after Kovalev started working on the issue of Soviet psychiatry, he ran into trouble. "In the beginning, the task seemed quite standard: to understand what was going on, prepare concepts for reform of normative acts, and take them to the Politburo for signing by Shevardnadze and the Minister of Health. Unexpected events that destroyed this scheme started from the very beginning, mostly because we were met with unusually strong resistance on the part of the Ministry of Health. The normal request to be able to study the existing instructions was met by an unexpected reaction from the relevant bureaucrats: 'there are no instructions,' they told us. But we knew they existed and not only because it couldn't be otherwise. We had copies, or rather quotes, from them that had reached us via rather detective methods."[144]

During his work on the case of Soviet political abuse at the Foreign Ministry, Andrei Kovalev also met the leaders of these practices, Georgi Morozov and Marat Vartanyan. In particular, the latter made a lasting impression. "The first time I met with them personally was in the office of the head of international affairs of the Ministry of Health of the USSR, E. Kosenko, who successfully continued to carry out this function in the Russian Ministry after the collapse of the [Soviet] Union. A silent Chief Psychiatrist of the USSR Ministry of Health, A. Churkin, also attended that meeting. I formulated the task ahead of us from the point of view of foreign policy, discussing in that context the professional diagnostic views of the leaders of punitive psychiatry. Vartanyan exploded: 'How can you talk about insufficiencies of our psychiatry, when the whole world is in awe?' I was not able to withstand such an overt hypocrisy and very undiplomatically taught him a lesson on the morality of the criticism towards us, [mentioning] the lists of victims of abuse of psychiatry and our expulsion from the World Psychiatric Association."[145]

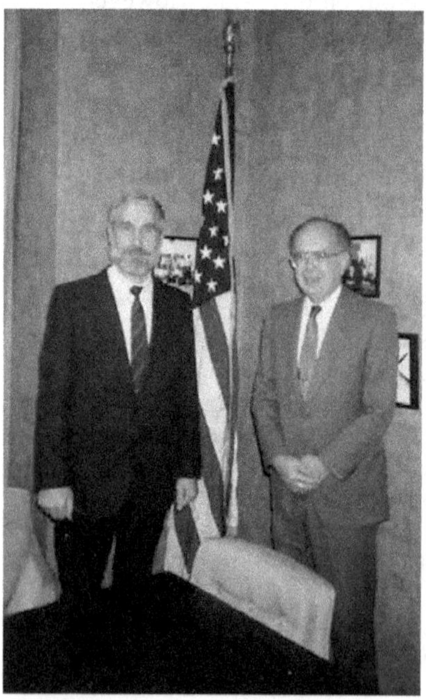

Anatoly Koryagin and Richard Schifter, 1988

[144] *Page from the Book of Condolences*, p. 6

[145] *Page from the Book of Condolences*, p. 4-5

Assistant Secretary of State Richard Schifter, convinced that any investigative or explorative mission should be carried out by psychiatrists rather than diplomats, sought the active involvement of the APA and contacted Ellen Mercer, who referred the issue to the Board of Trustees in June 1987. The Board of Trustees gave their approval in principle for the APA to become involved and allocated the sum of $15,000 to cover expenses. The Soviet Embassy was contacted, but no response followed. In subsequent discussions between the State Department and the Soviet Ministry of Foreign Affairs, it became clear that the Soviets would not allow the APA to undertake such a mission. Seeing that on this issue the Soviets would not budge, Schifter decided to adapt his strategy and seek APA involvement in an informal and unofficial way by asking the association to provide consultants to the State Department.

In March 1988, a Soviet official delegation visited the United States, accompanied by Gennady Milyokhin, the person responsible for international affairs at the Serbski Institute. Knowing that among the delegation members would be a psychiatrist who had specifically been asked to discuss involuntary psychiatric commitment, Schifter asked Ellen Mercer to suggest American psychiatrists who might participate. She suggested Dr. Loren Roth from Pittsburgh.[146]

The discussion proved to be fruitful and led to Loren Roth being invited to participate in roundtable human rights discussions in Moscow in April 1988. Although he traveled to Moscow as a private psychiatrist, it was clear to all sides that he had been delegated by the APA to do so. One of the proposals was to involve the National Institute of Mental Health (NIMH) in the potential US visit, something to which the Soviets reacted enthusiastically because they were eager to resume collaboration on mental health issues which had been discontinued after the Soviet invasion of Afghanistan. The compromise decision reached was that the undertaking would be a State Department mission with consultation from both NIMH and the APA.

In a memorandum to APA Medical Director Melvin Sabshin, Loren Roth noted how pressure on the Soviet psychiatric establishment was now

---

[146] Dr. Loren Roth is the Associate Senior Vice Chancellor, Health Sciences at the University of Pittsburgh. He was the former Chief Medical Officer of the University of Pittsburgh Medical Center. At the time described in this chapter (1988-9) he was Director of the Law and Psychiatry Program at WPIC and Psychiatric Team Leader of the U.S. Delegation to assess changes in Soviet Psychiatry.

coming from a very different side. "…It is clear that the winds of change… blow not from the West, but from the East. In effect, the Foreign Ministry is involved in a kind of internal political struggle with Soviet psychiatry. Soviet psychiatry is… being 'scapegoated,' but in a 'for internal consumption acceptable way' as having made errors in the past … which are now being fixed. Thus the psychiatrists get the blame for what has been, in most part, a political, KGB problem, even if some prominent psychiatrists, probably a minority, have been active and enthusiastic participants in the political abuse maters. They must now eat crow – but only Russian crow which is more digestible than American crow."[147] Still, no acknowledgement of past mistakes had been forthcoming, neither on the part of Soviet psychiatrists nor on the part of the Foreign Ministry: "While officially castigating the psychiatric establishment, the Foreign Ministry (and I assume 'higher ups') simultaneously still support it, de facto, in its old ways through its old leadership. Furthermore, I met no new leaders of Soviet psychiatry, with the exception of Dr. Churkin whose status is ambiguous."[148]

In his memorandum, Loren Roth outlined all the difficulties ahead, of which the political game between Soviet psychiatry and the Foreign Ministry was only one. "All this poses a most difficult question since we wish to be scientific and professional, yet the Soviets will attempt to stack the deck in every way." The road ahead would be a very difficult one, as without concrete scientific proof, the American visit could have a completely contrary effect and clear the way for a jubilant Soviet return to the WPA. "Because they have not been honest with us in admitting what they have done in the past, I believe they cannot be honest with us in the future vis-à-vis these examinations… Furthermore, Mr. Glukhov[149] made the following interesting remark concerning Soviet psychiatry: 'The past

147 Confidential memorandum of Loren Roth to Melvin Sabshin and Ellen Mercer, April 27, 1988, p. 2.

148 Confidential memorandum Loren Roth, p. 3. Eduard Shevardnadze confirmed in our interview that the issue had been discussed during a Politburo meeting and that it had been decided that the practice needed to end immediately. However, there was strong resistance, in particular from the KGB. He did not remember what the positioning of Chazov was with regard to this issue. Interview with Shevardnadze, October 15, 2009. According to Anatoly Adamishin, one of Shevardnadze's Deputy Foreign Ministers who was very much involved in human rights issues, Chazov's role was at first quite ambiguous but later a positive one. E-mail from Anatoly Adamishin, November 28, 2009.

149 Mr. Glukhov was Acting Head of the department for Human Rights and Humanitarian Affairs of the Soviet Foreign Ministry, as the formal head of the department, Yuri Borisovich Kashlev, had become head of the Soviet delegation to the CSCE Conference in Vienna. He was later succeeded by Yuri Reshetov.

was a silent movie, but the sound movie has yet to be written.' Clearly, the Soviet psychiatrists are unhappy."[150]

An additional problem Loren Roth foresaw was the tension between the political and the scientific agenda. Once direct scientific exchanges between American and Soviet psychiatrists were established, the ghost would be out of the bottle and it would be impossible to be put back, even if the visit as such would not provide the desired outcome: "Once an NIMH sponsored delegation goes to the USSR (whatever its findings), the point has been made that the Soviet Union is open; international experts are welcome; we are reasonable people; etc. It will be very difficult for anyone, including the APA, to dismiss that fact in the forum of world psychiatry. … If the consequences are negative, we have done an immoral act. Therefore, we must make certain that the outcome is positive. Otherwise what we are doing is not defensible."[151]

The head of the American delegation, Assistant Secretary of State Richard Shifter, managed to move psychiatry to the top of the agenda and, in spite of Soviet attempts to block this, have the issue discussed during a plenary session. The Soviet side consisted of a group of 25 Soviet officials, led by Richard Shifter's counterpart, Mr. Glukhov, and his deputy, Mr. Yuri Reshetov, "…(whom I call the 'bully'). Reshetov is blunt, barrel-chested, unfriendly, probably an alcoholic, and mean."[152] Chief psychiatrist of the USSR Ministry of Health, Aleksandr Churkin, represented the psychiatric field, and was later joined by Gennadi Milyokhin of the Serbski Institute.

The three-day visit, during which Loren Roth met Nikolai Zharikov and Georgi Morozov as well as a number of other Soviet psychiatrists, ended on a positive note. Clearly, disagreements with regard to the conditions under which a US visit would take place remained, but, in principle, both sides agreed that the door to further negotiations was open and that a visit might be feasible later that year.

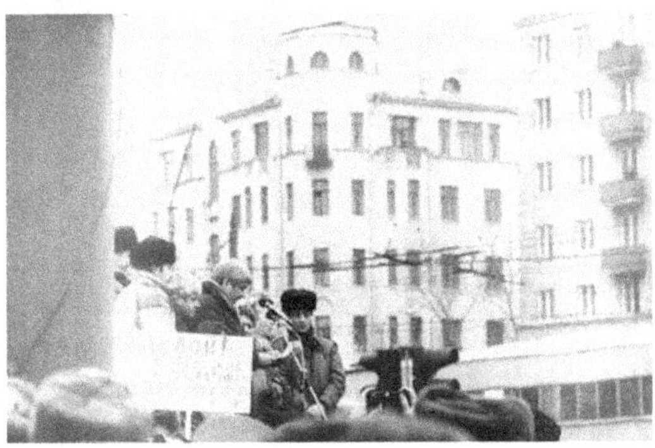

Democratic politician Yuri Afanasyev speaking at a demonstration in Moscow, 1990

150 Confidential memorandum Loren Roth, p. 4
151 Confidential memorandum Loren Roth, p. 5-6
152 Confidential memorandum Loren Roth, p. 11

Negotiations

Later than initially planned, a small delegation traveled to Moscow on 9-12 November 1988, in order to negotiate the terms of the agreement that would form the basis of the visit.[153] "What helped the successful outcome of the negotiations was the fact that the Chief Psychiatrist of the USSR Ministry of Health, A.A. Churkin, acknowledged cases of 'hyperdiagnosis' and 'unjustified long compulsory hospitalizations for forced treatment.' We should not forget that it was the diagnostic system that Soviet psychiatrists had developed themselves which made it capable to satisfy the most refined taste of a wirepuller, which appears the closest to what society demanded, and not the person… The word 'hyperdiagnosis' sounded, in that context, very nasty."[154] Dr. Roth made several trips along the way and his perseverance and hyperactivity alone must have driven the Soviets completely insane. At the same time, Andrei Kovalev's memoirs show that the latter developed a deep respect for Loren Roth and saw him as a "person who was committed to his cause and whom you could trust."[155] Undoubtedly, the psychiatric nomenklatura and the representatives of the USSR Ministry of Health did not share this view, yet they were so squeezed between the American State Department and the Soviet Foreign Ministry who had a common

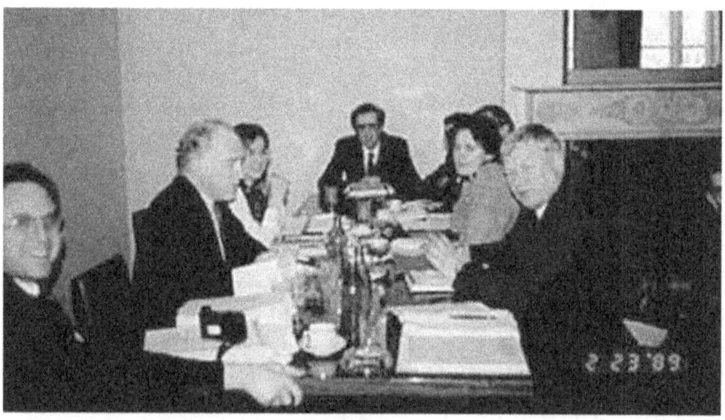

Negotiations in Moscow, February 1989. left Loren Roth and Bill Farrand. In the middle Andrei Kovalev. On the right Yuri Reshetov

---

153 The advance team consisted of Loren Roth, Darrel Regier, Sam Keith, Saleem Shah, and Ellen Mercer in addition to Bill Farrand of the US State Department.

154 *Page from the Book of Condolences*, p. 14

155 *Page from the Book of Condolences*, p. 14. The two maintained contact until 1996, and it was a letter to Loren Roth that enabled the author to trace Andrei Kovalev and establish contact.

agenda and were keen to end the political abuse of psychiatry in the USSR and remove it from the political agenda.[156]

A key element in the negotiations was the issue of a reciprocal visit to the United States. A confidential 45-page report by Ellen Mercer on the visit describes the negotiations in minute detail and shows that at every meeting this issue came to the fore. The Soviets insisted that their visit to the United States should be under the same conditions as the one being planned for the USSR; the US negotiators kept to the position that a positive outcome of the US visit to the USSR would certainly lead to an atmosphere that would contribute to a successful Soviet return visit, but that this did not automatically mean that all conditions would be identical. They would have to be negotiated. At the same time, however, the Soviet side used the possibility of an identical visit to the United States also as a means to try to soften the American conditions: "I believe the Americans are inclined to make an inspection visit – and I don't think the American psychiatrists will be satisfied if we go on the same conditions they propose for us."[157]

An additional issue was the complexity of the undertaking, as the Americans and, in particular, the National Institute for Mental Health (NIMH) were paying the expenses[158] and were keen to have a scientifically sound exercise, with all the preconditions it entailed. The fact that American conditions changed halfway through the negotiations evoked a rather angry reaction from Andrei Kovalev of the Foreign Ministry: "I appreciate the flexibility of the American side, but I'm surprised. When we speak of flexibility, it's only for the American side."[159]

Yet, in spite of occasional irritations on both sides, gradually an agreement was reached on all the details of the visit, and it seemed all was settled. "Just as we expected, the meeting was coming to an end with agreement on

156 This is confirmed by Andrei Kovalev, one of the main negotiators on the Soviet side. Interview with Andrei Kovalev, October 12, 2009.

157 Confidential USSR Trip Report, Ellen Mercer, November 8-13, 1988, p. 25

158 The overwhelming majority of funding for the project came from NIMH and according to estimates the project cost around $300,000.

159 Confidential USSR Trip Report, Ellen Mercer, November 8-13, 1988, p. 24. As Kovalev explained during my interview with him on October 12, 2009, "the issue was one of prestige. Of course it was clear that a Soviet visit to the United States would not take the form of an inspection, but in order to allow the Soviet Union not to lose face it was important to have this agreement on reciprocity. Farrand did not understand this, but for Schifter this was something he could completely adhere to."

all the necessary issues and the thoughts of the American team were turning to a bit of sightseeing in Moscow on our last day…. Mr. Kovalev said that it was very important to him to see if he had the right impression of what had happened here so that he could correctly report to his chief. He stated that his impression was that this is only the beginning of a large and mutual project that will begin in Moscow and continue in New York, Washington, etc. … He said: 'as we agreed, all relations between the United States and the Soviet Union are based on the principle of reciprocity. It is early to say when Soviet psychiatrists will visit the United States... [but] the principles of this visit will be the same as we just agreed for the American delegation in January'."[160]

Immediately, the atmosphere changed and a serious crisis was at hand. It seemed that all the work done over the past days and the agreements reached would be in vain and that the negotiations would be broken off: "it is not clear if the State Department is ready to be completely responsible for breaking the negotiations."[161]

"Mr. Kovalev continued by saying that on the first day of the meeting, we didn't know each other and our positions but movement in the direction of each other was possible. However, the representative of the State Department didn't change his position even an inch. … He stated that Mr. Farrand may be making a mistake by dealing with psychiatry as in the Dominican Republic rather than in a great power."[162] Andrei Kovalev remembers: "Yuri Reshetov, who was then the deputy head of my department, and the psychiatrists were already licking their teeth how they would search for political prisoners in American psychiatric hospitals."[163] … However, the representative from the State Department, R. Farrand, held a rather superficial position: no return visit, no reciprocity. 'How can there be reciprocity, when you have political abuse of psychiatry and we do not?' he asked. When everything seemed agreed upon and decided and the

160 Confidential USSR Trip Report, Ellen Mercer, November 8-13, 1988, p. 39. Looking back at that particular situation, Andrei Kovalev remembers that he had a free hand in the negotiations, provided there would be reciprocity. If that could not be achieved, the whole enterprise would falter and the KGB would block further steps. Letter of Kovalev to the author, October 15, 2009. The involvement of the KGB in all issues related to the negotiations, and in international diplomacy in general, was confirmed by Eduard Shevardnadze during our interview on October 15, 2009.

161 Confidential USSR Trip Report, Ellen Mercer, November 8-13, 1988, . p. 41

162 Confidential USSR Trip Report, Ellen Mercer, November 8-13, 1988, . p. 41

163 *Page from the Book of Condolences*, p. 15

members of the Soviet and American delegations started to get up to shake hands and exchange warm congratulations, I was forced to take the floor and, threatening the outcome of the negotiations, say that the visit will be carried out on the basis of reciprocity. Farrand exploded. ... I knew that the next day A.I. Glukhov [of the Foreign Ministry] would meet with the Assistant of the Secretary of State for Human Rights, R. Shifter, ... and I didn't doubt that this clever and sensitive diplomat would take a different position than his subordinate. That judgment proved to be correct."[164]

Sovietologist Peter Reddaway, selected to be a member of the US delegation, notes in his diary the continuous obstruction by Soviet psychiatrists. "When the Soviet psychiatrists (Ministry of Health – MoH) saw that the US group would be a much more serious and well-prepared one than any preceding group of visitors, it became wary and obstructive. However, the politically more powerful Ministry of Foreign Affairs (MFA) kept prodding the psychiatrists – sometimes even in front of the Americans – and in early November 1988 forced the MoH at last to agree to virtually all the US conditions."[165]

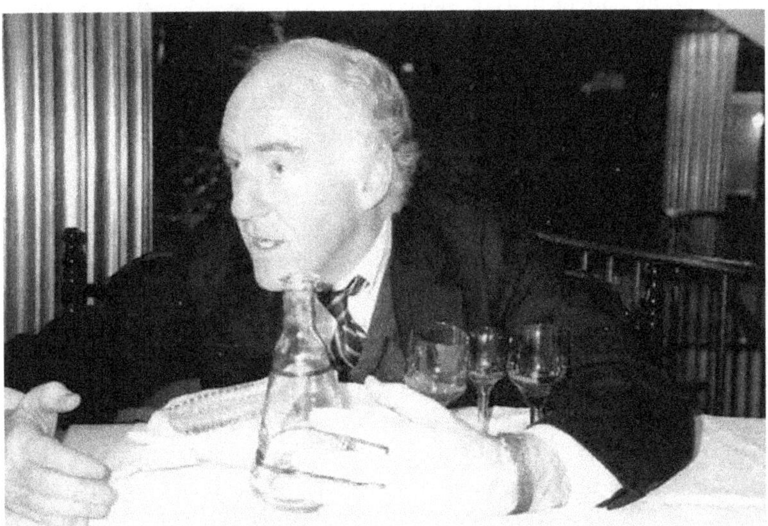

Bill Farrand

The reason for this should be sought, according to Reddaway, in the fact that the Soviets very much wanted the United States to agree on holding a

[164] *Page from the Book of Condolences*, p. 15

[165] *Confidential diary* of Peter Reddaway, April 12, 1989, p. 1

human rights conference in Moscow: "early November [1988] was the time that Soviet diplomacy was pulling out all the stops to get the West to hold a CSCE conference on human rights in Moscow in 1991 – hence the decision to agree to all our conditions. After the West responded positively to this and other concessions in late December, the Soviet psychiatrists, with the big diplomatic prize in the MFA's pocket, began backtracking on most of the promises they had made to us in November. In January-February it often seemed that – since we basically refused to compromise on the November agreement – the whole thing might collapse. But extra trips to Moscow by our negotiators… brought the MoH more or less into line."[166]

The two extra trips to remove these new obstacles were carried out by Bill Farrand of the State Department and Loren Roth. Roth remembers: "During this time ... Bill Farrand and I made two trips to Moscow. The second was on February 15, [1989,] ... The core issues then related to whether the Soviets or the Americans would go first [in examining patients] and whether the American side could examine patients without the Soviet side present, etc. We would not tolerate the Soviet side intimidating the patient or seeing the patient first, or alone for obvious reasons… Because many persons did not object to a Soviet psychiatrist being present while the American side went first, we arrived at a satisfactory resolution of both the human rights and the scientific issues. Both sides saw and heard the same thing, even with respect to the released patients."[167]

In his memoirs, Kovalev points to another reason for the constant obstruction on the Soviet side. "The issue was that the patients who interested the American psychiatrists in the first place had been diagnosed in the Serbski Institute. On their medical records was written 'secret.' The diagnoses had been written by Academicians and well-known professors. In the medical files, terrible things were encountered. For instance, they refused to discharge one of the patients from hospital until he would give up his religious convictions, for which he had been hospitalized. They wanted to hide all this and that's why they put the whole thing in the reverse."[168] In order to hide the most unpleasant documents, such as proof that high-level psychiatrists were involved, papers were ripped out of the files.[169] Subsequently, the Soviet psychiatric establishment used other tactics to try to obstruct the American visit. The files could not be photocopied, because the photocopiers at the Ministry had broken down; coincidentally, the same

166 *Confidential diary* of Peter Reddaway, p. 1-2
167 Letter from Loren Roth to the author, October 4, 2009
168 *Page from the Book of Condolences*, p. 16
169 Interview with Andrei Kovalev, October 12, 2009

counted for the copier at the Serbski Institute and the one in Vartanyan's office. Then a fire took place in Milyokhin's office, where the files were kept. He barely managed to save them from the fire. After this, they were stored in Andrei Kovalev's office, ready to be handed over to the Americans. By the time they were handed over, most of them had not yet been photocopied and thus the Americans received mostly original files.[170]

At some point, the Ministry of Health even decided at a meeting of all those involved (with undoubtedly included Morozov and Vartanyan) that no medical records would be handed over whatsoever. However, one of the officials at the Ministry of Health told Andrei Kovalev that the files could be handed over, and the latter called the American Embassy and an assistant came over to pick them up. "However, after the woman left with the files, I got a phone call from the same person at the Health Ministry who, this time, had a different tone. Instead of a conversation between acquaintances, it was an official conversation and he called my by my first name and patronymic. He informed me that the Ministry had decided not to hand over the files. I was shocked, it was clear I had been set up. I even checked the Criminal Code to see what punishment would be given for handing over official documents to a representative of a foreign country."[171] The situation was saved by Foreign Minister Eduard Shevardnadze, "who called Minister of Health Chazov and asked him to do everything possible to make the visit successful. Still, this chief Soviet 'medik,' as I was told by witnesses later, shouted on the eve of the visit that 'Kovalev is selling out the honor and dignity of the motherland'."[172]

With a week's delay, caused by some additional unexpected hurdles, the group of about 25 people traveled to the USSR on February 25, 1989. This group consisted of Bill Farrand of the State Department; Loren Roth as head of the psychiatric team; psychiatrists from the National Institute of Mental Health, including Darrel A. Regier, Scientific Director of the US Delegation, four émigré Soviet psychiatrists living in the U.S., and Harold Visotsky from Chicago as head of the hospital visit team. In addition, there were State Department interpreters, two attorneys, Ellen Mercer of the American Psychiatric Association and Peter Reddaway.[173]

---

170 Interview with Andrei Kovalev, October 12, 2009

171 Interview with Andrei Kovalev, October 12, 2009

172 *Page from the Book of Condolences*, p. 17.

173 The larger team consisted of forensic psychiatric experts (Joseph Bloom, M.D., John Monahan, Ph.D., Jonas Rappaport, M.D.); scientists from NIMH who formulated the standardized psychiatric interview (Director of the Division of Clinical Research at NIMH Darrel Regier, M.D., Sam Keith, M.D.,

Obstruction

Prior to the trip, a list of 48 names of patients and former patients was sent to the Soviets and they were asked to provide all case records provided that the individuals in question agreed to the release of their records. Eventually, these records were presented to the Americans - in either photocopy or (in most cases) in their original form. Yet when one reads the diaries of the members of the US delegation, one cannot avoid the impression that the obstruction continued to the very end of the visit. Patient records were not translated and not all were provided; much of what they did provide was handed over much later than promised, and thus the team had a hard time making use of all the information.[174] The Soviets demanded to examine all the patients themselves as well, to which the Americans agreed, and then also demanded to receive copies of all the videotapes of the examinations.

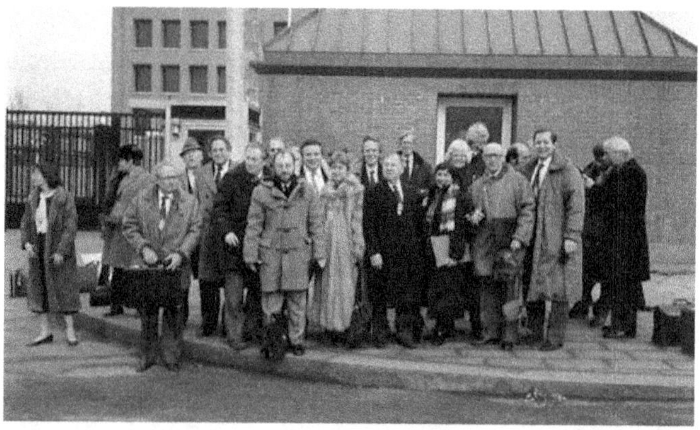

American Delegation in front of the US Embassy, March 1989

Robert Hirschfeld, M.D. and William Carpenter, M.D.); former Soviet psychiatrists living in the United States (Vladimir Levit, M.D., Felix Kleyman, M.D., David Lozovsky, M.D., Leon Stern, M.D.); attorneys (Joel Klein and Richard Bonnie); an expert in all aspects of the Soviet Union (Peter Reddaway); and leaders in international affairs in the APA (Harold Visotsky, M.D. and Ellen Mercer). In addition, the U.S. Department of State sent its representatives and six interpreters. Loren Roth, M.D. was the psychiatric team leader; the delegation leader was R. W. Farrand, Senior Deputy Assistant Secretary of State for Human Rights and Humanitarian Affairs and Darrel Regier M.D. was Scientific Director of the Delegation. The hosting organizations in the Soviet Union were the Ministry of Health and the Ministry of Foreign Affairs.

174 In fact, the Ministry of Health had not made any copies under the pretext that their photocopier had broken down, and thus the photocopies were made at the Ministry of Foreign Affairs. *Page from the Book of Condolences*, p. 17

Even more obstructive was the fact that the Soviets failed to produce all the patients on the list. Time and again they would claim that a patient could not be found or refused to be interviewed. "That is where we came in. We were in constant communication with both the Americans and with dissidents in Moscow, in particular Aleksandr Podrabinek who had become politically active again and was publishing an independent newspaper, *Express Khronika*. During telephone conversations with members of the American delegation … we collected information on the persons who, according to the Soviets, had disappeared without a trace or had refused to appear, and passed the information on to Podrabinek. He, in turn, went out to find them, and, via his network, the people were traced. Often it turned out that the people had been threatened or never even contacted, or had indicated that they wanted to be examined and the information had not been passed on by the Soviet authorities. This information was, in turn, again passed on to the American delegation, who, the next morning, confronted their Soviet hosts with this information. The Soviets were repeatedly speechless."[175]

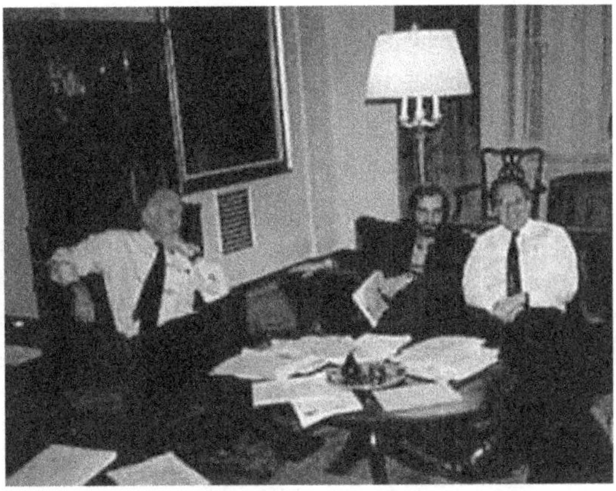

preparations in Moscow. l.t.r. Bill Farrand, Aleksandr Podrabinek, Loren Roth

The files of IAPUP are full of messages to the APA, in particular Ellen Mercer, reporting on the state of affairs in Moscow. All the potential patients were numbered and in communicating with Aleksandr (Sasha) Podrabinek, we worked only in codes. (1) Would mean that the person concerned definitely agreed to be interviewed by the American delegation; (2) meant maybe, (3) definitely not and (0) that the person was unknown. Messages were like "Sasha P[odrabinek] will check 19 and 44; 19 he'll know tomorrow whether the guy actually agrees or not, or disagree to consent, as the Soviets state. 44 is more difficult: where is the guy? Got the message on the second cable. I don't like it, and neither does Sasha. Two conditions are unacceptable, I'd say. What about the three earlier points, are they giving all the files in photocopy, and did they find all the others? Please call

175 *On Dissidents and Madness*, pp. 124-5

somewhat later – say 11.00 h. your time."[176] Other messages give the same idea: "Just a quick note, after talking to Sasha after talking to you. A. is not too ill, he agreed and wants to come with his wife. Sasha just spoke to her. K...... – G...... – N.......: they are (3), so no examination! ... Those who have a (1), Sasha is continuously in contact with them. They'll be there, even if Soviets say they can't be found or disagreed – except those who are inside of course; in that case Soviets don't want to show them."[177] Or, a bit later: "Very important news: Sasha P. has direct contact with no. 19 yesterday. He never refused an examination by the US delegation! They threatened him, tried to force him to refuse..."[178]

Day after day, Podrabinek would bring former psychiatric prisoners to the psychiatrists for their day-long examination beginning with the signing of a consent form, which they had never experienced in a Soviet examination, and a urine test. What we didn't know then was that also the Foreign Ministry was trying to find the "missing" patients and that the Soviet psychiatrists were thus pushed from two seemingly opposite sides. "One of the 'disappeared' patients we tried to find till four o'clock in the morning, sitting with Milyokhin and his group in his office at the Serbski Institute. We were told that he had been taken out of one hospital, but not delivered to the other. We found him only via the chief doctor of the hospital, where this patient had actually been taken. They probably fouled up the mood of this chief doctor, because we found him with his lover."[179] Interestingly, not only was the psychiatric establishment pressured by a common agenda of the American and Soviet Foreign Ministries, but also by the fact that both the Soviet Foreign Ministry and the dissidents were actively searching for patients the

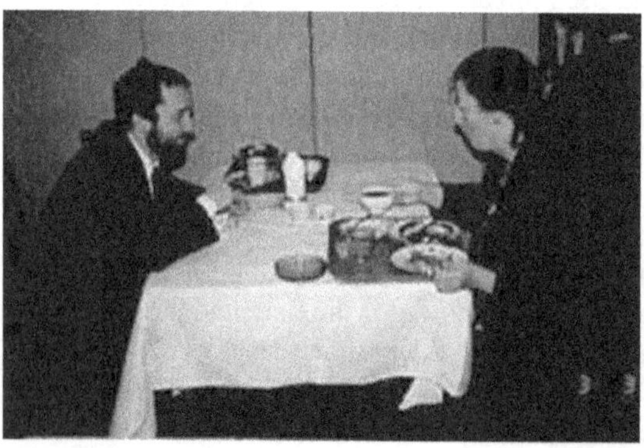

Aleksandr Podrabinek briefing the US delegation in Moscow, March 1989

---

[176] Urgent message to Ellen Mercer from Robert van Voren, no date. The content indicates that Mercer must have been in Moscow then. Maybe during the second preparatory visit?

[177] Fax to Ellen Mercer for Robert van Voren, "11 February, 1989, 5.30 Amsterdam time."

[178] Fax to Ellen Mercer, February 13, 1989, 13.30 Amsterdam time

[179] Page from the Book of Condolences, p. 18.

psychiatrists claimed to be untraceable or not willing to meet the American delegation.

Out of the list of 48 names, the Americans interviewed 27 people, all of whom were given standardized psychiatric interviews and forensic interviews. The interview process for each patient lasted approximately 4-6 hours. Family members or friends of the patients were also interviewed. Interviewing was performed by three interview teams - each team consisting of a Russian-speaking psychiatrist (a Soviet émigré living in the U.S.), a research scientist, a forensic psychiatrist or psychologist, and two interpreters. The Russian-speaking psychiatrist interviewed the patient in Russian and the interpreters translated into English for the research scientist and forensic specialist.[180]

At the same time, a hospital visit team traveled through the country and visited several psychiatric hospitals. "We were not required to name the hospitals the hospital visiting team would visit, including the Special Psychiatric Hospitals, until the delegation arrived in the USSR. This occurred, I recall vividly when Harold Visotsky and I, with some input from others, decided to visit Kazan, Chernyakhovsk Special Hospitals, as well as the Vilnius and Kaunas Hospitals. We announced this in small meeting with Reshetov in a rather dramatic way after we arrived in Moscow and he agreed."[181] The hospital visit team was allowed almost total access to the hospitals and grounds and was allowed to meet with many patients without the presence of the Soviets. Although these meetings were not psychiatric interviews, they provided relevant information on the type of cases interned in those hospitals and the conditions of treatment at each facility.

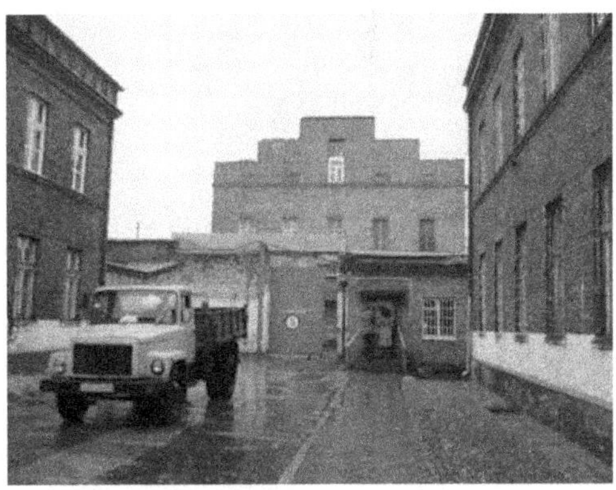

Chernyakhovsk forensic psychiatric hospital

The (confidential) reports on these visits are often heartbreaking, because of the fact that the Americans for the first time faced Soviet psychiatry in its true form, not only with regard to politi-

[180] The presence of émigré psychiatrists on the American delegation caused strong resistance on the part of the KGB, who refused to provide them with entry visas. Interview with Andrei Kovalev, October 12, 2009

[181] Letter from Loren Roth to the author, October 4, 2009

cal dissidents but to mental patients in general. Especially the visits to Kazan and Chernyakhovsk left a lasting impression, although also the open attitude of the new director of Chernyakhovsk Special Psychiatric Hospital was noted.[182] At the same time, the Soviets still tried to conceal the real situation (e.g. just before the delegation's visit, walls had been freshly painted, and quite a few members of the hospital visiting team noted fresh paint marks on their clothes) or influence the interaction between the Americans and their patients. One letter from Chernyakhovsk was especially noteworthy: "Respected delegation, we patients are very pleased and grateful for your visit to us. We ask you come to us more often – your visit makes it easier to live in these prisons. We very much want to tell you the true facts, which our administration in concealing from you. But all the patients are keeping quiet because they

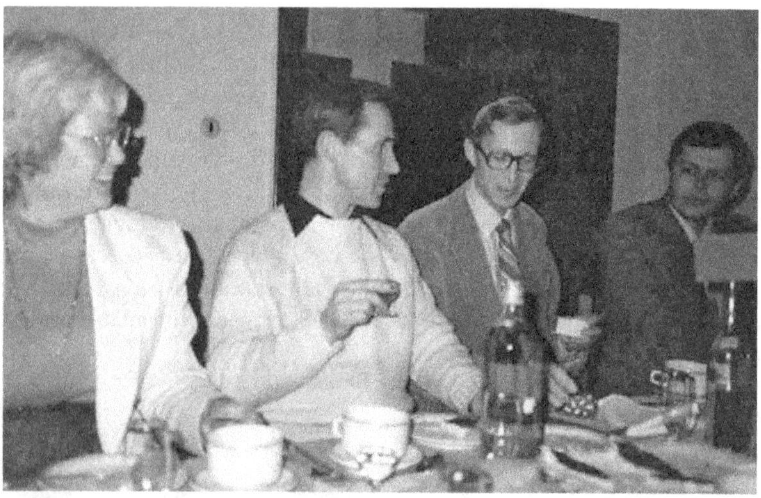

Chernyakhovsk hospital director Viktor Fukalov toasting to Ellen Mercer (l) and Peter Reddaway (r), March 1989

fear the consequences from their doctors. Simply for telling the truth they will give us injections after your departure… Thank you again for your visit to us. It was very nice to meet the professor who radiates such compassion. I would like to be treated in America – why not try such

182 Viktor Fukalov, who had been appointed Director of Chernyakhovsk just a few months prior to the American visit. Almost twenty years later he is repeatedly host to teams of experts of Global Initiative on Psychiatry, who work together with him and his staff on creating a more modern approach to treatment and rehabilitation in his hospital. Fukalov's openness and humanity is remarkable even for today's Russian standards.

an experiment? Or at least your professors could come here and get us discharged."[183].

In a letter sent to Ellen Mercer five months after the US visit, Viktor Fukalov, the director of the Special Psychiatric Hospital in Chernyakhovsk, described what effect the visit had on his hospital: "During several days after your departure the hospital looked like a disturbed bee-hive. ... Some of our doctors still have difficulty to understand, and they object to, the way the American colleagues talked with the patients, from whom the treating doctors were unceremoniously removed. Also many patients later expressed their dissatisfaction with the form and the contents of the questioning. By the way, many decided to keep silent; some were very much pleased and proud to have had the possibility to have contact with American specialists. There were also those who said they certainly were not doctors, but CIA agents.[184] Later in his letter, he expressed his desire to maintain contacts with American colleagues and thanked Ellen Mercer extensively for the books she sent upon her return to the USA.

In Lithuania, the hospital visit team encountered the rise of Lithuanian nationalism, a country which then seemed to be firmly rooted in the USSR but which a year later would declare independence, thereby initiating a process that would lead to the disintegration of the Soviet Union. In Vilnius, they visited the Republican Psychiatric Hospital in Naujoji Vilnia, some twenty minutes by car from the center of Vilnius, headed by Dr. Valentinas Maciulis who had been director since 1982. "We received the instruction from the Ministry of Health in Moscow about a week in advance, telling us to prepare for a visit by a US delegation," Valentin Maciulis remembers. "It was an interesting political time, perestroika was in full swing and we were increasingly independent. Our Communist Party had separated from the CPSU, we had our national movement here in Lithuania, Sajudis, and on top of that we didn't pay much attention to the things Moscow said, we followed our own course and reforms were here already under way. But this was different for us, because it concerned a delegation by Americans, a

183 *Additional observations on Chernyakhovsk SPH*, by Peter Reddaway, p. 141. This fear was not unfounded. The WPA delegation visiting the USSR in 1991 met one of the people who had been examined by the US delegation in 1989, and after the US visit his treatment had been increased: "...case 3, who complained to the US delegation in Kazan strict supervision hospital in 1989. The notes reported 'a change in the patient's condition' and the drugs were considerably increased." Report on the WPA visit in 1991, p. 21.

184 Letter of Viktor Fukalov to Ellen Mercer, August 1989. IAPUP correspondence files, 1988.

unique chance to meet people from the West, so we were delighted to have the possibility. Westerners had never been to our hospital before, until then we only had hosted a conference for psychiatrists from 'fraternal countries' such as Poland, Czechoslovakia and Hungary."[185]

The US delegation was well received. "We cleaned up the hospital, of course, and received them. For us it was a big event. They looked around freely, could see patients and medical files, and used my meeting room as a base… For us it was like a door opening to the outside world. Until then we knew nothing, we did not even receive the publications and models from the World Health Organization. Everything went to Moscow and was 'processed' there, adapted to the Soviet requirements as decided by the establishment in Moscow, and then presented to us as if they were their ideas."[186]

Also in Kaunas the atmosphere was pretty nationalistic. The director of the Kaunas Ordinary Psychiatric Hospital, Dr. Voldemaras Berneris, was even for Lithuanian standards outspoken and, contrary to Maciulis in Vilnius, rather skeptical about the delegation's visit because it had been planned by Moscow. In her dairy, Ellen Mercer notes: "The first thing that Dr. Berneris said was that we were late and asked if the Americans work on Saturdays. He stated that one must respect the host and that means that guests must respect the host. The team apologized for being late and indicated that the timing of the visit was not totally under our control. Dr. Visotsky evoked the names of Drs. Chazov and Churkin, which made matters only worse, as he indicated that not even Minister Chazov could break the union rules regarding weekend work. Dr. Berneris indicated that they would show Lithuanian hospitality in any event… He further stated, however, that the team was destroying the hosts because they have to work on Saturday and Sunday and they won't be able to go to church."[187]

What the Americans did not know at that time, and which would have given the meeting a special dimension, was the fact that Berneris had been one of the five members of the psychiatric commission led by Professor Jonas Surkus[188] who had posthumously found the Kaunas student Romas Kalanta to be suffering from "schizophrenia." Kalanta, a 19-year old student in Kaunas, immolated himself in 1972 in protest against the Soviet

185 Interview with Valentin Maciulis, October 20, 2009

186 Interview with Valentin Maciulis, October 20, 2009

187 Confidential diary by Ellen Mercer on her visit to Kaunas OPH, p. 1

188 Prof. Jonas Surkus, Professor at Kaunas University, was one of the leading psychiatrists in communist Lithuania. He died in 1998 at the age of 79.

occupation of Lithuania, a symbolic act very similar to that of Jan Palach in Prague after the Soviet occupation.[189]

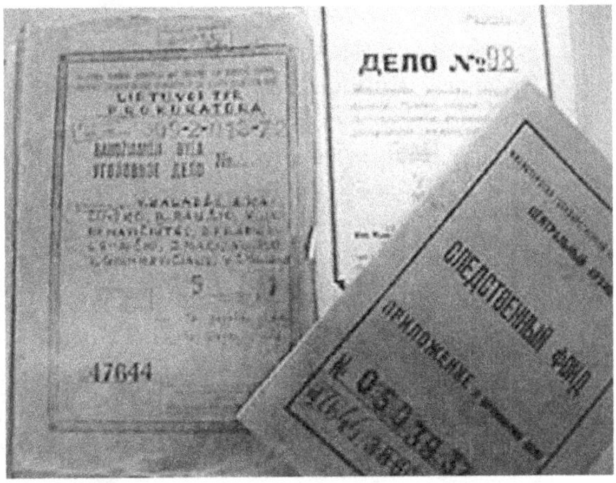

Kalanta file

Kalanta's death resulted in unusually heavy riots in Kaunas, which were mainly the result of the fact that the authorities decided to bury Kalanta as quickly as possible in order to avoid public unrest and by doing so, inadvertently caused exactly what they tried to avoid.[190] The city was temporarily blocked off from the rest of the country and surrounded by military, waiting for the order to intervene. The riots lasted several days and were eventually quelled by riot police resulting in arrests of demonstrators. The authorities, trying to explain why a young man would kill himself in such a way and in an attempt to avoid him becoming a national hero, first tried to find evidence of drug use. When no proof of drugs was found during a house search, they convened a number of top psychiatrists in the country to declare the deceased to be mentally ill. In a way, as Lithuanian psychiatrist Dainius Puras remembers, their diagnosis was not so strange. "In light of those times, being citizens of the Soviet Union and Soviet psychiatrists, they could not explain his behavior otherwise. He had written in one of his diaries that he dreamed that one day Lithuania would be free again. In 1972 that was just 'madness'; who could imagine that eighteen years later the country would declare independence?! The first commission underlined this remark in Kalanta's diary with red; this was clearly proof that there was something wrong with him. In addition, he had long hair, a clear sign

189 Jan Palach, a Prague student, was 21 years old when he set himself on fire in Wenceslas Square in Prague, on 16 January 1969. He was the first of a group of students to sign a suicide pact, but most of the others did not go through with their part, after the well-publicized pleas Palach made on his deathbed about the degree of pain they faced

190 See for instance the reference of 30 May 1972 by LSSR KGB Chairman J. Petkevičius on the self-immolation of Romas Kalanta and the subsequent events, document 19720530, to be found on www.kgbdocuments.eu

of schizophrenic defect – not able to take care of his own appearance. And thus they concluded that he was suffering from "schizophrenia."[191] In 1989, a commission led by Dr. Liaudginas Radavicius, with Dainius Puras being one of the members, studied the files extensively and interviewed friends and relatives of Kalanta. They came to the conclusion that there was no evidence that Kalanta had been suffering from any mental illness. The fact that Berneris had been involved in such a high-profile case and did not know whether the Americans were aware of that fact, might be another explanation for his expressive behavior.

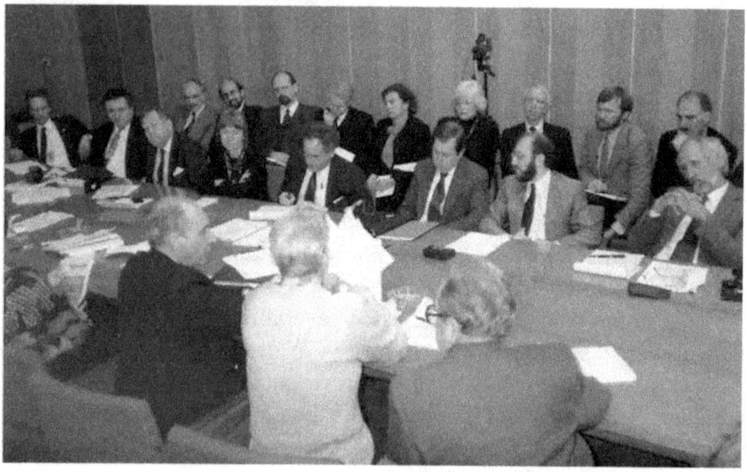

Concluding meeting between Soviet representatives and the US Delegation, Moscow, March 1989

After the visits to the various hospitals and the examination of alleged victims of political abuse of psychiatry, a joint meeting of both sides was held to discuss the experiences.[192] Each side had the opportunity to raise issues during this large meeting. Several of the Soviet psychiatrists starting giving long talks and were, in time, cut off by the Soviet chairman in the press of time. The talks were not always directly related to the issues at hand. The highlight of the presentations from the Soviet side came when the USSR Institute of State and Law's Professor S.V. Borodin and S.V. Polubinskaya spoke. The senior Borodin spoke first and basically negated

191 Interview with Dainius Puras, October 19, 2009. The commission was led by Professor Jonas Surkus of Kaunas; Professor J. Andriuskeviciene of Vilnius University; chief psychiatrist J. Gutmanas; Kaunas psychoneurological hospital director V. Berneris and his deputy D. Dauksiene.

192 This meeting was held on March 10, 1989, two days before the departure of the US delegation

all of the theories that the Soviet psychiatrists had supported and talked about the use of the law in such an inappropriate way. Following his talk, the Americans gave him a very long ovation, which clearly evoked emotion in this elderly man who had fought these battles for so long without result. The diaries of the team members show that an agreement between the two sides was still a far way off. The diary of Elmore Rigamer, head of the psychiatric services at the State Department, notes a very interesting discourse on one of the patients, a certain A.[193] "Dr. Keith discussed the patient A., stating that the activity of fighting for freedom is insufficient to make a diagnosis of schizophrenia and to warrant hospitalization for five years. Dr. Smulievich said that the patient had a schizoaffective illness, but the more he talked, the more confused and ambiguous his thoughts became. Dr. Smulievich described the patient A. as having pseudo-psychopathy which is not the same as chronic schizophrenia. His terminology is confused and appears to be influenced by a desire to fit it into a category that allows broad discretion in making dispositions. Smulievich then tried to describe what is psychopathic. 'In the Soviet system this is a person who has overvalued ideas. Yes, one can fight for freedom in a thousand and one ways but it should not be to the neglect of other areas of his life. A. fought for freedom and even wrote books about freedom, neglecting all other ideas in his life. His life became unbalanced, all of his interests were expressed in one area.' I wondered how he would diagnose an artist at the Bolshoi whose life is devoted to the perfection of the Ballet."[194]

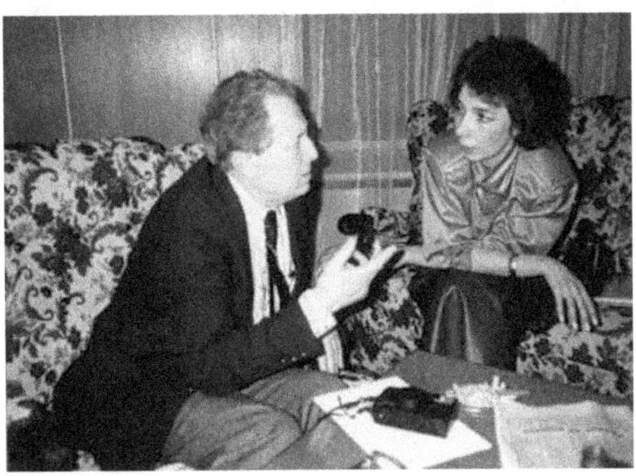

US Delegation member David Lozovsky with lawyer Svetlana Polubinskaya, March 1989

After a visit of more than two weeks, the delegation returned home and wrote its report. From confidential sources we at IAPUP knew that the report was pretty damaging to the Soviet authorities. Not only had the delegation established that there had been systematic political abuse of psychiatry, but also that this abuse had not ended, that there were

193 name withheld by the author because of medical confidentiality

194 Report by E. Rigamer on the joint meeting with the Soviets, March 10, 1989, p. 3-4

still victims of the political abuse in psychiatric hospitals and that the Soviet authorities – in particular the Soviet Society of Psychiatrists and Neuropathologists – still denied that psychiatry had been used as a method of repression.

As agreed, the Soviets had the right to write their commentary to the report, which should be published in conjunction. However, at that moment, Andrei Kovalev fell ill and during his absence a text was prepared by the Soviet psychiatric establishment and handed over to the US Embassy. "When I returned to work and found out, I read the text and the attached note, which was signed by Yuri Reshetov, who was at that time head of my department, and I was shocked. The medical part of the commentary was written in a completely confrontational manner and was simply blunt. This was very much different was the legal part, which had been put together by Professor S.V. Borodin and S.V. Polubinskaya. We redid the medical part together with specialists who had had nothing to do with the first version, and it took me a long time to convince Reshetov to replace the nonsense with the new text. In the end he agreed."[195]

But also on the Western side things did not go as opponents of Soviet political abuse of psychiatry had hoped for. Although the American visit to the USSR took place before the WPA Regional Symposium in Granada, during which the Soviets would be given ad-hoc membership of the WPA under rather mysterious circumstances, the report did not seem to have any effect on this decision, except maybe that the ad-hoc membership was rushed through the Executive Committee to precede the publication of the report. As Ellen Mercer said in an interview with the Canadian Broadcasting Corporation, "the Secretary General of the World Psychiatric Association has given the impression to a number of people here [in Granada] that he's really not particularly interested in the American report… that he doesn't seem to understand the significance of it… he doesn't seem to understand the thoroughness in which it was undertaken with very strict scientific procedures as formulated by our National Institute of Mental Health. I think it is unfortunate that he doesn't seem to be more interested in the report."[196]

In the opinion of IAPUP, the report had to be published as soon as possible, but for reasons unclear to us it was constantly postponed. We gradually got the feeling that the US Government didn't want the publication of the report to worsen the position of the Soviets and reduce their chances

[195] *Page from the Book of Condolences*, p. 23

[196] Interview with the CBC, March 1989. Text published in *Documents* 26, August 1989

to a return into the WPA. On July 12, 1989, Hearings were organized in the US Congress, where the author represented IAPUP. In my speech, I stressed that "our association also deeply deplores the fact that it has taken the American psychiatric delegation so long to publish its report. We feel that this factor very much helped the leadership of the World Psychiatric Association to bend the rules of the Statutes and Bylaws of its Association and to give the All-Union Society provisional membership of the WPA. The four months silence on the part of the American psychiatric delegation allowed the Soviets to pretend that nothing is wrong."[197] My remarks resulted in a fierce reaction on the part of Richard Schifter; yet, at that time to me his fierce reaction only confirmed the accuracy of my suspicions.

However, US delegation leader Loren Roth has a very simple explanation for the "delay": "The reason for the delay back there in 1989 when this was published was --from the perspective of the report authors - 'no delay at all.' This report was conceived of as a truly scientific publication ….The NIMH, which paid the main [part] for this trip would have nothing else. Most of the writing was done by Regier, Keith (NIMH), Bonnie and Roth, and by the visiting team that went to the hospitals in Kazan, Chernyakhovsk, Lithuania, etc. … I made several trips to Washington to do this. Such writing and revision and achieving "balance" plus civility took time, etc. Many of us knew the human rights issue was the underlying driving concern for us and for the State Department, but from the scientific perspective and writing this had to be done in such a traditional respectable format in accord with agreed upon facts and organization. I believe the diagnostic material was reviewed very carefully and had to be. The "delay" issue is an example of what you note I said and thought from the beginning. We had to do both science and human rights and sometimes one or another took precedence in the short run. We did not want to be accused of being unfair or ideological within our own internal judgment or conscience."[198]

Eventually the report was published in the *Schizophrenia Bulletin* in both English and Russian; however, due to the late date of publication, the impact on the events in Athens remained limited.[199] As far as I could establish, the report was never published in the Soviet Union.

For Andrei Kovalev, it was clear that the outcome of the US State Department visit should result in a revision of the law on psychiatric help. This opinion

---

197 Statement of Robert van Voren before a Hearing of the US Commission on Security and Cooperation in Europe, July 12, 1989

198 e-mail from Loren Roth to the author, October 1, 2009

199 *Schizophrenia Bulletin*, Supplement to Vol. 15, No. 4, 1989

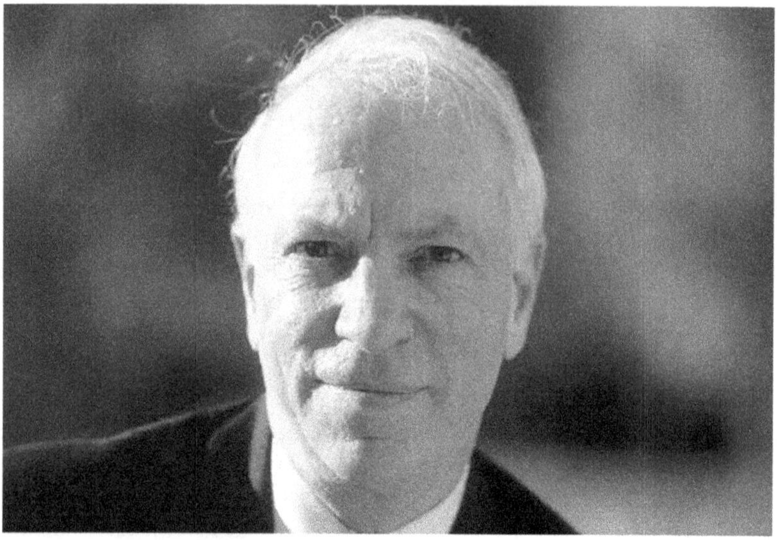

Richard Bonnie, 2007

was shared with his boss, Foreign Minister Eduard Shevardnadze. In the archive of the Central Committee of the CPSU is a document of August 8, 1989 with regard to the revision of the law on psychiatric help, signed by Shevardnadze, Health Minister Evgeni Chazov and Anatoly Logunov.[200] According to this document addressed to the Central Committee, the Ministry of Health and the Academy of Sciences of the USSR "during the implementation of the decision of the Central Committee of May 10, 1989, regarding Soviet-American contacts in the field of psychiatry ... came to the conclusion that possible changes in official instructions and other normative acts ... are not sufficient to fulfill the set tasks. The [existing] Regulation [on Psychiatric Help] does not fully exclude the possibility of arbitrary use of psychiatry, and also heightens the possibility of unjustified compulsory hospitalization in a psychiatric hospital."[201] According to the authors, a new Law on Psychiatric Help had to be developed: "All this will be one more step in the direction of taking psychiatry off the political agenda."[202]

---

200 Anatoli Alekseyevich Logunov, Director of the Institute of High Energy Physics at Serpukhov, rector of the Moscow state University (1977-1992), member of the CPSU Central Committee and vice president of the USSR Academy of Sciences (1974-1991).

201 *On the improvement of legislation with regard to psychiatric help,* document to point 21 of the minutes no. 171 of the Politburo, August 8, 1989.

202 *On the improvement of legislation with regard to psychiatric help,* August 8, 1989.

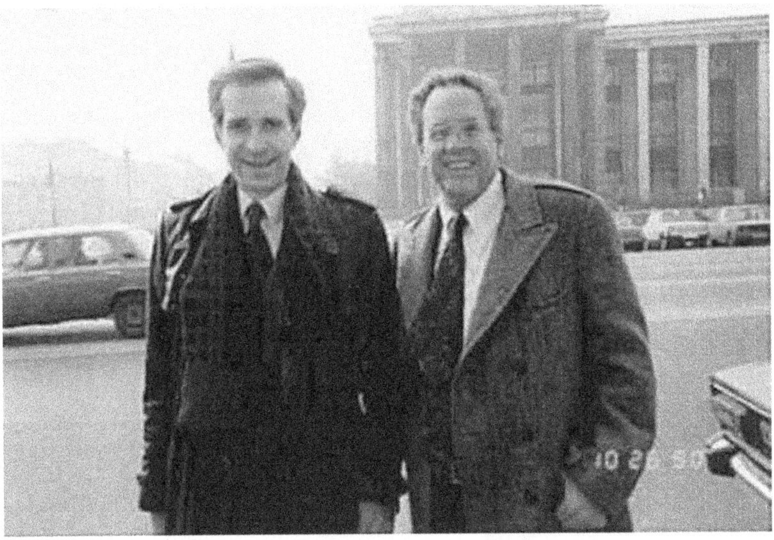

Andrei Kovalev and Loren Roth in Moscow, October 1990

However, things were not that easy. Even when the psychiatric establishment agreed that legal changes were unavoidable, resistance came from another corner. "Immediately following the visit, a note was delivered to the Central Committee of the CPSU with a draft decree in which it was explained why the adoption of the law was necessary. … Neither the physicians nor the lawyers at the Ministry of Justice could be against it. Strong resistance came from a rather unexpected direction. When the decree of the Central Committee was already, as they say, 'on the way out,' a special opinion regarding this was written by Politburo member Chebrikov, who from the beginning of perestroika chaired the KGB and was dismissed by Gorbachev at the first possible moment. I wrote the text of the reaction of [Foreign Minister] Shevardnadze to this missive. The Minister signed and went on holiday. Some time later, I was called in by the secretariat of the Minister and they showed me a new document by Chebrikov regarding this. The tone of the document was very unpleasant and I decided to write an adequate draft of the answer. Why not adopt a law when even the Ministry of Health and the leading lawyers at the Ministry of Justice … were convinced of its necessity? My draft was sent to Shevardnadze and in spite of his constantly delicate position, he signed the answer to this endless harassment. Chebrikov couldn't get anywhere and the law was eventually adopted."[203]

[203] *Page from the Book of Condolences*, p. 23-24

But Chebrikov and the totalitarian system of repression that he represented did not give up that easily. "Regarding the role of Chebrikov in setting up and maintaining punitive mechanisms speaks the fact that when the psychiatrists were put under control he, in spite of active resistance of the Foreign Ministry, managed to push through a document of the Ministry of Health, which allowed complete arbitrariness when there was even only a slight suspicion of alcoholism or drug abuse. Of course, this document was also prepared by the psychiatrists. I think society was saved from narcological repression only because of Chebrikov's dismissal."[204]

[204] *Page from the Book of Condolences*, p. 24

Chapter 28 – Granada

At the end of March 1989, the last WPA Regional Symposium before the World Congress in Athens took place in a town that appealed to everyone's imagination: Granada, one of the most beautiful towns in Andalusia, a South Eastern region of Spain, with the famous Alhambra, a garden complex dating back to Moorish times and still enticing enough to attract mass tourism throughout the year. Coming from a colder Northern European country, it also appealed to my desire to see sunshine and have good spring weather. After a cold, rainy and depressive grey January and February, the usual weather type for winter in The Netherlands, it was time to have sunshine, blue skies and sitting out on terraces sipping wine. Granada seemed to be the perfect place just for that. Unintentionally, I became part of the regular psycho-tourism that so often determines the number of participants in psychiatric congresses (which, I am sure, is no different for any other profession).

Ellen Mercer completely shared my emotions. Although from Washington D.C., and thus going through something that at least bore a real resemblance to what winter is supposed to be, she also felt the urge to have some sunshine and see spring in practice, as a sort of guarantee that better times were ahead. E-mail was still not regularity, so communication was mainly through fax or telephone conversation. Her question was straightforward and simple: what is the weather going to be? Enthusiastically I informed her that late March in Southern Spain could mean 25-30 degrees C, blue sky, sunshine all over. So better bring your summer clothes!

When my plane soared over the Sierra Nevada Mountains and started its landing at Granada airport, I immediately knew I was in for trouble. The sky was gray and heavily clouded and the hills around Granada were also unusually white, snowed under as a result of a cold spell. I didn't bring any winter clothes, but what was worse: Ellen undoubtedly brought her whole summer wardrobe. For many years after, I would have to listen to the long explanation how I had been the cause of a long-lasting battle with freezing temperatures and the absence of anything to shield herself against it.

However cold, Granada did keep its promise of extreme beauty. The Alhambra was an extraordinary experience, with beautiful gardens set in the hills interluded with Moor constructions, fountains and overlooks. Ever since, Ellen Mercer's miniature garden in Washington D.C. was named after the Alhambra.[205] The weather was not all that bad, actually, and I remember

---

205 See chapter 10, "Meeting Ellen Mercer"

we even set outside several times drinking wine with the President of the German Psychiatric Association, Johannes Meyer-Lindenberg, who turned out to be a very pleasant and intelligent man and was a connoisseur of Spanish wines and kitchen. His father had been ambassador to Spain, and part of his upbringing had been in the country we were now visiting.

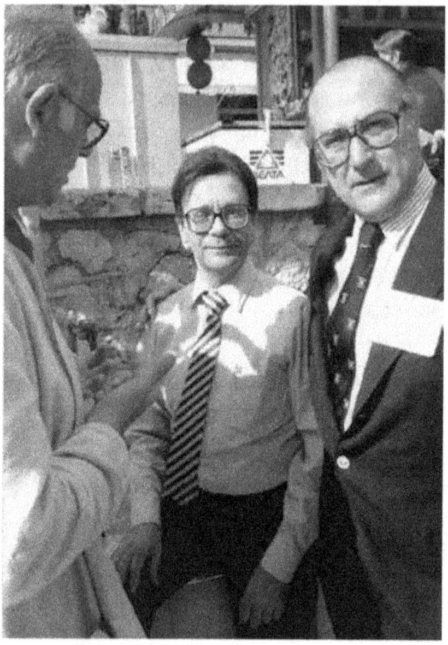

Johannes Meyer Lindenberg, Jorge Costa e Silva, Rodolfo Fahrer, Granada, March 1989

The days in Granada made Johannes a close and lasting friend of our organization. While sipping light "*Banda Azul*" red wine on a terrace next to the Alhambra, enjoying the few rays of sunshine and mastering the cold, we discussed the issue of Soviet political abuse of psychiatry and Johannes explained why the issue was so close to his heart. As a German, he felt a special responsibility, in particular, because members of his profession had either stood by in silence or actively participated in the Euthanasia program of the Nazi's, in the course of which the majority of German persons with mental disability or chronic mental illness were "euthanized" as part of the pathological desire to develop a "clean Aryan race."[206] The fact that many if not most of his colleagues had stood by without

[206] The so-called "Euthanasia" program was National Socialist Germany's first program of mass murder, predating the genocide of European Jewry, by approximately two years. The effort represented one of many radical eugenic measures that aimed to restore the racial "integrity" of the German nation. It endeavored to eliminate what eugenicists and their supporters considered "life unworthy of life": those individuals who--they believed--because of severe psychiatric, neurological, or physical disabilities represented at once a genetic and a financial burden upon German society and the state. According to Von Cranach in the course of the program 180,000 persons with mental illness or intellectual disability were murdered (Von Cranach, M., *In Memoriam*. Exhibition WPA XI World Congress on Psychiatry. Hamburg 1999). In a recent study in *The Schizophrenia Bulletin* E. Fuller Torrey and Robert Yolken conclude that between 220,000 and 269,500 individuals with schizophrenia were sterilized or killed. See *Psychiatric Genocide: Nazi Attempts to Eradicate Schizophrenia*, Schizophrenia Bulletin, Nov 2009. They also give figures of 200,000 to 275,000 persons with mental illness killed.

doing anything during this extermination process made Johannes feel doubly responsible and strong in his convictions that the profession must speak out and publicly voice its disagreement. For us, therefore, he was a natural ally. For Neumann, coming from the DDR, the German state that claimed that it bore no responsibility for the Nazi past and that it had made a clean break with Hitler's legacy (and at the same time accused West-Germany of not having done so), the positioning of Meyer-Lindenberg was almost blasphemy. In his report on the WPA Athens Congress, he angrily wrote that Meyer-Lindenberg "by the way, who played an outspoken anti-Soviet role and in a fascist way represented ethical principles (starting with the German experiences under fascism), turned himself energetically against a re-election of the DDR-representative."[207]

This, for Neumann, unusually aggressive attitude must been seen in the light of the complex political developments at the time. While the Athens World Congress took place, the political regime in the DDR was crumbling, and during the Athens World Congress, Erich Honecker was sacked as Party leader.[208] For Neumann this meant a very uncertain future, and undoubtedly a source of much anxiety.

On top of that, one should realize that relations between West German and DDR representatives were special and strained. The DDR delegates had to deal with a constant feeling of competition with their West German neighbors and, because of the latter's economic boom and world standing, also suffered from a certain inferiority complex. The West-Germans clearly looked down on their East-German neighbors and indeed felt superior, even if only subconsciously – one of the factors of the ongoing political tension between the two halves until this very day. Having known Johannes Meyer-Lindenberg personally, I have no doubt that he felt that Neumann was probably officially or unofficially an agent of an intelligence service and that at the time when the Communist regimes in the East were in trouble, electing a representative of a regime he despised would have been contrary to his convictions.

There was one more person who joined our ranks during this Granada trip, and also in this case it was Ellen Mercer who was the person to introduce him to us. Jorge Alberto Costa e Silva, a member of the WPA Executive

207 *Reisebericht* of Jochen Neumann on the WPA World Congress, October 1989, p. 5

208 Erich Honecker was forced to resign as Party leader on October 18, 1989. The General Assembly during which the Soviets were allowed to return to the WPA conditionally was held a day before, on October 17.

Committee, had decided to run for Presidency of the WPA and Granada was for him a good opportunity to promote himself and to convince potential delegates of national psychiatric associations and other influential psychiatrists that he was the right man for the job. Being a short energetic man from Brazil, he would walk around agitatedly waving his arms going from one to the other. His ticket was being from a Third World country (at that time Brazil did not have the standing as an emerging economic tiger) and a proponent of strong action in the field of human rights. Within the Executive Committee, he almost automatically voted alongside Melvin Sabshin, and thus his vote was usually against a return of the Soviet All-Union Society and in favor of a strong position with regard to medical ethics. However, he did not show a strong opinion of his own, and the question remains whether he was strong on human rights on his own accord or just because he felt that being with Mel Sabshin and sharing his views would be politically clever.[209]

A fact is that he very quickly became friendly with us, "us" being the IAPUP delegation and those who were circling around our group. "[He] knew exactly how to say the things that we wanted to hear and managed to wind us around his finger in no time. Within a few hours, I had become his good friend and, to my dismay, I was called shortly "Bobby" instead of Robert, a nickname that I have never used. When I met him at subsequent congresses he would come running in my direction, loudly exclaiming, "Oh, Bobby, so good to see you!" and would then embrace me with his short arms. It all seemed sincere, but, in fact, he had realized that our influence was considerable and that our support would greatly strengthen his chances of being elected to the presidency of the WPA."[210]

In Granada, an interesting development began whereby unofficial meetings were organized of representatives of organizations with potential voting power at the upcoming General Assembly of the WPA in Athens, during which we would discuss tactics with regard to the Soviet issue. Those discussions centered around the positioning of the various psychiatric associations and the chance of the Soviets to return in spite of their refusal to admit the systematic political abuse of psychiatry. The meeting showed how influential our

---

209 Based on interviews with Costas Stefanis, Jochen Neumann and Melvin Sabshin; all three agreed that Costa e Silva was more a follower than somebody with an opinion of his own. From the IAPUP correspondence files it becomes clear that he regularly asked IAPUP to contact its lawyer, Prof. Charles André Junod in Geneva, and check issues related to the voting structure, and proposed new Statutes and Bylaws of the WPA.

210 *On Dissidents and Madness*, p. 118

organization had become, because although we had officially no relationship to the WPA, we united an increasingly powerful group of people who did have an influence within the organization and who stood a good chance of deciding the position of the WPA when it would come to a voting in Athens.

Looking back, it is hard to imagine how an outside pressure group like ours could become so influential within an international scientific body. I asked Costas Stefanis in July 2009 during our first interview whether it didn't drive him crazy to think that an outside organization could have such an influence over the association he was leading. I hit the nail on its head. "Absolutely," he said, "it was maddening. Everything you said was taken as a sure fact and wherever I went I would encounter people belonging to your organization who would harass me with questions about my so-called 'clandestine negotiations' in Moscow. It was terrible."[211] The fact that by then the issue had become a matter of high-level diplomacy between the US State Department and the Soviet Ministry of Foreign Affairs must have made things even worse for Stefanis – the pressure was now on both sides, from pressure-groups below and politicians above, and he was trying to contain the situation like a rodeo-rider on a bull that went berserk.

The combination of having and ever increasing influence over WPA affairs and the need to be sure that the next Executive Committee of the WPA would be strong on the abuse issue and on other issues of medical professional ethics and human rights, made us an important element in any person's election campaign, and Costa e Silva was probably the first to realize this. He courted us, made us believe that he was the perfect candidate for the job and that, with him, our issue would be safe and well-defended. Almost a year before Granada, we started thinking about "our" slate for the new Executive Committee, trying to figure out who would be a good candidate for each of the positions up for election so that, for a change, we would find the next leadership on our side, and not against.

In the correspondence of IAPUP there are several documents related to this issue, from which it became clear that the organization actively solicited candidates and tried to find associations willing to nominate them. For instance, the minutes of an IAPUP-meeting in Brugge in June 1989 reads: "Various people known to oppose political abuse of psychiatry actively have been asked to be a candidate for the next WPA Executive Committee. Here follows a list (c=contacted, yes=agreed, nom. = nominated by a psych. association)

211 Interview Costas Stefanis, July 15, 2009

H. Visotsky (USA): c, yes, nom. Not Gen Secr. Or Pres.
A. Piotrowski (Poland): c, yes, nom.
J. Grigor (Australia) c, yes, nom.
J. Costa e Silva (Brasil) c., yes, nom?
G. Mustafa (Kenya) c., yes, nom. By Royal College?
M. Roth (Un. Kingdom):
F.H.L. Beyaert (NL):
F. Lieh-Mak (HongKong): "[212]

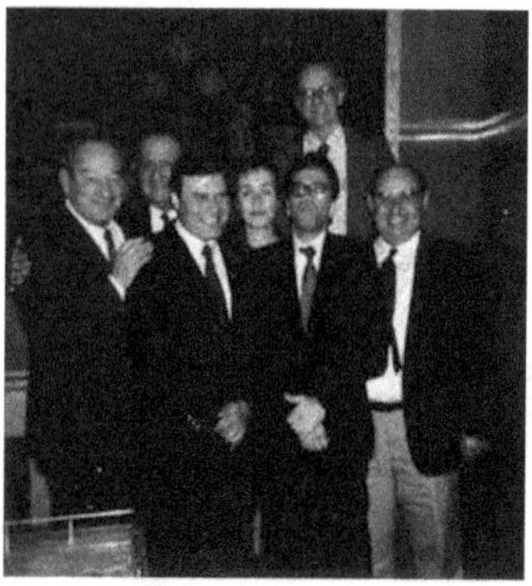

By the time we came to Granada in March 1989, we already had a pretty good idea whom to push for membership of the Executive Committee. Jorge Alberto Costa e Silva seemed to be the best candidate for President and so we agreed to support him. And, gradually, we found candidates for the other positions.

Celebrating Ellen Mercer's birthday, l.t.r. Fini Schulsinger, Melvin Sabshin, Costas Stefanis, WPA secretary Vibeke Munk, Jorge Costa e Silva and Jochen Neumann, in the back Neils Reisby

Ad-hoc membership for the Soviets

Initially, we were unaware of the fact that AUSNP President Nikolai Zharikov had also traveled to Granada, with the purpose of steering the All-Union Society into the WPA. Again, this was a move that was clearly orchestrated with Stefanis (and probably also Schulsinger): "Prof. Zharikov was present in Granada … and during a discussion round on the changes in Soviet psychiatry, he behaved in a way that was close to pure stupidity. Because of his not answering concrete questions and by repeating boring long platitudes, the participants in the meeting were completely frustrated and irritated. … The voting in favor of ad-hoc membership of the All-Union Society with a modest majority of 4 to 2 had almost failed because of a formality. The request for admission was only a copy of a letter on simple paper – even without a heading - and without a signature. Stefanis than quickly got himself a signature of Zharikov, who was somewhere in the neighborhood. The disregard of formalities and lack of being informed has not changed at all on the Soviet side."[213]

212 "Strictly Confidential", IAPUP-Meeting, Brugge, 18-19 June, 1988

213 *Reisebericht* of Jochen Neumann on the WPA EC Meeting, Granada, March-April 1989, p. 2. The All Union Society had sent a telegram to Schulsinger

The Soviet ad hoc admission was a *tour de force* of Stefanis and Schulsinger; that is clear both from Neumann's reports and the minutes of the Executive Meeting. The issue clearly dominated the meeting; yet, in the report the information is concentrated in a fairly long report with the following remark preceding it: "*Please note that the following text, which has been prepared by the President and the Secretary General, is meant to reflect the EC's discussion of ad-hoc membership of the all-Union Society, as it took place on several occasions during our meetings.*"[214]

According to the (carefully prepared) minutes, "in September 1988, an international group of five psychiatrists: Drs. J. Birley, R.G. Priest, Melvin Sabshin, Costas Stefanis and the Secretary General visited Moscow, invited for an exchange of scientific viewpoints. ... During the discussions, representative Soviet colleagues indicated an increasing interest in enrollment of the Soviet psychiatrists with the WPA. They were informed that the deadline for applications was one year before an ordinary General Assembly (i.e., in this case: 17 October 1988). The Soviet colleagues informed the visitors that the all Union Society... would have their annual assembly at the end of October 1988. On this occasion, the society would most likely split, resulting in an All Union Scientific Society for Psychiatrists, whereas the neuropathologists (neurologists) would form their own society. Then the All-Union Scientific Society of Narcologists and Psychiatrists would be in a position to ratify the application for enrollment. The Soviet colleagues asked whether it was likely that the WPA EC would accept formally to receive the application before the deadline, in which it was indicated that the final decision would be taken a few weeks later. The EC members present, and also the British colleagues, could not see any obstacles to such a procedure."[215]

---

on October 12, 1988, stating "Proceeding from necessity restore and promote unity and collaboration among national psychiatric societies directorial board members of all-union scientific society of neuropathologists and psychiatrists put question of enrolment with WPA final decision of board be sent nearest future." IAPUP correspondence files, 1988.

214 Minutes of the WPA EC, Granada, March-April 1989, p. 6

215 Minutes of the WPA EC in Granada, March-April 1989, p. 7. Interestingly, as we saw in Chapter 22, the annual meeting of the All-Union Society had been postponed till late October because of the power struggle between Georgi Morozov and Marat Vartanyan, who both wanted control over the society. During the visit to Moscow, Stefanis is said to have lobbied with Minister of Health Chazov for Vartanyan's candidate, Aleksandr Tiganov. Eventually, it was Morozov's candidate Nikolai Zharikov who won and succeeded Morozov as President. In other words, the power struggle in Moscow was more important than getting the application to the WPA in time before the deadline.

The minutes continued by stating that in October 1988, the EC had received a telegram from the All-Union Society with the formal application (however, with the same conditionality that the assembly still had to confirm the decision). "During its session in Washington, the EC unanimously agreed to interpret this as a valid application."[216] On January 6, the Soviets confirmed that following the split the decision had been "met with great support... Hereafter, the Secretary General ... requested the standard information on membership... The information was delivered by the President of the All Union Scientific Society... Prof. N. N. Zharikov, in Granada... By mistake, an unsigned copy was first given to the Secretary General. This was corrected the next day by Professor Zharikov, who handed over the signed original, in addition to which he also signed the copy."[217]

And now follows a nice euphemistic sentence: "A long discussion took place. During this discussion, there was no disagreement with regard to formalities concerning the Soviet application."[218] In fact, the discussions were harsh, and it was clear that the application of the All Union Society had been orchestrated and that without very active involvement of Stefanis and Schulsinger, the Soviets would still have messed things up. Melvin Sabshin abstained from voting, because he felt the outcome of the US State Department visit to the USSR should be studied first, and the report was due to be published within the next few months. Costa e Silva abstained from voting, because "he wanted to see a signed application on proper stationary first."[219] The fact that the minutes were so carefully doctored, trying to leave no place for misinterpretation or conflicting views, shows that both were well aware that they were skating on very thin ice indeed.

After the Granada meeting, and with confidentially transmitted questions from Costa e Silva faxed to Amsterdam, IAPUP consulted its Swiss legal advisor, Prof. Charles-André Junod, who was rather clear as to the validity of the Soviet ad-hoc admission. "A mere declaration of an intention to possible join the WPA does <u>not</u> constitute an application within the meaning

---

216 Minutes of the WPA EC in Granada, March-April 1989, p. 7. In the Stasi files is a copy of a telegram from Georgi Morozov to Prof Kühne in Jena, informing him that on October 10 the AUSNP had re-applied for membership of the WPA. See: HA XX 499, p. 84

217 Minutes of the WPA EC in Granada, March-April 1989, p. 8. Interestingly, no such original was found in the archives of the World Psychiatric Association.

218 Minutes of the WPA EC in Granada, March-April 1989, p. 8. Later in the minutes (p. 14) it says: "There had been a discussion, even though it might not be considered a full or exhaustive discussion by all EC members."

219 Minutes of the WPA EC in Granada, March-April 1989, p. 8

of… the Statutes and… the Bylaws. Accordingly, the telegram addressed by the All Union Society to WPA's Executive Committee on October 11th, 1988, does not constitute a formal application for membership, but rather some pre-announcement. … Therefore, the twelve month notice period provided for by the second paragraph of clause (5) of the Bylaws of WPA cannot be computed from the date of the above mentioned telegram."[220] In other words, the non-signed application from the All-Union Society (which was signed on the spot after Stefanis' intervention) was already too late for the time-span indicated in the Statutes and Bylaws, and thus had the same status as the application from the Independent Psychiatric Association, which was sent in several weeks before Granada. Yet they were not dealt with equally, as we shall see.

As the minutes of the Executive Committee meeting were carefully doctored, they also provided little indication of the prevailing atmosphere at the meetings. Thus we have to rely on the travel report by Jochen Neumann. This report, albeit short and factual, very clearly airs the atmosphere during the deliberations. Costas Stefanis was suffering from severe pains because of a slipped disk in his neck (on which he was later operated), but insisted on chairing the meetings.[221] "The atmosphere in the Executive Committee was unusually tense, and for the first time in a long period on the edge of personal conflicts. Stefanis, who was quite seriously ill, didn't want to have the chairmanship taken away from him and with his style of leadership,

---

220 Letter of Ch.A. Junod to Robert van Voren, April 18, 1989. The Minutes of the WPA EC meeting in Washington indicates that the EC was willing to accept it as such, however: "At the beginning of this session [on Wednesday October 12, 1989, 9 AM] a cable, dated October 11, 1989, from the All Union Scientific Society … was telefaxed to the Washington Hilton Hotel and delivered to the Secretary General. The application was an application from the Soviet society to enrol with the WPA, given that the decision of the board would be confirmed by the Assembly of Delegates at their Annual Meeting at the end of October 1988. The EC unanimously agreed to interpret the cable as a preliminary application until it was confirmed by the society's Assembly of Delegates. Thereafter, the EC would consider it as a formally correct application to be presented to the General Assembly." Minutes of the WPA EC, Washington D.C., October 1988, p. 4. Later in the minutes (p.15) it says: The EC has decided to conceive of this as a formal application." As far as Prof. Junod is concerned, this was therefore a wrong interpretation.

221 The minutes read: "The President opened the meeting. He had come to Granada although he had been in constant pain for weeks, due to two slipped discs, for which he was to undergo surgery shortly. He had felt obliged to come, because the agenda of the EC included issues of major importance for the WPA". Minutes of the WPA EC in Granada, March-April 1989, p. 2

even more unbearable than usual, he heated the atmosphere additionally."[222] Also Schulsinger was increasingly tense, in particular because he was increasingly under attack in the press, and some time before somebody had tried to break into his office. According to the Danish media, the man had been hired by the Scientology Church and had also planned to break into the office of the WPA Secretariat, hoping to find documents that would prove that Schulsinger was using the WPA for his own private purposes.[223] Looking back, it is almost certain that he suspected IAPUP to be linked with Scientology and that the burglary had in fact been the work of both organizations, because from that moment he used every opportunity to declare that IAPUP was "Scientology" and "CIA-inspired."[224] That he had no proof of these links, and could not have had any because no such links existed, was not of importance; a sort of paranoia had gripped him, and increasingly determined his behavior. In his travel report of August 1988, Neumann refers to the fact that IAPUP has threatened Schulsinger with legal action unless he stops his allegations that the organization is CIA and Scientology inspired. "The cause of it, are the repeated uncontrolled public remarks by Schulsinger that IAPUP was not a serious organization, financed from dubious sources, among others the CIA. Van Voren was allegedly a CIA associate or financed by the CIA. Regrettably one has to remark, that Schulsinger is developing a big personal ambition and would like to be elected President."[225]

Indeed, on August 3, 1989, I had written to Fini Schulsinger that "while in my presence you limited yourself to implying that our association is backed by a 'larger organization' (Amsterdam, October 1988) or receives its funds from dubious sources (Jerusalem, June 1989), I increasingly receive information that in my absence you allege that either our association is funded by the CIA or that I am in fact a CIA agent… I must … request you confirm to me, until latest August 10, 1989, that a) you shall, in the future,

222 *Reisebericht* of Jochen Neumann on the WPA EC Meeting, Granada, March-April 1989, p. 3

223 *Reisebericht* Jochen Neumann on the WPA EC Meeting in Copenhagen, August 1988, p. 4

224 For instance during a Conference of the International Academy on Law and Mental Health in Jerusalem on June 25-30, 1989, Schulsinger dismissed a presentation by the author by stating it was "unacademic and similar to that of the Scientology Church". He added that the budget of "that association" (meaning IAPUP) was even bigger than that of the WPA; "as far as the WPA is concerned we at least know where the money comes from," he said, "as far as this association is concerned we can only guess." See *Documents* 25, July 1989

225 *Reisebericht* of Jochen Neumann on the WPA EC Meeting August 1989, p. 7

strictly refrain from any such allegations, and also instruct accordingly any member of your WPA staff; b) you are making the necessary steps with a view to correct these libelous allegations wherever you have made them."[226]

Of course, Schulsinger never made any steps accordingly, and only informed IAPUP on August 8 "that I have not performed any illegal actions concerning you or your activities."[227] He indicated that all further communication should go via his lawyer. Indeed, any basis for human interaction had by now disappeared, and we would never speak again. Schulsinger's growing aggression would also determine his success as candidate for Presidency of the WPA in Athens.

Finally the preparations for the upcoming elections for the new Executive Committee, to take place during the General Assembly in Athens only six months later, already influenced the positioning of the individual EC members. And almost all had their ambitions. Schulsinger was opting for Presidency of the WPA, and – as noted before – found Stefanis in his way who refused to disclose his plans and created the impression that he might run for a second term (and considering the flawed relationship between the two he might have done this just to irritate his General Secretary). Costa e Silva was also running for Presidency, while Melvin Sabshin had not yet excluded the possibility of running for the same post himself, considering whether he could combine that post with his being Medical Director of the APA. Reisby, generally seen as an assistant to Fini Schulsinger and colorless, did not seem to have any outspoken ambitions, but Neumann, as we can see from his report, was also hoping to come back to the Executive Committee after Athens: "[I] was told by three main groups, that a continuation of membership of the Executive Committee by [me] was planned. It is a fact, that the reporter [Neumann] enjoys a rather high level of respect and is openly supported when speaking during "open sessions" of the Committee and Section advisors. He was told by Professor Montenegro that the Latin American countries have suggested a renewed membership of the Executive Committee for [me] and will provide their support. On the part of the APA (Ellen Mercer) I was told that they would also support [my] candidacy."[228]

---

226 Letter to Fini Schulsinger from Robert van Voren, August 3, 1989. The letter was written according to the instructions of IAPUP's lawyer, Prof. Charles André Junod, as worded in his letter to the author on July 26, 1989.

227 Letter from Fini Schulsinger, August 8, 1989

228 *Reisebericht* of Jochen Neumann on the WPA EC Meeting, Granada, March-April 1989, p. 4

But not all supported Neumann. In his reports he notes that the French are opposed ("but I have no knowledge of the reasons for this") and as we know also Johannes Meyer-Lindenberg did not want a DDR-representative back on the Executive Committee. In both cases this opposition had nothing to with Neumann personally but was simply because of the fact that he was a representative from the DDR, a country that was considered by then to be more Soviet than the Soviet Union and, on top of that, was at that moment even criticized by the Soviet leadership for being so immune to change.[229]

Independent Psychiatric Association

Interestingly, the changes in the Soviet Union had also resulted in a new competition for the All-Union Society. In March 1989, less than a month

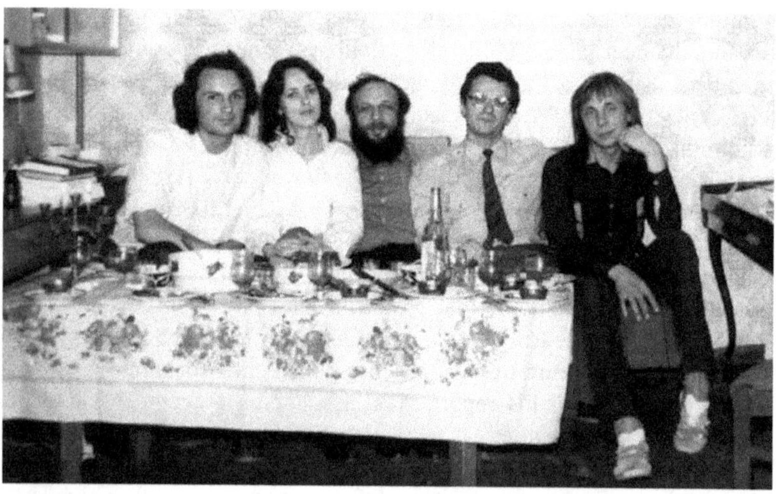

IPA Moscow, 1989. l.t.r. Robert van Voren, Christine Shaw, Viktor Lanovoi

[229] For instance on December 1, 1988, DDR Party leader Erich Honecker had addressed the Central Committee of the SED and declared: "The people of the DDR has achieved a standard of living as never before in its history. In principle it is higher than in the FRG." He rejected the new Soviet concept for society with the argument that "there is no valid model for all socialist countries." On January 19, 1989, at a meeting in Helsinki Honecker said: "The Wall will still be standing in 50, indeed in 100 years if the reasons for its existence have not yet been removed. It is indeed needed to protect our Republic from thieves, to say nothing of those who are glad of the chance to upset peace and stability in Europe." When Gorbachev visited the DDR on the occasion of the 40th anniversary of the DDR, citizens were shouting "Gorby, Gorby" and asking him to help them.

before the Regional Symposium in Granada, an "Independent Psychiatric Association (IPA)" had applied for membership of the World Psychiatric Association. It was the first crack in the wall of the monopoly of the All-Union Society over Soviet psychiatry. The IPA had been set up by a group of several dozen psychiatrists and psychologists in Moscow. The leader was a certain Viktor Lanovoi, a psychologist who was waiting for many years for an exit visa to Israel and had now developed the plan to establish a new psychiatric association. "He was surrounded by a group of psychiatrists and psychologists who supported his initiative. At that moment, the Soviet Union knew only one psychiatric association, the All-Union Society of Neuropathologists and Psychiatrists. There was no alternative. Setting up an alternative psychiatric association was the ultimate challenge, because this would break the monopoly of the All-Union Society.

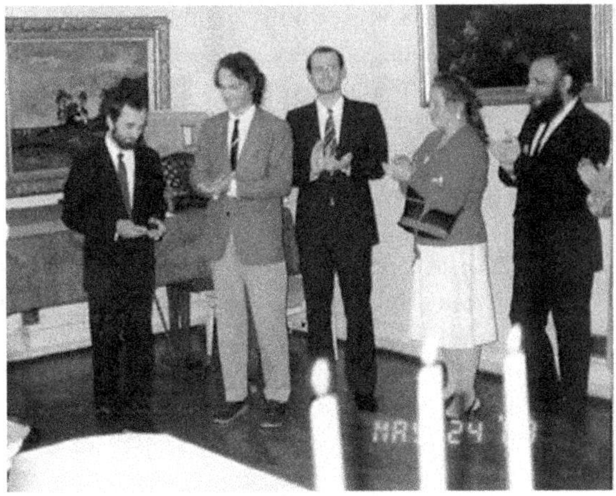

Aleksandr Podrabinek receives the Anatoly Koryagin Award at the Dutch Embassy in Moscow. L.t.r. Podrabinek, Van Voren, Konstantin Karmanov, Podrabinek's wife Alla and Viktor Lanovoi, May 24, 1989

Together with Ellen Mercer of the American Psychiatric Association (APA), we set ourselves to work. During several meetings the statutes of the Independent Psychiatric Association were developed and an activity plan was written. The APA functioned as an example, and Ellen provided an organizational chart that could be used by the initiative group. During a next visit, it turned out that they had used the example quite literally. The APA had within its structure at least forty commissions and departments, and that format had been copied in its entirety. However, the Independent Psychiatric Association had at that moment hardly forty members, and thus all the members were in more than one commission or department and were having multiple tasks. It was quite hilarious and cost us considerable effort to convince them to reduce it all to an acceptable structure."[230]

230 *On Dissidents and Madness*, pp. 115-6

Whether Lanovoi fully believed in the goals of the IPA, or saw his involvement as a means to force the Soviets to give him an exit visa to Israel, is difficult to say. Fact is, that as soon as the Soviets offered him and his wife a chance to immigrate to Israel, he took the offer. He was succeeded by Dr. Yuri Savenko, a psychiatrist, who would become the IPA's president for many years to come.

The IPA applied for WPA membership almost immediately after it's founding, but quickly ran into trouble with the WPA Secretary General, who refused the application on formal grounds. Just prior to the Granada meeting, Schulsinger informed the IPA that its application for membership had been received too late as WPA Statutes and By-Laws stipulated that applications for new membership must be received one year prior to the General Assembly meeting where they would be voted upon: "This may be an obstacle for your enrollment at the upcoming General Assembly in Athens, October 1989."[231] However, according to the newly proposed Statutes and By-Laws, applications must be received 6 months prior to General Assembly meetings, and on basis of those the IPA was not too late. The IPA had informed the WPA of its wish to join on March 9, and the original letter of application had been written on March 27, 1989. However, it had been delayed in transmission to the WPA due to the difficulties in getting the letter to the West. In addition, the All-Union Society had only announced their *intention* to decide to apply in November 1988, and their official application was submitted in Granada and was not even signed. If their application was accepted (and it was, as we saw above) it would be very hard to reject that of the IPA, especially if one wanted to avoid a new scandal.

Schulsinger was forced to backtrack. "The new Soviet society that was favored by the Americans was not yet accepted as ad-hoc member, because some formalities still need to be fulfilled. The Americans tried to prevent confirmation of the ad-hoc membership of the All-Union Society until the well-known investigation report of the American commission that visited the Soviet Union was not published. In the end… the ad-hoc membership was decided upon."[232] In a letter to WPA member societies Schulsinger justified the decision by stating that "just before the EC-meetings in Granada, the WPA Secretariat had received an application, dated 9 March 1989, in which a new society, the 'Independent Psychiatric Association' of the USSR applied for membership. As the

231 Letter from Fini Schulsinger to Viktor Lanovoi of the IPA, March 21, 1989.

232 *Reisebericht* of Jochen Neumann on the WPA EC Meeting, Granada, March-April 1989, p. 2-3

EC has unjustifiably been suspected of not keeping strictly to the rules for accepting applications, the EC found it difficult to deviate from the Bylaws at this occasion and accord ad hoc membership to this new Soviet society."[233]

On May 30, 1989 the application of the IPA for membership of the WPA was again faxed to the Secretariat of the WPA in Copenhagen. The association was now officially up for membership, to be decided by the General Assembly in Athens. In one of his reports, Jochen Neumann explains that WPA membership of this new association is almost unavoidable, even though it is clear that accepting them would be a "political decision. … M.Sabshin himself says that the group is a creation of the US Embassy in Moscow. The All-Union Society has, however, established official contacts with this group and by doing so recognized their existence."[234]

---

233 Letter by Fini Schulsinger to WPA member societies, April 27, 1989. In a letter to Jim Birley of the Royal College, dated June 16, 1989, Fini Schulsinger wrote that "the EC would have preferred to be able to grant this association ad hoc membership, but was hesitant at the end of March because of heavy accusations that we did break the time limit rules with regard to the All Union Scientific Society of Psychiatrists. Personally, I feel a little bit as a victim of a double-bind situation and can confirm Gregory Bateson's and other prophets' assumptions that such a situation provokes mental unrest."

234 HA XX 1386/2, p. 8

Part V

The Final Act

Chapter 29: Athens

I don't understand: how can one accept back in the WPA those who tortured before and do not acknowledge it today.

Semyon Gluzman

I departed for Athens three weeks before the World Congress. This seemed a bit early, but the idea was that I would prepare the grounds, activate the network of contacts in Greece (the foundation of which had been laid during the lecture tour of Anatoly Koryagin and myself) and prepare the local press for what was about to happen. I set up office in Hotel Caravel, close to the Hilton Hotel where, among others, the General Assembly would take place, and spent my days preparing for the "Big Event." On September 25, our office officially opened its doors.[1] "Because of Vladimir Bukovsky, we wound up in the Caravel Hotel. This hotel was owned either by *Nea Demokratia* or a person closely associated to the party. The director was a great admirer of Ronald Reagan and strongly anti-communist, and so we were warmly welcomed. For our stay in the hotel during the congress, we were offered a hugely discounted suite on one of the top floors that we could turn into our headquarters. The associate of Karamanlis, who had accompanied us on our lecture tour, was hired to be our local coordinator."[2] Kostas Karamanlis personally negotiated the special discount price that made it all affordable.[3]

I was accredited as correspondent of "Greece's Weekly," a weekly English language journal for foreigners, which allowed me to attend all press conferences by the WPA and eliminated the possibility that I would be made to leave. Leaflets had been translated into Greek for local consumption, and large quantities of promotional materials had been sent to Greece from the Netherlands. In spite of the fact that Greece was now a member of the European Union, it took considerable effort to get them released by customs. We had produced several leaflets, outlining the position of GIP, as well as two books that dealt with the history of Soviet psychiatric abuse and its nature.[4] I found most of our materials twenty years later in the Stasi

1 See the announcement in *Documents 27*, August 1989

2 *On Dissidents and Madness,* p. 121

3 IAPUP Correspondence, 1989

4 One of the leaflets gave background information on leading Soviet psychiatrists, a number of whom were in Athens personally; the other leaflets explained the position of IAPUP with regard to a return of the All-Union Society, outlining our conditions for such a return. The two books were *Soviet Psychiatric Abuse in the Gorbachev Era* and *On Totalitarian Psychiatry* by Semyon Gluzman.

files of Professor Karl Seidel, a member of the East-German delegation and at the same time an IM, who probably collected them in Athens and gave them to the Stasi.

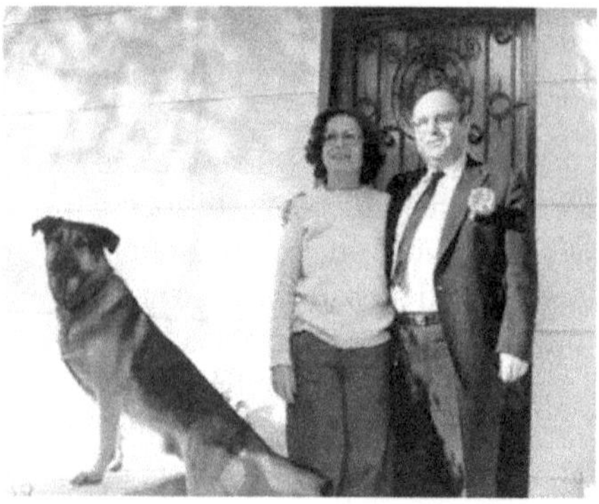

Jochen Neumann with Adela Stefanis, early 1989, Athens

Also Jochen Neumann informed the DDR-leadership of our extensive preparations and the influence we had managed to acquire. In his report on the meetings of the Executive Committee in Athens in August 1989, he described the various power groups among the membership of the WPA, and concludes: "And finally there are the groups that are directly or indirectly linked to IAPUP. This group, to which belong not only persons who are directly linked to IAPUP, but also other individuals who are currently important in psychiatry, politics and business, starts to exert its influence – also with considerable material resources… IAPUP possesses unusually extensive material and ideal reserves that suggest a broad support from influential and wealthy circles. IAPUP has announced internationally that in preparation of its activities it will move is headquarters from Holland to Athens during the World Congress and the General Assemblies (starting in early September), and it has made its bank account public that it will use for this purpose while being in Athens."[5]

After two weeks, my solitary confinement ended. The first to arrive was Christine Shaw from the United Kingdom who, for many years, had been the editor of the *Information Bulletin* of IAPUP. Christine was a historian specializing in Italian renaissance and, in the years prior to the Athens Congress, we worked closely together. In a way we were antipodes: I was a leftist-looking long-haired and chain-smoking activist, while she was a very British well-educated and mannered woman who spoke the most British English I had ever heard until then. Christine was also known because of her handwriting, which was so miniscule that you needed a magnifying glass to read it; she could fit a whole novel on one sheet of paper. Together we formed an excellent and very productive team, working very hard and with a lot of humor and dedication. The combination became even more unique when Ellen Mercer joined us. Being very American both

5 *Reisebericht* on the WPA EC Meeting, August 10-14, 1989, p. 2-4

outwardly and in her behavior, constantly intermitting her remarks with a lot of laughter, she added a special flavor to the group. In the spring of 1989, the three of us had traveled to Moscow to meet with dissidents and the Independent Psychiatric Association, a trip during which we had so much fun that sometimes my cheeks would be painful from laughter. We looked like the "Three Musketeers" who had entered hostile territory to conquer the enemy. The relaxed atmosphere in the Soviet Union, so much different from several years before when the country was stifled and political prisoners were languishing in camps, prisons and psychiatric hospitals, very much helped make this trip a memorable one. Of course, the Independent Psychiatric Association was harassed by the authorities, who rightfully saw it as a threat to their monopoly over Soviet psychiatry. Yet at the same time we could openly meet with dissidents like Aleksandr Podrabinek, and discuss the issue of Soviet psychiatric abuse and the WPA. The air of victory over totalitarianism was already in the air.

Jan Veldmeijer also arrived in Athens several days in advance. Like myself, Jan had been a courier for the dissident movement for quite a few years and was working with the Second World Center in Amsterdam, a sister organization that supported the democratic movement in the Soviet Union. He had gradually taken over the financial administration of IAPUP and was also assisting with all the logistics. The first task ahead was to organize a symposium on "Psychiatric Abuse on the Gorbachev Era," which was to take place in the Caravel Hotel the evening of October 14, right after the start of the World Congress. The target audiences were the Greek and international press, as well as the delegates of national psychiatric associations and all others who could influence the voting during the General Assembly. The Soviet delegation also was invited and several Soviet officials attended the meeting. For those days, it was a unique moment, when, in one meeting hall, one could find Aleksandr Karpov, the new chief psychiatrist of the USSR Ministry of Health who had replaced Aleksandr Churkin shortly before the World Congress, along with Semyon Gluzman and Anatoly Koryagin, the dissident psychiatrists who had both served many years in the Soviet Gulag because of their opposition against the political abuse. Others who attended included Algirdas Statkevicius, a Lithuanian psychiatrist and member of the Lithuanian Helsinki Committee who had spent several years incarcerated in the Special Psychiatric Hospital of Chernyakhovsk before moving to Chicago.[6] Karpov actively tried to engage in discussions with us that was, for that time, a very un-Soviet attitude that took us by surprise.

6 Statkevicius later returned to Lithuania and is currently living in Vilnius, where the author met him in 2008.

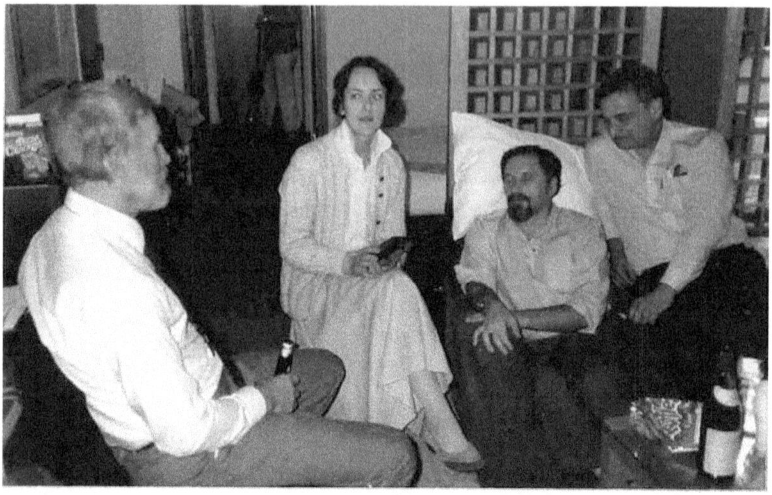

l.t.r. Anatoly Koryagin, Christine Shaw, Semyon Gluzman and Ion Vianu, Athens 1989

The rest of the IAPUP delegation arrived one by one during the days before the World Congress started. Our delegation consisted of members of the IAPUP Council of Representatives and delegates from various national member groups, as well as Anatoly Koryagin, Semyon Gluzman and Algirdas Statkevicius. Gluzman had arrived straight from Kiev on September 8, coincidentally on the same plane as the Soviet delegation.[7] It was his first international trip.

Our group was also joined by some of our newly found friends among the delegates to the World Congress, such as the German Society President and delegate Johannes Meyer-Lindenberg, with whom we had become friends in Granada half a year earlier. Other collaborators included Jim Birley, the President of the British Royal College of Psychiatrists and "a typically British intellectual with an excellent reputation, friendly and without any pretense, but at the same time direct and sharp when he had to be;" and Roelof ten Doesschate, the first Dutch delegate who really had an interest in the problem of Soviet psychiatry and who had been instructed to act as he saw fit.[8] This he immediately did: "On Tuesday evening, I participated in an informal meeting organized by

7 *From the secretariat*, in *Documents* 30, November 1989

8 *On Dissidents and Madness*, p. 128. See also Ten Doesschate's report on the Athens mission, p. 1: "Mandate for the Dutch Psychiatric Association delegate to the World Congress: the executive committee gives ten Doesschate the open mandate he asked for." IAPUP files.

IAPUP where I met some of the other delegates for the first time, in particular Johannes Meyer-Lindenberg (West Germany) and Jim Birley (United Kingdom), with whom I spent a lot of time in the coming days."[9]

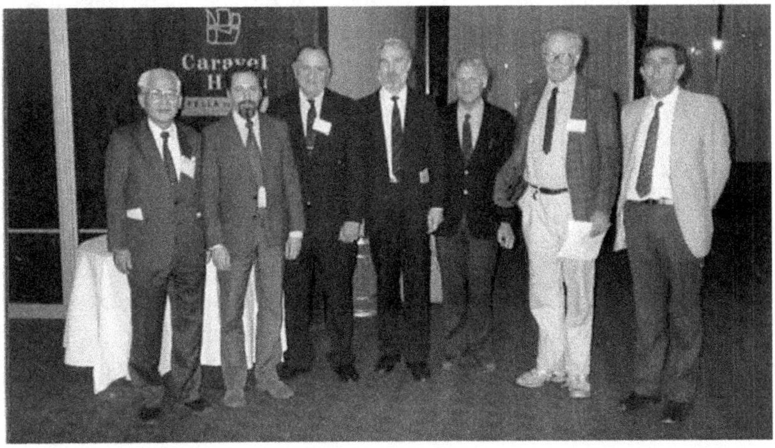

Athens, October 1989. L.t.r. Shogo Terashima, Semyon Gluzman, Melvin Sabshin, Anatoly Koryagin, Algirdas Statkevicius, Jim Birley and Roelof ten Doesschate

Around them circled many other participants and delegates to the General Assembly, who more or less identified themselves with "our cause." Some of them came to the regular brainstorming session in our office at the Caravel Hotel, that we organized from the very start of the World Congress and where the daily state of affairs was discussed. Standard items on the agenda were an assessment of the division of votes among the delegates with regard to the Soviet issue and what the chances were of "our" candidates for the Executive Committee.

The congress in Athens attracted almost ten thousand participants, among them a sizeable Soviet delegation led by Nikolai Zharikov, Marat Vartanyan, Pyotr Morozov and a whole list of psychiatrists, about twenty of them, who, as mentioned earlier, arrived on the same plane as Semyon Gluzman.[10] Most of them stayed out of the limelight, apart from Marat Vartanyan who flamboyantly walked around during the welcome reception of the World Congress and came up to talk to his "friend," Ellen Mercer, in spite of the fact that she was accompanied by several members of our group. "Speaking fluent English and grinning broadly, Vartanyan immediately mingled with

9 Report on the Athens Congress by Roelof ten Doesschate, p. 2, November 2, 1989. IAPUP archives.

10 See chapter 18, *Meeting Costas Stefanis*.

his Western 'friends,' explaining that as a 'democrat' he was always for perestroika within Soviet psychiatry, that the 1983 decision however was necessary because Soviet psychiatry was 'incriminated,' that the AUSNP was now prepared to return to the WPA but they would not be pleased with anything less than a complete and unconditional membership."[11]

The Gluzman approach

It was going to be a close call, that much was clear. The Soviet delegation benefited from the political climate. The democratization in the Soviet Union was, for many delegates, reason to vote in favor of a return of the Soviet All-Union Society. Here the hard-line reaction of Anatoly Koryagin could not be the necessary answer. The time of black and white was gone; this called for a subtle and balanced response. That answer could only be provided by Semyon Gluzman, and, thus, he moved from being a witness to becoming the most important actor in the game. This led to tensions with Anatoly Koryagin, who, until then, had been the center point of international attention and the spokesperson of those against a Soviet return.

The relationship between the two men was difficult from the very start, due to their different characters but also because of the fundamental difference in views and approaches. Gluzman was a philosopher, a man who in his own view had become a dissident "by coincidence," only because he had taken medical ethics seriously and had followed the Hippocratic Oath rather than the Oath of the Soviet Doctor. His ten years in camp and exile had not turned him into a revolutionary. Rather, it had mellowed him, and had led to his view that they were all products of the Soviet system, dissidents and henchmen alike, and that, in a way, he was freer than the guards on the watchtowers of the prison camps. In his book *On Soviet Totalitarian Psychiatry* he tried to understand the nature of Soviet psychiatry, why it deviated so much from world psychiatry and had become a tool of repression. He tried to *understand*, while Koryagin immediately *condemned*. Their positions were incompatible.

The letter that Gluzman wrote to members of the WPA in June 1989 was really the furthest he allowed himself to go. I myself remember vividly how much he struggled with the issue, whether to oppose a return of the All-Union Society and speak out openly, or to keep the arguments "scientific" and leave the political positioning to others. In the end, he agreed to add his voice to those against a return of the AUSNP, mainly because of the lack of any morality

[11] *From the secretariat*, in *Documents* 30, November 1989

on the part of the Soviet psychiatric establishment and their constant brazen denial that anything was wrong. In that sense, Gluzman shared the feelings of disgust that Jochen Neumann so often worded in his travel reports.

In his letter of June 18, 1989, Gluzman explains his positioning from the very first sentence: "Good and evil most often have the same color: grey - the color of ordinariness. From there come the self-deception, hopes and disbelief, especially at a distance, when the haze softens the contours of the face and appearance. Deficiencies can be seen from a direct, close view: a richness of crevices and spots is accentuated in detail. I am nearby, n the middle of it. But I will try to be objective in looking at the image."[12]

Gluzman continued to explain the extraordinary nature of the situation ahead. "What is happening today in our country is a miracle. It is unexpected, incomprehensible. But it is happening. Hopes have risen. Slowly the sick country is freeing itself from totalitarian ways of thinking, unable to self-analyze, deprived of moral tendencies." Yet, at the same time, "the totalitarian power … is alive and strong. And it resists. … Also psychiatry resists, the stagnant, self-isolated, poor and amoral totalitarian psychiatry. … How can one not resist? How can one not hate that unexpected destruction of everything which was habitual and peaceful, a destruction which is called 'glasnost and perestroika'?"

According to Gluzman, neither Morozov nor Vartanyan really wanted a return of the All-Union Society. "Isolation is more peaceful for them, more peaceful in all respects. Among others individuals covering up the real value (and sometimes the [real] author) of their 'scientific achievements'… But they are small wheels. They aren't asked. 'It is necessary. We have to return to the WPA!' That is the command."[13]

Gluzman then turned to the WPA. "The problem is you, is the WPA. Do you agree? Can you agree? Can you smile and shake the hand of a person who personally participated in psychiatric punishments of many mentally healthy people? Can you smile and shake the hands of men and women who, on the basis of suffering and despair of their mentally healthy fellow citizens, built their scientific and professional careers…" He continued: "I don't understand. Really, I don't understand: how can one accept back in the WPA those who tortured before and do not acknowledge it today. Don't you know that it is neither President Gorbachev, nor deputy Sakharov who

12 *Letter to Western Colleagues*, by Semyon Gluzman, published in *Documents* 25, July 1989

13 *Letter to Western Colleagues,* June 18, 1989

you want to accept back into the WPA, but the same Morozov, Zharikov, Vartanyan? Not the thousands of ordinary Soviet psychiatrists, who saw it all, understood it all, but were afraid to protest, but the fake scientists and hangmen, the stained, those without a conscience, the incompetent ones."

According to Gluzman, there was no way someone could pretend that the issue was not his or her concern. "The director who, sent by Hitler, performed Beethoven in Zürich, Paris or Budapest, became guilty of the most obscene lie, under the pretext that he was a musician and was involved in music and nothing else. Those are the words of Thomas Mann. The psychiatrists, who accept in their midst unconfessed hangmen, are guilty of the most obscene lie, under the pretext that they are psychiatrists and are busy with psychiatry and nothing else."

In conclusion, Gluzman showed how complex the issue was also for him, who had spent ten years in camp and exile because of his opposition to the political abuse, yet at the same time someone who had developed the ability to look at the issue from a distance. "I cannot give you any advice on how to behave," he wrote. I know only one thing for sure – how not to behave. In the past, doctors were tried in Nürnberg, guilty of the deaths of thousands of mentally ill people. The concept of totalitarian psychiatry was convicted there as well. I don't call for a trial or for vengeance. The most important are not the legal procedures. On top of that, hangmen usually do not recant. The thing that happened in Granada, and that can happen in Athens as well, has a name: complicity. Do you understand?"[14]

With his balanced letter, Gluzman had, unwittingly, made a masterful move. Eastern Europe was gripped in an ever-increasing sequence of political events and although at that moment it was unclear what the ultimate consequences would be, it was clear that times were changing fast and that the ordinary hard-line position no longer appealed to the larger (psychiatric) community. In his letter, Gluzman successfully integrated the doubts of many psychiatrists about how precisely these political developments should influence their decision regarding a Soviet return. By separating the Soviet psychiatric establishment (the "hangmen") from the rest of the country, and by indicating that it was not the country they were voting back into the WPA but the same group of people who had been in charge for the past decades, he managed to give the campaign against a Soviet return an enormous boost. However, for Koryagin it was all too philosophical,

14 *Letter to Western Colleagues,* June 18, 1989. When mentioning Granada Gluzman refers to the decision of the Executive Committee of the WPA to give the Soviet All-Union Society ad-hoc membership.

too blurry. Irritated by the "rising star" of Gluzman and his sophisticated approach, he gradually withdrew from the campaign, and most of the time he spent in the swimming pool of the Caravel Hotel.

The first clash

The first Extraordinary General Assembly convened on October 11, "in the big and expensive Intercontinental Hotel, in a beautiful ball room with enormous chandeliers and mirrors. The majority of delegates sleep in that hotel. In my hotel, the hot water was usually turned off after 8 PM and you have the knob in your hand when you try to open the door."[15]

The meeting was fully dedicated to the adoption of new Statutes and Bylaws of the WPA. This was the masterpiece of Jochen Neumann, who after preparatory work by Melvin Sabshin, had led a task force to prepare new statutes for the organization, intended to streamline its functioning and to make it more democratic.[16] The main criticism of the old structure was that a relatively small number of (exclusively Western) psychiatric associations dominated the voting power at General Assemblies and the smaller (mainly non-Western) societies had far too little say in the organization. In fact this was true and was still a reflection from the early days of the organization when it was a Western-dominated body. In addition, there was a serious lack of continuity because of the fact that the whole executive committee was voted in and dismissed *en bloc*; as a result, the organization was paralyzed for a considerable amount of time during the handover period (which could last up to a year). In addition, World Congresses once every six years were too infrequent, and the combination of both factors led to the proposal of having an increased Executive Committee with staggered voting, and a World Congress every three years.

The working group led by Melvin Sabshin had been set up in 1986, and submitted its recommendations to the Executive Committee in November 1987 in Warsaw.[17] The main recommendations had been to organize a World Congress every three years, staggered voting of the members of the

---

15 Report on the Athens Congress by Roelof ten Doesschate, November 2, 1989, p. 3. IAPUP archives.

16 Members of the task force were, apart from Jochen Neumann, Alfred Freedman (USA), Ahmed Okasha (Egypt), Shogo Terashima (Japan) and Ulysses Vianna (Brazil).

17 Members of the working group had been, apart from Melvin Sabshin, Alfred Freeman (USA), Felice Lieh-Mak (Hong Kong) and Juan Jose Lopez Ibor (Spain)

Executive Committee, and an increase of its membership from six to eight members with closely defined tasks and responsibilities and to initiate a process of regionalization of the WPA. The task force led by Neumann had incorporated most of the recommendations in their proposal for new WPA Statutes and Bylaws.

The proposed changes definitely made sense, and would enhance the efficacy of the organization. However, the "non-democratic nature" of the WPA had been for many years a constant argument by the Soviets and their allies as to why they had decided to resign from the WPA, and also why they refused to return to the organization.[18] This automatically made the proposed change in structure suspicious, and the fact that the task-force was led by an East German only made these suspicions even stronger. Of course, for the Soviets the changes in Statutes and Bylaws were important, because they could determine the voting power of those against a return of the All-Union Society. In the Stasi archives are several translations of requests from the KGB to the Stasi to inform them and to "check and confirm these indications [that Neumann is working on a revision of the Statutes] as well as to inform whether it is possible to carry out an operational check on the state of affairs and the content of these documents."[19] One document contains the concrete suggestion to organize a consultation of Neumann "with the Soviet delegation to the II Psychiatric Congress of socialist countries in Varna/Bulgaria (24-26.4.87). (Members of the Soviet delegation are Vartanyan, Kozlov and Morozov)."[20]

The eleven-hour session of the Extraordinary General Assembly turned out to be a showdown between the WPA Executive Committee and the member societies of the organization. Stefanis and Schulsinger were the most active members of the Executive Committee at this meeting, supported by a Parliamentarian who, as I later found out, was a close friend of Costas Stefanis, Antonis Vgontzas.[21] "The meeting was very badly contained by the chairman, Costas Stefanis; everybody spoke for hours about anything. And when the meeting didn't to in the direction that Stefanis wanted, a legal advisor sitting on his right was pushed forward to, with some unclear remarks about Swiss law, support the arguments of Stefanis."[22]

---

18 See, for instance, HAXX, 1386/2 p. 76

19 HAXX 1386/1, p. 37 and pp. 50-60; HAXX 1368/2, 17 and 18.

20 HAXX, 1386/1, p.45

21 I found out only in the course of writing this book and interviewed Vgontzas on September 3, 2009.

22 Report on the Athens Congress by Roelof ten Doesschate, November 2, 1989, p. 3. IAPUP archives.

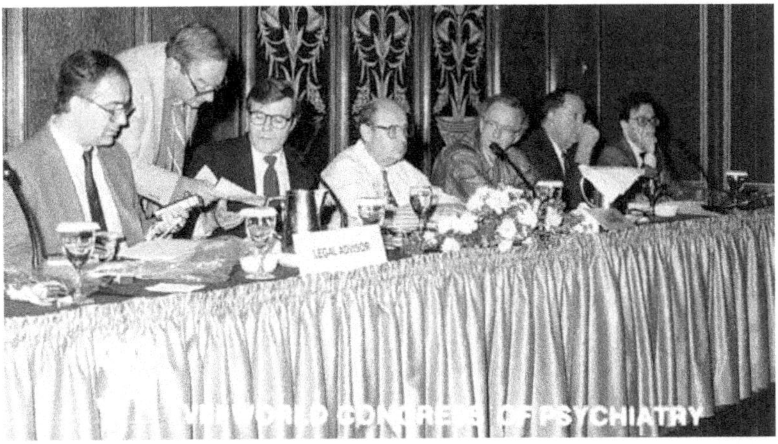

Athens General Assembly 1989 l.t.r. Antonis Vgontzas, Fini Schulsinger, Costas Stefanis, Jochen Neumann, Neils Reisby, Melvin Sabshin, Jorge Alberto Costa e Silva

Jochen Neumann, who for the past two years had worked very hard to prepare the draft of the Statutes and Bylaws and now saw his work discussed with the members of the WPA, was completely stressed and somewhat preoccupied as a result of the political developments in his country.[23]

[23] In the East-German city Leipzig so-called "Monday-demonstrations" had begun on 4 September 1989 after regular prayers for peace in the Nikolai Church, and eventually filled the nearby downtown Karl Marx Square. Many dissatisfied East German citizens gathered in the court of the church, and non-violent demonstrations began in order to demand rights such as the freedom to travel to foreign countries and to elect a democratic government. Informed by (West German) television and friends about the events, people in other East German cities begun repeating the Leipzig demonstration, meeting at city squares on Monday evenings. A major turning point were the events in the West Germany Embassy of Prague, where thousands of East Germans had fled to in September. West-German Foreign Minister Hans-Dietrich Genscher negotiated an agreement that allowed them to travel to the West, in trains that had to pass first through the GDR. The speech of Hans-Dietrich Genscher from the balcony was interrupted by a very emotional reaction to his announcement. When the trains passed Dresden central station in early October, police forces had to stop people from trying to jump on the trains. By 9 October 1989, just after the 40th anniversary celebrations of the GDR and two days before the first Extraordinary General Assembly, the gathering of demonstrators at the Nikolai Church had swelled to more than 70,000 (out of the city's population of 500,000), all united in peaceful opposition to the regime. The most famous chant became *Wir sind das Volk!* - "We are the people!" reminding their leaders that a democratic republic has to be ruled by the people, not by an undemocratic party claiming to represent them.

Antonis Vgontzas remembers: "Neumann was very nervous and anxious at the time of the General Assemblies. He was all the time going out to learn what was happening in his own country, trying to get some news. His mind was more in East-Berlin than in Athens, so to say."[24]

Being Anatoly Koryagin's interpreter, I also attended this General Assembly. In my report on the Athens events, published in the Documents of IAPUP, I showed very clearly my irritation about the role of Antonis Vgontzas: "They brought in a 'legal advisor' into the scenario who, like a parrot, reiterated the twists of the mind of the WPA President, Costas Stefanis, who consistently tried to prevent votes on resolutions with which he did not agree. This was apparent when a motion was raised to carry through a statutory alteration in which a two-thirds majority would be necessary to admit a new association. Stefanis, a major proponent of the unconditional return of the AUSNP… foresaw the danger that this would reduce the chances of the AUSNP and postponed the voting on the motion for hours. During this period, he was constantly supported by his 'legal advisor'. … The motion was never voted upon. The [Executive Committee], however, understood that the delegates could not be so manipulated and the 'legal advisor,' snapped at by the Australian delegate, kept quiet for the rest of the meeting."[25]

When reading the transcript of the tapes made during the Extraordinary General Assembly, one gets a more balanced picture of what actually happened, although this does not decrease the confusion, to the contrary. Indeed, the main issue on the table was the question whether the General Assembly could only vote on amendments that had been proposed by the Executive Committee or also on amendments coming from the floor. Jim Birley, the delegate from the United Kingdom, proposed to equalize the majorities needed for admission and expulsion: "Admission is being decided on a simple majority, now expelling… has to be made by a two-thirds majority. Now, I think this is inconsistent." Birley's motion caused considerable debate and confusion, and ultimately led to the involvement of Parliamentarian Vgontzas in the discussion. However, the tone of the meeting had been set, and after lunch the tension continued to build up.

The first explosion came when Stefanis implied that proposed alterations from the floor could not be voted upon unless they had been listed in the proposed changes to the Statutes and Bylaws as submitted by the Executive

---

24 Interview with Antonis Vgontzas, September 3, 2009

25 *Documents* 30, November 1989

Committee. That immediately evoked an angry reaction from Harold Visotsky, the US delegate: "Mr. President… our organization warned me that there might be surprises, which is why I walk around with a startled look on my face. However, … what did startle me was the interpretation of our council. This body, this assembly is the governing body. In they want to change all the constitution at this meeting, they can. The recommendations of the taskforce are just recommendations, and this body can take up item by item, because it is the governing body. Unless, I have a surprise that I am unaware of, that seems to be based in the constitution of this organization."[26]

Stefanis responded to Visotsky by stating "I fully respect what Dr. Visotsky has said that this is the governing body, and might do anything, might change the organization, might dissolve the organization, but… it requires a certain procedure..… [It] has to comply with the requirements that exists." The tape continues:

"*Meyer-Lindenberg*: In your letter of ...[unclear] it says to deal with proposals for alterations of the present WPA statutes, and this is the same in the draft agenda. That is exactly what we are dealing with, as far as I understand the language, and I would propose to continue that.

C[ostas]S[tefanis]: Well, it is, as far as I can read it, and I don't really want to start with this kind of adversary atmosphere… …

Birley: I am sorry to be difficult, Mr. Chairman, but this is a proposal for an alteration of the Bylaws that we are putting to you, and you are not allowing to be voted on. What you are saying is that the only proposals we can vote on are the proposals which we received from the executive. That is not constitutional under WPA law."[27]

Again, Vgontzas took the floor, explaining that in his view only alterations could be voted upon in articles for which alterations were proposed, which led to an angry intermission by the Canadian delegate, Rae-Grant: "Mr. President, this is our assembly, the assembly according to the present and the proposed constitution is the governing body of our association. We are being bogged down on minutia and niceties… I would suggest that the way out of this is not by law and legal opinions, but by a vote of the governing body of this organization, namely the general assembly. And I would call for a vote whether to uphold your ruling or to go ahead with the vote as it has been requested." The transcript then reads: "applause."[28]

---

26 Transcript of the Extraordinary General Assembly, October 11, 1989, p. 19

27 Transcript of the Extraordinary General Assembly, October 11, 1989, p. 20-21

28 Transcript of the Extraordinary General Assembly, October 11, 1989, p. 22

The tape transcript again records a long debate, opinions pro and contra, and a Stefanis who does not seem to be able to draw the discussion to a conclusion. At a certain moment he says:
"But you see how this situation is developing, when we deviate from the basic rules, but I do not know whether ... what I have proposed really serves ease of the tension or the other way around, intensifies the... and it is not clear to me, but anyway I think
Sabshin: You said you would call the vote
CS: Pardon me
Neumann: Not Varma again, either call for a vote or not."[29]

Clearly, also within the Executive Committee itself irritation was increasing because of the inability of the Chairman to come to a conclusion of the debate. Neumann's worst fears, as expressed in his travel report after the Granada meeting ("If Stefanis leads the General Assembly just as bad as the sessions of the Executive Committee and the All-Union Society will not become more disciplined and prepare itself with a clear concept, it will become a disaster."[30]) seemed to become reality. The debate continued, and every time Stefanis avoided putting the motion of Birley to the vote. Instead, the delegates were asked to vote on the question whether amendments to the statutes as proposed by the floor could be voted upon. The record reads:
"*CS*: be seated, the results of the voting will be announced. Yes votes that is to discuss all items 188, no votes 99, the total of votes 287, and for a two thirds majority is lacking by 34, it is 65.6 percent, it requires 66.3 percent, and despite the relative majority, the proposal is turned down."[31]

The result was an uproar among the delegates: why suddenly a two-third majority?! Amid the resulting confusion, the Australian delegate, John Grigor, asked Stefanis: "What change in the question did we just vote for, that requires a two thirds majority?
CS: We did not, we did not vote for any change.
Grigor: Well, why then did we not just require a simple majority vote?
(heavy whispering)
CS: John [Grigor], if I understand you correctly. The issue that you raise is the voting was not on a specific change, but on the possibility to change. That is right? And whether this required two thirds majority, that is the

---

29 Transcript of the Extraordinary General Assembly, October 11, 1989, p. 24. Neumann refers here to the Indian delegate, Dr. Varma, who throughout the meeting took the floor with long statements that often had little bearing on what was actually being discussed, as we will see later in this chapter.

30 Report Jochen Neumann on the WPA Executive Committee, April 1989, p. 4

31 Transcript of the Extraordinary General Assembly, October 11, 1989, p. 27

question. Wait for your answer. My answer.
It is, the answer is since this aimed at changing the statutes, it is implied that requires the same majority as the change of the statutes.
Grigor: Oh, dear me. I cannot accept that…"[32]

The discussion continued, now focusing on whether the voting on allowing propositions from the floor should require a simple or a two third majority. Confusion reigned. At some stage Neumann intervened: "Distinguished delegates, excuse me for being impolite, but I would like to draw your attention to the fact that our interpreters leave the room at 6 o'clock. And if we are not disciplined, we exclude some of our colleagues from the participation in the discussion because they need interpreters."[33] The meeting had been going on since 10.00 AM, with an intermission for just over one hour for lunch, and they had not yet been able to move even beyond the motion of Jim Birley.

Suddenly the meeting gathered speed. The proposed motion of Jim Birley seemed to be off the table, at least for the time being, and one by one the proposed changes in the Statutes were mentioned. When nobody reacted swiftly, they were immediately considered as having been accepted. Australian delegate John Grigor gave it another try "I think you have worn us down a bit by dehydration, but I do want to point out to the G[eneral] A[ssembly] that in my view, it is rather unfortunate that these amendments are presented in this way."[34] This also had no effect. When a delegate from Kuwait wanted to raise an issue about one of the previous articles, Neumann immediately responded: "We have passed it already now. It is out of order, we have passed it."[35]

The statutes were rushed through, article by article. Next were the Bylaws. The delegates agreed to consider them page-by-page, rather than article-by-article, at which point, the US delegate, Harold Visotsky, raised a not unimportant question:
"Are the statutes that we have just passed, now in force?
Stefanis: That will be a question in the end.
Visotsky: It is a question,. I know it is a question. I am asking you a question.
Stefanis: No, you want to this to be decided at this moment."[36]

32 Transcript of the Extraordinary General Assembly, October 11, 1989, p. 29
33 Transcript of the Extraordinary General Assembly, October 11, 1989, p. 31-32
34 Transcript of the Extraordinary General Assembly, October 11, 1989, p. 34
35 Transcript of the Extraordinary General Assembly, October 11, 1989, p. 34
36 Transcript of the Extraordinary General Assembly, October 11, 1989, p. 41

Eventually, after an intervention by Parliamentarian Antonis Vgontzas, it was made clear that the new Statutes and Bylaws would take effect immediately after this Extraordinary General Assembly.

The meeting dragged on for several more hours, only ending at 9.00 PM. The motion of Jim Birley was indeed never put to the vote. Somehow, it seemed Costas Stefanis has managed to avoid a decision on having a two-third majority obligatory for acceptance of a new member society. Such decision, if taken, would have effectively blocked a return of the All-Union Society. When reading the transcript of the session, it is hard to believe that this was not in the back of his mind.

The debate

The next day, a joint meeting of the Executive Committee and the Committee took place. According to the report on the Athens events in IAPUP's *Documents*, at least one of the issues on the agenda was the possible return of the All-Union Society. "...The Soviets had plenty of chances to describe the 'perestroika' and 'glasnost' within the realm of Soviet psychiatry. They explained that systematic political abuse of psychiatry had never taken place. The most 'incidental diagnostic mistakes' were made by 'individual psychiatrists'."[37]

The main counter-move that the Soviets had brought to Athens was a memorandum signed by Grigori Lukacher, a Moscow neuropathologist who was working in the Serbski as one of the department heads.[38] The statement optimistically started with the claim that "The All-Union Scientific Society considers it necessary to declare that it fully supports the policy of perestroika and those revolutionary changes that are taking place in our society."[39] In the document, the All-Union Society claimed that an "independent Commission" had been established, "which is composed of eight persons. It compromises psychiatrists, lawyers and social workers. ... The Commission is independent from the Health Ministry or any party or state organs."[40] The document further stated that "expressing its firm and

37 *Documents* 30, November 1989

38 In 1990 he is mentioned as doctor of medical sciences, professor and head of a unit at the Serbski Institute. He authored a book on neurological manifestations of alcoholism.

39 Statement by the All-Union Scientific Society of Psychiatrists, undated, disseminated in Athens by the Soviet delegation.

40 The names of the members of this Commission never became known, and it is in fact not known whether the Commission actually existed at all, or was just

resolute wish to put an end to isolated cases that took place in the past, of use of psychiatry for non-medical purposes, the All-Union … Society … declares that it is ready to give foreign experts on psychiatry, representing WPA, a possibility to visit and speak with any patient in the Soviet Union if a case occurs that cannot be solved by the national independent Commission. … The All-Union Society… devoted to the humane tradition of our health care, strongly condemns any instances of the use of psychiatry of non-medical purposes in our country…"[41]

Although some delegates felt the document was a step in the right direction, others were more negative and felt it fell short of what was considered to be the minimum condition to allow the Soviets to return: an admission that there had been systematic abuse of psychiatry for political purposes. Semyon Gluzman, on receiving a copy of Lukacher's statement, set himself to work and, on October 14, disseminated his detailed refutation of Lukacher's claims among the delegates to the WPA General Assembly, which he ended by saying that "I can assure you that the views I expressed above are shared by those Soviet psychiatrists who dare to express their disagreement with the official leadership of our psychiatry openly, as well as those who still fear to voice their opinions in public for fear of repression on the part of the psychiatric administration."[42]

The continued denial by the Soviets that anything had been fundamentally wrong angered an increasing number of delegates and, unwittingly, the Soviets were becoming their own worst enemy. Things started to look pretty bad for them and this had quite an effect on their presence in Athens. Most of the delegation was banned from the Congress, including Marat Vartanyan, and the main negotiator on the Soviet side became Yuri Reshetov, the deputy head of the Department of Human Rights of the Ministry of Foreign Affairs, who had been directly involved in the US State Department delegation to the USSR. The psychiatrists were pushed to the sideline – it was now the Foreign Ministry that decided what was needed to save face. Andrei Kovalev, who worked at Reshetov's department at the Ministry of Foreign Affairs, was not at all informed of what was happening in Athens and doubts whether Reshetov had to consult with the political leadership in Moscow all the time. In his view, Reshetov had relative freedom in his

---

something invented for the purpose. See also the Report by the WPA Team of the Visit to the Soviet Union, June 1991, p. 14

41 Statement by the All-Union Scientific Society of Psychiatrists, undated, disseminated in Athens by the Soviet delegation.

42 Gluzman's response was published in *Documents* 30, November 1989.

decisions, and did most if not all of the negotiations by himself.[43] This point was fully confirmed by former Foreign Minister Eduard Shevardnadze, who pointed out that Reshetov had his instructions and knew exactly what he had to achieve. "Not fulfilling the instructions would have meant the end of his career," he added with a smile. [44]

Four psychiatric associations suggested to the WPA leadership to organize a debate between the All-Union Society and their opponents, represented by Semyon Gluzman on behalf of the Independent Psychiatric Association. "We have the impression that a considerable number of the delegates is badly informed about the current situation in Russia and because of the euphoria over perestroika want to admit them without any conditions," wrote Roelof ten Doesschate in his report.[45] "We, the delegates from the BRD [West-Germany], Great Britain, and the Netherlands decided to organize an informal gathering, where both the 'official' Russians and the independent Russians can speak and answer questions."[46] It would be the only time that Gluzman spoke on behalf of this group, because their points of view differed considerably, but it was the only way in which a debate could be given a formal basis. Both associations from the USSR had applied for membership in the WPA, and although the All-Union Society had been given ad-hoc membership on rather dubious grounds (e.g. with an unsigned letter of application), at least this allowed a diplomatic way out of the predicament.

Negotiations started. Dutch delegate Roelof ten Doesschate writes in his report: "Noteworthy meetings were:
- With Costas Stefanis, in his beautiful suite in the Intercontinental, in order to get his agreement to organize such a meeting. A bit vaguely he expresses his support;
- With Semyon Gluzman, representative of the independent association, in order to discuss the preconditions of such a meeting and also the risks for them in the future. He wants to participate and considers the risks for himself to be acceptable.
- With M. Vartanyan about the participation of the AUSNP in this exchange. If they are able to participate in this with several representatives there is no objection. In the following days, we don't see Vartanyan, Morozov and

43 Interview with Andrei Kovalev, October 12, 2009

44 Interview with Shevardnadze, October 15, 2009.

45 Report on the Athens Congress by Roelof ten Doesschate, November 2, 1989, p. 4. IAPUP archives.

46 Report on the Athens Congress by Roelof ten Doesschate, November 2, 1989, p. 4. IAPUP archives.

other representatives of the AUSNP again and the negotiations go via Y.A. Reshetov…"[47]

Being Gluzman's interpreter, I was allowed to join the discussions. "Not present was the current General Secretary, Fini Schulsinger. Apparently, they had decided that his presence was not such a good idea, considering his earlier attacks on us. Present were WPA President Costas Stefanis, candidate for presidency Jorge Alberto Costa e Silva, executive committee member Felice Lieh Mak from Hong Kong, and Harold Visotsky as delegate of the American Psychiatric Association. On the other side was Semyon Gluzman with me as his interpreter. The latter was a precondition: I was not supposed to have an opinion and if I had one, I should keep it to myself. I was only to translate the thoughts of Gluzman; a ridiculous and rather insulting situation. Ridiculous because Gluzman and I constantly discussed tactics and politically shared, by now, the same views, as any normally thinking person would have understood. Insulting, because I was pushed in the corner as a sort of dog: come on, move it, under the table! It was, however, not the first time that this happened to me and I had learned to swallow, to pretend nothing was happening and just continue with what I intended to do."[48]

On the other side, negotiations with the Soviets were carried out by a small group of delegates under the leadership of Jim Birley. The group included the German delegate, Johannes Meyer-Lindenberg; the Dutch delegate, Roelof ten Doesschate; and Harold Visotsky on behalf of the APA. "The conditions which were stipulated by the Soviets changed from hour to hour. A mutual debate was excluded, first Zharikov and then Vartanyan were pushed forward from the Soviet side and then pulled back. Finally it was apparent that Gluzman faced a group of eight Soviets: seven psychiatrists plus Reshetov of the Ministry of Foreign Affairs."[49]

The debate took place during the evening of October 15, and turned out to be a complete fiasco, both for the Soviets on stage, and for the organizers of it, Stefanis and Schulsinger. Instead of having an open, honest and equal

47 Report on the Athens Congress by Roelof ten Doesschate, November 2, 1989, p. 4. IAPUP archives.

48 *On Dissidents and Madness*, p. 129

49 As far as the author remembers, on the Soviet side the team consisted of Modest Kabanov, Aleksandr Karpov, Pyotr Morozov, Yuri Reshetov, Nikolai Zharikov and three others. Unfortunately, no minutes of this meeting were in the documents provided by Jochen Neumann, nor found in the WPA archives. Quite possibly, the meeting was not recorded.

debate, the stage had been set quite symbolically: the eight Soviets were sitting on stage, leaving no place for Gluzman, who was, therefore, force to stand at the bottom of the stage, with myself as interpreter, at least a meter lower. The press had been banned from the meeting, sometimes removed from the hall by physical means by Stefanis and Schulsinger personally.[50] "There were eight against one, and optically a lost battle. Either this was done on purpose or the organizers had been incredibly short-sighted. A strange feeling took possession of us: here we could only win. It was the feeling of the underdog - the only way forward is up."[51] The agreed upon allotment of one hour for each side became half an hour for Gluzman and an hour and a half for the Soviet delegation. "With reddened and nervously twisted faces, the Soviets tried to deny that political abuse of psychiatry had taken place in their country. Reshetov, whose eyelid continuously dropped out of anger, repeated the line dictated by Moscow that 'under previous political circumstances, cases of abuse for non-medical purposes could have taken place,' while Chief Psychiatrist Karpov stated that he was surprised to hear that 'his colleague Gluzman' had been banned from psychiatry and that he would give him a job as a psychiatrist immediately, asserting subsequently that 'Gluzman is not even a psychiatrist'."[52]

In his response, Gluzman made again a masterful move. The center point of his counter-attack was an article in the journal *Kommunist*, a publication of the Central Committee of the CPSU, in which the unchanged conditions in Soviet psychiatry had been described in detail and strongly criticized. For the Soviet delegation this posed a serious problem, because *Kommunist* represented the official Party line and, for them, it was impossible to go against it. Gluzman was ominously waving the journal in front of the eyes of the Soviet representatives on stage, which had quite an effect on them, and concluded his remarks in the same balanced manner: "I think there is no need to assure the General Assembly that I sincerely want changes in Soviet psychiatry. My goal is not to discredit my fellow countrymen present here, but to cure that clearly sick phenomenon of psychiatric abuse, for which today's leadership of official Soviet psychiatry is personally responsible.... Whatever your decision is, it will be yours; it will be your decision alone. Psychiatry is not politics. It shouldn't be politics. And I hope that your decision will not be based on political motives. Morality should be the basis of your analysis and your conclusions. Remember: psychiatry in my country is only starting to change, and although there is a long way ahead to breach a morally oriented and legally based psychiatry,

50 *Documents* 30, November 1989

51 *On Dissidents and Madness*, p. 130

52 *Documents* 30, November 1989

we are nonetheless optimists. But we need your help. Your moral refusal to accept the evil and the lies, your rejection of the leadership of official Soviet psychiatry would help us. I appeal to your conscience."[53]

If the debate was organized to change the opinion of the delegates in favor of the Soviets, it failed. The opposite happened. It strengthened the opinion of the opponents that too little had changed in Soviet psychiatry to allow a return of the Soviet Society and that their statements were still dominated by lies.

Negotiations with Moscow

For Reshetov, representing the Soviet Foreign Ministry, the debacle during the Extraordinary General Assembly on October 15 must have been a clear signal that too little had been done to satisfy the demands of the delegates who opposed a return of the All Union Society. Negotiations continued, however not with the WPA Executive Committee but with the group of four delegates mentioned before, led by Jim Birley. These negotiations continued up to the General Assembly on October 17, and would continue even during the breaks between sessions. During the deliberations, Jim Birley would return to this issue twice, pointing out that "all my negotiations … has not been with a single psychiatrist in the association, it has all been done by somebody who is not a psychiatrist, and is not even a member of the association, so you can see how they are an autonomous, professional body."[54] As Harold Visotsky later noted in his confidential report of the Athens Congress, "in surveying the groups of both friendly and neutral societies, it was my impression that a vote to admit the USSR without conditions (as recommended by the current executive committee) would be extremely close. In consultation with Drs. Lieh Mak and Costa e Silva, I met with Mr. Reshetov, accompanied by Dr. Lieh Mak and, later, Dr. Alan Beigel, to inform him that because of our strong showing in the election of the executive committee, we would vote against admission of the All-Union Society unless they accepted conditions for admission."[55]

The General Assembly took place in a large congress hall of the Hotel Intercontinental in Athens. In the back of the meeting hall sat, on the left

53 Statement by Dr. Semyon Gluzman, WPA Extraordinary General Assembly, October 15, 1989. In *Documents* 30, November 1989.

54 Transcript of the General Assembly of the WPA, Athens, October 17, 1989, p. 30.

55 Notes by Harold Visotsky, late October-early November. IAPUP archives, p. 4

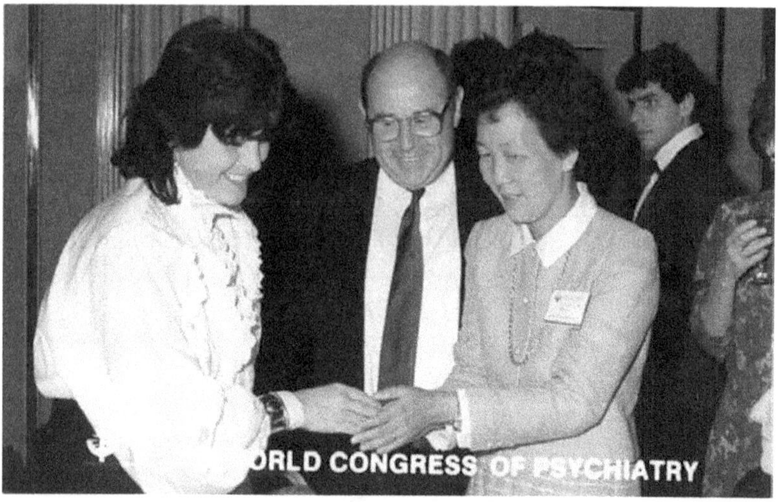

l.t.r. Monika Neumann, Jochen Neumann and Felice Lieh Mak, 1989 Athens World Congress

hand side, Anatoly Koryagin, honorary member of the WPA and former political prisoner, with me next to him as interpreter. On the other side of the aisle sat, more or less at the same height, Nikolai Zharikov as delegate of the Soviet delegation and Pyotr Morozov as his interpreter.[56]

The sessions started with the election of the new Executive Committee, first the President, followed by the President-Elect, the General Secretary and the other offices. Among the candidates for President were the outgoing General Secretary, Fini Schulsinger, and "our" candidate, Jorge Alberto Costa e Silva. Stefanis strongly urged the candidates not to take the floor for a nomination speech, but this evoked a lengthy debate among the delegates whether it was democratic not to allow candidates to speak:
"*CS*: I wish this discussion will not be protracted in defining democracy in the cradle of democracy, as John Grigor has mentioned. And now, may I ask Dr. Varma who is first among those who wanted to take the floor. And we keep an order. I repeat my plea, as short as possible.
Varma: Mr. President, I wanted to take the floor not to speak about myself, but to speak about the issue that was before the House: whether the candidates should have an opportunity to speak or not. If you permit I was to speak about that.
CS: I did not get it.

56 Later, after a break, Zharikov had been exchanged by the Soviets for Tiganov.

Varma: I am still referring to Dr. Grigor's point that was supported by the delegate from Canada and so on: whether the candidates should be righted to speak in this forum or not. I wanted to express an opinion about that.
CS: But, Dr. Varma, please, it is over, it is over, it is over."[57]

Then Schulsinger took the floor. He started to speak calmly, but soon became increasingly agitated when discussing his motives in relation to the Soviet issue. "Since it was known that I could be a candidate for President, twisted and invented information about my motives and activities has been spread by a certain group in its bulletin, and maybe otherwise.[58] This is not the first time groups have tried to stigmatize me with twisted or untrue information. Scientology has also used such methods. I feel that such attempts are interfering with my personal integrity, and I do not want to step down from my integrity and defend myself though I must say that my activities to have contact with the All Union Society about future collaboration has been three times, they have all been reported to the EC and appeared in the minutes.... I shall be brief and, in conclusion, inform you that I think the all Union Society has met the criteria for readmission from the 1983 G[eneral] A[ssembly] resolution. However ... I think it will be necessary for the GA ... to adopt a resolution which will take the Soviet society on their word and oblige the EC to collaborate with them and have access to information from the Soviet Union..."[59]

The transcript then reads "applause"; however, I remember vividly that many people in the audience were surprised by the aggressive tone in Schulsinger's statement and his reference to the Scientology Church. This eventually was reflected in the allocation of votes, because Schulsinger received only 47 votes from 9 societies, whereas Costa e Silva received 223 votes from 29 societies. Costa e Silva was to be the next President of the WPA.

Now the other officers were elected, one by one. Felice Lieh-Mak became President-Elect, the first woman to lead the World Psychiatric Association, with 271 votes from 31 countries in her favor. Juan Jose Lopez Ibor from Spain followed as the new General Secretary, collecting 268 votes from 37 countries. Then the other officers were elected. The composition of the group was very much in accordance with the hopes of the opponents of Soviet psychiatric abuse and the slate IAPUP had promoted, and very much criticized by Jochen Neumann in his travel report: "The election

57 Transcript of the General Assembly of the WPA, Athens, October 17, 1989, p. 8
58 Schulsinger here clearly referred to IAPUP
59 Transcript of the General Assembly of the WPA, Athens, October 17, 1989, p. 9

of the Executive Committee resulted, as expected, in a completely pro-US Executive Committee… President for the next three years is Costa e Silva, Rio, an extremely wealthy Brazilian bourgeois, a complete APA-marionette. He had traveled [to Athens] already as future President with his complete following including a big limousine with driver, a second car for special purposes and 3 secretaries. President is Lieh Mak, Hong Kong. She is a moral person, belongs to the national bourgeoisie in Hong Kong, has become big scientifically in New York and is fully pro-America. General Secretary is Lopez Ibor, Madrid, a moral person, but very much right wing. His father belonged to the inner circle of Franco in Spain. His father and he himself are close to the Argentinean generals. Secretary for finance is Grigor, Melbourne, a moral person, but extremely right wing, pro-American, anti-Soviet. Secretary for meetings is Visotsky, APA Chicago. Secretary for the Committee is Cazzullo, Milan, a bourgeois opportunist and businessman with intelligence.

Secretary for publications in Furedi, Budapest, and a Hungarian businessman who on basis of his relationships with higher circles has gathered a great wealth and with this wealth is counted to the pro-Western protagonists. Secretary for Sections in Beigel, Tucson/USA."[60]

The descriptions of the elected officers by Neumann did not so much reveal a pro-Communist or anti-Western positioning, as his frustration with the fact that as a candidate for an Executive Committee he himself had hardly received any vote and that his presence on the international scene herewith seemed to come to an end. An attempt by John Grigor to have him elected to the Committee of the WPA was blocked by Neumann himself on procedural grounds.[61] On top of that, the uncertain political situation in the DDR probably very much increased his anxiety, and with that his frustration. In his travel report he continues: "Colleagues from about 30 (!) countries apologized to the DDR-delegate that they could not vote for him… Terashima (Japan) apologized with tears in his eyes… A Greek colleague stated openly: 'You have paid for your integrity'."[62]

---

60 *Reisebericht* by Jochen Neumann on the WPA World Congress, Athens, October 1989, p. 3-4
Grigor received 270 votes from 34 societies; Visotsky 291 votes from 35 societies; Cazzullo 242 votes from 28 societies; Furedi 224 votes from 25 societies and Beigel 211 votes from 19 societies.

61 Transcript of the General Assembly of the WPA, Athens, October 17, 1989, p. 20

62 *Reisebericht* by Jochen Neumann on the WPA World Congress, Athens, October 1989, p. 4

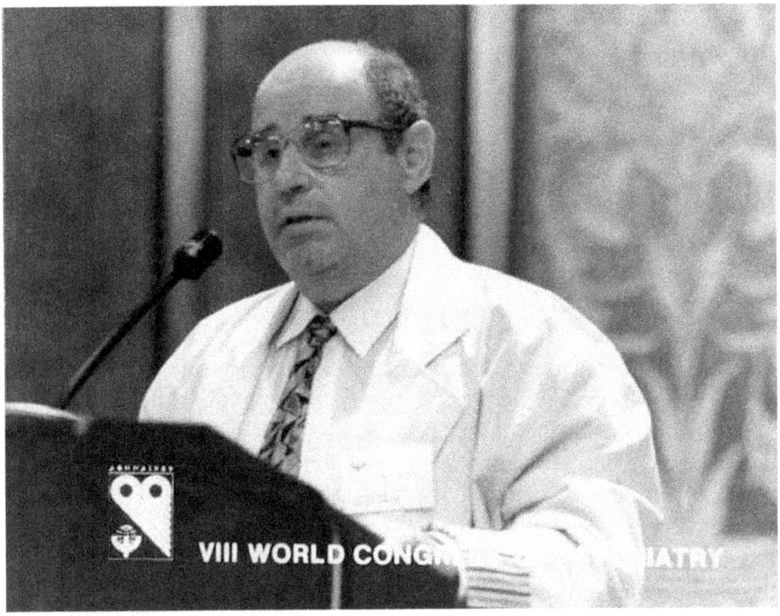

Jochen Neumann at the Athens WPA World Congress, 1989

The elections of the new Executive Committee had, in fact, been predetermined well in advance. IAPUP was not the only organization that had been busy with the development of a slate that would defeat the current Executive Committee. Harold Visotsky makes clear in his notes that all was prepared in advance, and Roelof ten Doesschate writes in his notes that "During a lunch in the harbor of Piraeus, where delegates from the larger countries with about half of the votes were present, the ultimate list was decided upon, keeping in mind the capacities and domiciles of the candidates."[63]

The Soviets re-enter

By the time the elections were over, it was well into the evening and the delegates had been in session, with short intermissions, since 14.30 PM. Still the regional representatives of the WPA had to be elected, which also took considerable time, and when the issue of admission of new member societies into the WPA was presented, it was after 22.00 h. in the evening, and the delegates were quite exhausted. On top of that, the threat of interpreters

63 Report on the Athens Congress by Roelof ten Doesschate, November 2, 1989, p. 5. IAPUP archives.

walking out of the meeting was hanging like a sword of Damocles over those present. The key issue – the possible return of the All-Union Society – had to be rushed through the General Assembly. Whether this was the result of bad chairmanship or a matter of tactics, is a question that probably will never be answered. At that time we were convinced of the latter.

In the mean time, negotiations with the Soviets had continued outside the General Assembly. "During the break, Reshetov was given a choice: either to acknowledge the political abuse of psychiatry, or to see the AUSNP not being re-admitted. Reshetov had to make up his mind on the spot."[64] When the Assembly finally reached the Soviet item on the agenda, Costas Stefanis read out the 1983 resolution, which had stated that "The World Psychiatric Association would welcome the return of the All-Union Society … to membership of the Association, but would expect sincere cooperation and concrete evidence beforehand of amelioration of the political abuse of psychiatry in the Soviet Union." The British delegate, Jim Birley, immediately took the floor. "I would like to point out that there is a problem about this; this situation as we are looking for concrete evidence of the amelioration of the political abuse of psychiatry in the Soviet Union. And the society has a considerable problem in doing anything about this because they have never recognized or admitted that such political abuse has ever occurred. So just at present, we are logically in a position where we cannot possibly expect the society to have done anything about something which did not exist."[65]

A discussion followed, which was cut short by Melvin Sabshin who turned to the Soviet delegation in the audience: "I would like to ask the ad hoc members of the All Union Society that are present the following question: if in any action that the assembly takes tonight, that we in the assembly could state, that there <u>has</u> been an acknowledgement of political abuse of psychiatry in the Soviet Union. Would the Soviet delegates, ad hoc delegates, object to our use of such a phrase in whatever action we might take?
CS: So this is a proposal
Sabshin: it is a question, Sir, I am asking a question.
CS: It is a proposal rather, addressed to the Chair, in order to ask the delegate of the ad hoc member, the All Union Society, whether he is willing to answer this question, posed by Dr. Sabshin. May I ask, who. Yes, Dr.Morozov."[66]

64 *Documents* 30, November 1989

65 Transcript of the General Assembly of the WPA, Athens, October 17, 1989, p. 25

66 Transcript of the General Assembly of the WPA, Athens, October 17, 1989, p. 25

Pyotr Morozov got up, and said: "Could I make a statement on behalf of the delegation, my vice-president is here."[67] After having received permission from Stefanis he read out a hand written statement, in which the All-Union Society … "publicly acknowledge that previous political conditions in the USSR created an environment in which psychiatric abuses occurred for non-medical reasons, including political." He added that "victims of abuse shall have their cases reviewed in the USSR"; that "the Registry shall not be used against psychiatric patients"; that "the All-Union Society unconditionally accepts Review Instrument as was unanimously accepted by the WPA General Assembly"; that the All Union Society supports the changes in the Soviet law" and, finally, that "the All-Union Society encourage an enlightened leadership in the psychiatric professional community in my country."[68]

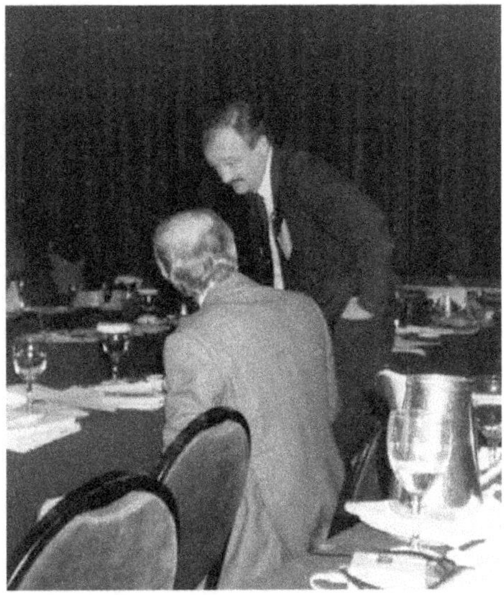

Pyotr Morozov (standing) at the WPA General Assembly, Athens, 1989

Stefanis thanked Morozov and suggested to submit it as a document.
"P[yotr] M[orozov]: Yes, of course, it is in handwriting, it could be typed and submitted.
CS: yes, Dr. Sabshin. Dr. Morozov. The last point was not heard.
Morozov: The All-Union Society encourages an enlightened leadership in the psychiatric professional community in my country.
The floor: We would like to hear the first point.

67 Transcript of the General Assembly of the WPA, Athens, October 17, 1989, p. 26. Morozov here refers to Aleksandr Tiganov, who had replaced Nikolai Zharikov as the Soviet delegate.

68 Transcript of the General Assembly of the WPA, Athens, October 17, 1989, p. 26. Harold Visotsky notes in his report on the Athens Congress: "I prepared the draft of a statement to be read by the representatives of the All-Union Society (…) The… statement is my draft language, but the final draft essentially had all of the above elements and was read to the Assembly by Dr. Peter Morozov…" See Harold Visotsky's report on the Athens Congress, p. 4-5, IAPUP archives.

CS: The first point you would like to have it repeated. Very slowly, yes. Dr. Morozov, I am apologizing for having you on the floor again, but…
Morozov: the All-Union Society … publicly acknowledge that previous political conditions in the USSR created an environment in which psychiatric abuses occurred for non-medical reasons, including political."[69]

The assembly then moved to a discussion as to how to proceed. There were a considerable number of resolutions on the table with regard to the Soviet issue, but the statement read by Morozov had altered the situation. The delegates voted to have the text included in any future resolution concerning Soviet membership; 313 votes were cast in favor, 28 against, with 2 abstentions.

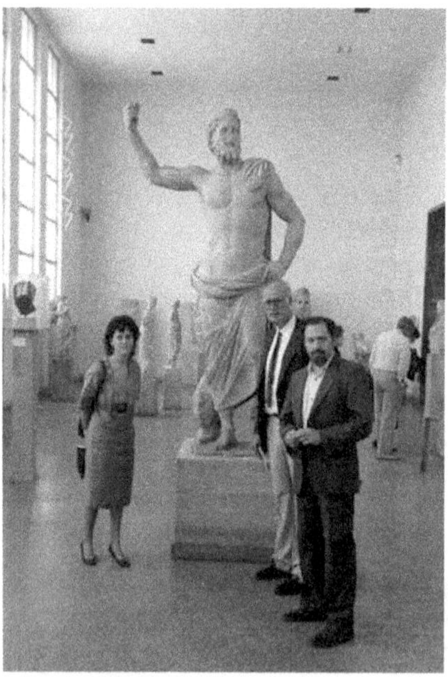

Johannes Meyer-Lindenberg and Semyon Gluzman, Athens 1989

Johannes Meyer-Lindenberg took the microphone and read an emotional plea to the delegates not to close their eyes and turn away from their responsibility. "Exploiting psychiatry for political purposes was one of the many crimes committed during the National Socialist regime in Germany with regard to both psychiatric patients and healthy individuals. As president of the German Society of Psychiatrists and Neurologists, I would particularly like to stress this fact to make you feel the weight of our responsibility when discussing these issues."[70] He then turned to the Soviet issue and said: "Lately, the Soviet part has been more open in admitting facts of misusing psychiatry for political purposes. This relative openness and the fact that it has become possible to follow events in the Soviet Union allow us to say that some reforms apparently are on the way. However, reports from the Soviet Union show that the misuse of psychiatry ... still continues. Certain responsible government structures and psychiatrists are still there,

69 Transcript of the General Assembly of the WPA, Athens, October 17, 1989, p. 26-7

70 Transcript of the General Assembly of the WPA, Athens, October 17, 1989, p. 29

still in control, while those who try to restore the ethical principles of psychiatry are still being discriminated against. ... Since psychiatry's ethics are obligatory for everybody, we simply cannot be satisfied with the first steps Soviet psychiatry is making in the right direction and see them as some kind of guarantee that sooner or later the misuse of psychiatry will stop. The only way in which we can influence the process of conducting reforms and help psychiatrists restore their professional pride is to arduously keep demanding that the following conditions be observed: no misuse of psychiatry may take place and psychiatry as a science must aim at restoring and preserving patients' health."[71]

Meyer-Lindenberg concluded: "We have moral obligations. As long as there are cases of forced hospitalization of dissidents in the Soviet Union or any other country, we must use our authority to put an end to this. I am fully convinced that if we do not use the power of moral influence, we will have to share moral responsibility for the fate of victims and their suffering."[72]

After Meyer-Lindenberg, Jim Birley stressed again that the Soviets were represented in Athens by a diplomat, and not by a psychiatrist. The Australian delegate, John Grigor, added that "we also know that the leadership has not changed, that we sat here all week listening to the non-medical delegation being prepared to make admissions, which the psychiatrists until tonight could not make without prevarification and modification."[73] A long discussion followed, intermitted by requests from Costas Stefanis to keep the remarks short, as time was running out and soon they would be without interpreters. Felice Lieh Mak, just elected as President-Elect, suggested a resolution that included the statement read by Morozov, and then adding that within one year the Review Committee should visit the USSR and that if evidence of continued political abuse of psychiatry were to be found, a special meeting of the General Assembly should be convened to discuss suspension of membership of the Soviets.

Jim Birley, clearly frustrated by the direction in which the discussion was going, again pointed out who was in charge on the Soviet side: "what good are we doing to the WPA to admit a society which up till half an hour ago never even mentioned that it was aware of political abuse, there was

71 Transcript of the General Assembly of the WPA, Athens, October 17, 1989, p. 29

72 Transcript of the General Assembly of the WPA, Athens, October 17, 1989, p. 29

73 Transcript of the General Assembly of the WPA, Athens, October 17, 1989, p. 30

actually a piece of paper there recognizing it written in the handwriting of Harold Visotsky.[74] ... This society is run by the Politburo, it is run by a foreign office department. They have no independence. When I asked them whether they were able to speak for themselves at the press conference, they said they did not. When I negotiated with them about the statement, I negotiated with the Foreign Office. They are totally unlike any other society in this room which has its own independence and is run by its own president."[75]

It was again Melvin Sabshin who found a political way out of the predicament. He returned to the proposed resolution by Felice Lieh Mak, and said that "what Dr. Lieh Mak has indicated comes close to where I find myself, but I wonder, Dr. Lieh Mak, if you might be willing to accept that this is a motion to admit under conditions, emphasize: under conditions." It tuned out to be the best possible compromise. In the end, 291 votes were cast in favor, 45 against, with 19 abstentions. The Soviets had been readmitted to the WPA under conditions.[76]

The meeting was now coming to an end. It was well after midnight, the interpreters had already left, and only a number of remaining items on the agenda had to be pushed through. Among these was the admission to membership of the Independent Psychiatric Association, which passed swiftly with only six abstentions. The General Assembly ended at 0.45 in the morning.[77]

Anatoly Koryagin was deeply shocked. He hadn't thought that the

---

74 Birley here referred to the fact that the Soviet statement had actually been written by the American delegate, as the Soviets were not able to put anything on paper.

75 Transcript of the General Assembly of the WPA, Athens, October 17, 1989, p. 30. Apart from negotiating with Reshetov on an admission that a systematic political abuse of psychiatry had taken place in the USSR, he also negotiated an apology from the All-Union Society for the letter of January 30, 1983, in which the Soviets had resigned from the WPA and voiced accusations against the Royal College, the APA and the WPA. In the apology, signed by Dr. Pyotr Morozov, it said: "[The letter] was emotional and incorrect. The All-Union Society expresses its regrets to the WPA, to the American Psychiatric Association and to the Royal College of Psychiatrists." Letter addressed to Jim Birley and signed on October 17, 1989, with copies to Stefanis and Harold Visotsky.

76 Transcript of the General Assembly of the WPA, Athens, October 17, 1989, p. 42

77 Transcript of the General Assembly of the WPA, Athens, October 17, 1989, p. 49

Soviets would be allowed to return and considered the statement by the Soviets as completely insincere and hypocritical. Accepting a compromise was not an option for him, Out of anger, he renounced his honorary membership of the WPA on the spot, in spite of attempts by many to change his mind.[78] Also Neumann was unhappy. In his travel report he wrote that "to [my] personal taste, the acknowledgements and concessions went a bit too far, but it is not up to us to judge. The leader of the Soviet delegation was an experienced diplomat of the Foreign Ministry, Dr. Yu. Reshetov."[79]

The Soviet delegation returned to Moscow jubilantly. "Morozov, Zharikov and Vartanyan, arriving at Moscow's Sheremetyevo airport upon their return from Athens being somewhat drunk, asserted that the AUSNP had achieved full membership and that no acknowledgement (of abuse) had been made."[80] In an interview with a Soviet television crew, Vartanyan answered to the question whether there had been any conditions to a Soviet return: "No, that is wrong information, which you received from somewhere. There were no conditions. We set the conditions. That is, we proposed… eh... the Executive Committee of the WPA to come to us on an official visit to the Soviet Union within a year."[81] The next day, the government newspaper *Izvestiya* carried a report on October 19, stating that the AUSNP had been granted full membership (without mentioning any of the conditions), while "the recently founded Independent Psychiatric Association received the status of a temporary member (until the next General Assembly, to take place in three years from now)."[82] The spreading of disinformation on the part of the Soviets had clearly not yet ended. Only on October 27, 1989, *Meditsinskaya Gazeta* reported the conditions put by the WPA General Assembly.[83]

---

78 In a letter to the WPA General Secretary, Koryagin officially renounced his Honorary Membership on November 8, 1989 with a short text: "On 17th October 1989 the All Union Society of Psychiatrists and Narcologists of the USSR, which counts among its members criminal psychiatrists, guilty of psychiatric anuses for political purposes, was readmitted to the World Psychiatric Association. As I do not wish to be a member of an organization together with that kind of persons, I renounce the honorary membership of the World Psychiatric Association, which I held since 1983."

79 *Reisebericht* of Jochen Neumann on the Athens World Congress, October 1989, p. 5

80 *Documents* 30, November 1989

81 *Documents* 31, December 1989

82 *Izvestiya*, October 19, 1989

83 "The USSR again member of the WPA", *Meditsinskaya Gazeta*, October 27, 1989

For Jochen Neumann the return to East-Berlin was less jubilant. The same day the General Assembly ended, Erich Honecker was removed from power and succeeded by Egon Krenz. Three weeks later, on November 9, 1989, the Berlin Wall came down. Neumann's life would never be the same.

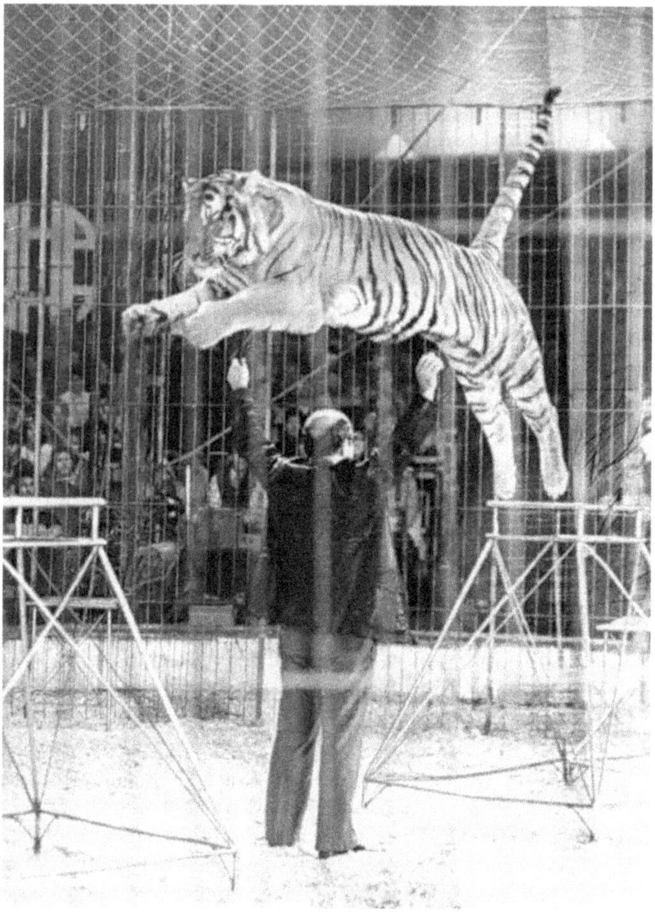

Neumann with a Siberian tiger, Leipzig, 1978

Part VI

The Curtains Close

Chapter 30 - Aftermath

When the ideological façade crumpled in 1989 or 1991, it was plain to see: outside the tiny fraction of former dissidents, Soviet citizens knew no rule save that of selfishness.

Tzvetan Todorov[1]

We are relishing our victory whereas the communists, even yesterday our jail keepers, taste the bitterness of defeat. But at the same time, conscious as we are of this victory, we feel that, in a strange way, we are losing.

Adam Michnik[2]

Even though the party was a bit spoiled by the article in *Meditsinskaya Gazeta* of October 27, in which the conditions put to a Soviet return were quoted, the psychiatric establishment very actively and successfully maintained the image of the injured child that had been punished unfairly. In an interview with *Sotsialisticheskaya Industriya*, while discussing the outcome of the Athens Congress, USSR Chief Psychiatrist Aleksandr Karpov found a subtle way not to lie directly, but to bend the truth to such an extent that Soviet psychiatry was again portrayed as a victim of an international slanderous campaign:

"Aleksandr Sergeyevich… there are various rumors: some say that we were ousted from the World Psychiatric Association, others assert that we left it.

A: The decision was voluntarily. The fact is that we did not work together with the former leadership of the WPA. It wasted all its energy not on building bridges of mutual understanding, but on searching for abuse in Soviet psychiatry." …

Q: So your return to the WPA happened rather painlessly?

A: Not exactly. From the very first day of arrival in Athens, the delegation collided with a very well organized campaign against it. IAPUP… was especially zealous in this. At numerous press conferences, they accused us of violating human rights… Our compatriot, S. Gluzman, especially invited to Greece, poured oil onto the fire. He circulated a declaration on inhumane treatment in our clinics.

---

1 Tzvetan Todorov, *Hope and Memory*, p.45

2 In Michnik, Adam: *Post-communist Europe and the difficulties of democracy.* Published in Five Years Gorbachev, Amsterdam, 1990. p. 110

Q: Nevertheless, it is probably not accidental that such an opinion was formed on Soviet psychiatry?
A: Of course, there have been cases wherein people who did not need to be hospitalized ended up in our hospitals. They could have been observed at home, completely ambulatory. But this is not with any kind of evil intent. We have our share of incompetent workers, as does any profession. We do try to get rid of them."[3]

On the part of the opponents of an unconditional return of the All-Union Society, the assessments varied from very negative to optimistic and upbeat. Anatoly Koryagin had, as indicated before, been shocked and refused to remain an Honorary Member of the WPA.[4] Also Semyon Gluzman disliked the decision, but mainly because he felt the WPA General Assembly had refused to take a moral stand and had refused to understand that they voted in people like Morozov and Vartanyan and not like Gorbachev and the more enlightened leaders of the USSR. In a letter to IPA President Savenko, he wrote the day after the vote: "All the complications and unpleasantries of the situation here you can't imagine. The leadership of the All-Union Society has shown all its colors, the chief psychiatrist turned out to be the diplomat Reshetov."[5] Harold Visotsky remarked in his report on the Athens Congress that "this outcome did not satisfy everyone,"[6] and in a note to the

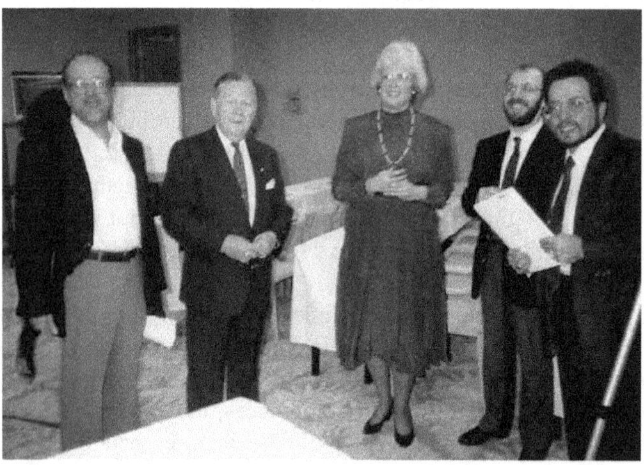

Saleem Shah, Harold Visotsky, Ellen Mercer, Felix Kleyman, Leon Stern, 1988

3 *Sotsialisticheskaya Industriya*, October 31, 1989
4 See chapter 28
5 Letter of Semyon Gluzman to Yuri Savenko, President of the IPA, October 18, 1989. IAPUP archives.
6 Report by Harold Visotsky on the Athens Congress, p. 5, IAPUP archives.

author, he added: "Perhaps there could have been better outcomes – but I think we have a vigilant Executive Committee and will have a tough Review Committee."[7]

While *Meditsinskaya Gazeta* had made public that conditions were put to the Soviet return to the WPA, the fact that the Soviet delegation had admitted to political abuse of psychiatry remained unknown to the Soviet public until November 1989, when Radio Liberty/Radio Free Europe correspondent Wayne Brown described in *Moskovskie Novosti* what had happened in Athens.[8] The full text of the statement was published by Pyotr Morozov more than two months later, in February 1990, in a trial edition of a new journal, Vrach.[9] However, the journal had a very small print run. Only on October 24, 1990, would the *Meditsinskaya Gazeta* publish the full text after Jim Birley had been handing out copies to journalists in Moscow.[10]

In the meantime, President Aleksandr Tiganov of the All-Union Society tried to alter the text itself by writing a letter to Schulsinger, proposing some "precisions" in the text of the resolution that had been passed by the General Assembly. One of these "precisions" was the fact that "the word 'abuse' should be used in plural, the word 'political' should be removed in 'political conditions' to avoid repetition and the word 'occurred' changed to 'may have occurred'."[11] These "precisions" resulted in an altogether different text, namely that 'conditions' created an environment in which psychiatric abuse 'may have occurred'. Tiganov' s attempt to rewrite history was unsuccessful; Schulsinger responded that the text remained the way it was ("It is my personal conviction that there is no substantial difference between what was presented to the General Assembly and the precisions proposed by you") and ended his letter with offering his congratulations to the AUSNP for their re-entry into the WPA.[12] It is unclear whether he sincerely believed there was no real difference in the text, or that it was a sarcastic way of telling Tiganov to forget it. However, for Jim Birley his response was reason enough to write to the new WPA President, Costa e Silva, and ask the latter "to make an enquiry to ask the All Union Society

[7] Note from Harold Visotsky to Robert van Voren, probably late October-early November 1989. IAPUP correspondence files, 1989

[8] *Moskovskie Novosti*, No. 48, November 25, 1989, p. 12

[9] *Vrach*, February 1990

[10] *Report on the WPA Visit to the USSR*, 9-29 June 1991, p. 3

[11] Letter by Tiganov of November 1, 1989, published in *Documents* 33, February 1990

[12] Letter by Fini Schulsinger, November 9, 1989, published in *Documents* 33, February 1990

whether they have in fact accepted the original statement, as it stands, and whether this has been ratified by one of their recent meetings."[13] He also made clear that he fully disagreed with Schulsinger's statement: "it seems to me that there are important differences."

Disinformation remained an important tool of the Soviet psychiatric establishment, on one hand trying to nullify the image that they had acknowledged political abuse of psychiatry in the past and that conditions had been put on their return to the WPA and, on the other hand, trying to create the impression that the Independent Psychiatric Association had not been given full membership, but a provisional or temporary one. Also the fact that the report of the US State Department delegation's report still had not been published in the USSR[14] was used to diminish its importance and play down the conclusions. In particular, the same chief psychiatrist, Aleksandr Karpov, repeated the claim that, in fact, the Americans had not found any evidence of political abuse. "They examined thirty people. The difference in diagnoses were, at times, substantial, but they did not manage to discover one person who was hospitalized for political reasons."[15] "The main conclusion made by the Americans was that recent cases of placing Soviet citizens in psychiatric hospitals for political purposes have not been observed."[16]

With regard to the Independent Psychiatric Association (IPA), the artificially created uncertainty about their membership triggered the new President of the WPA, Costa e Silva, to write a letter to Yuri Savenko, Chairman of the IPA, stressing that his association had been accorded full membership of the WPA. "I hereby wish to congratulate you with this result and to express my sincere hope for a fruitful collaboration with your association."[17]

Diversion

Also other methods were used by the Soviets to create a lack of clarity or cause confusion. More than a year earlier, on June 30, 1988, the Toronto *Globe and Mail* published an article entitled "The horrors of Soviet psychiatry," an article written by Mikhail Tsaregorodtsev, who was presented as "a

13 Letter from Jim Birley to Costa e Silva, March 1, 1990.

14 The Russian version was never published in the USSR.

15 *Sotsialisticheskaya Industriya*, October 31, 1989

16 *Izvestiya*, October 20, 1989

17 Letter by Jorge Alberto Costa e Silva to Yuri Savenko, January 20, 1989. Published in *Documents* 33, February 1990.

writer who practices psychiatry part-time at a state-run clinic in Moscow. He served six years as a military psychiatrist attached to the Red Army."[18] The article had quite an impact, because it was written by a completely unknown Soviet psychiatrist yet published in a Western newspaper, and left no doubt that Soviet psychiatry was rotten to the core. Tsaregorodtsev turned out to be the founder and director of the "International Independent Research Center on Psychiatry" in Moscow, which from the very beginning would often be confused with the Independent Psychiatric Association.

Observers became concerned when Tsaregorodtsev started handing out documents confirming that the bearer was not mentally ill, without carrying out a proper psychiatric examination.[19] In some cases, the documents were pre-printed and only the name had to be filled in. The Moscow Working Commission and, later, the Independent Psychiatric Association had examined dozens of people who either had been victim of political abuse of psychiatry or were threatened by a "political hospitalization" in order to have proof that the hospitalizations had been or would be for non-medical purposes. Tsaregorodtsev's documents pretended to have the same value, yet were clearly of a totally different nature. Also, Tsaregorodtsev disseminated lists of alleged victims of political abuse of psychiatry. This, in turn, evoked angry reactions from the Soviet authorities that information on political abuse of psychiatry was "slanderous," whereby the (incorrect) information of Tsaregorodtsev was used as proof.

The rising suspicions were confirmed in August 1988, when the *Meditsinskaya Gazeta* published an article under the title "Our man in the Atlanta Constitution" in which it was reported that Tsaregorodtsev was, in fact, a former criminal, who had been arrested in 1975 at the age of 38 while in his second year as a medical student at the Moscow Semashko Medical Stomatological Institute. The reason for his arrest was that he was intoxicated and drugged a young girl, Sveta, and raped her. "Later, friends carried the still-unconscious Sveta out of the apartment to the loft. Here the inhabitants only discovered her on the next day, delivered her to the hospital, but it was already too late: not having regained consciousness, Sveta died of 'poisoning by preparations of a morphine type'; Tsaregorodtsev was arrested."[20]

Tsaregorodtsev was taken to the Serbski Institute and was diagnosed as being mentally ill and, therefore, unaccountable and sent for

18 *Globe and Mail*, June 30, 1988

19 See, for instance, Documents 35, April-May 1990

20 "Our Man in Atlanta Constitution", *Medisinskaya Gazeta*, August 19, 1988

compulsory psychiatric treatment to a mental hospital.[21] Apparently he did not spend a long time there because, in 1976, he was examined by a military medical commission but probably not accepted because according to the available information, he was re-examined in 1978 and only then declared to be fit for military duty. That same year, he went back to continue his studies at the Semashko Institute. Soon after, it seems, he committed his next offense. "...In an intoxicated state, [he] struck his wife with a knife in the shoulder. Once again, a criminal case was opened but an expert commission pronounced him unaccountable regarding the incriminating activities. The criminal case against him was closed."[22] However, in 1979, Tsaregorodtsev was again examined at the Kashchenko Psychiatric Hospital (for another violation of the law but it is unclear whether that was related to the stabbing of his wife) and found to be mentally ill. In spite of all this, he finished his studies the Semashko Institute in 1983.[23]

The *Meditsinskaya Gazeta* also revealed the reasons behind this strange turn of events. The father of Tsaregorodtsev, Gennadi Ivanovich Tsaregorodtsev, was head of the Department of Philosophy of the Academy of Medical Sciences,[24] and undoubtedly pulled all the possible strings to avoid having his son convicted for rape and murder. And it was Deputy Minister S.Y. Chikin who, in 1978, signed a declaration "I do not object" that allowed the return of Tsaregorodtsev Jr. to the Semashko Institute.[25]

But that was not all. It turned out that Tsaregorodtsev Sr. was a good friend of Marat Vartanyan and, when considering this information, all the pieces of the puzzle came together. It became clear as to why the Soviet psychiatric establishment purposely mixed the Independent Psychiatric Association with the organization of Tsaregorodtsev Jr., even in Athens on the eve of the General Assembly, and it also explained why Tsaregorodtsev had such extraordinary access to the Soviet media. It is quite likely that he was used as a ploy to create confusion and give the authorities the pretext to

---

21 *Meditsinskaya Gazeta,* December 28, 1988. According to confidential sources the Serbski Institute had a "hidden" department for cases involving children and relatives of the top nomenklatura.

22 "Our Man in Atlanta Constitution", *Medisinskaya Gazeta*, August 19, 1988

23 *Meditsinskaya Gazeta,* December 28, 1988

24 See the *Spravochnik* (guide) of the USSR Academy of Medical Sciences of 1976, p. 89

25 *Meditsinskaya Gazeta,* December 28, 1988. Needless to say, All the facts in the newspaper were confirmed by the Ministry of Health of the RSFSR and the Procuracy of the Russian RSFSR

claim that all the information on cases of political abuse of psychiatry was nothing more than "slander."

By the time the Athens meeting was over, the trump card of Mikhail Tsaregorodtsev was played and his real identity was sufficiently exposed. Yet the establishment had another trump card up their sleeve.

At the end of 1989, a sudden split occurred within the Independent Psychiatric Association. It happened quite unexpectedly, and took many by surprise, even those who were closely connected to the IPA. The instigator of the split was a young man, Konstantin Karmanov, who had been a victim of political abuse of psychiatry and who had functioned for quite a while as "executive secretary" of the association.[26] Even before the Athens Congress, Karmanov had made use of the absence of Yuri Savenko to act completely independently, publishing materials that seriously violated medical confidentiality and eventually trying to alter the status of the IPA which would have resulted in his becoming the highest authority within the organization.[27] Luckily, Karmanov was stopped in time and the damage was repaired. "After the World Congress in Athens, attempts were made by the Soviet authorities to split the IPA, to expel the most active members from the association and thereby effectively neutralize it. This was done in close cooperation with the Ministry of Health. The attempt to take over the IPA failed and those who participated in this clearly orchestrated plan were expelled.[28] Since then, the breakaway group, although involving very few psychiatrists, claimed to be the genuine IPA and the member of the WPA and is openly supported in this by the Soviet authorities. Recently, this breakaway group was given legal status in the USSR, while such a status was denied to the actual IPA."[29]

The "breakaway" IPA was led by a Dr. Leonid Kytaev-Smyk, with Konstantin Karmanov being executive secretary. Indeed, Aleksandr, chief psychiatrist of the USSR Ministry of Health, had immediately recognized

26 Karmanov, an economist by profession, was said to have studied at the Moscow Institute for International Relations, a very prestigious educational institute that attracted it students almost exclusively from the nomenklatura.

27 *Documents* 35, April-May 1990

28 Some members were expelled on December 5, 1989, while Konstantin Karmanov and his 'comrade in arms' Oleg Ukhov were expelled on the eve of the Athens World Congress, on October 8, 1989. See Documents 35, April-May 1990

29 Press release of IAPUP of April 2, 1990, published in *Documents* 34, March-April 1990

this IPA and facilitated its legal registration.[30] It turned out to be a political mistake that would haunt him until the end of his job at the Ministry in 1991 (when the Soviet Union was dissolved). Outgoing General Secretary of the WPA Fini Schulsinger also hastened to recognize the breakaway IPA as the real WPA member, only to be overruled by the incoming President Costa e Silva.[31] On March 5, 1990, Costa e Silva wrote a letter to Karpov making clear that the only IPA that was a member of the WPA was the one headed by Yuri Savenko. "We would appreciate your assistance in facilitating the registration of this association as soon as possible."[32] On September 6, 1991, WPA Secretary General Lopez Ibor informed Yuri Savenko of the unanimous decision of the Executive Committee that "his" IPA would from then on be considered as the WPA member admitted in Athens.[33]

Later, it turned out that Karmanov was also linked to Tsaregorodtsev and that he and (former IPA member) Oleg Ukhov had been co-founder with Tsaregorodtsev of an "Association of Victims of Psychiatric Repression."[34] Apparently, the authorities were planning the development of a next trump card.

Power struggle continues

In the mean time, the scheming within the psychiatric establishment continued unabatedly, with Marat Vartanyan trying to take over the leading role from his prime enemy Georgi Morozov, who had given up his position as President of the AUSNP in 1988 (but had been immediately elected as Honorary President of the AUSNP) and was supposed to retire as Director

30 *Izvestiya*, March 16, 1990. With Chazov still being Minister at that time, it is quite conceivable that behind the scenes Marat Vartanyan was involved in this as well.

31 In the minutes of the May 1990 handover meeting of the WPA EC in Hong Kong it says that "the WPA Secretariat [in Copenhagen] had only received correspondence from the IPA headed by Drs. Leonid Kitayev-Smyk and Constantin Karmanov, and had considered that as the WPA Member society… (…) The Secretary general [Schulsinger] found it logical and formally correct that the IPA board members who had actually continued to keep up the relationship with the WPA in straight continuation of Dr. Lanovoi's initiatives, were also considered as representatives of the "IPA" that was adopted as a WPA member in Athens." WPA EC Minutes, Hong Kong, May 1990, pp. 3-4

32 Letter of Jorge Alberto Costa e Silva to Aleksandr Karpov, March 5, 1990, published in *Documents* 34, March-April 1990

33 Letter from Lopez Ibor to Savenko, September 6, 1991

34 Press release of IAPUP of April 2, 1990

of the Serbski Institute in 1990, after having turned 70 years of age. His retirement was reported in September 1990,[35] but it was also reported that he had immediately become "Honorary Director" of the Serbski Institute and that he retained his office. Politically Morozov was weakened because of his bad reputation as a result of the political abuse. The Party apparatus in Moscow, where he worked part-time as head of the health department, tried to stay clear from him in order not to be hit by the resulting flak.

For a while, Vartanyan seemed to be going strong. His protector, Evgeni Chazov, was slowly positioning himself to become the President of the Academy of Medical Sciences for which elections were planned in 1990. The current President, Valentin Pokrovsky, had been "elected" three years before to this position after having been pre-selected by Chazov and was a rather weak figurehead.[36] He could easily be controlled and did not oppose Vartanyan's election to full Academy membership in 1988. Chazov had also abolished the Scientific Council of the Ministry of Health and handed over its functions to the Academy. If he had become its new President, he would have acquired a strong power base. For Vartanyan it seemed his protection would continue for many years to come.

However, things went differently. On March 29, 1990, Chazov stepped down as Minister of Health after a car accident in which one of his arms was wounded.[37] The wounds were serious but certainly not incapacitating; however, they formed a perfect pretext to leave the Ministry and prepare himself for the Academy. In his election campaign, he favored a strong Academy independent from the Ministry of Health; a position exactly opposite from his position as Minister, when he made the Academy completely subject to his Ministry. This complete turn-around caused opposition among some of the Academicians, and his demagogic and arrogant style did not help his popularity. To make things worse, Pokrovsky refused to not run for a second term, causing a serious obstruction to

---

35 See *Documents* 38, September 1990

36 Valentin Pokrovsky is described in the book *Betrayal of Trust* as "a seemingly jolly man who enjoyed his vodka and readily hugged visitors, Pokrovsky was, several sources insisted, very close to the KGB." Pokrovsky actively participated in a witch hunt organized by the KGB against virologist Viktor Zhdanov, who was forced appear become a commission of the Academy of Medical Sciences in spite of having suffered a stroke several days earlier. A few days after the commission session, he died and was replaced by Pokrovsky's son, Vadim. See *Betrayal of Trust*, pp. 185-6

37 He was replaced by the politically rather weak Igor Denisov, former Director of the Medical Institute in Ryazan and a deputy of Chazov.

Chazov's plans. In the end, Chazov failed; the Academicians decided to choose the colorless Pokrovsky over Chazov,[38] and with Chazov's demise Vartanyan suddenly found himself without his main political protector.

Yet he did not give up. Being a professional opportunist and schemer, he had understood that after Athens, the flags were blowing in a different direction, and quickly he adjusted himself to the new political situation. He presented his All-Union Research Center on Mental Health (ARCMH) as the real motor of reform in the country and set up a number of bogus organizations, such as the "Association in Defense of Mental Health Care and Help to the Mentally Ill" and a "Society for the Humanization of Psychiatry."[39] At the same time, he organized a conference on psychoanalysis in Moscow, sponsored by his friend and fellow Armenian Martin Azarian[40] from the United States. However, he made sure that those who were really involved in psychoanalysis in Moscow were not invited. Interestingly, previously, Vartanyan had denounced psychoanalysis as a "bourgeois invention."[41]

Aleksandr Tiganov replaced Morozov's clone Nikolai Zharikov in 1989 as President of the AUSNP. Zharikov had made a complete fool of himself in Granada and also in Athens, and had been replaced by Tiganov half way through the General Assembly.[42] Tiganov was generally known as being not a bad psychiatrist but completely dependent on Marat Vartanyan, and his election was a big victory for the latter. However, the end for Vartanyan came quite unexpectedly from another side. For many years, he had been suffering from kidney ailments, and now it turned quickly worse. On July 12, 1993, Vartanyan died, at age 62, the end of a turbulent yet very disputed life.

---

38 *Meditsinskaya Gazeta*, June 8, 1990. Pokrovsky would remain President of the Academy until 2006.

39 The deputy director of the "Association in Defense of Mental Health Care," a certain Kozlov, turned out to be a KGB colonel when in September 1990 psychiatrist Gennadi Milyokhin was not allowed on a plane from Chelyabinsk to Moscow for being too drunk. Kozlov pulled out his KGB identity card, after which Milyokhin was allowed on board. See *Documents* 38, September 1990

40 See also *Psychiatric News*, February 2, 1990. Martin Azarian, who was President of International University Press, a publishing company specializing in books about psychoanalysis and psychiatry, had extensive business contacts in Moscow. He died in October 2001

41 Travel notes Peter Reddaway, June 1990

42 Personal observation of the author, who, as interpreter for Anatoly Koryagin, attended the General Assembly and was sitting in the same row as the Soviet delegation.

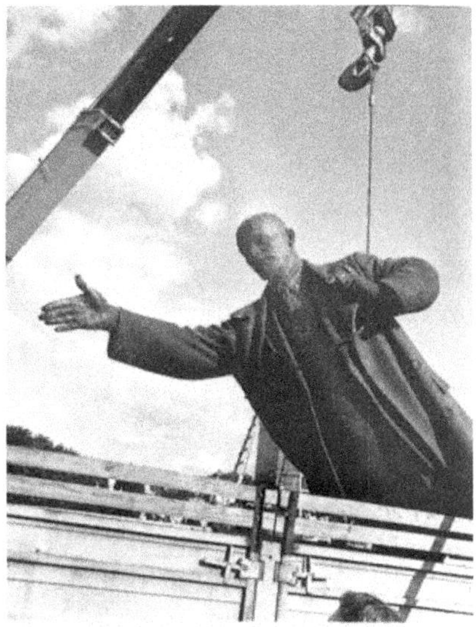

Lenin dismantled in Vilnius, 1991

The AUSNP slowly withered away, with all energy being spent on politicking, scheming, and trying to survive. By January 1991, it had changed its name to the Federation of Societies of Psychiatrists and Narcologists of the USSR, a completely empty name because no such federation existed and most Soviet republics had either their own psychiatric association or were in the process of establishing one.

One more assessment

One of the conditions for a return of the All Union Society to the WPA had been the acceptance of a follow-up visit by a WPA team that would check whether political abuse of psychiatry had indeed ended. Due to the fact that the new WPA Executive Committee met for the first time only in May 1990 in Hong Kong, it took quite a while to get the organizing process off the ground. The initial date suggested for the visit was March 1991. Dr. Jim Birley, who had been the British delegate to the WPA, was appointed Chairman of the Negotiating and Visiting Teams.

Several months later, in October 1990, a negotiating team, consisting of Jim Birley, Loren Roth (who had been the leader of the US visiting team in 1989) and Parameshvara Deva from Malaysia traveled to Moscow to prepare the grounds for the actual visit. They reached an agreement, which was signed by Jim Birley on November 5, 1990, and Nikolai Zharikov on behalf of the All-Union Society two weeks later.[43] The visit itself took place later than envisaged and was postponed by the All Union Society because of a lack of hard currency. In the end, the team arrived on June 9, with the expenses of the undertaking being almost fully covered by the WPA itself.[44] The Soviet contribution was limited merely to the provision of three

43 See Report of the WPA mission of June 1989, p. 38. According to the final agreement there were two options: the delegation would either only focus on psychiatry or on both psychiatry and narcology. Zharikov signed only the part regarding psychiatry on November 22, 1990, because they either did not get permission from the USSR Ministry of Internal Affairs to allow the WPA delegation to visit the institutions for drug addicts, or actually never asked for it.

44 The team consisted of Jim Birley (leader of the delegation); Loren Roth,

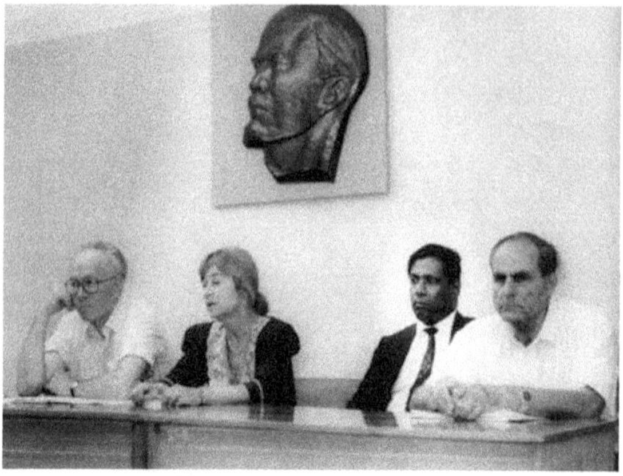

WPA delegation to the USSR, l.t.r. Jim Birley, interpreter, Parameshvara Deva, Gery Low-Beer

drivers and a bus. The team stayed in Moscow for three weeks. The first week was used for preparations and translating patient records; during the second week interviews with selected patients were held, and during the last week hospitals were visited in Moscow and Ukraine (several in Kiev and the Special Psychiatric Hospital in Dnepropetrovsk).

For the Soviets, the visit proved to be far from an overwhelming success. Not only did the team find additional evidence of political abuse of psychiatry and the extensive misdiagnosis of patients, but the collaboration with the All Union Society was, to say the least, faulty and the Soviets often quite obstructive. Information was provided far too late or not at all; information on six patients that had been selected by the Independent Psychiatric Association was not provided at all.[45] When the team arrived at Moscow airport, there was no official representative present to help the delegation bring in their equipment; and when the All Union Society was asked to have somebody accompany the team to the airport upon departure, they simply refused.[46]

The team examined ten patients, and had asked the Soviets in advance to make sure that the treating psychiatrist would be available. In fact no attempt was made to do so, and no arrangements had been made in Moscow

Parameshvara Deva (Kuala Lumpur), four Russian speaking psychiatrists (Gery Low-Beer from London, Vladimir Levit, Alla Levit and Feliks Kleyman from the US), Driss Moussaoui from Casablanca, Otto Dörr from Santiago, the US lawyer Richard Bonnie, two secretaries and three interpreters.

45 The Presidium of the All-Union Society decided on February 19, 1989, that it would be unable to provide any documentation on these cases. As argument was used that the names had been provided at "too short notice." However, with the visit being postponed for three months from March till June 1989, this argument could not be maintained and functioned only as a pretext for obstruction. See the report of the WPA mission of June 1989, p. 4.

46 Report of the WPA mission of June 1989, p. 5.

to provide accommodation for these psychiatrists. Eventually, psychiatrists who were made available were sometimes fully uninformed. Most had been warned only 24 hours in advance, and had not read any documents explaining the mission of the visit. Of the ten patients seen, only 6 had doctors who had previously seen them.

But also the attempts to make patients available were sloppy in the least, and in some cases completely obstructive. In one case, the team was told "by Dr. Milyokhin that his village, far from Moscow, was difficult to contact on the telephone and calls had to be booked at least 24 hours ahead. In fact we got through to him on the hotel phone within 2 hours. He told us, and his wife confirmed, that apart from a general statement in April that the Team was coming (time not specified) he was given no other information. He was most eager to see us and was interviewed, with his wife, later than the other cases, traveling to Moscow at his own expense."[47]

In another case, the message to a patient "had changed to presenting himself to the [Serbski] Institute rather than to the Hotel [where the Team was living and working]. When he arrived with his friend, he finally saw a doctor Lasovoi who told him that there was no WPA Commission in Moscow and that he should go back to his home some 200 miles away. Their enquiries about accommodation for the night were met by a suggestion that they

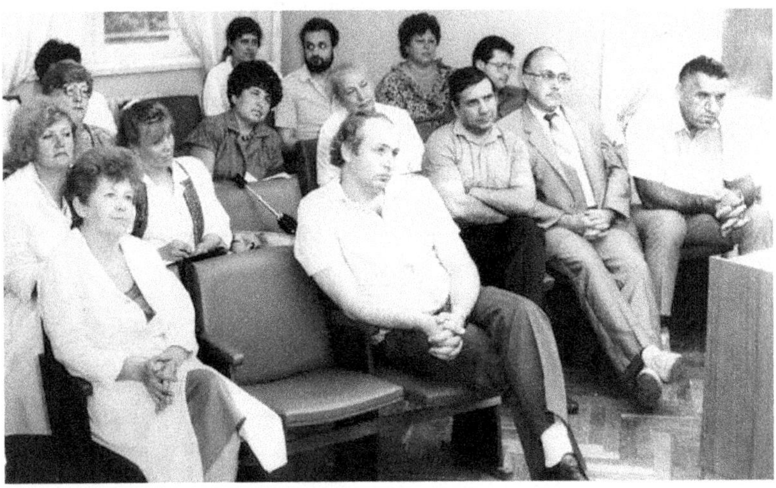

Ukrainians psychiatrists listening to the WPA delegation. In the front in the middle Dr. Yuri Yudin, Chief Psychiatrist of Ukraine, and right from him Dr. Oleg Nasynnik, Chief Psychiatrist of Kiev

47 Report of the WPA mission of June 1989, p. 8.

'sleep under the stars'."[48] But that was not all. When the person returned home, police broke into his apartment under the pretext that they were looking for a murder suspect, and he was taken down to the police station for questioning, and threatened "not to talk to the US psychiatrists."[49]

The diagnostic outcome of the mission was quite significant. Soviet psychiatrists had previously diagnosed all ten people as suffering from schizophrenia. Only in one case was the diagnosis confirmed; the team was confident that none of the other 9 ever suffered from schizophrenia. For five persons, they found no evidence of any mental illness whatsoever. One person was rather depressed (the result of his living circumstances). "Two others might have experienced mood swings which could have been pathological, but were probably short-lived. One person raised some discussion of a choice between hypomania or specific delusional disorder."[50] Of the six persons who were hospitalized in a Special Psychiatric Hospital, four of the cases were clearly of a political nature and of these four, three had never been mentally ill.[51]

The anger about the lack of support on the Soviet side and their constant obstruction can still be clearly felt when reading the conclusions in the team's report to the WPA Executive. A lot of time, money and effort had been put in this undertaking, and it seemed the Soviets considered this as something the WPA needed, not they themselves: "With respect to our Team's Visit, which was by invitation from the All Union Society, we found that in its planning and in assuring its success in compliance with the agreed Protocol, enlightened and efficient leadership was conspicuously absent. ... In Athens the All Union Society made two main commitments to the WPA: First, to fulfill the undertakings which it made in its Statement and secondly to act as an efficient and professional host for the visit of the WPA Team. The WPA should consider whether or not these two commitments have been fulfilled."[52]

The Team's anger was fully shared by the WPA Executive Committee. In an unusually angry letter to the Presidium of the All-Union Society, WPA General Secretary Juan José Lopez Ibor even threatened to start the process of suspension or expulsion. In a letter to Aleksandr Tiganov, the new chairman of the All Union Society (or, as the now called

48 Report of the WPA mission of June 1989, p. 8.
49 Report of the WPA mission of June 1989, p. 8.
50 Report of the WPA mission of June 1989, p. 9-10
51 Report of the WPA mission of June 1989, p. 10
52 Report of the WPA mission of June 1989, p. 33

themselves, the Federation of Societies of Psychiatrists and Narcologists of the Commonwealth of Independent States), he explained that the WPA delegation had not found any evidence of new cases of political abuse of psychiatry and that therefore convening a Extraordinary General Assembly of the WPA was not necessary but that, "nevertheless, the Executive Committee cannot overlook the strong evidence of lack of cooperation from your society in the planning and the fulfillment of the visit." He continued that "the poor level of cooperation, support and hospitality to the delegation… is contrary to what we expected from colleagues and caused considerable inconveniences and costs to the WPA… The AUSNP made a Statement in the General Assembly that included five items. Several have not yet been fulfilled. Therefore, the Executive Committee has unanimously agreed that it will not recommend continuing membership of your society in June 1993… unless you can produce convincing evidence that … all the statements and compromises made by the AUSNP delegation in Athens to the General Assembly have been met."[53]

The report on the letter in the minutes of the Acapulco meeting of the Executive Committee in November 1991 was followed by a dry but very telling remark: "[WPA General Secretary] Prof. Lopez Ibor Jr. informs that he has requested the constitution of the [AUSNP] and of the Psychiatrists and Narcologists Federation Council. The question was raised to clarify whether the Psychiatrists and Narcologists Societies Federation Council represents a conglomerate of member societies, because if it is so, each of them could become a member society of WPA."[54] However, it was already too late. Less than two months after the Team's visit to the USSR, a coup against Mikhail Gorbachev had been carried out. The coup failed, and was followed by the implosion of the Soviet Union. As a result, the All Union Society was left without a country to represent. By the time Lopez Ibor sent his letter to the AUSNP, the organization was nothing more than a piece of paper anyway. In October 1992, the USSR Federation of Psychiatrists and Narcologists officially resigned from the WPA.[55]

Alternatives

After the problems with the "breakaway" IPA were solved, the Independent Psychiatric Association faired reasonably well and became a stable factor in Soviet psychiatry. The biggest problem was the lack of growth of its

53 Minutes of the WPA EC Meeting, Acapulco, November 1991, p. 8
54 Minutes of the WPA EC Meeting, Acapulco, November 1991, p. 9-10
55 Letter from Juan Jose Lopez Ibor to Jim Birley, October 23, 1992.

membership, which continued to hover around not more than fifty, and the rather elitist positioning of its leadership. They believed that they had the exclusive right to be considered "ethical" and had a tendency to have the same monopolist attitude as their opponents.

The real opposition to the AUSNP came from the other Soviet republics, and from within the Russian Federation itself, where one after the other national psychiatric associations were set up. Even before the World Congress of the WPA, an Estonian Society of Psychiatrists had applied for membership, an association set up as early as 1988,[56] but the General Assembly decided to put the application on hold. "This is a question of how to deal with regionalization within the country. If you want to leave it for a while until the new EC thinks about the whole issue of regionalization within the same country, then I think it would be wise for the time being. Consider the application still standing but no decision to be taken, unless you think otherwise. It has been agreed."[57]

In 1990, a small initiative group consisting of Dr. Dainius Puras, Dr. Gintautas Daubaras, and Dr. Liaudginas Radavicius founded the Lithuanian Psychiatric Association (LPA), and in 1992 the LPA received ah-hoc membership status of the WPA.[58] In January 1991 Semyon Gluzman managed to establish a Ukrainian Psychiatric Association. From the very start he took a different approach than the Independent Psychiatric Association, trying to avoid a "dissident" association but instead incorporating as many of the leading figures as possible, provided they were not active and knowing participants in the repression machinery and support the notion that reform was necessary. In this way, he managed to win over the chief psychiatrist of Ukraine, Yuri Yudin, the chief psychiatrist of Kiev, Oleg Nasynnik, Professor Valery Kuznetsov from Kiev and even the chief psychiatrist of the Ministry of Internal Affairs, M. Ryaboklyach.[59] "For these gentlemen, this was far from being a small step because the Soviet Union was still the Soviet Union and Gluzman was a well-known opponent of Soviet psychiatry who had served a sentence of ten years because of his views. To a certain degree,

56 Letter of Ants Anderson to Robert van Voren, October 26, 1989

57 Costas Stefanis at the General Assembly. Transcript of the General Assembly of October 17, 1989, p. 45

58 Letter from Juan Jose Lopez Ibor to Jim Birley, October 23, 1992.

59 The Ministry of Internal Affairs (MVD) was considered part of the state security system, administered camps and prisons, guarded Special Psychiatric Hospitals (which in 1988 had been transferred to the Ministry of Health, but still for security were dependent on the MVD) and had in Stalin time even been part of the same structure as the KGB – NKVD.

he was still considered as an 'enemy of the people' and to join him in his efforts was for the above-mentioned persons a difficult and, above all, courageous decision. That Gluzman subsequently appeared with an anti-Soviet activist like me made it undoubtedly even more difficult."[60] At the founding congress of the Ukrainian Psychiatric Association, a statement was adopted, which said that "today's psychiatry is our country is to a great extent dehumanized and in service of personal and non- professional interests of the government, whose institutions are incapable of ensuring the defense of human rights and the economic development of our society. The result is that the loss of priority of the moral-ethical and spiritual aspects [in psychiatry] started with the activities of doctors, including psychiatrists. This manifested itself with inevitable regularity in cases of psychiatry for goals which have nothing to do with health and welfare."[61]

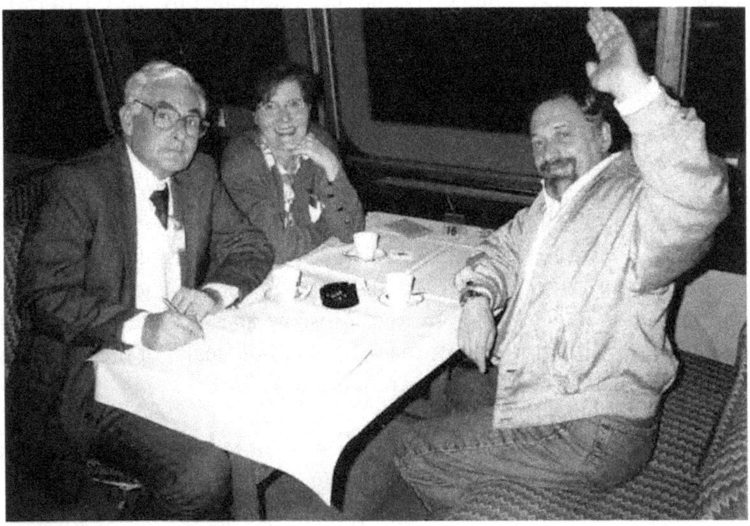

Claus Einar and Erika Langen with Semyon Gluzman, early 1990s

Even in Leningrad, the second largest city and former capital of Russia, hundreds of psychiatrists joined the Leningrad Psychiatric Society, later named St. Petersburg Psychiatric Association, out of protest against the continued dominance of the old nomenklatura over psychiatry in Russia. Their dissatisfaction came to light in February 1990, when the Leningrad Society of Psychiatrists adopted an appeal to the All Union Society, which was tabled at a meeting of the expanded board of the AUSNP on March

60 *On Dissidents and Madness*, p. 142

61 "Announcement to the psychiatric community of Ukraine" translation printed in *Documents* 39, October 1990.

26, 1990. In the letter, the Leningrad Society complained that "the activity of the current Presidium of the All Union Society of Psychiatrists does not correspond to the spirit of reforms taking place in the country today. It is characterized by passivity, avoidance of many vitally important problems of psychiatry or attempts to decide them secretly… … So far nothing has been reported to republican and regional societies on the conclusion of the commission of American psychiatrists who inspected Special Psychiatric Hospitals in our country in March 1989. The Soviet response to these conclusions is unknown to a broad mass of members of the Society. The necessary information and evaluation of the conclusions of the Eighth Congress of the World Psychiatric Association have not been given. … There are rumors of some kind of 'conditions' on which the return of our Society were allegedly based that has disturbed the practicing psychiatrists in our country. These rumors have not been dispelled by the board of the All Union Society of Psychiatrists until today."[62]

The appeal continued with the statement that "dissatisfaction with the activity of the Board of the All Union Society promoted the emergence in the USSR of independent psychiatric associations, one of which was recently unconditionally accepted as a full member of the World Psychiatric Association… The composition of the board of the All Union Society is characterized by a concentration of all power in the hands of three Moscow institutions on a Union level. Of the 23 members of the presidium of the board of the society, 20 are from Moscow and of those, 18 are from institutions directly subordinate to the Ministry of Health of the USSR and the Academy of Medical Sciences of the USSR."[63]

The appeal resulted in strong reactions from the Moscow psychiatrists. Marat Vartanyan "expressed perplexity regarding the Leningrad psychiatrists' lack of information on the Athens congress, since V.A. Lebedev and M.M. Kabanov participated in it." In its decision, the presidium stated that "The style of the petition does not do justice to its authors, a number of proposals in the petition do not correspond with reality."[64] Nothing was done to try to keep the Leningrad psychiatrists on board and, as a result, they went their own way. For many years, the St. Petersburg Psychiatric Association (as it was renamed the moment Leningrad changed into St. Petersburg) was

62 Korsakov Journal of Psychiatry and Narcology, no.8, 1990. Reprinted in translation in *Documents* 39, October 1990.

63 Korsakov Journal of Psychiatry and Narcology, no.8, 1990. Reprinted in translation in *Documents* 39, October 1990.

64 Korsakov Journal of Psychiatry and Narcology, no.8, 1990. Reprinted in translation in *Documents* 39, October 1990.

chaired by Professor Vladimir Tochilov, a former student of Yuri Nuller. Nuller, a professor of psychiatry and pharmacology at the Bekhterev Institute and a close friend of many dissidents including Gluzman, served eight years in Kolyma under Stalin, and was widely respected as an honest ethical person and a great scientist. Until his death in 2004, the association maintained a course independent of Moscow.[65]

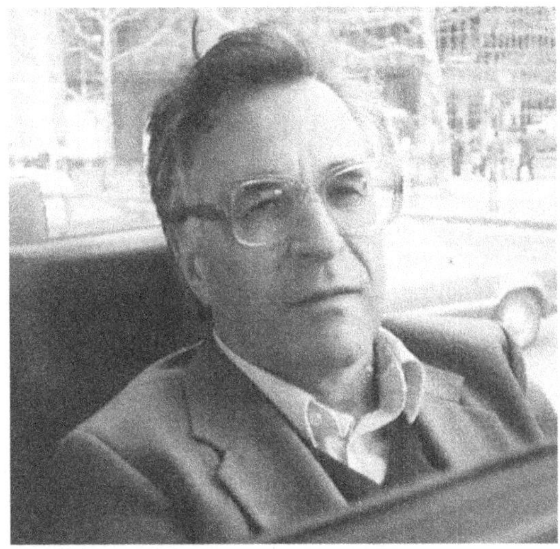
Yuri Lvovich Nuller

Following the collapse of the Soviet Union in August 1991, psychiatric associations were established in all newly independent republics. In October 1992, the Executive Committee of the WPA accepted the Kazakh Psychiatric Association, Latvian Psychiatric Association, and the Lithuanian Psychiatric Association as ad-hoc members.[66]

In Russia, next to the IPA and the St. Petersburg Psychiatric Association, a Russian Society of Psychiatrists was established as a separate legal entity, not as a successor to the All Union Society, and applied for membership in the WPA in October 1992.[67] In August 1996, the successor organization to IAPUP, Geneva Initiative on Psychiatry, brought a delegation of 75 representatives from Eastern Europe and the former USSR to the WPA World Congress in Madrid. The delegation consisted of many Presidents or delegates from new associations that had applied for membership of the WPA or were hoping to see their ad hoc membership status changed into full membership.

65 On Yuri Nuller see *On Dissidents and Madness*, pp. 177-179

66 Letter from Juan Jose Lopez Ibor to Jim Birley, October 23, 1992.

67 Letter from the Russian Society of Psychiatrists to Lopez Ibor, October 12, 1992. The Society claimed to have 500 members.

Chapter 31- Siegerjustiz and its consequences

Emancipate yourselves from mental slavery;
None but ourselves can free our mind.
Bob Marley, Redemption Song

West Germany took over its Eastern sister and quickly sent the country to the dustbin of history. Many former East Germans feel they were victims of "Siegerjustiz," victor's justice, without any respect for what had been and what was built with the energy of many citizens who were convinced that they were building an "other Germany." These feelings greatly reduced the happiness following the fall of the regime and the opening of the gates to the West and became the source of a lot of discontent in the years following *Die Wende*.

Indeed when one looks how the files of the Stasi were used to "cleanse" society from those who collaborated with the regime, one cannot escape the feeling that it was a rather one-sided affair. Of course, the enormous number of cases that were dealt with made equal treatment much more difficult; yet, some of the basic rules could have been set differently. Alleged former Stasi agents (both those who were professional agents and the unofficial IM) were not allowed to see their own files, which following the end of the DDR regime were managed by what were called the "*Gauck Behörde*".[68]. Yet the very same files were used to draw up documents certifying whether someone was "clean" or not. Many felt that secondary circumstances were not sufficiently taken into account or the fact that one was blackmailed, pressured or otherwise forced to collaborate. This was particularly painful because this confrontation with a "democratic institution" did not really strengthen their belief in democratic society. To the contrary, it strengthened the feeling that West Germany had taken over their country without any consideration of its history and socio-political background.

The reports by the *Gauck Behörde* had considerable consequences for many of the former agents and IM. When the outcome was that a person indeed had been a collaborator, the document - that turned their lives completely upside down and ruined many careers - could not be contested because of the inability to access one's own files. The persons concerned often lost their positions or part of their pension, suffered from psychological aftereffects and social isolation. On top of that, the consequences were not equal for

---

68 Named after the director Joachim Gauck. Since Marianne Birthler took over the leadership of the files in 2000, they are called *Birthler Behörde*.

all professions. Teachers who lost their job because of their collaboration with the Stasi were not able to work as teachers again and, thus, lost their profession altogether. Doctors who worked in government institutions, on the other hand, still had the possibility of going into private practice and, thus, had a way out of the situation. Many of the interviewees in the analysis by Kerz-Rühling and Plänkers were dismayed about this inequality, and felt that if the treatment had been more equal and just (and thus not only based on files) it would have been easer to live with the consequences.[69]

It is, therefore, not strange that after *Die Wende* some of the IM felt victimized, in particular when their collaboration with the Stasi was revealed without taking the specific circumstances into account, including if they were forced to collaborate. It was forgotten that much of the information in the files had been recorded by the *Führungsoffizier*, and not by the informer him/herself. And the *Führungsoffizier* had his own reasons to exaggerate, to show more effect of his operation that there actually might have been. He had a plan to fulfill, like any other sector of the socialist economy, so what guarantee is there that the information in the files is an exact record of what truly happened? Also, quite a few IM did not even know that the category of "*Inoffizieller Mitarbeiter*" of the Stasi even existed, or they had agreed to collaborate out of fear and were completely surprised that now they were classified as an IM. Many kept their collaboration secret after 1989 out of fear of disclosure as such to family or society and hoped that their files would disappear. Only a few had the courage to disclose their collaboration on their own accord. In some cases, this did not lead to any consequences; in other cases, however, they lost their jobs and became social outcasts. Quite a few IM suffered severe psychological distress, physical or even mental illness after having been disclosed after 1990.[70]

The question of how to deal with dictatorial pasts and those who participated in maintaining the regimes is an issue that many societies faced and there is no easy solution. In many of the Eastern European countries the lustration process has been slow or virtually non-existent, partially because files were unavailable (e.g. the KGB managed to take most files from the Baltic countries to Moscow and is still able to use them as a means for blackmailing politicians) or because those in power had a personal interest in keeping things hidden.[71]

69 *Verräter oder Verführte*, p. 231, 235

70 *Verräter oder Verführte*, p.17, 30, 145

71 See, for instance, Mark S. Ellis, *Purging the past: The Current State of Lustration Laws in the Former Communist Bloc*, Law and Contemporary Problems, Vol. 59, No. 4

In South Africa, a Truth and Reconciliation Commission was established, chaired by Bishop Desmond Tutu.[72] While the Commission definitely contributed substantially to the easing of the pain in society and allowing former enemies to live side by side in one country and in relative peace, it never managed to do full justice to what had happened. The Commission was empowered to grant amnesty to those who committed abuses during the apartheid era, as long as the crimes were politically motivated, proportionate, and there was full disclosure by the person seeking amnesty. To avoid victor's justice, no side was exempt from appearing before the Commission. The Commission heard reports of human rights violations and considered amnesty applications from all sides, from the apartheid state to the liberation forces including the African National Congress. Many witnesses gave testimony about the secret and immoral acts committed by the Apartheid Government, the liberation forces including the ANC, and other forces for violence that many say would not have come out into the open otherwise. Presented in October 1998, the Commission report condemned both sides for committing atrocities. Out of 7112 petitioners, 849 were granted amnesty; 5,392 people were refused amnesty and were supposed to be tried in a court of law. In reality, however, only a few individuals were eventually tried and, thus, still managed to get away with their actions.

In many Eastern European countries, in particular former Soviet republics, it was virtually impossible to list all those who collaborated with the regime. After 75 years of communism, basically everybody collaborated in one way or another. Many children and adolescents joined the *Pioneer* and *Komsomol*[73] organizations, and it was essential to join the Party for many careers. The rest was a slippery slope – in order to live quietly and undisturbed and be an active part of society, compromises had to be made, some small, some bigger. The only way out was to separate oneself from society, to live on an "island" and have as little as possible to do with the outside world. Some became dissidents and made a clear separation with communist society and its structures, even though in the life of dissidents, there is also the eternal necessity to maintain the thin line between self-preservation and collaboration. For instance, in the 1980s many political prisoners were called in by the KGB at the end of their term of camp or

72 The work of the TRC was accomplished through three committees: The Human Rights Violations Committee investigated human rights abuses that occurred between 1960 and 1994; The Reparation and Rehabilitation Committee was charged with restoring victims' dignity and formulating proposals to assist with rehabilitation; and The Amnesty Committee considered applications from individuals who applied for amnesty in accordance with the provisions of the Act.

73 The communist youth organizations in the USSR.

exile and asked to sign a document promising to refrain from political activity. Not signing meant a new arrest and a new term of imprisonment, signing meant giving in to the KGB. So people negotiated, tried to agree to a text that allowed them to go free, yet at the same time preserve their self-respect. Only a few were strong enough to refuse any compromise.[74]

As a result, in the former Soviet Union, very few people lost their positions because of their participation with the "old regime." Especially in the Russian Federation, the legal successor to the USSR, lustration of senior Communist Party and KGB officials was staunchly resisted and has never been implemented. Many of the people concerned have remained in power. In fact, most of the modern Russian politicians started their careers in the Soviet Union. Galina Starovoitova first proposed a law project on lustration to the Parliament in December 1992, but it was never passed.[75] People basically just repositioned themselves and continued like before. An attempt to put the Communist Party of the Soviet Union (CPSU) on trial, propagated by a number of dissidents including Vladimir Bukovsky, faltered and ended all attempts to disclose the crimes of the previous regime. The archives of the KGB that had been partially accessible for researchers, were closed again, and the same counts for the archives of the CPSU.[76]

Also in the limited field of psychiatry, very little lustration took place. For instance, Georgi Morozov lost his position as Director of the Serbski Institute in Moscow, but was named "Honorary Director" and succeeded by a student of his, Tatyana Dmitrieva, who allowed Morozov (who was also "Honorary President of the All Union Society") to use the Institute as his base and hardly altered his influence on post-Soviet psychiatry.[77] It

---

74 *On Dissidents and Madness,* p. 99

75 Galina Starovoitova (1946-1998), a Deputy of the Duma and a highly respected progressive politician, was killed in St Petersburg, one of the first political murders under the Putin regime.

76 A large part of the archives of the Communist Party (preserved now in state archives such as Archive of the President of the Russian Federation, Russian State Archive of Contemporary History, Russian State Archive of Socio-Political History and State Archive of the Russian Federation), including almost all documents of its Central Committee, remains classified.

77 Tatyana Borisovna Dmitrieva (1951-2010), graduated from the State Medical University in Ivanovo in 1975 and worked as an intern in the Serbski Institute from 1976-1978. Defended her dissertation in 1990 and succeeded Georgi Morozov as Director, which she remained until her death on March 1, 2010, with a short interval in 1996-1998, when she was Minister of Health of the Russian Federation. For many years and until her death she was also Chief Psychiatrist of the Russian Federation.

was more a political move, on the eve of the Athens World Congress of the WPA, then a clear break with the Soviet past. The Independent Psychiatric Association in Moscow, which IAPUP helped establish, demanded a purge among psychiatrists, yet it was very difficult to imagine who should be purged: those who signed diagnoses of Soviet dissidents causing them to be hospitalized in psychiatric hospitals? But then who to blame - these psychiatrists, who often signed these diagnoses because they believed these people were really mentally ill, or their teachers, who had taught them Soviet psychiatry, instead of the psychiatry taught outside the USSR? Semyon Gluzman, the founder of the Ukrainian Psychiatric Association in 1991, was very clear on his position: he opposed any lustration and was convinced that such a process would never bring justice to the victims and would only make it even more difficult to build a humane and ethical mental health care service in the country. Instead, he incorporated all the leading psychiatrists in his country Ukraine, who agreed to open the windows and doors to the outside world. The result was a strong psychiatric association, which in the 1990s brought about real improvements in the state of affairs in mental health care service delivery in the country, as well as in the rest of the region.[78]

Yet the big difference between the Soviet Union and most of the other socialist states and East Germany was the fact that the DDR was taken over by a second German state and soon ceased to exist altogether. And the justice system that was put in place was the West-German one, with

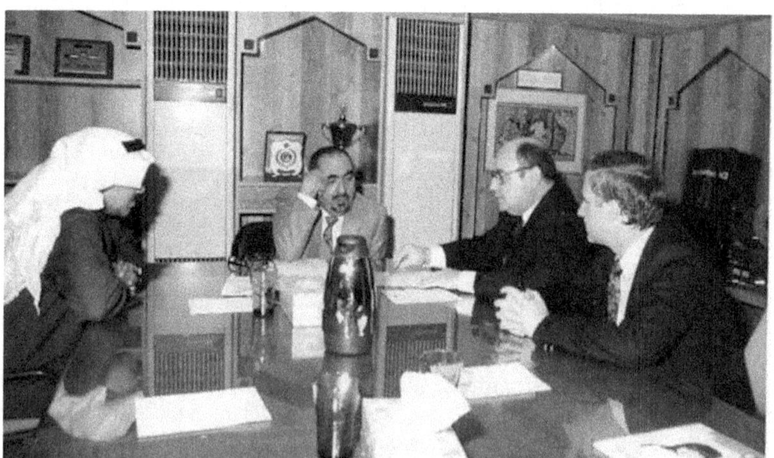

Jochen Neumann with the Minister of Health of Kuwait, Kuwait City, 1985

[78] *On Dissidents and Madness*, pp. 192-200

people judging the past who had not been part of it themselves, but who looked upon the East German state as an aberration of history, something that should not have existed. This created a lot of antagonism, a sense of not being taken seriously, a feeling that "the other Germany" tried to eradicate their state from history as soon as possible. Many did not share the jubilation in the West – for them the state that had been closely linked to Ronald Reagan's "Evil Empire" had been their home, and in spite of the many shortcomings, they still felt a sense of pride in it.

In the case of Jochen Neumann, these feelings were no different. At 53 years of age, he was at the peak of his career and Director of the Hygiene Museum in Dresden; from one day to the next, this career came to an end. "I had just reached the age when one starts to produce," he told me during our first meeting in February 2009. "I had been accumulating knowledge, having a life experience, and had reached the point when I could start to produce results. And that is when it all ended; I never had the chance."

Chapter 32 – Victors and Losers

The humanity of humans meets its fate, and in each age that fate is special and distinct from previous ages. The only common feature is that it is invariably heavy.

Vasili Grossman[79]

You, who return home,
And after closing the door
Say "good evening"
You don't know how it feels
To come through the door in silence.

Octavian Paler[80]

Wars have victors and losers. So did our "war," the fight against the political abuse of psychiatry in the Soviet Union. We won and enjoyed our victory. Soon after the collapse of communism, we started our work to rebuild psychiatry, to develop humane and ethical mental health care services in the former Soviet Union. We realized that the only possible barrier against a return of the political abuse of psychiatry was to build an independent, self-respecting and ethical psychiatric profession. We had to start from scratch, in many ways even first pulling down the old structures before having the opportunity of putting up new ones. By the year 1994-1995, we were heavily involved in the process of setting up non-governmental organizations in mental health, in mobilizing not only professionals but also family members and even users. We set up a Network of Reformers in Psychiatry, formally founded at a meeting in Bratislava in September 1993 and which, in the course of a few years, became the backbone of the reform movement in mental health in much of Eastern Europe and the former Soviet Union.[81]

Psychiatrists in the DDR were not part of this movement, and looking backwards this might have been a mistake. We assumed that the German Federal Republic took care of them and that they did not need any support on our part; yet now, 15-20 years later, one wonders whether integrating them into our Network would have helped them preserve a feeling of self-respect and independence from their West German colleagues. Instead, West Germany swallowed them up and made them part of the all-German psychiatric professional organizations and institutions, after the obligatory

[79] from Vasily Grossman, *The Sistine Madonna*

[80] Paler, Octavian: *Poems*. Albatros, Bucuresti, 1998

[81] For more information on these activities and the Network of Reformers see *On Dissidents and Madness*, chapters 17, 19, 20 and 22.

purges that left virtually all leading positions in East German mental health care delivery occupied by West Germans.

One wonders whether this turn of events has any footing in the concept of justice. Yes, many leading East German psychiatrists had been IM of the Stasi, and "our" Jochen Neumann had been one of them. Yet the West German takeover of the country made them non-persons within their own country and, at least some of them – and Jochen Neumann certainly belongs to that category – had done their work for the MfS honestly, with conviction, and while maintaining their principles. This is the paradox that cannot be addressed objectively: while being secret agents, they adhered to principles and norms so strictly that many of the persons living in the "free West" would have found it difficult to abide. So how does one judge their actions, their decisions and, actually, what gives us the right to judge them and determine whether they are good or bad?

The easiest concept is that of black and white, considering all those who collaborated with the MfS as perpetrators, as participants in a repressive regime that had a nearly perfect system of control over its citizens. A good example of this positioning is in the book "*Stasiland*" by Anne Turner, who tries to analyze the system of control through interviews with both victims and perpetrators but who, throughout her book, shows a predisposition towards the people she interviewed: the victims being victims, the perpetrators being perpetrators. It excludes the option of a perpetrator being either a victim or an honest person stuck in a system that got lost in a stampede of total control; or of a victim being an unpleasant personality who assumed the role of a victim merely because circumstances allowed him or her to use this role for his or her own benefit. Without having the experience of seeing both sides and having gone through a painful process of understanding how I, myself, was used time and again by persons who gave me the impression of being an ally only because it fit their long-term plans, I probably would have followed the same line of thought. Yet now I know it is not complete, it is not doing justice to what really happened. Life was much more complex than this and both sides had its victors and losers, its true believers and opportunists, who just used the opportunity for their own good.

Loneliness

Jochen Neumann turns out to be a loser in many respects. He was part of a system in which he believed and, as a result, turned out to be on the wrong side of history. He lost his country, the one he helped build over a period of forty years, a country in which he believed. Even though his international exposure made him understand how much was wrong, how much had become an aberration of the initial intentions and how much the State had gradually become a monster, it was a painful process for him. It was an ultimate moment of self-reflection when one has to acknowledge that much of the energy and efforts invested in an ideal have turned out to be in vain.[82]

In the early 1990s, a documentary film was broadcast on Dutch television, titled "The Bridge." It was a program based on interviews with former and current communists, people who had basically dedicated their lives to build a communist society and now saw the communist ideal crumble and whither away. It was a painful and moving documentary, because some of those interviewed had to acknowledge during the interview that all had been in vain and that, as a result, their lives had been rather worthless. Others, however, could not make that step and still maintained their belief in the system, even though it was clear that they knew it was all a hollow ideal with no remaining substance.

Half a year after the fall of the Berlin Wall, Neumann writes that "apart from the fact that I am convinced that I personally did nothing dirty and belonged to the group that wanted to do something good ... I feel myself complicit and, to a high degree, burdened with fellow guilt, the reason why I withdrew myself to a certain degree and I refrain from declamatory statements in response to the new developments."[83] And in a letter in February 1991, he adds: "I have decided to disappear from public life as much as possible and I will for the time being stick to that position. I become restless, however, by the fact that there are also former colleagues and "fellow fighters," who thought and acted like me but who present themselves now with great success as protagonists of the new developments. Thus, I am not fully sure whether I am not turning myself into something exotic, someone who is only disturbing the peace of mind of others."[84]

An article published in the American Journal of Psychiatry in October 1991 leaves no doubt that Neumann was fully aware of what had caused the collapse of the Communist system. In his view, the economic disaster was only part of the reason. "Rather, it was the psychological conditions of public life (e.g. total surveillance; spoon-feeding; absence of a right to a say; restrictions of all kinds; lack of freedom of thought, culture,

---

82 As Ellen Mercer remembers, "after the Berlin Wall came down, I received a package from Jochen with a piece of the Wall in it and a note saying that he cut it out of the Wall himself. It is still one of my treasures."

83 Letter to Dr. Steffen Haas, June 25, 1990.

84 Letter to Professor Bach in Dresden, February 15, 1991.

and religion; and special rights for privileged groups) that had become unbearable."[85] And then he voices the emotions that so much counted for himself: "The vast majority of citizens … were forced to live with a sociologically split ego. The decency, dignity, discipline and order that were demonstrated to the outside were in stark contrast to the accumulated inner emotions, fears, worries, pain, and even anger and hatred."[86] The article is remarkably straightforward and candid; it painted a picture of the challenges that Eastern European psychiatry faced after the collapse of the Communist system that was not at all different than the views of IAPUP and its successor organization, Geneva Initiative on Psychiatry.

With his ideal, Jochen Neumann also lost his career; from being one of the most influential DDR-psychiatrists with a wide international network, he turned into a non-entity, somebody who disappeared from the international psychiatric scene almost from one day to the next, evaporated, as if he had never been. In a letter to Costas Stefanis in August 1992, Neumann writes that he has been out of work since February 1992. "And there is hardly a chance," he adds. "Nearly 200 times I applied for a job (as a doctor, as a salesman for pharmaceuticals, as travel guide, as real estate agent and more). For some people I am politically spotted [tainted], for others I am too old (the main reason for refusals) and for the rest overqualified." In his letter, Neumann asks Stefanis for advice: there has been a job opportunity in Saudi Arabia; should he take it? However, the letter remained unanswered.[87]

Ironically, Neumann was, in a way, also a loser because he was principled and refused to budge and forsake the principles he believed in. He could have gone along with the tide; he could have tried to share the profit in these early months after the fall of the Berlin Wall. Many of the actors of the old regime managed to share the wealth that had been accumulated secretively and, by doing so,

85 *Psychiatry in Eastern Europe Today: Mental Health Status, Policies, and Practices*, by Jochen Neumann. In American Journal of Psychiatry, 148:10,, October 1991, p. 1386

86 *Psychiatry in Eastern Europe Today: Mental Health Status, Policies, and Practices*, p. 1388

87 After *Die Wende* Neumann worked from 1990 until 1992 as medical director and chief doctor of the psychiatric clinic in Ueckermünde, after which he left for Saudi Arabia. There he was for five years Consultant Neuropsychiatrist and Medical Director of the Al-Amal Hospital in Riyadh as well as Clinical Assistant Professor for Medicine (Psychiatry) at the King Saud University in Riyadh. After his return from the Middle East he worked from 1998 until 2001 as chief doctor of the psychosomatic department and consulting chief doctor of the neurological department of the Lindenallee clinic in Bad Schwalbach. In 2001 Jochen Neumann retired.

guaranteed their future economic base. Yet to the contrary, indignated as he was, hurt by the way the failure of the system hurt his own morality, Jochen Neumann decided to take immediate distance from them and cut all links, thereby excluding any possibility of a financial or economic reward.

And, finally, his greatest loss was probably the loss of his family, of his wife and daughter, who lost her understanding of her father and with whom the relationship remains both troubled and superficial until this very day.

When reading his private memoirs, this last issue seems to stand out most, determining his sense of self-respect, place in life and the value of everything around him. Throughout these memoirs, which have been written over a period of more than ten years and are sometimes very personal and private, one can feel the loneliness that has become the main component in Jochen Neumann's life. Both when living in Germany, a country that is not his and that has swallowed the country he lived for, and while being in exile in Saudi Arabia, Neumann airs a deep feeling of loneliness, of being superfluous, done with, put on the garbage heap of history. "Riyadh, August 28, 1995. Mood is very bad. Disappointment without boundaries."[88] The only satisfaction he gets is from his work in Riyadh and the compliments from his Saudi bosses. "They considered me rigid, reliable, hardworking and professional," he remembers.[89] Or as he writes in a letter of February 26, 1995: "…he values my professionalism very much and when he wants to show their respect, he says that in his view I am very much like Hitler."[90]

What is worse is that his sense of worthlessness, his all-encompassing feeling of not belonging anywhere and not being needed anywhere and by anybody, makes him want to end his life. He never expresses it directly, but it is there, from one page to the next, it is so omnipresent that it is almost unbearable to read. In 2002, he writes a letter to a friend in Germany, explaining his last wishes, the testament of a lonely and disenchanted man.

And still two years later, 15 years after the fall of the Berlin Wall, he writes: "Alone, you are alone, left over, mostly inadvertently. You don't belong anywhere anymore. Although you are biologically still mostly intact and also mentally, the existence takes place in a vacuum, without any social or psychological coordinates. You are not needed anymore, nowhere. If you would depart, a period would have to pass before you would be found after some time and more by coincidence… Nobody would miss you. Without

88 Note of August 28, 1995

89 Interview with Jochen Neumann, July 30, 2009

90 Note of February 26, 1995

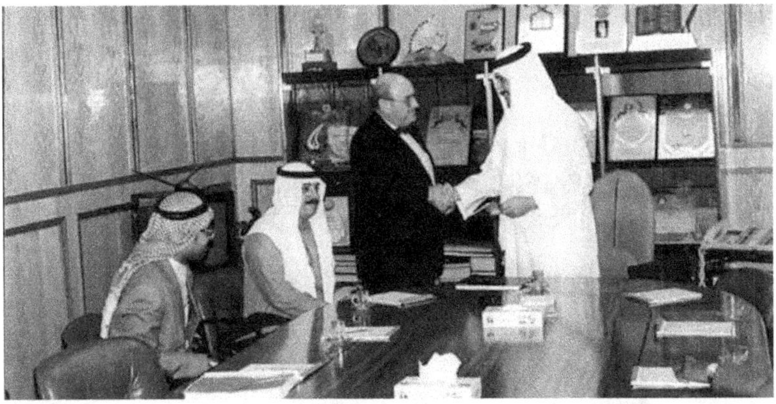
Jochen Neumann in 1997 in Riyadh with the Minister of Health Prof. Dr. Ali Shubokschi

family, without a home country. It is not surprising that you more and more often wonder whether life still makes sense. ... After a short but deep crisis, I decided to go for the year 2005. Without self-pity, without optimism. 2004 was a bad year. Nothing, absolutely nothing went well, and something went even really badly. We will wait another year."[91]

And also the year 2005 still doesn't bring any alleviation in his mental state. In September 2005, he writes: "No past, no identity, no tasks, no goals, no use, no criticism voiced (to say nothing about praise), hardly any communication, less and less contacts and de facto no family... ... And then also without a home country... I am just *on the road, solo*. Quo vadis? Towards sunset."[92]

It is finally the development of this book that brings about a fundamental change in Neumann's mindset. To his surprise, somebody is interested in his story, and to his happiness, old friends like Mel Sabshin and Ellen Mercer (with whom he maintained a very basic correspondence throughout the years) are keen to meet him, to talk to him. Initially he talks hesitantly; his e-mail reactions are slow and reserved. But, gradually, he starts to enjoy the process and when the first joint interview session with Mel Sabshin takes place, it seems he has made his turn around. He hands over a CD with his most private personal notes, among which are those quoted in this chapter, and after one of the hours-long interviews, he sits back and philosophizes a bit, and then suddenly remarks: "Maybe I should go to a WPA meeting again, just to see how things are nowadays." He hadn't been to any of them for almost twenty

91 *Silvester 2004*, note by Jochen Neumann, January 1, 2005
92 Note of September 13, 2005

years, since his last appearance at a WPA Regional Symposium in Hong Kong in May 1990.[93] It was as if, after twenty years, he allowed himself to voice this desire again, to reconnect to the world that was seemingly lost forever.

Still, in general terms, the feeling of loss and uselessness prevails, even until today and in spite of the process of contributing to the writing of this book. In September 2009 he remarks: "I don't think of the future. I have no future.

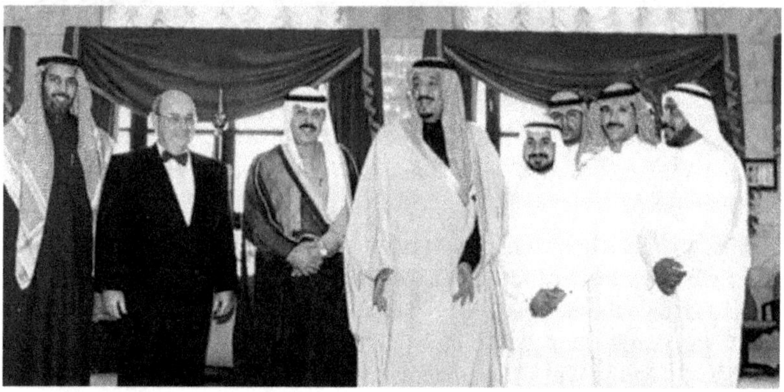

Neumann at a meeting with the Governor of Riyadh, HRH Prince Salman bin Abdul Aziz

If I think of the present, I am overtaken by pure anger; if I think of the past, I am engulfed by an endlessly deep sadness. Under the current socio-political circumstances, my professional achievements in life, which I accomplished independently from my political convictions and can be proven, are materially valued with a pension of 1355 euro. That is a shame and it also hurts, but the worst are the *lost dreams*. They have evaporated with the end of the DDR and *its* socialism. It is not the DDR that I mourn. It is the illusions that connected me to the country till the end; or rather, that *I* connected with it, the vision (delusion) of a bright future, of peace, of equal opportunities, culture, health and education for all, fraternity everywhere. What has been left is the complete emptiness without any confidence in current developments."[94]

93 In the WPA archives is a letter from WPA Secretary Vibeke Munk to Felice Lieh Mak, President Elect of the WPA, in which she writes: "Jochen Neumann called me yesterday from a turbulent East Germany. He asked me to convey the following to you: He was pleased to receive your invitation, which he accepts.... He will investigate how a DDR-citizen may obtain a visa for Hong Kong.... He resigned from his post as Director of the Hygiene Museum and has not left me a new address, but promised to call me regularly." Letter dated December 1, 1989.

94 Bruckstücke *Narratives, Personales*, September 2009, p. 1

Part VII

Conclusion

Lessons Learned. Any Lessons Learned?

No moral benefit can accrue from always identifying with the "right side" of history; it can only arise when writing history makes the writer more aware of the weaknesses and wrong turns of his or her own community. Morality is by definition disinterested.

Tzvetan Todorov[1]

Looking back, the issue of Soviet political abuse of psychiatry had a lasting impact on world psychiatry, as well as on the World Psychiatric Association. The issue triggered extensive discussions on medical ethics and the professional responsibilities of physicians (including psychiatrists), resulting in the Declaration of Hawaii of the World Psychiatric Association and subsequent updated versions.[2] Also many national psychiatric associations adopted such codes, even though adherence was sometimes merely a formality and sanctions for violating the code remained absent.

One cannot escape the feeling that at the beginning of their term in 1983, when setting themselves the task to bring the Soviets back into the WPA, President Costas Stefanis and General Secretary Fini Schulsinger did not realize that soon they would find themselves to be mere peons in a geo-political game between East and West with little control over the situation. They seem to have been caught up in a situation where they were not only following their own goals and convictions but were, at the same time, pressured from below by pressure groups like IAPUP, from inside by a

1 Tzvetan Todorov, *Hope and Memory*, p.145

2 The Declaration of Hawaii was adopted in 1977 by the WPA General Assembly at the 6th World Congress of Psychiatry in Honolulu, Hawaii and amended at the 7th Congress in Vienna in July 1983. The declaration stipulates, among others, that "the psychiatrist must never use his professional possibilities to violate the dignity or human rights of any individual or group and should never let inappropriate personal desires, feelings, prejudices or beliefs interfere with the treatment. The psychiatrist must on no account utilize the tools of his profession, once the absence of psychiatric illness has been established. If a patient or some third party demands actions contrary to scientific knowledge or ethical principles the psychiatrist must refuse to cooperate." The WPA subsequently adopted a Madrid Declaration in 1996, "To reflect the impact of changing social attitudes and new medical developments on the psychiatric profession." This Madrid Declaration was approved by the General Assembly of the World Psychiatric Association in Madrid in 1996, and enhanced by the WPA General Assemblies in Hamburg in 1999, in Yokohama in 2002, and in Cairo in 2005. For more information see www.wpanet.org

growing number of their member associations, and eventually from above, by the Ministries of Foreign Affairs of the USA and USSR, who, to a large degree, took the issue into their own hands and solved it as part of the process of détente. In particular, the extreme reactions of Prof. Schulsinger show a man who lost control not only over the situation but also over his own emotions. However, in a way everybody who took part in the events described in this book was caught up in the same theatre play called "Cold War," which influenced and, to a large degree, formed their views, convictions and subsequent actions, and convinced them that the truth was only on their side.

The years 1983-1989 made absolutely clear that psychiatry is politics, whether one likes it or not. The WPA leadership said they tried to keep politics out of psychiatry, yet the result of their actions and their dealings with the Moscow psychiatric leadership was exactly the opposite: it opened the door to carefully orchestrated interventions by the political leadership in Moscow, supported by active involvement of the secret agencies Stasi and KGB. At the same time, the goal of the opponents of political abuse of psychiatry to take politics out of psychiatry was equally unsuccessful. Their work was also an element in the Cold War between East and West and, equally in their case, "higher forces" undoubtedly had their influence.

After the fall of the Berlin Wall, it became clear that the political abuse of psychiatry in the Soviet Union was only the tip of the iceberg, the indicator that much more was fundamentally wrong. This much more realistic image of Soviet psychiatry became visible only after the Soviet regime started to loosen its grip on society and subsequently lost control over the developments and finally completely disintegrated. It showed that the actual situation was much more painful and that many more people had been effected. Millions of people were treated and stigmatized by an outdated hospital-based and biologically-oriented psychiatric service. Living conditions in hospitals were bad, sometimes even awful (yet in a way also reminiscent of the daily life of many regular Soviet citizens), and human rights violations were rampant.[3]

With the fall of Communism in Eastern Europe in the late 1980s, most of the systematic practices of using psychiatry to suppress political opponents ceased to exist. Some cases surfaced in Central Asia, notably in Turkmenistan and, more recently, in Uzbekistan. Also in Russia, individual

---

3 For a more extensive description of the situation the Soviet psychiatry by the author *see On Dissidents and Madness*, chapters 14 and 19-21.

cases of political abuse of psychiatry continue to take place. The ranks of the victims over the last years have included women divorcing powerful husbands, people locked in business disputes and citizens who have become a nuisance by filing numerous legal challenges against local politicians and judges or lodging appeals against government agencies to uphold their rights. However, there appears to be no systematic governmental repression of dissidents by means of the mental health system. Instead, citizens today fall victim to regional authorities in localized disputes, or to private antagonists who have the means, as so many in Russia do, to bribe their way through the courts.

Unfortunately, looking at those in charge in Russian psychiatry twenty years after the Athens WPA congress, it is hard to avoid the conclusion that Zharikov's assertion of 1989: "I think it is... a victory"[4] is, in fact, very close to the truth. Although for several years the positions of the Soviet psychiatric leaders were in jeopardy, especially after the implosion of the Soviet Union and during the first years of the Yeltsin rule, one can now safely conclude that they managed to ride out the storm and retain their powerful positions. In addition, they also managed to avoid an influx of modern concepts of mental health care delivery and a fundamental change in the structure of mental health care services in the Russian Federation. All in all, Russia seems to be the country where the impact of mental health reformers has been the least. Even the reform efforts undertaken in places like St. Petersburg, Kaliningrad and Tomsk have faltered or were encapsulated when centrist policies under Vladimir Putin brought them back in line. By and large, we are still looking at Soviet psychiatry in Russia and the fact that they recently published a fifth edition of a textbook on forensic psychiatry that was authored by the 88-year old Georgi Morozov and the above-mentioned 88-year old Nikolai Zharikov is one only of the painful reminders of this tragic situation.[5]

One of the conditions put to the All Union Society in Athens in 1989 was a democratic change of leadership of the All Union Society. The society ceased to exist in the early nineties following the disintegration of the USSR and a new Russian Society of Psychiatrists took its place. However democratic the election of its officers might be, this new body proved to be in no way a challenge to the dominant position of the psychiatric Academicians and Institute directors, who all owe their positions to the

4 Nikolai Zharikov in an interview to the Sverdlovsk television studio upon return from the World Congress in Athens, at Moscow Sheremetyevo airport

5 To the original text a section on compulsory treatment was added by Dr. V. Kotov.

psychiatric nomenklatura of the 1970s and 1980s. Age, however, plays a factor with, for instance, Nikolai Zharikov being 88, former Serbski Deputy Director Yuri Aleksandrovsky being 78,[6] and Georgi Morozov being 88, and said to be confined to his apartment on Kutuzovsky prospekt in Moscow and oblivious of most of the things that happen around him. It is not difficult to see a certain similarity to the Soviet leadership at the beginning of the 1980s, yet there is little hope that a "psychiatric Gorbachev" will emerge and that, when a younger generation takes the lead, much will change. Their power base is a continuation of the present status quo and their refusal to make radical changes is often combined with mercantile and sometimes quite cynical attitudes.

The tragedy is that the new political wind in Russia provides little hope of a change for the better. To the contrary, since the turn of the century, the number of places with an enlightened leadership is dwindling and they are under severe pressure to accept the inevitable. As far as the past is concerned, many of the current leaders of Russian psychiatry have revoked the earlier confession read at the 1989 WPA General Assembly that psychiatry in the Soviet Union had been abused systematically for political purposes. They now prefer to mention "individual cases of "hyper-diagnosis" or "academic differences of opinion."[7] Russian psychiatry is, naturally as in any other country, a mirror of Russian society and, also in that respect, there is little hope much will change for the better in the years to come.

Going into detail with regard to the situation in the various former Soviet republics would require a separate book but, in general terms, one has to conclude that the hope for a renaissance in the field of psychiatry in the New Independent States did not materialize. This assessment is made in spite of the many projects that were undertaken, of the commitment of many reform-minded psychiatrists and other mental health professionals, and of the development of a multitude of mental health related non-governmental organizations (NGOs). In that respect, the picture is definitely better than in 1988, when the only mental health related "NGO" was the All Union Society whose letterhead was printed with "Ministry of Health of the USSR" at the top, thereby making clear how "non-governmental" the organization actually was. There is now a wide network of professional organizations, relative/family organizations and user groups whose influence on the development of mental health care services is larger in some countries than in others but, in some cases, considerable. However, in many former

6 Aleksandrovsky retired several years ago.

7 Dmitrieva, D., *Alyans Prava i Miloserdiya*, Moscow, Nauka, 2001, pp. 116-130

Soviet republics, the training of new generations of psychiatrists is still in the hands of those who earned their positions by their allegiance to the psychiatric establishment or, at least, by a lack of resistance and bringing about change. This, regrettably, impedes full-scale mental health reform.

The political abuse of psychiatry in the Soviet Union was a unique experience and cannot be compared with, for instance, the systematic political abuse of psychiatry in the People's Republic of China. [8] The Soviet Union was, to a very high degree, a closed society and it was possible to keep international developments at bay. The fact that the security organs saw and used psychiatry as a handy means of repression made it even more isolable to external influences. The issue became an important factor during the Cold War of the 1970s and 1980s, and it was the process of détente that helped terminate the practice. To end the abuse was a decision taken at the highest political level, a necessary step in the process of rapprochement between the Soviet Union and the United States. Unfortunately, when the practice stopped, the political interest in bringing about a fundamental change in psychiatry and its leadership as a whole waned. In the case of China, we are looking at a totally different situation, a society that is much less insulated against external influences, a country much less centralized and a mental health field much less dominated by one small group of psychiatric leaders. In addition, China is much less responsive to external criticism than the Soviet Union ever was. The campaign that was mounted to end the political abuse of psychiatry in the Soviet Union would never have the same impact in the case of China.

What rests is the question of whether the drive to expel the All Union Society from the World Psychiatric Association, which inadvertently led to its decision to withdraw, was the right move and had the desired effect. For me, this question is of considerable importance, because here my role of author of this study is mixed with that of one of the main actors in the events, and one that maintained a rather maximalist position throughout the whole period. Interestingly, when starting to work on this book, I had serious doubts whether the IAPUP campaign had the right focus. Time is needed to take more distance, to soften one's positions, and the arguments of those who opposed expulsion gathered more weight. However, in the course of writing the book, I regained some of my earlier convictions.

Many Eastern European psychiatrists, or at least Eastern European psychiatric leaders, were opposed to expulsion or suspension of Soviet

8 See, for instance: Van Voren, R.: *Comparing Soviet and Chinese Political Psychiatry*; in: The Journal of the American Academy of Psychiatry and the Law, volume 30, number 1, 2002

membership, because it badly affected their position within the world psychiatric community. Their position was certainly not automatically linked with a pro-Soviet position. Professor Pal Juhasz, to whose memory this book is dedicated, is just one of many examples in which a strong dislike for his Soviet "brethren" was combined with an equally strong opposition to a Soviet expulsion. Also Jochen Neumann, one of the main characters in this book, remained totally against a Soviet exclusion and in favor of their return, even though little love was lost between him and the Soviet psychiatric establishment and at the end of his term he was convinced that the systematic political abuse in the USSR had indeed taken place. For them the World Psychiatric Association provided a window to the outside world, a welcome and very necessary counter-balance against the influence of Soviet psychiatry from the East. And the forced political "unity" of the Eastern Bloc resulted in their marginalization in world psychiatry as well, a side effect we probably did not take sufficiently into account.

However, at the same time, it is clear that change took place only because of the constant publicity about the political abuse of psychiatry and the ongoing pressure on Western governments to put and keep the issue on the political agenda when dealing with the Soviet Union. This pressure eventually resulted in the issue being raised by the US Government when developing the agenda of rapprochement in the late 1980s. If it hadn't been for the work of a number of Western psychiatric associations and groups like IAPUP, the political abuse of psychiatry in the USSR would never have been turned into a priority area and the Soviets would never have been pushed to end the practice. In short, ending the political abuse of psychiatry was not so much a decision by Soviet leaders out of moral or human rights considerations (although some Soviet diplomats undoubtedly had moral objections to these practices) but for pragmatic reasons – they realized it was an issue that would block progress in areas that were much more important to them.

This leads us to the moral side of the issue. As Semyon Gluzman pointed out in his letter to Western colleagues, "How can one accept back in the WPA those who tortured before and do not acknowledge it today."[9] Aside from political or diplomatic considerations, there is also an important moral case to be made. In fact, when looking at the evidence presented in this book, one can safely conclude that Soviet psychiatry did not change fundamentally and that any compromise or acknowledgement was made under severe political pressure both by the international community and

---

9 Letter to Western colleagues, Semyon Gluzman, June 18, 1989

the Soviet leadership. All statements made by the Soviets were made half-heartedly and followed by a variety of attempts to hide, annul or diminish the impact and a constant struggle to remain in power and change as little as possible. On one hand, it is a lucky coincidence that the Soviet Union disintegrated and the All Union Society was left without a country to represent. However, just like in general Soviet/Russian politics, those in control managed to ride out the storm and return to their positions of power as soon as the woes of political change subsided and everything gradually slid back into its old mould.

Morally, though, world psychiatry did manage to recover some of its standing by making clear that political misuse of the psychiatric profession is not acceptable and that it has the duty to make a stand and exclude those who violate fundamental standards of medical professional ethics. In the end, the WPA General Assembly of October 1989 did not welcome the Soviet AUSNP back with open arms but, instead, put conditions on the return of this member society because of the fact that their moral stand had not changed. In that sense, the Athens decision can be seen as a victory, one of morality over reason, and one of long-term thinking over politically opportunistic expediency. I still believe our campaign was a just one, and our objections to an unconditional return of the All-Union Society morally correct. If not for our active opposition, one can wonder whether the positioning of the WPA General Assembly would have been the same with conditions put to their return.

In spite of that concluding observation, the outcome of this research does not provide me with a definite answer to my question whether opposing Soviet membership of the WPA was the best possible approach. The picture that emerged has mellowed my views in many respects, but has also resulted in upsetting moments and sometimes in a sudden sense of disgust when seeing a fuller picture of the complicity of the Soviet psychiatric elite and their protectors. But then again, history is such that never a definite answer emerges and seeking that answer inevitably leads to more questions; answers are, in a way, nothing more than a reflection of today's moral, ethical and historical points of view. I hope my odyssey will help the reader form his or her own conclusions, based on his or her own specific concepts, views on history and the processes behind it. If I have been able to add the human dimension, the complexity of factors that form the foundation of historical processes, and the limitation on judging behavior and decisions on basis of today's norms and values, my work will not have been in vain.

Post Scriptum

The writing of this book was for those closely involved in it not only a unique experience but sometimes also a very emotional affair. For the author, it was a confrontation with his activist past, when subtleties were overshadowed by campaign needs and opponents were often reduced to caricature notions of "hangmen" and their "fellow-travelers." Little did we know or care about the reasons a person took a different position than ours, or became entangled in the use of psychiatry as a means of repression.

Probably the most telling example of this attitudinal shift is the relation that developed between the author and Jochen Neumann, the former leading DDR psychiatrist and informal agent of the Stasi, the Communist believer who belonged to the higher echelons of the East-German SED. Just over twenty years ago, our shoulders brushed in the corridors of a conference center in Washington D.C., enemies on either side of the barricade. Now we sit together, talk about the past, compare experiences and memories,

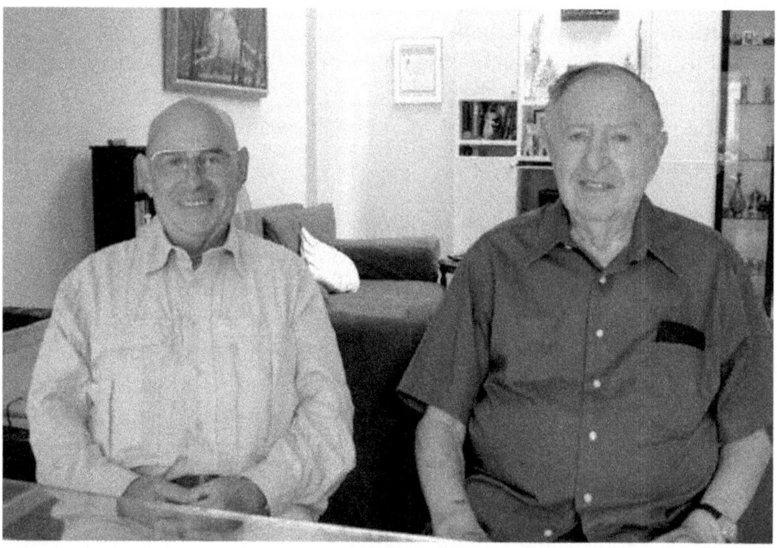

Jochen Neumann and Melvin Sabshin July 2009

and feelings of friendship and mutual respect determine our interaction. "Isn't it remarkable," he observes during one of our meetings, "that my worst enemy is writing my gravestone."
The issue of a "last testament" is never directly discussed during our sessions

and also not during the collective meetings with Ellen Mercer, Jochen Neumann and Melvin Sabshin, nor during my long talks with Costas Stefanis. But, at the same time, it is always in the air. My interlocutors are of progressing age and most are not in good health. It is clear that what will now be committed to paper is probably their last chance to have their say. It gives an extra dimension to the meetings, an extra pressure to put the wording exactly right and make sure the presentation of their recollections is one they can live and die with.

How complex this all is becomes particularly clear during the last collective sessions with Ellen Mercer, Jochen Neumann and Melvin Sabshin. A first full draft of the manuscript was on the table and I wanted from both main characters in the book a "go ahead." I know it is my book, my version of the historical events it describes but in the course of writing it has become a collective enterprise, a joint undertaking. Their opinion is to me at least

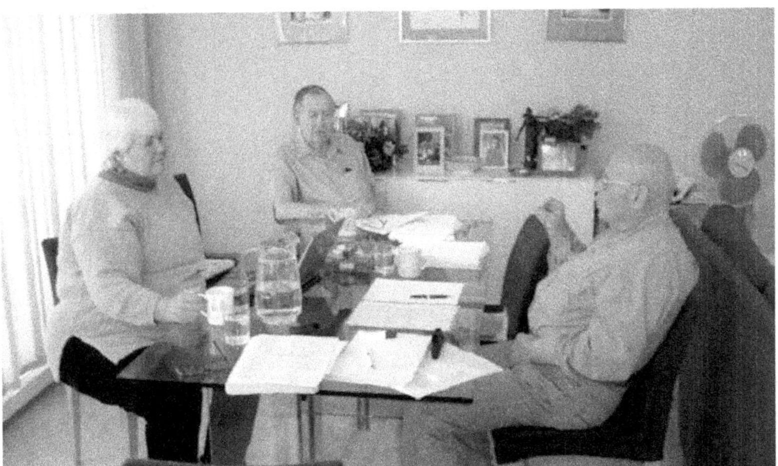

l.t.r. Ellen Mercer, Melvin Sabshin, Jochen Neumann, December 2009

as important as my own, even though, in the end, it is my decision to leave it as it is or alter the text.

One of the most important issues of contention is the question of who won and who lost. It is not an issue raised by Jochen Neumann, who in the end lost not only his country, but also his belief, career and family. He has no problem with the image of a loser, and agrees with my perception that, in the end, the Soviet psychiatric nomenklatura won. It triggers, however, a sharp reaction from Mel Sabshin who fundamentally disagrees with that notion. In his view, we did not lose, and the Soviet psychiatric establishment did not win. We achieved a moral victory and brought the political abuse of psychiatry to an end. In his view, we are the ones who won the battle with the Soviets suffering a moral defeat.

It is a difficult discussion. After long hours of going back into the past we all are tired, the issues we discussed are complex and, at moments, also painful. The knowledge that over twenty years have passed since these events took place and that our collective explorations will soon be coming to an end adds another dimension to the atmosphere in the room. The past year has affected us all; it has deeply influenced some of our thinking and created a new reality that needs time to digest. And so we cannot come to a conclusion as to who was victor and who was loser. We leave it as an open ended question.

List of Abbreviations

APA – American Psychiatric Association

ARCMH – All Union Research Center on Mental Health

AUSNP – All Union Society of Neuropathologists and Psychiatrists (after 1988: All Union Society of Narcologists and Psychiatrists)

BRD – *Bundesrepublik Deutschland*, West Germany

CIA – Central Intelligence Agency

CPSU – Communist Party of the Soviet Union

CSCE – Conference on the Security and Cooperation in Europe

DDR – *Deutsche Demokratische Republik* (German Democratic Republic, GDR)

DSM – Diagnostic and Statistical Manual, the classification of mental disorders developed by the American Psychiatric Association

DVpMP – *Deutsche Vereinigung gegen politischen Missbrauch der Psychiatrie* (German society against the political abuse of psychiatry)

FBI – Federal Bureau of Investigation

FDJ – *Freie Deutsche Jugend*, the Communist Youth Movement in the DDR

GDR – German Democratic Republic (DDR - *Deutsche Demokratische Republik)*

GIP – Geneva Initiative on Psychiatry (later: Global Initiative on Psychiatry)

HCUA – House Committee on Un-American Activities of the US Senate

IAPUP – International Association on the Political Use of Psychiatry (later: Geneva Initiative on Psychiatry)

ICD – International Classification of Diseases, developed by the World Health Organization

IM – *Inoffizieller Mitarbeiter* (unofficial collaborator or agent of the Stasi)

IPA – Independent Psychiatric Association

IPPNW – International Physicians for the Prevention of Nuclear War

KGB – *Komitet Gosudarstvennoi Bezopasnosti* (Committee for State Security)

KVP – *Kasernierte Volks Polizei*, military units of the Volkspolizei in the DDR\

LPA – Lithuanian Psychiatric Association

MfS – *Ministerium für Staatsicherheit* (Ministry of State Security, Stasi)

MVD – *Ministerstvo Vnutrennykh Del*, Ministry of Internal Affairs of the USSR

NIMH – National Institute for Mental Health in Washington D.C.

NKVD – *Narodnyi Kommisariat Vnutrennikh Del*, the People's Commissariat for Internal Affairs, the predecessor to the KGB

NSDAP – National Sozialistische Deutsche Arbeiter Partei (National Socialist German Workers' Party, the Nazi Party)

NVA – Nationale Volks Armee

PPI – Psychosomatic and Psychiatric Institute (Chicago, IL)

RAF – Royal Air Force

RSDLP – Russian Social Democratic Labor Party

SA – Sturm Abteilung (Storm Detachment)

SBZ – *Sowjetisch Besetzten Zone* (Soviet Occupied Zone)

SED – *Sozialistische Einheits Partei* (Socialist Unity Party, the Communist Party of the DDR)

SMERSH – Acronym of SMERt' SHpionam (Death to Spies) were the counter-intelligence departments in the Soviet Army formed in late 1942

UPA – Ukrainian Psychiatric Association

USSR – Union of Soviet Socialist Republics

WHO – World Health Organization

WPA – World Psychiatric Association

Bibliography

Abuse of Psychiatry in the Soviet Union; Hearing before the subcommittee on human rights and international organizations of the Committee on Foreign Affairs and the Committee on Security and Cooperation in Europe. US House of Representatives, Washington D.C., 1983

Adamishin, A., and Schifter, R.: *Human Rights, Perestroika and the end of the Cold War*. United States Institute of Peace Press, Washington DC, 2009

Alpert, Nachum: *The Destruction of Slonim Jewry*. Holocaust Library, New York, 1989

Andrew, Ch. And Gordievsky, O.: *Comrade Kryuchkov's top secret files on Foreign KGB operations*. Stanford University Press, Stanford, 1993

Andreyev, Catherine: *Vlasov and the Russian Liberation Movement*. Cambridge University Press, Cambridge, 1987

Anonymous authors: *Psychiatry, psychiatry and society*. Unpublished manuscript, 1995

Aretz, Jürgen & Stock, Wolfgang: *Die vergessenen Opfer der DDR*. Bastei-Lübbe, Bergisch Gladbach, 1997

Behnke, Klaus & Fuchs, Jürgen: *Zersetzung der Seele*. Rotbuch Verlag, 1995

Bentley, Eric (ed.): *Thirty Years of Treason*. Thunder's Mouth Press/Nation books, New York, 2002

Bloch, Sidney and Reddaway, Peter: *Russia's Political Hospitals*. Gollancz, London, 1977

Bloch, Sidney and Reddaway, Peter: *Soviet Psychiatric Abuse - The Shadow over World Psychiatry*. Gollancz, London, 1984

Bonnie, R., and Polubinskaya, S.: *Unraveling Soviet Psychiatry*. The Journal of Contemporary Legal Issues, Vol. 10, 279, 1999

Borodin, S.V. et.al.: *O psikhiatricheskoi Pomoshchi i Garantiyakh Prav Grazhdan pri ee Okazanii*. Respublika. Moscow, 1993

Böll, H, & Kopelew, L.: *Waarom hebben wij op elkaar geschoten?* De Prom, Baarn, 1982

Bracher, Karl Dietrich & Funke, Manfred: *Deutschland 1933-1945; Neue Studien zur nationalsozialistischen Herrschaft*. Bundeszentrale für politische Bildung, Bonn, 1992

British Medical Association: *Medicine betrayed*. Zed Books, London, 1992

Brown, Sarah Hart: *Standing against Dragons*. Louisiana State University Press, Baton Rouge, 1998

Bukovsky, Vladimir: *To Build a Castle, my Life as a Dissenter*. André Deutsch Publishers, London, 1978

Chistyakova, E. (ed.): *S Chuzhogo Golosa*. Moskovskii Rabochii, Moscow, 1982

Chronicle of Current Events No. 57. Amnesty International, London, 1981

Clogg, Richard: *A Concise History of Greece*. Cambridge University Press, Cambridge, 1992

Cranach, Michael von: *In Memoriam*. DGPPN, 1999

Detlef, Joseph: *Von Angeblichen Antisemitismus der DDR*. Kai Homilius Verlag, Berlin, 2008

Diner, Hasia R.: *The Jews of the United States*. University of California Press, Berkeley, 2004

Dinnersteun, Leonard: *Anti-Semitism in America*. Oxford University Press, Oxford/New York, 1994

Dmitrieva, Tatyana: *Alyans Prava i Miloserdiya*. Nauka, Moscow, 2001

Dmitrieva, Tatyana, and Kondratiev, F.V. (eds.): *Ocherki Istorii*. Sersbki Institute, Moscow, 1996

Documents on the Political Abuse of Psychiatry in the USSR 1-42. IAPUP, Amsterdam, 1987-1991

Dobrynin, Anatoly: *In Confidence.* Times Books, New York, 1995

Ellis, Mark S.: *Purging the past: The Current State of Lustration Laws in the Former Communist Bloc.* Law and Contemporary Problems, Vol. 59, No. 4, 1996

Engelmann, Berndt: *Im Gleichschritt Marsch.* Steidl Verlag, Göttingen, 1993

Engelmann, Berndt: *Bis alles in Scherben Fallt.* Steidl Verlag, Göttingen, 1993

Engelmann, Berndt: *Wir haben ja den Kopf noch fest auf dem Hals.* Steidl Verlag, Göttingen, 1993

Fatih Tayfur, M.: *Semipheral Development and Foreign Policy: The cases of Greece and Spain.* Ashgate, Burlington, 2003

Felshtinsky, Yuri and Pribylovsky, Vladimir: *The Age of Assassins – The Rise and Rise of Vladimir Putin.* Gibson Square, London, 2008

Fireside, Harvey: *Soviet Psychoprisons.* Norton, New York, 1982

Fritze, Lothar: *Täter mit gutem Gewissen.* Böhlau Verlag, Köln, 1998

Fröhlich, Sergej: *General Wlassow; Russen und Deutsche zwischen Hitler und Stalin.* Markus, Köln, 1987

Fulford, K.W.M., Smirnov, A.Y.U, and Snow, E.: *Concepts of Disease and the Abuse of Psychiatry in the USSR.* British Journal of Psychiatry, volume 162, pp. 801-810, 1993

Funder, Anna: *Stasiland.* Granta Publications, London, 2003

Garrett, Laurie: *Betrayal of Trust.* Oxford University Press, Oxford, no date

Gieseke, Jens: *Der Mielke-Konzern; Die Geschichte der Stasi 1945-1990.* DVA, München, 2006

Gieseke, Jens: *Der Traurige Blick des Hauptmanns Wiesler*. Zeitgeschichte Online, April 2006

Gindilis, Viktor: *Epizody iz Sovetskoi Zhizni*. OGI, Moscow, 2008

Gitelman, Zvi: *A Century of Ambivalence*, Indiana University Press, Bloomington, IN, 2002

Gluzman, Semyon: *On Soviet Totalitarian Psychiatry*, IAPUP, Amsterdam, 1989

Gonzalez, Evelyn: *The Bronx*. Columbia University Press, New York, 2004

Greenbaum, Masha: *The Jews of Lithuania*. Gefen Publishing House, Jerusalem, 1995

Grigorenko, Pjotr: *Erinnerungen*. Bertelsmann, Ulm, 1981

Hattig, Suzanne, et.al.: *Geschichte des Speziallagers Bautzen 1945-1956*. Michel Sandstein Verlag, Dresden, 2004

Hattig, Suzanne, et.al.: *Stasi Gefängnis Bautzen II*. Michel Sandstein Verlag, Dresden, 2008

Helmchen, Hanfried: *Psychiater und Zeitgeist; zur Geschichte der Psychiatrie in Berlin*. Pabst, Lengerich, 2008

Herst, Mathias: *Antisemitismus und Antizionismus in der DDR*. GRIn Verlag, Norderstedt, 2006

Kazanetz, Etely: *Differentiating exogenous psychiatric illness from schizophrenia*. Archives of General Psychiatry, Volume 36, July 1979

Kochan, Lionel (ed.): *The Jews in Soviet Russia since 1917*. Oxford University Press, Oxford, 1978

Kerz-Rühling, I., and Pläkers, T.: *Verräter oder Verführte - Eine psychoanalytische Untersuchung Inoffizieller Mitarbeiter der Stasi*. Ch.Links, Berlin, 2004

Koppers, A.: *A Biographical Dictionary on the Political Abuse of Psychiatry in the USSR.* IAPUP, Amsterdam, 1990

Korotenko, A & Alikina, L.: *Sovetskaya Psikhiatria: Zabluzhdeniya i Umysel.* Sfera, Kiev, 2002

Koryagin, A.: *The involvement of Soviet psychiatry in the persecution of Dissenters.* British Journal of Psychiatry, volume 154, pp. 336-340, 1989

Kovalev, Andrei: *Page from the Book of Condolences.* unpublished memoirs

Lewis, Lionel S.: *Cold War on Campus.* Transaction Publishers, New Brunswick/London, 1996

Loos, Dr. H.: *Psychiatrie braucht Öffentlichkeit.* Deutsches Ärzteblatt, Jg. 103, Heft 51-52, 2006

Lown, Bernard: *Prescription for Survival.* Berrett-Koehler Publishers, San Francisco, 2008

Maser, Werner: Das Dritte Reich; *Alltag in Deutschland von 1933 bis 1945.* Verlag Bublies, Schnellbach, 1998

Medvedev, Roj en Zjores: *Wie is er Gek?* Manteau, Amsterdam, 1973

Merskey, Harold, and Shafran, Bronislava: *Political hazards in the diagnosis of ,sluggish schizophrenia'.* British Journal of Psychiatry, volume 148, pp. 247-256, 1986

Miller, Barbara: *Narratives of Guilt and Compliance in Unified Germany.* Routledge, London/New York, 1999

Mohr, Clarence L., and Gordon, Joseph E.: *Tulane; the emergence of a Modern University 1945-1980.* Louisiana State University Press, Baton Rouge, 2001

Morré, Jörg: *Speziallager des NKWD.* Brandenburgische Lndeszentrale für politische Bildung, Potsdam, 1997

Müller, Thomas R. et.al.: *Psychiatrie in der DDR.* Mabuse Verlag, Frankfurt am Main, 2006

Müller-Enbergs, Helmut: *Inoffiziele Mitarbeiter des Ministeriums für Staatssicherheit. Teil 1: Richtlinien und Durchführungsbestimmungen.* Ch. Links, Berlin, 2001

Neumann, Jochen: *Reiseberichte* - reports to the DDR leadership on his foreign travels. unpublished reports 1982-1989

Neumann, Jochen: *Bruchstücke* - memoirs, essays, diary. Emmending, 1992-2005

Neumann, Jochen: *Psychiatry in Eastern Europe Today: Mental Health Status, Policies, and Practices.* American Journal of Psychiatry, 148:10, Washington DC, 1991

Neumann, Jochen: *Beiträge zur Biologischen Psychiatrie.* VEB George Thieme, Leipzig, 1982

Neumann, Greger, Littmann, Ott: *Psychiatrischer Untersuchungskurs.* VEB George Thieme, Leipzig, 1981

Neumann, Seidel, Wunderlich: *Psychopharmakotherapie mit Ausgewählten Antikonvulsiva.* Deutsches Hygienemuseum der DDR, Dresden, 1983

Neumann, Nickel: *Das Wachtum des Hirnstammes.* Hirzel Verlag, Leipzig, 1974

Naimark, Norman M.: *The Russians in Germany: A History of the Soviet Zone of Occupation, 1945-1949.* Harvard University Press, Cambridge, MA, 2005

Novikov, Jurij: *Andrei Sneznevskij - seine wege und Irrwege in der sowjetischen Psychiatrie.* Schriftenreihe der Deutschen Gesellschaft für Geschichte der Nervenheilkunde, band 3, 1997

Oltmanns, Reimar: *Spurensuche auf Verbrannter Erde.* Books on Demand GmbH, Norderstedt, 2009

Onken, Marlies: *Als Arzt wie als Staatsbürger.* unpublished dissertation, Göttingen, 2002

Payk Theo R.: *Psychiater. Forscher im Labyrinth der Seele.* Kohlkammer, Stuttgart, 2000

Podrabinek, Aleksandr: *Punitive Medicine.* Karoma, Ann Arbor, 1980

Posel, Deborah, and Simpson, Graeme: *Commissioning the Past.* Witwatersrand University Press, Johannesburg, 2003

Pravo i Psikhiatriya. Yuridicheskaya Literatura, Moscow, 1991

Pross, Christian: *Wir tragen die Diktatur in uns*; in Morawe, P.: Zwischen den Welten. Nomos, Baden-Baden, 2004

Pross, Christian: *Zersetzung*; in Birck, A., et.al: Das Unsagbare. Springer, Berlin, 2002

Puls Reform: Yuristy i politology pazmyshlyayut. Progress, Moscow, 1989

Quoirin, Marianne: *Agentinnen aus Liebe.* Eichborn, Frankfurt/Main, 1999

Reddaway, Peter: *Confidential Diary on the Visit by US Psychiatric Delegation to the USSR.* unpublished diary

Report of the US Delegation - Soviet Response. Schizophrenia Bulletin, National Institute of Mental Health, Washington DC, 1989

Richter, Holger: *Die operative Psychologie des Ministeriums für Staatssicherheit der DDR.* Mabuse Verlag, Frankfurt/Main, 2001

Richter, Dr. Eva A.: *Zwischen Feigheit und Gewinnsucht.* Deutsches Ärzteblatt, Jg 99, Heft 21-32, 2002

Richter, Dr.Eva A: *Die meisen IM-Ärzte bespitzellten Kollegen.* Deutsches Ärzteblatt, Jg 104, Heft 48, 2007

Richter-Kuhlmann, Dr. Eva A.: *Die Anwerbestrategie der Stasi.* Deutsches Ärzteblatt, Jg. 102, Heft 9, 2005

Richter-Kuhlmann, Dr. Eva A. and Weil, Dr. F.: *Ich stand hinter der DDR.* Deutsches Ärzteblatt, Jg. 103, Heft 18, 2005

Rosenberg, Schulsinger & Strömgren: *Psychiatry and its Related Disciplines - the next 25 years.* WPA, Copenhagen. 1986

Rundbrief 1/97. Deutsche Vereinigung gegen politischen Missbrauch der Psychiatrie, 1997

Rundbrief 2/98. Deutsche Vereinigung gegen politischen Missbrauch der Psychiatrie, 1998

Rundbrief 1/99. Deutsche Vereinigung gegen politischen Missbrauch der Psychiatrie, 1999

Rundbrief 4/99. Deutsche Vereinigung gegen politischen Missbrauch der Psychiatrie, 1999

Sabshin, Melvin: *Changing American Psychiatry*. American Psychiatric Press, Washington D.C., 2008

Salvaggio, John: *New Orleans' Charity Hospital*. Louisiana State University Press, Baton Rouge, 1992

Schrecker, Ellen W.: *No Ivory Tower; McCarthyism and the Universities*. Oxford University Press, Oxford, 1986

Schultz, George: *Turmoil and Triumph*. Scribner, New York, 1993

Simon, Annette: *Psychoanalytische Reflexionen zur Funktion der „Stasiunterlagen-Behörde"*. Forum der Psychoanalyse 2, Berlin, 2006

Simon, Annette: *Das Leben und die anderen*. Forum der Psychoanalyse 2, Berlin, 2007

Smith, Theresa: *No Asylum*. New York University Press, New York, 1996

Smulevitch, A.B.: *Slowly progressive schizophrenia - myth or clinical reality*. British Journal of Psychiatry, Vol. 155, pp. 166-177, 1989

Sotsial'naya i Klinicheskaya Psikhiatriya. issue 2-1994

Soviet Political Psychiatry - The Story of the Opposition. IAPUP, London, 1983

Stefanis, C., and Reisby, N.: *The involvement of the World Psychiatric Association in the issue of the political abuse of psychiatry*. Acta Psichiatrica Scandinavica, Volume 87, Issue S370

Süss, Sonja: *Politisch Missbraucht?* Ch. Links, Berlin, 1998

Süss, Walter: *Konzeption eines Forschungsprojekts zur Zusammenarbeit der osteuropäischen Geheimdienste, insbesondere von MfS und KGB.* Workshop"Zur Bedeutung von MfS-Firschung und stasi Akten für die Zeitgeschichtforschung, Berlin, November 26, 2004

Todorov, Tzvetan: *Facing the Extreme.* Metropolitan Books, New York, 1996

Todorov, Tzvetan: *Hope and Memory.* Princeton University Press, Princeton, 2003

Torrey, E. Fuller and Yolken, Robert: *Psychiatric Genocide: Nazi Attempts to Eradicate Schizophrenia.* Schizophrenia Bulletin, November 2009

Turashvili, David: *Flight from USSR.* Bakur Sulakauri Publishing, Tbilisi, 2008

Twomey, Bill: *South Bronx.* Arcadia Publishing, Charleston SC, 2002

Van Voren, Robert: *Soviet Psychiatric Abuse in the Gorbachev Era.* IAPUP, Amsterdam, 1989

Van Voren, Robert: *Koryagin: A Man Struggling for Human Dignity.* IAPUP, Amsterdam, 1987

Van Voren, Robert: *On Dissidents and Madness.* Rodopi, Amsterdam/New York, 2009

Vgontzas, Antonis: *Anamesa sti mikri kai megali istoria* (of small and big stories in history). Ekdotikos Organismos Livane, Athens, 2007

Wanitschke, Matthias: *Methoden und Menschenbild des Ministeriums für Staatssicherheit der DDR.* Böhlau Verlag, Köln, 2001

Weil, Francesca: *Ich habe doch niemandem geschadet.* Deutsches Ärzteblatt, Jg. 102, Heft 39, 2005

Weil, Francesca: *Ärztliche Ethik mit neuem Inhalt gefühlt.* Deutsches Ärzteblatt, Jg. 103, Heft 23, 2006

Weil, Francesca: *Zielgruppe Ärzteschaft*. V&R Unipress, Göttingen, 2008

Wilkening, Christina: *Ich Wollte Klarheit - Tagebuch einer Recherche*. Aufbau, Berlin, 1992

Wolfram, Neumann & Wieczorek: *Psychologische Leistungstests in der Neurologie und Psychiatrie*. VEB George Thieme, Leipzig, 1989

Woods, Jeff: *Black Struggle, Red Scare*. Louisiana State University Press, Baton Rouge, 2004

Wynn, Alan: *Notes of a Non Conspirator*. Andre Deutsch, London, 1987

Films and DVD's

Das war die DDR. Kapitel 1-7. Berlin, 1993

Die Firma: Das Ministerium für Staatssicherheit. 2007

Klemke, Christian and Lorenzen, Jan. M.: *Alltag einer Behörde*. Satzgeber

Interviews

Interview with Yosé Höhne-Sparborth, May 9, 2009, Hollandsche Rading

Interview with Andrei Kovalev, October 12, 2009, Brussels

Interview with Valentinas Maciulis, October 20, 2009, Vilnius

Interview with Ellen Mercer, June 27, 2009, Washington .D.C.

Interview with Ellen Mercer, June 28, 2009, Washington .D.C.

Interview with Jochen Neumann, March 26, 2009, Berlin

Interview with Jochen Neumann, June 3, 2009, Berlin

Interview with Jochen Neumann, July 29, 2009, London

Interview with Jochen Neumann and Melvin Sabshin, July 29, 2009, London

Interview with Ellen Mercer, Jochen Neumann and Melvin Sabshin, December 1-2, 2009, London

Interview with Dainius Puras, October 19, 2009, Vilnius

Interview with Elena Raes-Mozhaeva, June 6, 2009, Utrecht

Interview with Melvin Sabshin, February 11-12, 2009, London

Interview with Melvin Sabshin, April 20, 2009, London

Interview with Melvin Sabshin, July 29, 2009, London

Interview with Norman Sartorius, April 16, 2009, Geneva

Interview with Norman Sartorius, October 2, 2009, Geneva

Interview with Eduard Shevardnadze, October 15, 2009, Tbilisi

Interview with Costas Stefanis, July 15, 2009, Athens

Interview with Costas Stefanis, November 15, 2009, Athens

Interview with Antonis Vgontzas, September 3, 2009, Athens

Archives

Archive of the Stasi (Biothler Behörde), Berlin

Jochen Neumann's diaries, Deutsches Tagebucharchiv, Emmending

Jochen Neumann's travel reports for the DDR authorities, Hollandsche Rading/Vilnius

FBI files on Melvin Sabshin, New Orleans and Washington D.C.

Archives of the International Association on the Political Use of Psychiatry, Hilversum

Archival materials from the Secretariat of the Central Committee of the CPSU, collected and posted by Vladimir Bukovsky, web-based

Private archives of Ellen Mercer, Washington D.C.

Private archives of Peter Reddaway, Washington D.C.

Private archives of Loren Roth, Pittsburgh, PA

Private archives of Robert van Voren, Hollandsche Rading/Vilnius

Archives of the World Psychiatric Association, Geneva

Archive of Memorial, Moscow (photographs Irina Kaplun)

Photographs

The photos in this book are from the following sources:
Aleksandr Avramenko: p. 28
Global Initiative on Psychiatry archives: p. 5, 102, 110, 116, 117, 123, 126, 142, 146, 147, 148, 150, 156, 163, 166, 177, 179, 180, 204, 217, 230, 252, 254, 255, 257, 271, 305, 327, 328, 343, 345, 367, 379, 381, 400, 401, 433, 451, 452, 459
Memorial (Moscow): p. 168, 173
Ellen Mercer: p. 161, 243, 246, 249, 314, 353, 354, 356, 364, 371, 382, 390, 394, 410, 411, 434, 442, 457
Jochen Neumann: p. 52, 90, 92, 200, 222, 226, 234, 238, 264, 265, 277, 281, 284, 288, 291, 292, 293, 294, 295, 296, 333, 336, 339, 352, 408, 417, 428, 431, 438, 464, 471, 472
Peter Reddaway: p. 378, 383
Loren Roth: p. 368, 374, 375, 376, 387
Melvin Sabshin: p. 13, 32, 36, 63, 65, 69, 77, 85, 186, 189, 192,
Robert van Voren: p. 2, 26, 40, 96, 143, 175, 209, 361, 377, 482, 483

Index of Names

Index of Subjects

www.ingramcontent.com/pod-product-compliance
Lightning Source LLC
Chambersburg PA
CBHW051149180926
51611CB00001B/4
* 9 7 8 9 0 4 2 0 3 0 4 8 0 *